Anesthesiology Self-Assessment and Board Review: BASIC Examination

Jeff Gadsden, MD, FRCPC, FANZCA
Associate Professor
Department of Anesthesiology
Duke University
Durham, North Carolina

Dean R. Jones, MD, FRCPC
Clinical Assistant Professor
Department of Anesthesiology,
    Pharmacology, and Therapeutics
University of British Columbia
Vancouver, Canada
Regional Medical Director and Regional
    Department Head
Department of Anesthesiology
Fraser Health Authority
Surrey, Canada

New York Chicago San Francisco Athens London Madrid Mexico City
Milan New Delhi Singapore Sydney Toronto

Anesthesiology Self-Assessment and Board Review: BASIC Examination

1 2 3 4 5 6 7 8 9 DSS 21 20 19 18 17 16

ISBN 978-0-07-182919-9
MHID 0-07-182919-9

Notice

Medicine is an ever-changing science. As new research and clinical experience broaden our knowledge, changes in treatment and drug therapy are required. The authors and the publisher of this work have checked with sources believed to be reliable in their efforts to provide information that is complete and generally in accord with the standards accepted at the time of publication. However, in view of the possibility of human error or changes in medical sciences, neither the authors nor the publisher nor any other party who has been involved in the preparation or publication of this work warrants that the information contained herein is in every respect accurate or complete, and they disclaim all responsibility for any errors or omissions or for the results obtained from use of the information contained in this work. Readers are encouraged to confirm the information contained herein with other sources. For example and in particular, readers are advised to check the product information sheet included in the package of each drug they plan to administer to be certain that the information contained in this work is accurate and that changes have not been made in the recommended dose or in the contraindications for administration. This recommendation is of particular importance in connection with new or infrequently used drugs.

This book was set in Adobe Garamond Pro by Aptara, Inc.
The editors were Brian Belval and Regina Y. Brown.
The production supervisor was Rick Ruzycka.
Production management was provided by Dinesh Pokhriyal, Aptara, Inc.
The cover designer was Dreamit, Inc.
RR Donnelley Shenzhen was printer and binder.

Catalog-in Publication Data is on file for this title at the Library of Congress.

To Corie—my wife, best friend, and soul mate. Thank you for inspiring me, making me laugh, and mostly for supporting me through all of the late nights and weekends that it took to finish this project—I owe you a lot of date nights.

To my wonderful kids Duke, Reef, Holt, and Gigi—I love being your daddy and hope that we can always learn and grow together.

JG

To Elena, Alessandra, and Dylan—My inspiration. Thank you for all of your support and patience.

To Dr. Margaret Wood—I am indebted to your mentorship and support. Thank you.

DJ

Contents

PART 3: PHYSICS, EQUIPMENT, MONITORS, AND MATHEMATICS

PART 4: CLINICAL ANESTHESIA TOPICS

Preface

In response to the ever-expanding scope of medical knowledge that anesthesiology trainees are expected to master by the end of their training, the American Board of Anesthesiology recently implemented a staged examination process. This is designed to ensure that trainees have a firm command of the scientific basis underpinning the specialty by the conclusion of their second postgraduate year before switching their focus to the more advanced, clinical subspecialty topics.

Preparing for a high-stakes exam such as the ABA BASIC Examination is stressful, and time is always at a premium during residency training. In our years as educators (and in our own personal experience as residents), we have always found high-quality multiple-choice questions to be an invaluable aid to focus study and gain confidence. However, most current question banks primarily focus on clinical topics meant to help you pass the "final" written exam (now known as the ADVANCED Exam). The purpose of this question book is to serve as a "one-stop shop" to supplement your primary reading for the BASIC Exam. These 800+ questions have been designed and written to specifically match the BASIC Exam's content outline so that every area is comprehensively covered. Each question is accompanied by an in-depth explanation of why the answer is right, but often more importantly, why the other distractors were wrong. Each explanation is also referenced to a primary text and/or journal article.

The book has been organized into 30 chapters contained in four main sections:

- Part 1: Anatomy and physiology
- Part 2: Pharmacology
- Part 3: Physics, equipment, monitors, and mathematics
- Part 4: Clinical anesthesia topics

We hope that you will use these questions to study, refine your knowledge, test yourself, and ultimately sail through the BASIC Exam with ease. We also hope that this book will serve as a means to review important day-to-day topics quickly throughout the remainder of your training. Congratulations on beginning your training in the exciting specialty of anesthesiology, and all the best on the BASIC Exam!

Jeff Gadsden, MD, FRCPC, FANZCA
Dean R. Jones, MD, FRCPC

Acknowledgments

The Authors and Publisher would like to thank the following individuals for their review of the manuscript:

Benjamin Dunne, MD
Stephanie Jones, MD
S. Kendall Smith, MD, PhD

PART 1

Anatomy and Physiology

CHAPTER 1

Basic Anatomy

1. You are attempting to place a central line in the left internal jugular vein. Which structure is most likely to lie between the common carotid artery and the vertebral artery?

   (A) internal jugular vein
   (B) thyroid gland
   (C) transverse process of C6
   (D) nerve root of C7
   (E) thoracic duct

2. Which of the following best describes Chassaignac's tubercle?

   (A) the anterior tubercle of C5 transverse process
   (B) the posterior tubercle of C5 transverse process
   (C) the anterior tubercle of C6 transverse process
   (D) the posterior tubercle of C6 transverse process
   (E) the anterior tubercle of C7 transverse process

3. When choosing the correct interspace for a T5-6 epidural, which of the following would be the best surface landmark for initial orientation?

   (A) the spinous process of C5
   (B) the spinous process of C7
   (C) the spinous process of T4
   (D) the spinous process of T6
   (E) the spinous process of L4

4. Identify the structure indicated by the letter (B) in Figure 1-5:

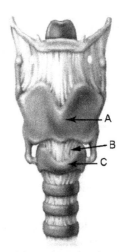

FIG. 1-5. Anatomy of the larynx and trachea. (Reproduced with permission from Hung O, Murphy MF. *Management of the Difficult and Failed Airway*. 2nd ed. New York, NY: McGraw Hill; 2012.)

   (A) thyrohyoid ligament
   (B) cricothyroid membrane
   (C) thyroid cartilage
   (D) cricoid cartilage
   (E) corniculate cartilage

5. Auscultation is performed on the right posterior chest at the level of T4, revealing crackles. Which of the following best describes the affected pulmonary lobe?

   (A) right upper lobe
   (B) right middle lobe
   (C) lingual
   (D) right posterior lobe
   (E) right lower lobe

6. With respect to the Figure 1-7, which of the following statements best describes the relationship between the cardiac silhouette and underlying cardiac anatomy?

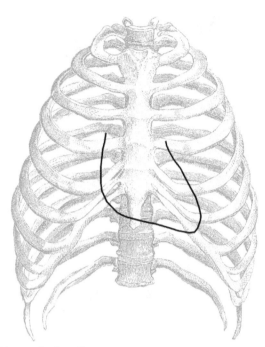

FIG. 1-7. Cardiac silhouette and rib cage.

(A) The left border of the heart is formed primarily by the left atrium.

(B) The left border of the heart is formed primarily by the left ventricle.

(C) The inferior border of the heart is formed primarily by the right atrium.

-(D) The right border of the heart is formed primarily by the right ventricle.

(E) The right border of the heart is formed by both the right and left atria.

7. Which of the following best describes the recommended locations to auscultate the aortic and mitral valves?

(A) aortic at left 2nd intercostal space; mitral at 2nd right intercostal space

(B) aortic at right 2nd intercostal space; mitral at 2nd left intercostal space

- (C) aortic at left 2nd intercostal space; mitral at apex

(D) aortic at right 2nd intercostal space; mitral at apex

(E) aortic at left 2nd intercostal space; mitral at left sternal edge

8. Which of the following best describes the anatomical relations of the subclavian vein when considering it as an approach for central venous cannulation?

(A) The vein is anterior to the subclavian artery.

(B) The vein is inferior to the subclavian artery.

(C) The vein is superior to the subclavian artery.

-(D) The vein passes over the first rib posterior to the anterior scalene muscle.

(E) The vein is lateral to the brachial plexus.

9. A line connecting the two iliac crests should pass through which vertebral level?

(A) T12

(B) L2

-(C) L4

(D) S1

(E) S2

10. Useful landmarks for identifying the caudal space include which of the following?

-(A) iliac crests

(B) ischial tuberosities

(C) sciatic notch

(D) sacral cornua

(E) S4 spinous process

11. Which of the following best describes the order of structures found just proximal to the wrist, from lateral (radial side) to medial (ulnar side)?

(A) radial artery, radial nerve, median nerve, ulnar artery, ulnar nerve

(B) radial nerve, radial artery, median nerve, ulnar artery, ulnar nerve

(C) radial artery, radial nerve, median nerve, ulnar nerve, ulnar artery

(D) radial nerve, radial artery, median nerve, ulnar nerve, ulnar artery

(E) radial artery, median nerve, radial nerve, ulnar artery, ulnar nerve

12. Which of the following best describes the location of the posterior tibial nerve?

    (A) posterior to the medial malleolus
    (B) anterior to the medial malleolus
    (C) posterior to the lateral malleolus
    (D) lateral to the Achilles tendon
    (E) adjacent to the dorsalis pedis artery

13. Which ONE of the following matching pairs of spinal roots and dermatomal regions is correct?

    (A) C8; posterior aspect of the thumb
    (B) T5; axilla
    (C) L1; umbilicus
    (D) L3; dorsal aspect of the foot
    (E) S1; popliteal fossa

14. You wish to perform a screening motor exam on a patient. Which ONE of the following matched pairs of nerve roots and corresponding muscle actions is correct?

    (A) C5-6; elbow flexion
    (B) C5; thumb opposition
    (C) L1; hip flexion
    (D) L5; knee extension
    (E) S2; ankle dorsiflexion

Note: Questions 15–17 refer to the computerized tomography (CT) image of the chest (Figure 1-16).

15. The arrow labeled "1" is pointing to:

    (A) the aortic arch
    (B) the ascending aorta
    (C) the descending aorta
    (D) the common carotid artery
    (E) the pulmonary trunk

16. The arrow labeled "2" is pointing to:

    (A) a peribronchial lymph node
    (B) bronchus intermedius
    (C) the left mainstem bronchus
    (D) the azygous vein
    (E) the esophagus

17. The arrow labeled "3" is pointing to:

    (A) the superior vena cava
    (B) the inferior vena cava
    (C) the descending aorta
    (D) the left pulmonary artery
    (E) the right pulmonary artery

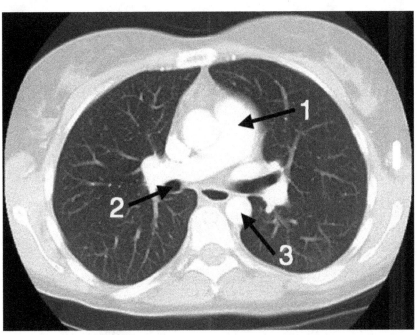

FIG. 1-16. Axial computed tomography (CT) of the chest (unlabeled).

18. The chest X-ray pictured is MOST compatible with which of the following diagnoses (Figure 1-18)?

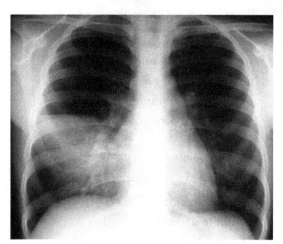

FIG. 1-18. Posterior-anterior (PA) chest X-ray.

(A) right upper lobe consolidation
(B) right middle lobe consolidation
(C) right lower lobe consolidation
(D) right-sided lung cancer
(E) atelectasis

19. Which of the following is the most likely diagnosis based on the image shown in Figure 1-19?

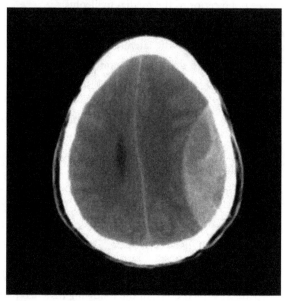

FIG. 1-19. Axial computed tomography (CT) slice of the head.

(A) meningioma
(B) astrocytoma
(C) subdural hematoma
(D) epidural hematoma
(E) subarachnoid hematoma

20. Match the numbered anatomical structures labeled on this sagittal MRI of the head to the available lettered choices (Figure 1-20).

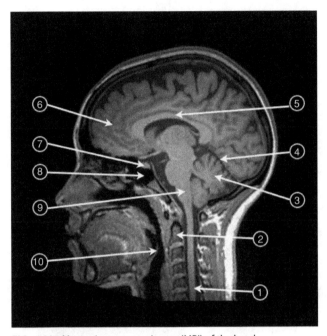

FIG. 1-20. Magnetic resonance image (MRI) of the head.

(1) _____   (A) CEREBELLUM   (K) MIDBRAIN

(2) _____   (B) PONS   (L) PITUITARY GLAND

(3) _____   (C) PARIETAL LOBE   (M) LATERAL VENTRICLE

(4) _____   (D) SPINAL CORD   (N) THALAMUS

(5) _____   (E) CORPUS CALLOSUM   (O) TENTORIUM

(6) _____   (F) ARCH OF ATLAS (C1)   (P) FRONTAL LOBE

(7) _____   (G) CAVERNOUS SINUS   (Q) EPIGLOTTIS

(8) _____   (H) MEDULLA   (S) CEREBELLAR TONSIL

(9) _____   (I) VOCAL CORDS   (T) SPHENOID SINUS

(10) _____   (J) ODONTOID PROCESS   (U) OPTIC NERVE

21. The lateral flexion-extension cervical spine X-rays shown Figure 1-21 MOST clearly demonstrate:

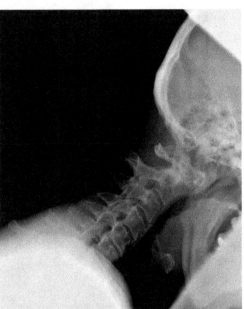

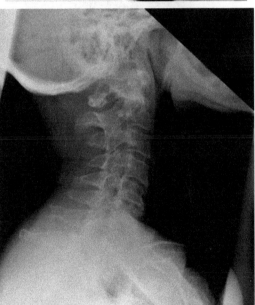

FIG. 1-21. Flexion/extension cervical spine X-rays.

(A) a C7 spinous process fracture

(B) spondylolisthesis

(C) osteoarthritis with decreased range of motion

(D) a vertebral body "step-off"

(E) atlantoaxial subluxation

Note: Questions 22 and 23 refer to the plain film of the lumbar spine (Figure 1-23).

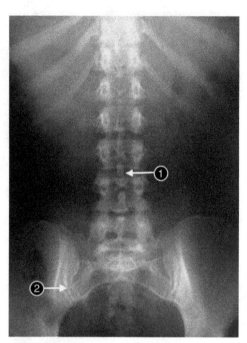

FIG. 1-23. Anterior-posterior X-ray of the lumbar spine.

22. In Figure 1-23, the arrow labeled "1" is pointing to which of the following structures?

   (A) spinous process of L2
   (B) L2/3 intervertebral disc
   (C) spinous process of L3
   (D) L2/3 facet joint
   (E) spinous process of L4

23. In Figure 1-23, the arrow labeled "2" is pointing to which of the following structures?

   (A) iliac crest
   (B) sacral foramina
   (C) sciatic notch
   (D) sacral hiatus
   (E) sacroiliac joint

24. Which of the following best describes the clinical diagnosis that can be made from the MR image seen in Figure 1-24?

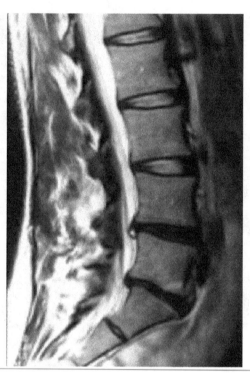

FIG. 1-24. Sagittal magnetic resonance (MR) image of the lumbar spine.

   (A) L4 compression fracture
   (B) spondylolisthesis
   (C) L2-L3 herniated disc
   (D) L3-L4 herniated disc
   (E) L4-L5 herniated disc

Note: Questions 25 and 26 refer to the magnetic resonance image (MRI) (Figure 1-25).

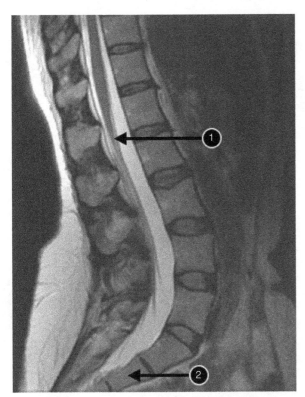

FIG. 1-25. Sagittal magnetic resonance (MR) image of the lumbar spine.

Note: Questions 27–30 refer to the ultrasound image of the anterior neck (Figure 1-26).

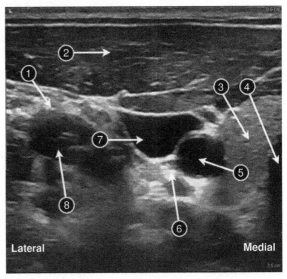

FIG. 1-26. Ultrasound image of the anterior neck taken in a transverse orientation.

25. In Figure 1-25, the arrow labeled "1" is pointing to which of the following?

(A) an epidural hematoma
(B) an epidural abscess
(C) the L5 vertebral foramen
(D) the conus medullaris
(E) the filum terminale

26. In Figure 1-25, the arrow labeled "2" is pointing to which of the following?

(A) L5 vertebral body
(B) L5-S1 disc
(C) S1 vertebral body
(D) sacral foramen
(E) S2 vertebral body

27. In Figure 1-26, which of the following labeled arrows most closely points to the thyroid gland?

(A) 1
(B) 3
(C) 4
(D) 6
(E) 8

28. In Figure 1-26, which of the following labeled arrows most closely points to the internal jugular vein?

(A) 4
(B) 5
(C) 6
(D) 7
(E) 8

29. In Figure 1-26, which of the following labeled arrows most closely points to the approximate location of the vagus nerve?

    (A) 1
    (B) 3
    (C) 4
    (D) 6
    (E) 8

30. In Figure 1-26, which of the following labeled arrows most closely points to the approximate location of the phrenic nerve?

    (A) 1
    (B) 2
    (C) 3
    (D) 6
    (E) 8

Answers and Explanations: Basic Anatomy

1. You are attempting to place a central line in the left internal jugular vein. Which structure is most likely to lie between the common carotid artery and the vertebral artery?

   (A) internal jugular vein
   (B) thyroid gland
   (C) transverse process of C6
   (D) nerve root of C7
   (E) **thoracic duct**

The internal jugular vein (IJV) lies in the carotid sheath and is most often lateral and anterior to the carotid artery and vagus nerve (Figure 1-1). It originates at the jugular foramen of the skull and terminates behind the clavicle upon joining with the subclavian vein to form the brachiocephalic vein. The IJV overlies much of the carotid artery in a significant number of patients—advancement of the needle inadvertently thought the vein may result in arterial puncture, especially if the needle is directed with a medial angulation.

Posterior to the carotid sheath and its contents lie the transverse processes, scalene muscles, nerve roots, and vertebral artery and vein. Vertebral artery puncture and cannulation resulting from excessively deep needle advancement has been reported during attempted IJV cannulation. This is also a potential risk during interscalene brachial plexus block, as the vertebral vessels lie close to the nerve roots.

The thoracic duct emerges from the thorax between the esophagus and the pleura. It forms an arch posterior to the carotid sheath and in front of the vertebral vessels before traveling inferiorly and opening into the angle of the junction of the internal jugular and subclavian veins. Needle injury to the thoracic duct is a rare but reported complication of left-sided central venous access (both IJ and subclavian veins), which may result in chylothorax or lymphocutaneous fistula.

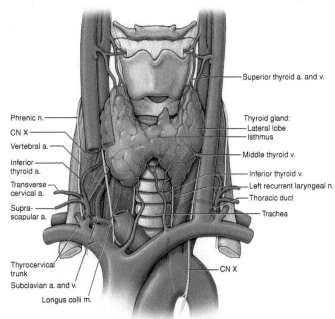

FIG. 1-1. Anatomy of the neck. Note the relative position of the carotid artery, the internal jugular vein, and the thoracic duct. (Reproduced with permission from Morton DA, Albertine K, Foreman KB: *The Big Picture: Gross Anatomy,* 1st Ed. New York, NY: McGraw Hill; 2011.)

Ref: Jacob S. *Human Anatomy: A Clinically-Orientated Approach.* 1st ed. London, UK: Churchill Livingstone; 2007.

2. Which of the following best describes Chassaignac's tubercle?

    (A) the anterior tubercle of C5 transverse process

    (B) the posterior tubercle of C5 transverse process

    (C) **the anterior tubercle of C6 transverse process**

    (D) the posterior tubercle of C6 transverse process

    (E) the anterior tubercle of C7 transverse process

Chassaignac's tubercle is the eponym for the large, anterior tubercle of the transverse process of the sixth cervical vertebra (Figure 1-2). It can be palpated medial to the sternocleidomastoid muscle at the level of the cricoid cartilage. Its immediate anterior relation is the carotid artery, which can be compressed against the tubercle quite easily when carotid massage is being employed for supraventricular tachycardia.

Chassaignac's tubercle is also a useful landmark for regional anesthetic procedures, such as stellate ganglion block. The stellate ganglion is a sympathetic ganglion formed by the fusion of the inferior cervical ganglion with the first thoracic ganglion (Figure 1-2). A common method of stellate ganglion block involves palpation of the C6 tubercle followed by gentle lateral retraction of the carotid artery. A needle is then directed to contact the tubercle and local anesthetic injected. While the location of the stellate ganglion is typically more inferior (antero-lateral to the vertebral bodies of C7 and/or T1), it is more difficult to access directly and the easy palpation of

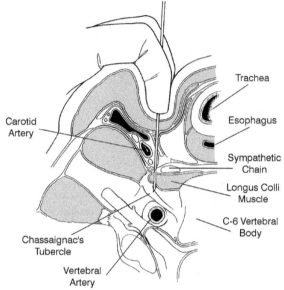

FIG. 1-2. Anatomical relationships of the stellate ganglion and the cervical transverse processes. (Reproduced with permission from Warfield CA, Bajwa ZH. *Principles and Practice of Pain Medicine*, 2nd ed. New York, NY: McGraw Hill; 2004.)

the C6 bony landmark makes it a safer location to insert a needle. With sufficient volume (e.g., 20 mL), the local anesthetic should spread inferiorly to block the stellate ganglion. Landmarking for deep cervical plexus block (e.g., to provide anesthesia for carotid endarterectomy) is also accomplished using Chassaignac's tubercle.

Typical cervical vertebrae (C3-C6) have short transverse processes with both anterior and posterior tubercles; each transverse process is perforated by a foramen transversarium, through which pass the vertebral artery and vein (Figure 1-3). The C7 transverse process has a

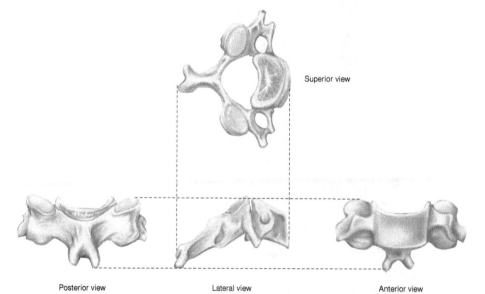

Superior view

Posterior view   Lateral view   Anterior view

FIG. 1-3. Cervical vertebrae. Front, back, side, and axial views. (Reproduced with permission from Mattox KL, Moore EE, Feliciano DV. *Trauma.* 7th ed. New York, NY: McGraw Hill; 2012.)

rudimentary (or sometimes absent) anterior tubercle, and the vertebral artery and vein lie outside the smaller foramen transversarium.

Ref: Mattox KL, Moore EE, Feliciano DV. *Trauma.* 7th ed. New York, NY: McGraw Hill; 2012.

3. When choosing the correct interspace for a T5-6 epidural, which of the following would be the best surface landmark for initial orientation?

(A) the spinous process of C5

(B) **the spinous process of C7**

(C) the spinous process of T4

(D) the spinous process of T6

(E) the spinous process of L4

While it is possible to palpate spinous processes at many levels, the most prominent and most easily palpable is C7 (also named vertebra prominens). This forms a convenient reference point to "count down" to the desired level when performing thoracic epidural or paravertebral anesthesia. The spinous processes of the thoracic spine may be easily palpable, but without a reference point it is difficult to be certain of the approximate level. Another convenient landmark is the inferior angle of the scapula, which is usually located at the same level as the T7 spinous process (Figure 1-4).

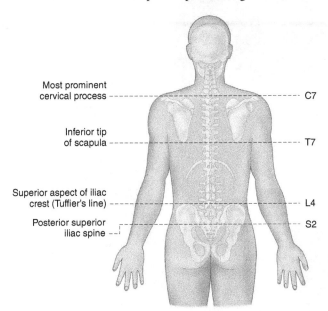

FIG. 1-4. Surface landmarks identifying spinal levels. (Reproduced with permission from Butterworth JF IV, Mackey DC, Wasnick JD. *Morgan and Mikhail's Clinical Anesthesiology.* 5th ed. New York, NY: McGraw Hill; 2013.)

Ref: Butterworth JF IV, Mackey DC, Wasnick JD. *Morgan and Mikhail's Clinical Anesthesiology.* 5th ed. New York, NY: McGraw Hill; 2013.

4. Identify the structure indicated by the letter (B) in Figure 1-5:

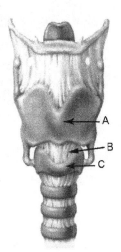

FIG. 1-5. Anatomy of the larynx and trachea. (Reproduced with permission from Hung O, Murphy MF. *Management of the Difficult and Failed Airway.* 2nd ed. New York, NY: McGraw Hill; 2012.)

(A) thyrohyoid ligament

(B) **cricothyroid membrane**

(C) thyroid cartilage

(D) cricoid cartilage

(E) corniculate cartilage

On the anterior surface of the larynx, the thyroid cartilage (A) and cricoid cartilage (C) of the larynx are connected by the cricothyroid membrane (B). This membrane is approximately 2 to 3 cm wide and about 1 cm high. The vocal cords have their anterior attachments approximately 1 cm above the upper border of the cricothyroid membrane. Accessing the airway through this membrane (i.e., cricothyrotomy) should therefore keep the operator well away from these critical structures. The only arterial structures of note are the cricothyroid arteries, branches of the superior thyroid arteries. These tend to course on the superolateral aspect of the membrane. Therefore, in making an incision with a knife, keeping as inferior as possible in the membrane and limiting the lateral extension of the incision is good practice (although in the heat of the moment, trust me—if you're doing a cricothyrotomy, injury to small vessels is not your primary concern). About 40% of people have a pyramidal thyroid lobe that extends superiorly in the midline and therefore may be injured during cricothyrotomy.

Ref: Hung O, Murphy MF. *Management of the Difficult and Failed Airway.* 2nd ed. New York, NY: McGraw Hill; 2012.

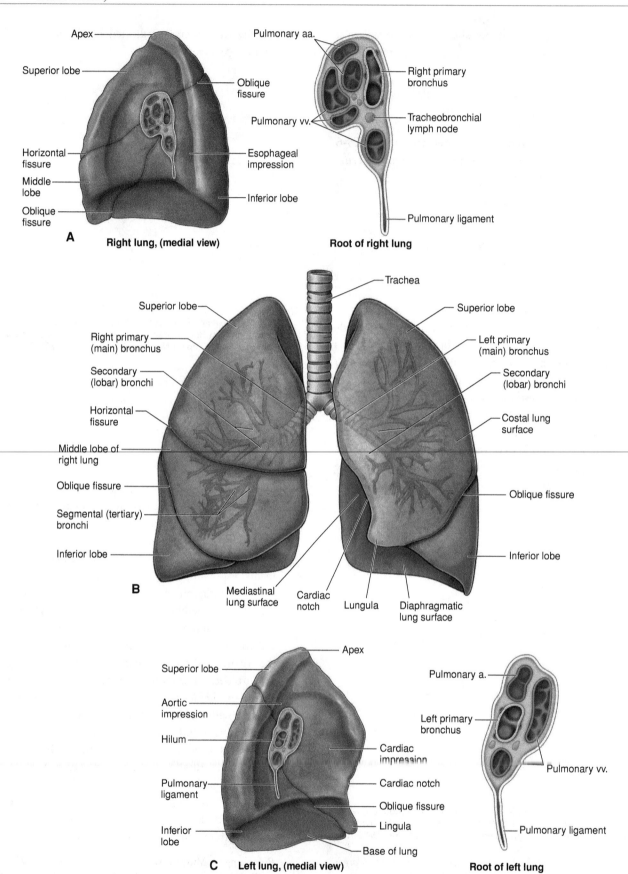

FIG. 1-6. A. Right lung in medial view. **B.** Bronchial tree and lungs. **C.** left lung in medial view. (Reproduced with permission from Morton DA, Albertine K, Foreman KB. *The Big Picture: Gross Anatomy*. 1st ed. New York, NY: McGraw Hill; 2011.)

5. Auscultation is performed on the right posterior chest at the level of T4, revealing crackles. Which of the following best describes the affected pulmonary lobe?

   (A) right upper lobe
   (B) right middle lobe
   (C) lingual
   (D) right posterior lobe
   (E) **right lower lobe**

Auscultation of the chest requires an understanding of the underlying pulmonary anatomy. The lower lobes of both lungs extend superiorly up to the level of the T3 spinous process (Figure 1-6). All but the topmost areas of the back therefore represent underlying lower lobes. In the left chest, the entire anterior portion is comprised of the left upper lobe, while the right anterior chest is primarily right upper lobe, with a small contribution from the right middle lobe. The oblique fissures run anteroinferiorly to superoposteriorly, and thus auscultation on the side of the chest may detect abnormal breath sounds in any of the lobes, depending on the level.

The lingula is the inferior division of the left upper lobe. There are no posterior lobes in either lung.

Ref: Morton DA, Albertine K, Foreman KB. *Gross Anatomy: The Big Picture.* 1st ed. New York, NY: McGraw Hill; 2011.

6. With respect to the Figure 1-7, which of the following statements best describes the relationship between the cardiac silhouette and underlying cardiac anatomy?

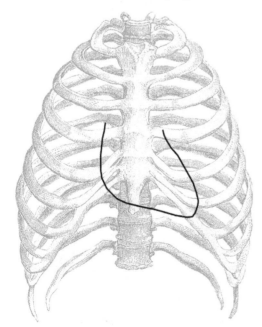

FIG. 1-7. Cardiac silhouette and rib cage.

   (A) the left border of the heart is formed primarily by left atrium.
   (B) **the left border of the heart is formed primarily by left ventricle.**
   (C) the inferior border of the heart is formed primarily by right atrium.
   (D) the right border of the heart is formed primarily by right ventricle.
   (E) the right border of the heart is formed by both the right and left atria.

The left heart border is made up almost entirely of the left ventricle, while the inferior border comprises the apical portion of the left ventricle and the right ventricle. The right heart border is primarily right atrium (Figure 1-8).

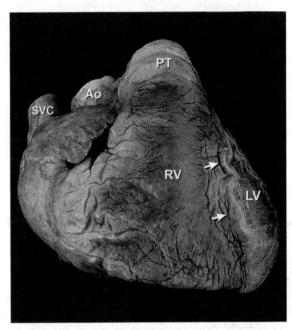

FIG. 1-8. Orientation of the heart in situ. The right and left ventricles form the inferior and left borders, respectively. The apical portion of the left ventricle also contributes to the inferior border. The right atrium forms the majority of the right border. Arrows correspond to anterior AV groove. (Reproduced with permission from Fuster V, Walsh R, Harrington R. *Hurst's The Heart.* 13th ed. New York, NY: McGraw Hill; 2011.)

Ref: Fuster V, Walsh R, Harrington R. *Hurst's The Heart.* 13th ed. New York, NY: McGraw Hill; 2011.

7. Which of the following best describes the recommended locations to auscultate the aortic and mitral valves?

   (A) aortic at left 2nd intercostal space; mitral at 2nd right intercostal space
   (B) aortic at right 2nd intercostal space; mitral at 2nd left intercostal space
   (C) aortic at left 2nd intercostal space; mitral at apex

(D) **aortic at right 2nd intercostal space; mitral at apex**

(E) aortic at left 2nd intercostal space; mitral at left sternal edge

The cardiac valves are clustered relatively closely in the mediastinum, but because of their position behind the sternum, they best heard at different locations. These are (Figure 1-9):

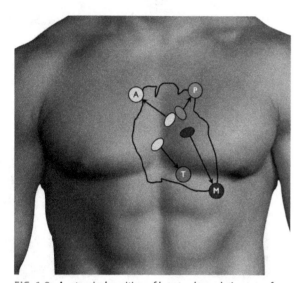

FIG. 1-9. Anatomical position of heart valves relative to surface landmarks. Arrows point to where each valve sound is heard best on the chest wall during auscultation. A = aortic valve, M = mitral valve, P = pulmonic valve, T = tricuspid valve.

Aortic valve: right 2nd intercostal space
Pulmonic valve: left 2nd intercostal space
Mitral valve: apex
Tricuspid valve: left inferior sternal edge

> **Ref:** Fuster V, Walsh R, Harrington R. *Hurst's The Heart.* 13th ed. New York, NY: McGraw Hill; 2011.

8. Which of the following best describes the anatomical relations of the subclavian vein when considering it as an approach for central venous cannulation?

(A) **The vein is anterior to the subclavian artery.**

(B) The vein is inferior to the subclavian artery.

(C) The vein is superior to the subclavian artery.

(D) The vein passes over the first rib posterior to the anterior scalene muscle.

(E) The vein is lateral to the brachial plexus.

The subclavian vein is the continuation of the axillary vein. It lies anterior to the subclavian artery beneath the clavicle, and passes over the first rib immediately medial to the anterior scalene muscle, which separates the vein from the artery (Figure 1-10). When performing subclavian vein cannulation, a needle directed too posteriorly may enter the subclavian artery. Likewise, a needle directed too deep may pass between the first and second ribs and result in a pneumothorax. For this

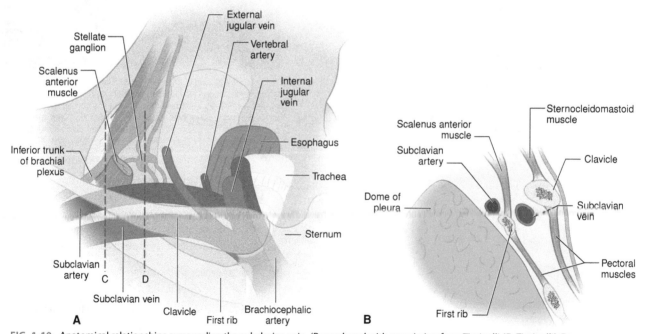

FIG. 1-10. Anatomical relationships surrounding the subclavian vein. (Reproduced with permission from Tintinalli JE. *Tintinalli's Emergency Medicine: A Comprehensive Study Guide.* 7th ed. New York, NY: McGraw Hill; 2011.)

reason, most descriptions of the technique advise performing the skin puncture at the junction of the lateral 1/3 and medial 2/3 of the clavicle and directing the needle towards the sternal notch, aiming to stay close to the inferior aspect of the clavicle.

Ref: Tintinalli JE. *Tintinalli's Emergency Medicine: A Comprehensive Study Guide.* 7th ed. New York, NY: McGraw Hill; 2011.

9. A line connecting the two iliac crests should pass through which vertebral level?

   (A) T12
   (B) L2
   (C) L4
   (D) S1
   (E) S2

The line connecting the iliac crests (intercristal line) has been described as typically crossing the vertebral level of L4, although it may be at the L4-L5 disc space, the L3-L4 disc space, or another level altogether (Figure 1-11). The precision of manually estimating the vertebral level has been shown to be poor compared with standards such as MRI or ultrasonography, and estimates are frequently off by one or two entire levels. The reason for this relates to the variability of the soft tissue overlying the iliac crests and the difficulty in precisely locating the osseous landmarks. When considered *radiographically*, the intercristal line does cross the L4 vertebra.

    In the thoracic spine, the inferior angle of the scapulae are approximately at the level of the T7 spinous process, although this is also not completely reliable.

Ref: Longnecker DE, Brown DL, Newman MF, Zapol WM. *Anesthesiology.* 2nd ed. New York, NY: McGraw Hill; 2012.

10. Useful landmarks for identifying the caudal space include which of the following?

   (A) iliac crests
   (B) ischial tuberosities
   (C) sciatic notch
   (D) sacral cornua
   (E) S4 spinous process

Surface landmarks for performing caudal anesthesia are relatively straightforward. The needle must pass through the sacral hiatus to access the sacral portion of the epidural space. The sacral hiatus is a midline defect resulting from the unfused laminae of S4 and S5 and is covered by the sacrococcygeal ligament. This may be

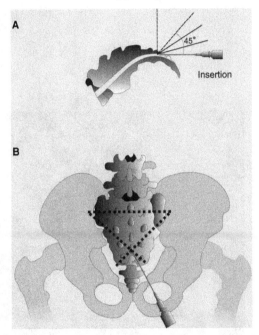

FIG. 1-12. A: Caudal approach: Angle of needle insertion required to enter the caudal canal. **B:** Landmarks. (Reproduced with permission from Hadzic A. *NYSORA Textbook of Regional Anesthesia and Acute Pain Medicine.* 1st ed. New York, NY: McGraw Hill; 2007.)

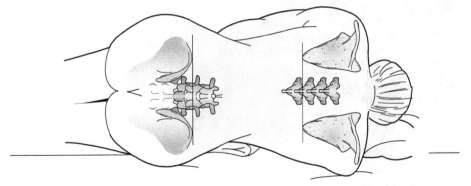

FIG. 1-11. A line connecting the two iliac crests should pass through the vertebral body of L4. A line connecting the two angles of the scapulae should pass through T7. (Reproduced with permission from Longnecker DE, Brown DL, Newman MF, Zapol WM. *Anesthesiology.* 2nd ed. New York, NY: McGraw Hill; 2012.)

felt as a depression just proximal to the coccyx, bounded on either side by two bony prominences, the sacral cornua. The hiatus forms an equilateral triangle with the posterior superior iliac spines, another helpful landmark (Figure 1-12).

Ref: Hadzic A. *NYSORA Textbook of Regional Anesthesia and Acute Pain Medicine.* 1st ed. New York, NY: McGraw Hill; 2007.

11. Which of the following best describes the order of structures found just proximal to the wrist, from lateral (radial side) to medial (ulnar side)?

(A) radial artery, radial nerve, median nerve, ulnar artery, ulnar nerve

(B) **radial nerve, radial artery, median nerve, ulnar artery, ulnar nerve**

(C) radial artery, radial nerve, median nerve, ulnar nerve, ulnar artery

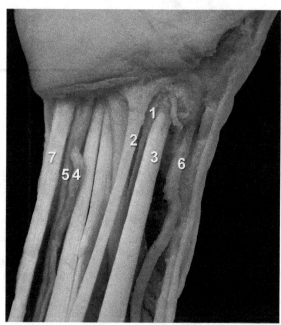

FIG. 1-13. Anatomy of the right wrist. 1 = median nerve, 2 = flexor palmaris longus, 3 = flexor carpi radialis, 4 = ulnar artery, 5 = ulnar nerve, 6 = radial artery, 7 = flexor carpi ulnaris. (Reproduced with permission from Hadzic A. *Hadzic's Peripheral Nerve Blocks and Anatomy for Ultrasound Guided Regional Anesthesia.* 2nd ed. New York, NY: McGraw Hill; 2012.)

(D) radial nerve, radial artery, median nerve, ulnar nerve, ulnar artery

(E) radial artery, median nerve, radial nerve, ulnar artery, ulnar nerve

Ref: Hadzic A. *Hadzic's Peripheral Nerve Blocks and Anatomy for Ultrasound Guided Regional Anesthesia.* 2nd ed. New York, NY: McGraw Hill; 2012.

12. Which of the following best describes the location of the posterior tibial nerve?

(A) **posterior to the medial malleolus**
(B) anterior to the medial malleolus
(C) posterior to the lateral malleolus
(D) lateral to the Achilles tendon
(E) adjacent to the dorsalis pedis artery

The posterior tibial nerve is one of five nerves that innervate the foot:

1. Posterior tibial nerve (branch of the tibial nerve). Innervates heel and sole of the foot, as well as most of the bones, ligaments and muscles of the foot. Located posterior to medial malleolus, adjacent to posterior tibial artery.

2. Superficial peroneal nerve(s) (branches of common peroneal nerve). Innervate dorsum of foot. Located superficially on extensor surface of ankle.

3. Deep peroneal nerve (branch of the common peroneal nerve). Innervates webspace of first and second toe. Located anterior to tibia, adjacent to dorsalis pedis artery.

4. Sural nerve (formed by joining of medial sural cutaneous nerve [from tibial nerve] and lateral sural cutaneous nerve [from peroneal nerve]). Innervates lateral aspect of foot. Located superficially and immediately lateral to the Achilles tendon.

5. Saphenous nerve (branch of femoral nerve). Innervates medial malleolus and variable amount of medial portion of foot. Located anterior to medial malleolus.

Ref: Hadzic A. *Hadzic's Peripheral Nerve Blocks and Anatomy for Ultrasound Guided Regional Anesthesia.* 2nd ed. New York, NY: McGraw Hill; 2012.

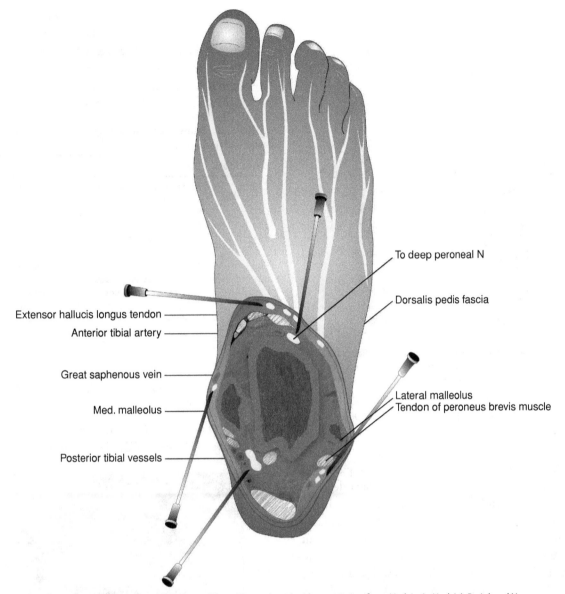

FIG. 1-14. Innervation of the ankle joint and foot. (Reproduced with permission from Hadzic A. *Hadzic's Peripheral Nerve Blocks and Anatomy for Ultrasound Guided Regional Anesthesia*. 2nd ed. New York, NY: McGraw Hill; 2012.)

13. Which ONE of the following matching pairs of spinal roots and dermatomal regions is correct?

(A) C8; posterior aspect of the thumb

(B) T5; axilla

(C) L1; umbilicus

(D) L3; dorsal aspect of the foot

(E) S1; popliteal fossa

The sensory innervation of the skin of the body (except for the face) is organized in a straightforward and logical pattern based on spinal nerve roots (Figure 1-15). The thorax and abdomen are easiest to understand, since the intercostal nerves wrap around circumferentially on either side, producing "bands" of dermatomal coverage.

As each spinal root emerges from the intervertebral foraminae, a small dorsal ramus branches off posteriorly to supply the dorsal aspect of the trunk (i.e., the spinal midline and the couple of inches either side of it).

The much larger ventral ramus (what we typically think of as the intercostal nerves) continues on to innervate the lateral and anterior aspects of the trunk *in addition to* the limbs. I'll repeat that. The cervical, brachial and lumbosacral plexi are formed by the *ventral* roots only. This is why there are no anterior C6, C7, or C8 dermatomes on the anterior chest wall—it skips from C5 right to T1. The ventral roots and their branches are exclusively devoted to the upper limb. In contrast, the dorsum of the body is sequentially

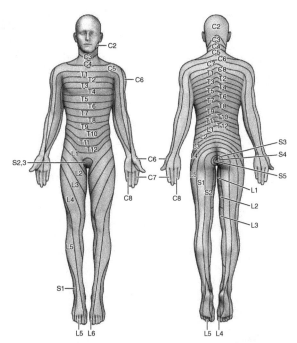

FIG. 1-15. Dermatomal innervation of the body. (Reproduced with permission from Diwan S, Staats P: *Atlas of Pain Medicine Procedures.* New York, NY: McGraw Hill, 2014.)

innervated from C2 right through to S5. Don't worry about the sensory territory of C1, he's strictly a motor nerve supplying several muscles in the neck.

Okay, so what's the deal with the weirdo pattern of innervation of the lower limb? During fetal development, the limb buds emerge from the tubular embryo, "dragging" respective nerves with each myotome. Early on, the sole of the developing foot faces forward, but over time, the limb undergoes a complete medial rotation so that the knee is facing forward and the sole towards the posterior. This rotation drags the already developed dermatomes with the underlying tissues, so that a "barber-pole" pattern emerges, like diagonal stripes running down from laterally to medially.

Ref: Morton DA, Albertine K, Foreman KB. *Gross Anatomy: The Big Picture.* 1st ed. New York, NY: McGraw Hill; 2011.

14. You wish to perform a screening motor exam on a patient. Which ONE of the following matched pairs of nerve roots and corresponding muscle actions is correct?

   (A) C5-6; elbow flexion
   (B) C5; thumb opposition
   (C) L1; hip flexion
   (D) L5; knee extension
   (E) S2; ankle dorsiflexion

You don't need to be the world's best neurologist to be a safe anesthesiologist. You do, however, need to know how to look for nerve root problems. Here's one common way to test for motor function. The power of the isometric contraction against resistance can be graded against the contralateral limb. Memorize this list and move on.

TABLE 1-1. Maneuvers for testing motor function of selected nerve roots.

Nerve roots	Diagnostic maneuver
C5-6	Arm flexion against resistance (musculocutaneous nerve)
C6-7	Wrist extension against resistance (radial nerve)
C8	Grip strength (median nerve)
T1	Finger abduction (fanning) against resistance (ulnar nerve)
C8-T1	Thumb opposition against resistance (median nerve)
L2-L3	Hip flexion against resistance (femoral nerve)
L3-4	Knee extension against resistance (femoral nerve)
L4-5	Ankle dorsiflexion against resistance (peroneal nerve)
L5-S1	Knee flexion against resistance (sciatic nerve)
S1-S2	Ankle plantarflexion against resistance (tibial nerve)

Ref: Hadzic A. *NYSORA Textbook of Regional Anesthesia and Acute Pain Medicine.* 1st ed. New York, NY: McGraw Hill; 2007.

Note: Questions 15–17 refer to the computerized tomography (CT) image of the chest (Figures 1-16–1-17).

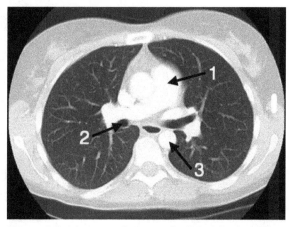

FIG. 1-16. Axial computed tomography (CT) of the chest (unlabeled).

15. The arrow labeled "1" is pointing to:

   (A) the aortic arch
   (B) the ascending aorta
   (C) the descending aorta
   (D) the common carotid artery
   (E) the pulmonary trunk

16. The arrow labeled "2" is pointing to:

    (A) a peribronchial lymph node

    (B) **bronchus intermedius**

    (C) the left mainstem bronchus

    (D) the azygous vein

    (E) the esophagus

17. The arrow labeled "3" is pointing to:

    (A) the superior vena cava

    (B) the inferior vena cava

    (C) **the descending aorta**

    (D) the left pulmonary artery

    (E) the right pulmonary artery

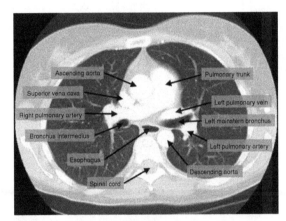

FIG. 1-17. Axial computed tomography (CT) of the chest (labeled).

Ref: Chen MYM, Pope TL, Ott DJ. *Basic Radiology.* 2nd ed. New York, NY: McGraw Hill; 2011.

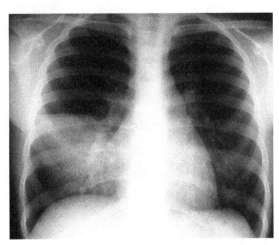

FIG. 1-18. Posterior-anterior (PA) chest X-ray.

18. The chest X-ray pictured is MOST compatible with which of the following diagnoses (Figure 1-18)?

    (A) right upper lobe consolidation

    (B) **right middle lobe consolidation**

    (C) right lower lobe consolidation

    (D) right-sided lung cancer

    (E) atelectasis

This chest X-ray shows airspace consolidation in the right middle lobe. The horizontal fissure is clearly seen separating the affected area from the right upper lobe. The costophrenic angle and diaphragm are also clearly seen, indicating a lack of consolidation in the lower lobe. Air bronchograms can be seen. Atelectasis may also appear as a wedge-shaped or linear opacity, but there is typically associated volume loss and ipsilateral shift, features not seen on this radiograph. There is no obvious lung cancer seen.

Ref: Chen MYM, Pope TL, Ott DJ. *Basic Radiology.* 2nd ed. New York, NY: McGraw Hill; 2011.

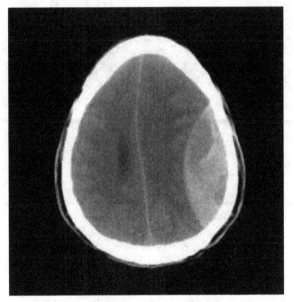

FIG. 1-19. Axial computed tomography (CT) slice of the head.

19. Which of the following is the most likely diagnosis based on the image shown Figure 1-19?

    (A) meningioma

    (B) astrocytoma

    (C) subdural hematoma

    (D) **epidural hematoma**

    (E) subarachnoid hematoma

This head CT shows a convex, lens-shaped hyperdense mass that is characteristic of an epidural hematoma.

Some midline shift is also seen with compression of the ipsilateral lateral ventricle. Cranial epidural hematomas usually result from a blow to the head that causes separation of the periosteal dura from the bone and shearing of the interposed blood vessels. These are most commonly seen in the temporoparietal region, with the middle meningeal artery being the most common culprit vessel. Subdural hematomas, in contrast, typically appear as concave hyperdensities.

Ref: Chen MYM, Pope TL, Ott DJ. *Basic Radiology.* 2nd ed. New York, NY: McGraw Hill; 2011.

20. Match the numbered anatomical structures labeled on this sagittal MRI of the head to the available lettered choices (Figure 1-20).

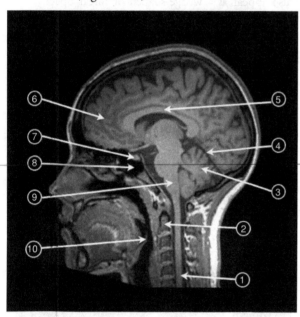

FIG. 1-20. Magnetic resonance image (MRI) of the head.

(1) _____   (A) CEREBELLUM   (K) MIDBRAIN
(2) _____   (B) PONS   (L) PITUITARY GLAND
(3) _____   (C) PARIETAL LOBE   (M) LATERAL VENTRICLE
(4) _____   (D) SPINAL CORD   (N) THALAMUS
(5) _____   (E) CORPUS CALLOSUM   (O) TENTORIUM
(6) _____   (F) ARCH OF ATLAS (C1)   (P) FRONTAL LOBE
(7) _____   (G) CAVERNOUS SINUS   (Q) EPIGLOTTIS
(8) _____   (H) MEDULLA   (S) CEREBELLAR TONSIL
(9) _____   (I) VOCAL CORDS   (T) SPHENOID SINUS
(10) _____   (J) ODONTOID PROCESS   (U) OPTIC NERVE

1D, 2 J, 3 A, 4 O, 5E, 6P, 7 L, 8 T, 9 H, 10Q

Ref: Chen MYM, Pope TL, Ott DJ. *Basic Radiology.* 2nd ed. New York, NY: McGraw Hill; 2011.

21. The lateral flexion-extension cervical spine X-rays shown Figure 1-21 MOST clearly demonstrate:

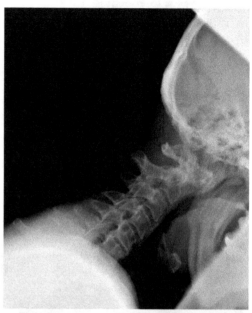

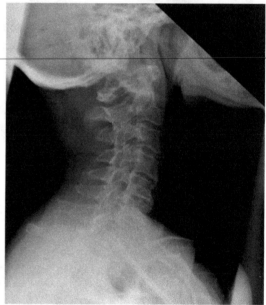

FIG. 1-21. Flexion/extension cervical spine X-rays.

(A) a C7 spinous process fracture
(B) spondylolisthesis
(C) osteoarthritis with decreased range of motion
(D) a vertebral body "step-off"
(E) atlantoaxial subluxation

Atlantoaxial subluxation is defined as the posterior movement of the odontoid process into the vertebral foramen of the C1 vertebra with neck flexion, thereby narrowing the spinal canal. This is caused by laxity of

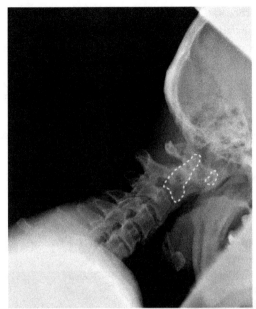

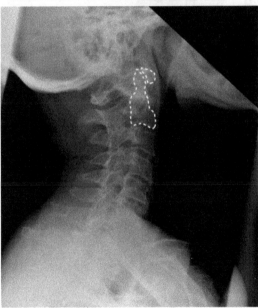

FIG. 1-22. Flexion/extension cervical spine X-rays showing excessive widening of the predentate space.

(Figure 1-22). The space between the odontoid process and the posterior aspect of the anterior tubercle of C1 (the "predentate space") should be negligible in extension. In flexion, a widening of the space by 3 mm or less in adults (5 mm or less in children) is considered normal. Abnormally wide predentate spaces should prompt a referral to a neurosurgeon for further evaluation. Patients scheduled for surgery with severe rheumatoid arthritis or symptomatic Down syndrome patients should have screening X-rays performed.

Ref: Longnecker DE, Brown DL, Newman MF, Zapol WM. *Anesthesiology.* 2nd ed. New York, NY: McGraw Hill; 2012.

Note: Questions 22 and 23 refer to the plain film of the lumbar spine (Figure 1-23).

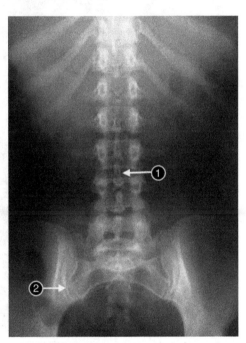

FIG. 1-23. Anterior-posterior X-ray of the lumbar spine.

the transverse ligament that normally holds the odontoid process in place against the anterior arch of C1 and restricts posterior movement. Subluxation may be so severe that it causes impingement of the spinal cord, leading to motor and/or sensory symptoms, as well as bowel/bladder or other myelopathic symptoms. Conditions associated with increased laxity include Down syndrome, rheumatoid arthritis, systemic lupus erythematosus, psoriatic arthritis, neurofibromatosis and trauma.

The diagnosis can be made with lateral cervical spine radiographs in both flexion and extension

22. In Figure 1-23, the arrow labeled "1" is pointing to which of the following structures?

(A) spinous process of L2

(B) L2/3 intervertebral disc

(C) spinous process of L3

(D) L2/3 facet joint

(E) spinous process of L4

Ref: Chen MYM, Pope TL, Ott DJ. *Basic Radiology.* 2nd ed. New York, NY: McGraw Hill; 2011.

23. In Figure 1-23, the arrow labeled "2" is pointing to which of the following structures?

    (A) iliac crest
    (B) sacral foramina
    (C) sciatic notch
    (D) sacral hiatus
    (E) **sacroiliac joint**

    Ref: Chen MYM, Pope TL, Ott DJ. *Basic Radiology.* 2nd ed. New York, NY: McGraw Hill; 2011.

24. Which of the following best describes the clinical diagnosis that can be made from the MRI seen in Figure 1-24?

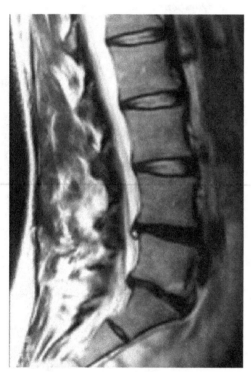

FIG. 1-24. Sagittal magnetic resonance (MR) image of the lumbar spine.

    (A) L4 compression fracture
    (B) spondylolisthesis
    (C) L2-L3 herniated disc
    (D) L3-L4 herniated disc
    (E) **L4-L5 herniated disc**

    In this sagittal MRI of the lumbar spine, the first two sacral vertebral bodies can be visualized most caudally, followed by the vertebral bodies of L5 through L2. The vertebral body of L1 is partially seen. There are no obvious bony deformities such as fracture within these structures. Likewise, significant displacement of any of the vertebrae (e.g., spondylolisthesis) is not apparent. Normal-appearing intervertebral discs are observed between L1-2, L2-3, and L3-4. However, there is significant posterior disc herniation of the L4-5 disc resulting in compression of the thecal sac. The L5-S1 disc is also bulging into the spinal canal to a lesser extent. MRI is the modality of choice to diagnose disc herniation.

    Ref: Chen MYM, Pope TL, Ott DJ. *Basic Radiology.* 2nd ed. New York, NY: McGraw Hill; 2011.

Note: Questions 25 and 26 refer to the magnetic resonance image (MRI) (Figure 1-25).

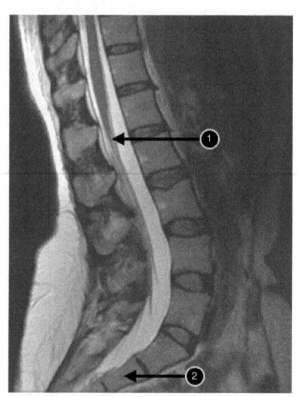

FIG. 1-25. Sagittal magnetic resonance (MR) image of the lumbar spine.

25. In Figure 1-25, the arrow labeled "1" is pointing to which of the following?

    (A) An epidural hematoma
    (B) An epidural abscess
    (C) The L5 vertebral foramen
    (D) **The conus medullaris**
    (E) The filum terminale

26. In Figure 1-25, the arrow labeled "2" is pointing to which of the following?

(A) L5 vertebral body

(B) L5-S1 disc

(C) S1 vertebral body

(D) sacral foramen

(E) **S2 vertebral body**

In this sagittal MRI, the spinal cord and nerve roots can be seen as dark structures in the spinal canal outlined against the bright CSF background. The arrow labeled "1" is pointing toward the terminal portion of the spinal cord, the conus medullaris. The spinal cord typically ends at the level of the L1 vertebral body in adults (in this image, it appears to end at the L1-2 disc space). In infants, it ends at approximately L3. The clinical implication for this is clear—spinal anesthesia should be performed at a level sufficiently distal to the L1 space so as to minimize the risk of contacting the conus with the needle. Given that practitioners are notoriously poor at correctly estimating level by surface landmarks such as iliac crests (may be mistakenly off by as many as two levels), it may be prudent to routinely place the needle at L4-5 or L5-S1.

The sacrum can be distinguished from the lumbar spinal elements due to its fused nature. No intervertebral discs can be observed between segments S1 and S2 in this image (just a small space), whereas substantial discs are seen between all lumbar vertebrae. Of note, the dural sac typically ends at about S1 in adults (S3 in infants).

The filum terminale is a delicate strand of fibrous tissue (of pial origin) that extends from the conus medullaris to the end of the spinal canal (filum terminale internus), and then through the sacral epidural space (filum terminale externus) where it attaches to the coccyx.

Ref: Chen MYM, Pope TL, Ott DJ. *Basic Radiology.* 2nd ed. New York, NY: McGraw Hill; 2011.

Note: Questions 27–30 refer to the ultrasound image of the anterior neck (Figure 1-26).

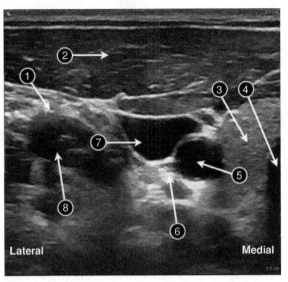

FIG. 1-26. Ultrasound image of the anterior neck taken in a transverse orientation.

1 = Approximate location of phrenic nerve running along anterior surface of anterior scalene muscle
2 = Sternocleidomastoid muscle
3 = Thyroid gland
4 = Airspace within trachea
5 = Internal carotid artery
6 = Approximate location of the vagus nerve within the carotid sheath
7 = Internal jugular vein
8 = Anterior scalene muscle

27. In Figure 1-26, which of the following labeled arrows most closely points to the thyroid gland?

(A) 1

(B) **3**

(C) 4

(D) 6

(E) 8

28. In Figure 1-26, which of the following labeled arrows most closely points to the internal jugular vein?

(A) 4

(B) 5

(C) 6

(D) **7**

(E) 8

29. In Figure 1-26, which of the following labeled arrows most closely points to the approximate location of the vagus nerve?

    (A) 1
    (B) 3
    (C) 4
    (D) 6
    (E) 8

30. In Figure 1-26, which of the following labeled arrows most closely points to the approximate location of the phrenic nerve?

    (A) 1
    (B) 2
    (C) 3
    (D) 6
    (E) 8

This image is one commonly acquired for ultrasound-guided internal jugular vein (IJV) cannulation. It is obtained by placing a linear ultrasound transducer in a transverse orientation just lateral to the cricoid cartilage and sliding medial and lateral to center the IJV. The vein is distinguished from the nearby carotid artery in four ways:

1. The IJV is typically lateral and superficial to the carotid artery.

2. The vein is often triangular or irregularly shaped, whereas the carotid artery is round. With increasing pressure on the skin with the ultrasound transducer, the vein can be made to collapse, whereas the artery will not.

3. An awake patient can be asked to perform a Valsalva maneuver, which will greatly increase the cross-sectional area of the vein.

4. The color Doppler function can be used to confirm brisk pulsatile flow in the artery but not the vein. However, this can be misleading in some cases where transmitted pulsations through the vessel walls also render the flow in the IJV pulsatile.

With the IJV target confirmed, a needle is directed out-of-plane (i.e., straight down from above), passing through the sternocleidomastoid muscle. The operator watches closely for the indentation of the anterior wall of the vein by the needle, and after a "pop" is felt, the needle tip should be visible within the lumen of the IJV, and venous blood aspirated to confirm placement. Most operators will then set the transducer down, and use the nondominant hand to advance a wire through the needle. Confirmation of the wire location in the IJV can be performed using ultrasound prior to dilation and cannula insertion.

Ref: Carmody KA, Moore CL, Feller-Kopman D. *Handbook of Critical Care and Emergency Ultrasound.* New York, NY: McGraw Hill; 2011.

CHAPTER 2

Central and Peripheral Nervous System Anatomy and Physiology

1. Which of the following pathways is involved in the transmission of pain?

   (A) corticobulbar tract
   (B) corticospinal tract
   (C) lateral spinothalamic tract
   (D) dorsal columns
   (E) medial lemniscus

2. A patient has a lesion involving one half of the spinal cord (Brown-Sequard syndrome). Which of the following best describes the expected deficit?

   (A) contralateral weakness
   (B) ipsilateral impaired vibratory sensation
   (C) contralateral impaired sense of joint position
   (D) ipsilateral impaired pain sensation
   (E) contralateral loss of all sensation

3. The cerebral cortex is made up of 6 lobes. Which of the following lobes is involved in "fight-or-flight" responses?

   (A) frontal
   (B) parietal
   (C) corpus callosum
   (D) insula
   (E) limbic

4. Which of the following parts of the cerebellum is involved in propulsive movements such as walking?

   (A) the vermis
   (B) paleocerebellum
   (C) neocerebellum
   (D) archicerebellum
   (E) flocculonodular system

5. Which of the following structures acts as a major outflow of the basal ganglia?

   (A) caudate
   (B) putamen
   (C) globus pallidus
   (D) subthalamic nucleus
   (E) red nucleus

6. Control over the transition from inspiration to expiration is located in which of the following areas?

   (A) nucleus of the tractus solitarius
   (B) ventral respiratory group
   (C) dorsal respiratory group
   (D) medullary respiratory center
   (E) apneustic center

7. The respiratory pattern of inspiration and expiration can be influenced by the carotid and aortic arterial chemoreceptors. Afferent fibers of the glossopharyngeal and vagus nerves project this information primarily to which of the following areas?

   (A) nucleus tractus solitarius
   (B) ventral respiratory group
   (C) botzinger complex
   (D) apneustic center
   (E) pontine respiratory group

8. The anatomic location of the **reticular formation** includes all of the following areas EXCEPT:

   (A) thalamus
   (B) midbrain
   (C) pons
   (D) medulla oblongata
   (E) locus ceruleus

9. The vertebral arteries pass through the foramen magnum of the skull and form which of the following blood vessels?

   (A) anterior cerebral artery
   (B) anterior communicating artery
   (C) posterior cerebral artery
   (D) posterior communicating artery
   (E) basilar artery

10. Which of the following veins or venous sinuses of the head typically drains into the external jugular vein?

   (A) occipital vein
   (B) superior sagittal sinus
   (C) pterygoid plexus
   (D) cavernous sinus
   (E) great cerebral vein (of Galen)

11. In the adult, the inferior end of the spinal cord, or conus medullaris, is typically at what level of the vertebral column?

   (A) L2
   (B) L3
   (C) L4
   (D) L5
   (E) S1

12. A medial branch block is often performed in the diagnosis of facet joint pain in the spine. The "medial branch" is the mainly sensory component of which branch of a spinal nerve?

   (A) dorsal ramus
   (B) ventral ramus
   (C) rami communicantes
   (D) dorsal root ganglion
   (E) ventral root

13. The T4 dermatome level typically corresponds to which of the following?

   (A) nipple
   (B) umbilicus
   (C) anterior aspect of neck
   (D) posterior aspect of thumb
   (E) anterior aspect of thigh

14. A patient undergoes an open abdominal aortic aneurysm repair with supra-renal aortic cross-clamping. Postoperatively, the patient is noted to have paraplegia with preserved proprioceptive sensory function. If the spinal cord injury was due to placement of the aortic cross-clamp, which of the following spinal arteries was likely interrupted?

   (A) anterior sulcal artery
   (B) posterolateral spinal artery
   (C) anterior spinal artery
   (D) anterior medial spinal artery
   (E) great radicular artery

15. During the second stage of labor, a patient notes significant perineal pain. Sensory innervation of the perineum originates from which of the following nerves?

   (A) lumbosacral trunk
   (B) superior hypogastric plexus
   (C) hypogastric nerve
   (D) pelvic splanchnic nerves
   (E) pudendal nerve

16. At approximately the L3/4 level, an epidural catheter is placed for management of labor pain. The epidural catheter does not function as expected: onset of analgesia is delayed and the analgesia is patchy in distribution. Where is the likely location of the catheter?

   (A) intervertebral foramina
   (B) subarachnoid space
   (C) subdural space
   (D) epidural space
   (E) epidural vein

17. Which of the following proposed anatomic boundaries of the posterior epidural space is correct?

   (A) rostral boundary = sacral hiatus
   (B) caudal boundary = base of the skull
   (C) posterior boundary = interspinous ligament
   (D) lateral boundary = pedicle
   (E) anterior boundary = spinal cord

18. The oculomotor nerve (cranial nerve III) provides parasympathetic innervation of the eye via which of the following ganglia?

(A) geniculate ganglion
(B) sphenopalatine ganglion
(C) otic ganglion
(D) ciliary ganglion
(E) submaxillary ganglion

19. During preoperative anesthetic assessment, a patient feels unwell and "faints." Neurally mediated syncope may be caused by which of the following?

(A) diabetes
(B) volume depletion
(C) supraventricular tachycardia
(D) ocular pressure
(E) myocardial ischemia

20. Various ganglia provide autonomic innervation to the head. Which of the following ganglia contains preganglionic sympathetic fibers?

(A) submaxillary
(B) ciliary
(C) sphenopalatine
(D) otic
(E) superior cervical

21. Activation of receptors in the carotid sinus activates a reflex arc termed the baroreceptor reflex (baroreflex). Which part of this reflex is correctly identified?

(A) Low blood pressure increases the number of baroreceptor action potentials.
(B) Afferent nerve fibers travel from the carotid sinus via the vagus nerve to the medulla.
(C) In the medulla, the nucleus of the tractus solitarius (NTS) releases GABA.
(D) Tonic discharge of sympathetic nerves is inhibited.
(E) Resultant change includes vasoconstriction and tachycardia.

22. In the spinal cord, which of the following components of the sympathetic nervous system forms the white rami communicantes?

(A) preganglionic neuron
(B) postganglionic neuron
(C) collateral ganglion
(D) spinal nerve
(E) sympathetic ganglion

23. Afferent nociceptors respond to various harmful stimuli. In order to respond to stimuli, which type of peripheral nociceptor requires activation by inflammatory mediators?

(A) silent
(B) polymodal
(C) thermoreceptor
(D) mechanoreceptor
(E) chemoreceptor

24. Pain stimuli, via Aδ fibers, travel to subdivisions of gray matter within the spinal cord. In an uninjured spinal cord, in which lamina of the dorsal horn do Aδ fibers terminate?

(A) lamina I
(B) lamina III
(C) lamina IV
(D) lamina VI
(E) lamina VII

DIRECTIONS: For each functional description (questions 25–29), select ONE lettered structure that is most closely associated with it. Each lettered structure may be selected once, more than once, or not at all.

(A) amygdala
(B) basal ganglia
(C) cerebral cortex
(D) cerebellum
(E) hippocampus
(F) hypothalamus
(G) internal capsule
(H) medulla
(I) pons
(J) reticular activating system
(K) thalamus

25. This portion of the limbic system is located in the medial aspect of the temporal lobe. It is important for converting short-term memory to long-term memory, and for spatial navigation.

26. This diffuse collection of neurons are responsible for regulating arousal behavior.

27. This is a 2- to 3- mm-thick layer of gray matter covering the gyri and sulci, responsible for complex functions such as memory, language, abstraction, and judgment.

28. A group of nuclei situated at the base of the forebrain that are associated with voluntary motor control.

29. A large band of white matter providing a thoroughfare for axons leaving and entering the cerebral cortex.

30. A healthy 30-year-old man is receiving general anesthesia for a sinus procedure. During the case, he becomes light and bucks on the endotracheal tube. His next blood pressure reading from the cuff is 175/90 mm Hg (baseline 120/80 mm Hg). What is the effect of this increase in systemic blood pressure on his cerebral blood flow (assuming no change in intracranial pressure)?

    (A) cerebral vasodilation with increased cerebral blood flow

    (B) cerebral vasodilation with decreased cerebral blood flow

    (C) cerebral vasoconstriction with increased cerebral blood flow

    (D) cerebral vasoconstriction with decreased cerebral blood flow

    (E) cerebral vasoconstriction with no change in cerebral blood flow

31. Which of the following statements about cerebral blood flow (CBF) is TRUE?

    (A) CBF averages 150 mL/100 g/min of brain tissue.

    (B) White matter has a higher CBF compared to gray matter.

    (C) CBF increases logarithmically with increases in $PaCO_2$.

    (D) CBF is unresponsive to changes in PaO_2 above 60 mm Hg.

    (E) Volatile anesthetics produce a dose-dependent decrease in CBF.

32. Regarding cerebral blood flow (CBF), "inverse steal" refers to which of the following?

    (A) decreased relative CBF to pathologic areas during hypocapnia

    (B) increased relative CBF to pathologic areas during hypercapnia

    (C) increased relative CBF to pathologic areas during hypocapnia

    (D) decreased relative CBF to normal areas during hypocapnia

    (E) increased relative CBF to normal areas during hypercapnia

33. Which of the following statements best reflects the relationship between cerebral metabolic rate for oxygen ($CMRO_2$) and cerebral blood flow (CBF)?

    (A) CBF remains constant until a threshold minimum level of is $CMRO_2$ is reached.

    (B) CBF increases proportionally as $CMRO_2$ decreases.

    (C) CBF decreases proportionally as $CMRO_2$ increases.

    (D) CBF decreases proportionally as $CMRO_2$ decreases.

    (E) CBF is independent of $CMRO_2$.

34. You are providing anesthesia for a patient with long-standing moderate hypertension that is poorly controlled. Which of the following ranges of mean arterial pressure BEST represents the limits of autoregulation of cerebral blood flow in this patient?

    (A) 50 mm Hg and 100 mm Hg
    (B) 50 mm Hg and 125 mm Hg
    (C) 50 mm Hg and 150 mm Hg
    (D) 75 mm Hg and 150 mm Hg
    (E) 75 mm Hg and 175 mm Hg

35. Which of the following statements regarding cerebral ischemia is TRUE?

    (A) The penumbra area of an ischemic insult is the area most affected by the lack of oxygen.
    (B) Global ischemia is defined as interruption of cerebral blood flow to one entire cerebral hemisphere.
    (C) Ischemic depolarization occurs when cerebral blood flow is diminished to 30 mL/100 g/min.
    (D) Cell death in ischemia involves activation of the AMPA receptor by glutamate and the influx of calcium into the cell.
    (E) Autoregulation of cerebral blood flow is maintained at the affected area during focal but not global ischemia.

36. Which of the following statements regarding glucose and cerebral ischemia are TRUE?

    (A) Hyperglycemia has been demonstrated to be harmful for both focal and global ischemia.
    (B) Hyperglycemia has been demonstrated to be harmful in focal but not global ischemia.
    (C) Hyperglycemia has been demonstrated to be harmful in global but not focal ischemia.
    (D) Dextrose-containing solutions are safe to use in brain-injured patients due to the small amount of sugar present.
    (E) Patients with brain injury, stroke, or brain tumor should be managed with intensive insulin therapy to ensure tight glycemic control.

37. Which of the following cerebral autoregulation curves shown in Figure 2-9 best describes the traumatically injured brain?

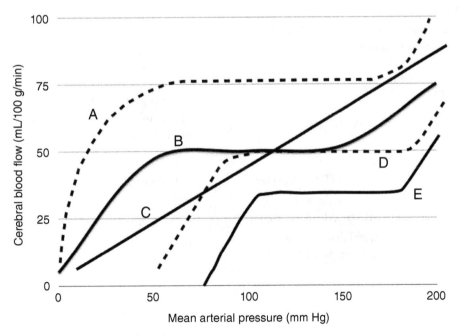

FIG. 2-9. Cerebral autoregulation curves.

38. Where in the central nervous system is cerebrospinal fluid (CSF) produced?

    (A) cerebral aqueduct
    (B) cisterna magna
    (C) fourth ventricle
    (D) choroid plexus
    (E) interpeduncular cistern

39. Which of the following statements regarding cerebral spinal fluid (CSF) is TRUE?

    (A) The total volume of CSF is approximately 250 mL.
    (B) CSF is produced by the arachnoid granulations of the lateral ventricles .
    (C) The pressure in the CSF with the patient sitting is approximately 20 to 30 cm H_2O.
    (D) CSF is formed at a rate of approximately 60 mL/hr.
    (E) CSF circulation exhibits nonpulsatile flow.

40. Which of the following regarding the blood-brain barrier (BBB) is TRUE?

    (A) The BBB regulates the CSF and brain interstitial potassium level.
    (B) The BBB is readily permeable to plasma glutamate.
    (C) The main barrier structure in the BBB is the basement membrane of the capillaries.
    (D) The BBB is immature at birth and takes 3 to 4 months to fully develop.
    (E) The only cells capable of crossing the BBB in the healthy brain are neutrophils.

41. Which one of the statements regarding transport across the BBB is TRUE?

    (A) CO_2 must dissociate into HCO_3^- and H^+ before crossing the BBB.
    (B) Hydrogen ions readily diffuse across the BBB.
    (C) Glucose is transported by the GLUT-5 transporter.
    (D) Lipid soluble drugs with a molecular weight < 400 Da can cross the BBB by diffusion.
    (E) Drugs with a high (> 8) number of hydrogen bonds in aqueous solution cross the BBB readily.

42. In traumatic brain injury, which of the following mechanisms best describes the mechanism for breakdown of the BBB?

    (A) Astrocytes secrete transforming growth factor-β.
    (B) Lipopolysaccharide promotes disruption of the tight junctions via free radicals and interleukins.
    (C) Production of bradykinin releases IL-6 from astrocytes, leading to opening of the BBB.
    (D) Accumulation of amyloid-β.
    (E) Reduction in the efficacy of P-glycoprotein.

43. A patient is admitted to the critical care unit with a closed head injury. The admitting resident leaves orders to hyperventilate the patient with a goal $PaCO_2$ of 25 mm Hg. Which of the following is the likely consequence to this therapeutic decision?

    (A) a rise in CSF bicarbonate levels
    (B) a reduction in CSF bicarbonate levels
    (C) an elevation in CSF potassium levels
    (D) a reduction in CSF sodium levels
    (E) a reduction in CSF pH

44. Blood and CSF are sampled at the same time from a patient. Which of the following solute values would you expect to be equal for both CSF and plasma?

    (A) $PaCO_2$
    (B) K^+
    (C) Ca^{2+}
    (D) Glucose
    (E) Osmolality

45. Assuming a normothermic brain can tolerate 4 minutes of ischemia, what is the approximate expected duration of ischemia that can be tolerated at 27°C?

    (A) 5 minutes
    (B) 6 minutes
    (C) 9 minutes
    (D) 12 minutes
    (E) 15 minutes

46. Which of the following is LEAST likely to promote cerebral protection during anesthesia for patients with ischemic brain injury?

    (A) propofol
    (B) etomidate
    (C) dexmedetomidine
    (D) lidocaine
    (E) xenon

47. You are administering anesthesia for a patient undergoing coronary artery bypass. Which of the following is the BEST agent to use to induce preconditioning of the brain against ischemia?

    (A) propofol
    (B) thiopental
    (C) fentanyl
    (D) isoflurane
    (E) ketamine

48. Which of the following anatomic segments forms the inferior (distal) end of the spinal cord?

    (A) cervical enlargement
    (B) lumbosacral enlargement
    (C) conus medullaris
    (D) cauda equina
    (E) filum terminale

49. A cross-section of the spinal cord shows an "H" of gray matter surrounded by white matter. Which portion of the spinal cord gives rise to preganglionic fibers of the autonomic nervous system?

    (A) anterior horn
    (B) intermediolateral horn
    (C) posterior horn
    (D) dorsal column
    (E) ventral column

50. The gray matter of the spinal can be divided into a number of different layers or laminae (Rexed's laminae). Which of the following laminae gives rise to the lower motor neurons that innervate the arms and legs?

    (A) I
    (B) II
    (C) V
    (D) VI
    (E) IX

51. A deep tendon reflex (an example of a spinal reflex) involves which of the following components?

    (A) stretch of extrafusal muscle fibers in muscle spindles
    (B) activation of afferent Ia fibers
    (C) activation of alpha motor neurons by interneurons
    (D) activation of gamma motor neurons by interneurons
    (E) contraction of intrafusal muscle fibers

52. The afferent limb of the oculocardiac reflex is which of the following nerves?

    (A) III
    (B) V
    (C) X
    (D) VII
    (E) II

53. Ascending fibers of the spinothalamic tract travel in which of the following areas of the spinal cord?

    (A) central canal
    (B) ventral column
    (C) lateral column
    (D) dorsal column
    (E) dorsal gray column

54. Descending fibers of the corticospinal tract travel mainly in which of the following areas of the spinal cord?

    (A) central canal
    (B) ventral column
    (C) lateral column
    (D) dorsal column
    (E) dorsal gray column

55. A patient is undergoing a complex scoliosis repair. Which of the following monitors may potentially indicate ventral (anterior) spinal cord ischemia?

    (A) SSEP
    (B) MEP
    (C) BAEP
    (D) EEG
    (E) VEP

56. Which of the following correctly identifies the number of subunits in a nicotinic acetylcholine-gated ion channel?

    (A) 2
    (B) 3
    (C) 4
    (D) 5
    (E) 7

57. The mature type of nicotinic receptor is characterized by which ONE of the following?

    (A) They are densely concentrated in the folds of the synaptic clefts.
    (B) They are expressed at extrajunctional sites in response to burn injury.
    (C) They contain a γ subunit in place of an ε subunit.
    (D) They have a relatively long open time compared with immature nicotinic receptors.
    (E) They are upregulated in myasthenia gravis.

58. Which of the following statements regarding the resting potential of neurons is TRUE?

    (A) A high external concentration of K^+ ions maintains a resting potential of -90 mV.
    (B) A high internal concentration of K^+ ions maintains a resting potential of -70 mV.
    (C) A high external concentration of Ca_2^+ ions maintains a resting potential of -90 mV.
    (D) A high internal concentration of K^+ ions maintains a resting potential of -55 mV.
    (E) A high internal concentration of Na^+ ions maintains a resting potential of -90 mV.

59. Which of the following statements regarding the electrochemistry of action potentials in neurons is TRUE?

    (A) The threshold potential is -90 mV.
    (B) Potassium efflux is the initiating event in the action potential.
    (C) Voltage-gated potassium channels are slower to open than sodium channels.
    (D) Hyperpolarization (or "undershoot") is the result of sodium channels remaining in an open state.
    (E) Hyperkalemia decreases the excitability of neurons.

60. Which of the following is TRUE regarding the refractory period of action potentials?

    (A) During the absolute refractory period, only electrical stimuli can produce another action potential.
    (B) It is impossible to produce another action potential during the relative refractory period in humans.
    (C) The relative refractory period is twice as long as the absolute refractory period.
    (D) Voltage-gated potassium channels are open during both refractory periods.
    (E) The absolute refractory period follows the relative refractory period.

61. Which of the following BEST describes orthodromic conduction?

    (A) conduction in both directions along an axon
    (B) conduction along only myelinated axons
    (C) conduction from the cell body of a nerve to its axonal terminals
    (D) conduction along the axon towards the cell body
    (E) conduction of impulses along only unmyelinated axons

62. Which of the following regarding saltatory conduction of action potentials is TRUE?

    (A) Saltatory conduction requires more energy than continuous conduction.
    (B) Saltatory conduction is twice as fast as continuous conduction.
    (C) The distance between Nodes of Ranvier is up to 4 mm.
    (D) The concentration of voltage-gated sodium channels at a Node of Ranvier exceed that of unmyelinated axon by a factor of up to 100 times.
    (E) Saltatory conduction is so-named because of the sodium (e.g., salt ~ saltatory) channels that facilitates its propagation.

63. Which of the following is a neurotransmitter that takes part in presynaptic inhibition?

    (A) gamma-aminobutyric acid (GABA)
    (B) glutamate
    (C) norepinephrine
    (D) glycine
    (E) aspartate

64. Which of the following neurotransmitters binds to N-methyl-D-aspartate (NMDA) receptors in the central nervous system?

    (A) acetylcholine
    (B) norepinephrine
    (C) GABA
    (D) glutamate
    (E) substance P

65. Which of the following is a biochemical precursor to epinephrine?

    (A) isoproterenol
    (B) dihydroxy-phenylalanine
    (C) glutamine
    (D) tryptophan
    (E) acetyl-CoA

66. Which of the following sequences correctly identifies the steps in muscle fiber excitation-contraction coupling?

    (A) motor neuron discharge ▶ binding of acetylcholine to nicotinic receptors ▶ increased Na^+ and K^+ conductance in motor end-plate membrane ▶ generation of action potential in muscle fibers ▶ binding of calcium to troponin C ▶ formation of cross-linkages between actin and myosin.
    (B) inward spread of depolarization along T tubules ▶ binding of acetylcholine to nicotinic receptors ▶ release of Ca^{2+} from sarcoplasmic reticulum ▶ generation of action potential in muscle fibers ▶ binding of calcium to troponin C ▶ formation of cross-linkages between actin and myosin.
    (C) motor neuron discharge ▶ inward spread of depolarization along T tubules ▶ increased Na^+ and K^+ conductance in end-plate membrane ▶ generation of action potential in muscle fibers ▶ binding of calcium to troponin C ▶ formation of cross-linkages between actin and myosin.
    (D) motor neuron discharge ▶ binding of acetylcholine to nicotinic receptors ▶ increased Na^+ and K^+ conductance in end-plate membrane ▶ generation of action potential in muscle fibers ▶ release of Ca^{2+} from troponin ▶ formation of cross-linkages between actin and myosin.
    (E) generation of action potential in muscle fibers ▶ generation of end-plate potential ▶ increased Na^+ and K^+ conductance in end-plate membrane ▶ generation of action potential in muscle fibers ▶ binding of calcium to troponin C ▶ formation of cross-linkages between actin and myosin.

67. The molecular mechanism of muscle contraction involves "thin filaments" sliding over "thick filaments." Known as the sliding filament theory, the "thin filament" refers to:

    (A) actin
    (B) myosin
    (C) tropomyosin
    (D) troponin C
    (E) sarcoplasmic reticulum

68. Which of the following statements regarding nociception is TRUE?

    (A) Most nociceptors are either Meissner corpuscles or Pacinian corpuscles.

    (B) Nociceptive afferent fibers are comprised primarily of Aβ and C-fibers.

    (C) Polymodal nociceptors can respond to both pressure and extremes of temperature.

    (D) C fibers conduct at a rate of 12 to 35 m/s.

    (E) Eating a Carolina Reaper pepper will activate TRPM8 receptors.

69. Substance P acts on which receptor type?

    (A) NMDA

    (B) AMPA

    (C) cholinergic

    (D) serotnergic

    (E) neurokinin-1

70. Which of the following statements regarding wide dynamic range neurons is TRUE?

    (A) They serve only noxious stimuli.

    (B) They are primarily responsible for the windup phenomenon.

    (C) They are a third-order neuron.

    (D) They are most abundant in lamina II.

    (E) They are efferent neurons.

71. Which of the following regarding the substantia gelatinosa is TRUE?

    (A) It is the most ventral of all the Rexed laminae.

    (B) It is also known as lamina V.

    (C) It receives primarily Aδ afferents from the periphery.

    (D) It is the site of opioid induced modulation of pain transmission.

    (E) It contains cell bodies of the preganglionic sympathetic neurons.

72. Which of the following neural structures is involved in the transmission of pain impulses to higher levels of the central nervous system?

    (A) fasciculus gracilis

    (B) ventral posterior lateral nucleus

    (C) fasciculus cuneatus

    (D) medial lemniscal tract

    (E) lateral corticospinal tract

73. Which one of the following pain treatment modalities is best explained by Melzack and Wall's gate control theory of pain modulation?

    (A) dorsal column stimulation

    (B) amitriptyline

    (C) carbamazepine

    (D) transcutaneous lidocaine patches

    (E) pregabalin

74. Supraspinal descending inhibitory pathways that modulate pain transmission are mediated primarily through:

    (A) substance P

    (B) calcitonin gene-related peptide (CGRP)

    (C) glycine

    (D) glutamate

    (E) norepinephrine

75. Which of the following regarding visceral pain is TRUE?

    (A) Visceral nociceptive afferents are primarily B fibers.

    (B) Viscera contain "silent" nociceptors that are minimally responsive at baseline.

    (C) Visceral afferent input makes up >40% of total spinal cord afferent input.

    (D) Vagal afferents project to the cuneate nucleus.

    (E) Afferent first-order neurons enter the spinal cord at a specific level and synapse immediately with a single second order neuron at that same level.

76. Which of the following statements regarding pain and affective disorders is TRUE?

    (A) Pain severity is more predictive of functional limitation than fear of movement or re-injury.

    (B) Approximately 10% of chronic pain patients suffer from depression.

    (C) Chronic pain patients are more likely to express anger than nonchronic pain patients.

    (D) Internalization of anger is associated with pain intensity.

    (E) Anxiety is not prevalent in patients with fibromyalgia.

77. Which of the following statements regarding the influence of gender on pain perception is TRUE?

    (A) Men are more likely to be diagnosed with temporomandibular disorders and migraine headaches.

    (B) Women report overall increased pain severity than men.

    (C) Estrogen functions to decrease analgesic requirements.

    (D) Red hair and fair skin in women are a marker for increased sensitivity to pain.

    (E) Sociocultural elements likely play a role in any perceived differences.

78. In the autonomic nervous system (ANS), all preganglionic neurons release which of the following neurotransmitters?

    (A) acetylcholine

    (B) norepinephrine

    (C) adenosine triphosphate (ATP)

    (D) substance P

    (E) neuropeptide Y (NPY)

79. Classically, which of the following adrenergic receptors is considered an "autoreceptor," thereby playing a role in ANS negative feedback?

    (A) α_1

    (B) α_2

    (C) β_1

    (D) β_2

    (E) β_3

80. At postganglionic sympathetic nerve endings, the termination of action of norepinephrine is due mainly to:

    (A) metabolism by monoamine oxidase (MOA).

    (B) metabolism by catechol-O-methyltransferase (COMT).

    (C) metabolism by DOPA decarboxylase.

    (D) reuptake by uptake-1 mechanism.

    (E) reuptake by uptake-2 mechanism.

81. At a noradrenergic synapse, which of the following enzymes is the rate-limiting step in the production of norepinephrine?

    (A) phenylalanine hydroxylase

    (B) tyrosine hydroxylase

    (C) L-DOPA decarboxylase

    (D) dopamine-β-hydroxylase

    (E) phenylethanolamine-N-methyltransferase

82. Botulinum toxin ("Botox") has a number of medical indications and side effects related to muscle weakness. How does botulinum toxin affect cholinergic transmission?

    (A) blocks the transport of choline from the extracellular space into the nerve terminal

    (B) blocks the synthesis of acetylcholine in the nerve terminal

    (C) blocks transport of acetylcholine into vesicles at the nerve terminal

    (D) blocks the influx of Ca^{2+} into the nerve terminal

    (E) blocks exocytosis of acetylcholine into the synaptic cleft

83. Which of the following autonomic nervous system neurons principally release norepinephrine?

    (A) preganglionic neurons

    (B) parasympathetic postganglionic neurons

    (C) sympathetic postganglionic neurons innervating sweat glands

    (D) sympathetic postganglionic neurons innervating skeletal muscle blood vessels

    (E) sympathetic postganglionic neurons innervating systemic veins

84. Acetylcholine's actions on parasympathetic postsynaptic receptors are terminated mainly by:

    (A) pseudocholinesterase
    (B) butyrylcholinesterase
    (C) acetylcholinesterase
    (D) reuptake of acetylcholine by autoreceptors on the presynaptic membrane
    (E) downregulation of muscarinic receptors on the postsynaptic membrane

85. At parasympathetic ganglia, acetylcholine acting on nicotinic receptors will lead to the activation or influx of which of the following second messengers or ions?

    (A) Na^+
    (B) Cl^-
    (C) cAMP
    (D) IP_3
    (E) DAG

86. Which of the following provides sympathetic nervous system innervation to the head and neck?

    (A) cranial nerve III
    (B) cranial nerve X
    (C) splanchnic nerve
    (D) inferior cervical ganglion
    (E) celiac ganglion

87. The autonomic nervous system is influenced by many higher CNS centers. The rostral ventrolateral medulla (RVLM) plays a role in regulation of peripheral vascular tone. Descending neurons from the RVLM modulate preganglionic sympathetic neurons by releasing which one of the following neurotransmitters?

    (A) glutamate
    (B) GABA
    (C) acetylcholine
    (D) norepinephrine
    (E) dopamine

88. A patient with a spinal cord injury (SCI) suffers from autonomic dysreflexia. Which of following statements best explains why the patient is potentially at risk of hypertensive crises?

    (A) SCI interrupts peripheral baroreceptor activation.
    (B) SCI interrupts ascending sensory input to sympathetic nerves.
    (C) SCI interrupts descending inhibitory input to sympathetic nerves.
    (D) SCI interrupts descending activation of parasympathetic nerves.
    (E) SCI interrupts ascending sensory input to parasympathetic nerves.

89. Which type of nerve fibers are responsible for the transmission of afferent input regarding cold tissue temperature throughout the body?

    (A) Aα fibers
    (B) Aβ fibers
    (C) Aδ fibers
    (D) B fibers
    (E) C fibers

90. The primary thermoregulatory control center is located in the:

    (A) spinothalamic tract.
    (B) pons.
    (C) reticular activating system.
    (D) hypothalamus.
    (E) anterior pituitary gland.

91. The "set point" is best described by which of the following concepts?

    (A) the temperature of the input to the hypothalamus where the output is zero
    (B) the point at which sweating begins during heating
    (C) the point at which further vasodilation cannot occur
    (D) the point below which shivering begins
    (E) an exciting moment in a tennis match

92. Which of the following mechanisms of heat production most accurately describes the EARLIEST thermoregulatory response to cold?

    (A) neuroendocrine release of dopamine
    (B) shunting of blood away from visceral organs
    (C) vasoconstriction
    (D) shivering
    (E) neuroendocrine release of thyroxine

93. Which of the following is NOT a factor in the increased risk for hypothermia in neonates?

    (A) a large skin-to-surface-area ratio
    (B) increased thermal conductance of the skin
    (C) higher evaporative losses
    (D) immature thermoregulatory responses
    (E) nonfunctional shunts in the fingers and toes

94. The synthesis of acetylcholine is catalyzed in the terminal of cholinergic nerves by which of the following enzymes?

    (A) choline acetyltransferase
    (B) choline methyltransferase
    (C) acetylcholinesterase
    (D) pseudocholinesterase
    (E) specific cholinesterase

95. Release of acetylcholine from synaptic vesicles into the synaptic cleft is dependent on the influx of which ion?

    (A) sodium
    (B) potassium
    (C) calcium
    (D) magnesium
    (E) hydrogen

96. Spontaneous, small-amplitude depolarizing potentials at the neuromuscular junction are typically seen:

    (A) with an upper motor neuron lesion.
    (B) with normal quantal release of acetylcholine.
    (C) after fasciculations when using succinylcholine.
    (D) in Lambert-Eaton syndrome.
    (E) in hypercalcemia.

97. Which of the following statements regarding the neuromuscular junction is TRUE?

    (A) Acetylcholine binds to one specific subtype of muscarinic cholinergic receptor.
    (B) Cholinergic receptor activation results in the influx of potassium ions in the muscle cell.
    (C) Calcium efflux through the acetylcholine receptor channel is necessary for the generation of end-plate potentials.
    (D) Cholinergic receptors in the neuromuscular junction have two acetylcholine binding sites.
    (E) Junctional folds in the motor end plate serve to reduce the exposure of cholinergic receptors to acetylcholine.

98. Prejunctional nicotinic receptors located on motor nerve endings are responsible for:

    (A) decreasing the uptake of choline into the cell.
    (B) increasing the release of acetylcholine via positive feedback mechanism.
    (C) modulating the calcium influx following depolarization.
    (D) decreasing the rate of fusion of vesicles with the plasma membrane.
    (E) hyperpolarizing the membrane to prevent further release of acetylcholine.

99. Which of the following statements regarding neuromuscular anatomy and function is TRUE?

    (A) Each muscle fiber is typically innervated by 5 to 10 individual axons.
    (B) Nerve endings on slow-twitch muscles are larger and more complicated than those on fast-twitch muscles.
    (C) The motor unit for the extraocular muscles contains more muscle fibers than the motor unit for the quadriceps muscles.
    (D) The synaptic cleft is approximately 20 to 50 nm wide.
    (E) Acetylcholinesterase is synthesized in the liver and transported to the synaptic cleft.

Answers and Explanations: Central and Peripheral Nervous System Anatomy and Physiology

1. Which of the following pathways is involved in the transmission of pain?

   (A) corticobulbar tract
   (B) corticospinal tract
   (C) lateral spinothalamic tract
   (D) dorsal columns
   (E) medial lemniscus

   The lateral spinothalamic tracts are involved in the transmission of pain, temperature, and touch. As pain fibers enter the spinal cord, they typically cross over to form the lateral spinothalamic tract, meaning that ascending pain transmission carries sensation from the contralateral side.

   Descending pathways involved in control of the motor system include the corticospinal, corticobulbar, corticopontine, rubrospinal, reticulospinal, vestibulospinal, and tectospinal tracts. The dorsal column system is involved in ascending transmission of fine touch, proprioception, and two-point discrimination. The fibers originate in the skin, joints, and tendons and end in the dorsal column nuclei (nucleus gracilis and nucleus cuneatus). A crossed fiber bundle, the medial lemniscus, then projects from these nuclei to the contralateral thalamus. The ventral posterolateral (VPL) thalamic nuclei then send sensory information to the somatosensory cortex.

   Refs: Waxman SG. *Clinical Neuroanatomy*. 27th ed. New York, NY. McGraw Hill, 2013.
   Hammer GD, McPhee SJ. *Pathophysiology of Disease: An Introduction to Clinical Medicine*. 7th ed. New York, NY: McGraw Hill; 2014.

2. A patient has a lesion involving one half of the spinal cord (Brown-Sequard syndrome). Which of the following best describes the expected deficit?

   (A) contralateral weakness
   (B) ipsilateral impaired vibratory sensation
   (C) contralateral impaired sense of joint position
   (D) ipsilateral impaired pain sensation
   (E) contralateral loss of all sensation

   Brown-Sequard syndrome involves:
   - Ipsilateral weakness (due to transection of the corticospinal tract).
   - Ipsilateral loss of joint position and vibratory sense (due to transection of the posterior column).
   - Contralateral loss of pain and temperature sense approximately 1 or 2 levels below the lesion (due to transection of the spinothalamic tract.
   - Other signs include unilateral and segmental radicular pain and muscle atrophy.

   Ref: Hammer GD, McPhee SJ. *Pathophysiology of Disease: An Introduction to Clinical Medicine*. 7th ed. New York, NY: McGraw Hill; 2014.

3. The cerebral cortex is made up of 6 lobes. Which of the following lobes is involved in "fight-or-flight" responses?

   (A) frontal
   (B) parietal
   (C) corpus callosum
   (D) insula
   (E) limbic

   The cerebral cortex is made up of the frontal, parietal, temporal, occipital, insular, and limbic lobes:

   1. Frontal lobe: motor cortex and areas for abstract reasoning, judgment, creativity, and social behavior.

2. Parietal lobe: somatosensory cortex

3. Occipital lobe: primary visual cortex

4. Temporal lobe: primary auditory cortex

5. Insula: is thought to contribute to interoceptive awareness (e.g., awareness of body states such as your own heartbeat), motor activities such as swallowing, and emotions.

6. Limbic lobe: part of the limbic system.

The limbic lobe is made up of the parahippocampal gyrus, cingulate gyrus, and subcallosal gyrus. The limbic system contains the limbic lobe and the hippocampus, dentate gyrus and amygdala. It is involved in the following behaviors: feeding, "fight or flight" responses, aggression, and emotion. The corpus callosum contains myelinated and unmyelinated fibers and connects the two cerebral hemisphere.

Ref: Waxman SG. *Clinical Neuroanatomy.* 27th ed. New York, NY: McGraw Hill; 2013.

4. Which of the following parts of the cerebellum is involved in propulsive movements such as walking?

(A) the vermis

(B) **paleocerebellum**

(C) neocerebellum

(D) archicerebellum

(E) flocculonodular system

Anatomically, the cerebellum is divided into two hemispheres connected by the vermis. Each hemisphere is further divided into:

- Archicerebellum, which is formed by the flocculus, nodulus, and connections (flocculonodular system). This part of the cerebellum is involved with maintaining equilibrium and has connections with the vestibular system.

- Paleocerebellum, which is involved with propulsive movements such as walking or swimming.

- Neocerebellum, which is involved with the co-ordinating fine movement.

Ref: Waxman SG. *Clinical Neuroanatomy.* 27th ed. New York, NY: McGraw Hill; 2013.

5. Which of the following structures acts as a major outflow of the basal ganglia?

(A) caudate

(B) putamen

(C) **globus pallidus**

(D) subthalamic nucleus

(E) red nucleus

The extrapyramidal system is important for control of movement and posture. The extrapyramidal system includes the basal ganglia, substantia nigra, subthalamic nucleus, red nucleus, and brain stem reticular formation. The basal ganglia are made up of the caudate nucleus, putamen, and globus pallidus. The major site of input to the basal ganglia is via the striatum (caudate and putamen). Excitatory corticostriate inputs come from various parts of the cerebral cortex. In turn, the caudate and putamen project inhibitory inputs to the internal part of the globus pallidus (GPi). The GPi sends inhibitory outputs to the thalamus. The thalamus completes the feedback loop with projections back to the cerebral cortex. Another feedback loop involves the substantia nigra. Inputs travel from cerebral cortex, to striatum (caudate and putamen), to substantia nigra, and back to striatum. The pars compacta area of the substantia nigra projects dopaminergic neurons to the striatum. This is known as the nigrostriatal projection. Degeneration of the pars compacta substantia nigra alters activity of the basal ganglia and causes Parkinson's disease. Overall, both the globus pallidus and substantia nigra act as the major outflows of the basal ganglia.

Ref: Waxman SG. *Clinical Neuroanatomy.* 27th ed. New York, NY: McGraw Hill; 2013.

6. Control over the transition from inspiration to expiration is located in which of the following areas?

(A) nucleus of the tractus solitarius

(B) ventral respiratory group

(C) dorsal respiratory group

(D) medullary respiratory center

(E) **apneustic center**

Spontaneous respiratory activity is maintained in areas of the medulla and the pons. The medullary respiratory center is composed of the dorsal respiratory groups (DRG) and the ventral respiratory groups (VRG). The DRG is located in the nucleus of the tractus solitarius (NTS) and consists generally of inspiratory neurons. The VRG contains both inspiratory and expiratory neurons. The pons contains the apneustic center, which can be considered the area of control over the transition from inspiration to expiration. (A lesion at this level of the pons can cause apneustic breathing, which is likely due to sustained activity of the medullary neurons with prolonged inspiration and occasional expiration.)

Ref: Levitzky MG. *Pulmonary Physiology.* 8th ed. New York, NY: McGraw Hill; 2013.

7. The respiratory pattern of inspiration and expiration can be influenced by the carotid and aortic arterial chemoreceptors. Afferent fibers of the glossopharyngeal and vagus nerves project this information primarily to which of the following areas?

   (A) **nucleus tractus solitarius**
   (B) ventral respiratory group
   (C) botzinger complex
   (D) apneustic center
   (E) pontine respiratory group

Afferent fibers of the glossopharyngeal and vagus nerves project primarily to the nucleus of the tractus solitarius (NTS). Spontaneous respiratory activity is maintained in areas of the medulla and the pons. The medullary respiratory center is composed of the dorsal respiratory groups (DRG) and the ventral respiratory groups (VRG). The DRG is located in the nucleus of the tractus solitarius (NTS) and consists generally of inspiratory neurons that project to contralateral spinal cord and maintain diaphragm activity via the phrenic nerve. The VRG contains both inspiratory and expiratory neurons. Within the VRG is a group of neurons called the Botzinger complex which may act as a "pacemaker" area for respiratory rhythm. The pontine respiratory group (PRG), or pneumotaxic center, is located in the upper pons. It serves to fine tune respiration and influences the apneustic center (also located in the pons). The apneustic center can be considered the area of control over the transition from inspiration to expiration.

Refs: Ropper AH, Samuels MA, Klein JP. *Adams and Victor's Principles of Neurology.* 10th ed. New York, NY: McGraw Hill; 2014.
Levitzky MG. *Pulmonary Physiology.* 8th ed. New York, NY: McGraw Hill; 2013.

8. The anatomic location of the **reticular formation** includes all of the following areas EXCEPT:

   (A) **thalamus**
   (B) midbrain
   (C) pons
   (D) medulla oblongata
   (E) locus ceruleus

The reticular formation is a complex group of neurons in the tegmentum of the medulla oblongata, pons, and midbrain. The reticular formation also includes nuclei such as the locus ceruleus, raphe complex, and parabrachial nucleus. Ascending projections from the reticular formation involve the lateral hypothalamic area and nonspecific thalamic nuclei. The thalamic nuclei then project throughout the cerebral cortex.

The locus ceruleus is within the reticular formation at the level of the pons. It is involved in the sleep/wake cycle. Medications such as dexmedetomidine act as noradrenergic neurons in the locus ceruleus. The reticular formation plays a role in maintaining generalized arousal, and regulation of respiration, blood pressure, and heart rate. The descending reticulospinal pathway is also involved in modulation of spinal reflexes. The term reticular activating system is sometimes used, reflecting the important role the reticular formation plays in arousal.

Ref: Waxman SG. *Clinical Neuroanatomy.* 27th ed. New York, NY: McGraw Hill; 2013.

9. The vertebral arteries pass through the foramen magnum of the skull and form which of the following blood vessels?

   (A) anterior cerebral artery
   (B) anterior communicating artery
   (C) posterior cerebral artery
   (D) posterior communicating artery
   (E) **basilar artery**

The basilar artery is formed by the fusion of the two vertebral arteries after they pass through the foramen magnum of the skull (Figure 2-1). The major cerebral arteries all originate from the circle of Willis. The circle of Willis is supplied by the left and right internal carotid arteries and the basilar artery. The anterior cerebral artery originates from the internal carotid artery. The anterior communicating artery connects the two anterior cerebral arteries. The posterior cerebral artery originates from the basilar artery and is also supplied via the posterior communicating artery, which connects the internal carotid artery to the posterior cerebral artery.

Ref: Waxman SG. *Clinical Neuroanatomy.* 27th ed. New York, NY: McGraw Hill; 2013.

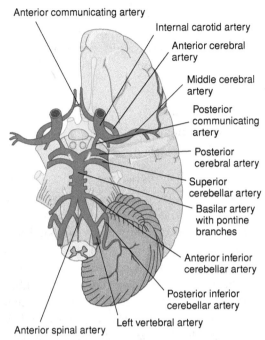

Anterior communicating artery

Internal carotid artery

Anterior cerebral artery

Middle cerebral artery

Posterior communicating artery

Posterior cerebral artery

Superior cerebellar artery

Basilar artery with pontine branches

Anterior inferior cerebellar artery

Posterior inferior cerebellar artery

Left vertebral artery

Anterior spinal artery

FIG. 2-1. Circle of Willis and principal arteries of the brain stem. (Reproduced with permission from Waxman SG. *Clinical Neuroanatomy.* 27th ed. New York, NY: McGraw Hill; 2013.)

10. Which of the following veins or venous sinuses of the head typically drains into the external jugular vein?

   (A) occipital vein
   (B) superior sagittal sinus
   (C) **pterygoid plexus**
   (D) cavernous sinus
   (E) great cerebral vein (of Galen)

The pterygoid plexus receives venous drainage from the superficial face. It contributes to the retromandibular vein that descends and divides into a posterior branch and then joins the external jugular vein (it also has an anterior branch that drains into the internal jugular vein). The venous sinuses are found between the inner and outer layers of dura. The inferior sagittal sinus and great cerebral vein (of Galen) form the straight sinus. The straight sinus, superior sagittal sinus, and occipital vein form the confluence of the sinuses, which in turn drains into the transverse sinus, the sigmoid sinus, and then the internal jugular vein (Figure 2-2).

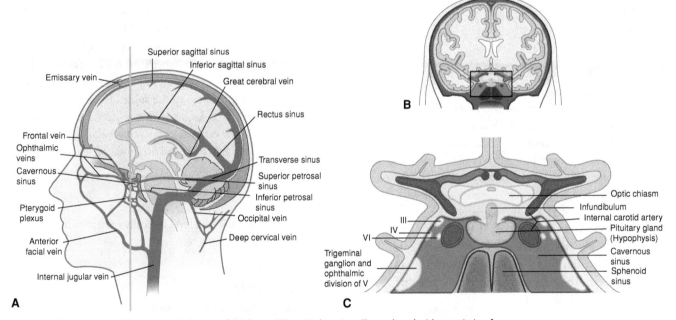

Superior sagittal sinus

Inferior sagittal sinus

Emissary vein

Great cerebral vein

Rectus sinus

Frontal vein

Ophthalmic veins

Cavernous sinus

Transverse sinus

Superior petrosal sinus

Inferior petrosal sinus

Pterygoid plexus

Occipital vein

Deep cervical vein

Anterior facial vein

Internal jugular vein

A

B

Optic chiasm

Infundibulum

Internal carotid artery

Pituitary gland (Hypophysis)

III

IV

VI

Trigeminal ganglion and ophthalmic division of V

Cavernous sinus

Sphenoid sinus

C

FIG. 2-2. Organization of the veins and sinuses of the brain. **(A)** sagittal section. (Reproduced with permission from Waxman SG. *Clinical Neuroanatomy.* 27th ed. New York, NY: McGraw Hill; 2013.) **(B)** coronal section cut along the plane shown by the line in (A). (Modified and reproduced with permission from Poirer J, Gray F, Escourolle R. *Manual of Basic Neuropathology.* 3rd ed. WB Saunders, 1990.) **(C)** Expanded view of the cavernous sinus and surrounding structures. (Reproduced with permission from Waxman SG. *Clinical Neuroanatomy.* 27th ed. New York, NY: McGraw Hill; 2013.)

The cavernous sinuses surround the sella turcica at the base of the brain. Many important structures traverse the cavernous sinus including the internal carotid artery, oculomotor nerve, trochlear nerve, abducens nerve, ophthalmic branch of trigeminal nerve, and trigeminal ganglion. The superior and inferior petrosal sinuses drain the cavernous sinus, eventually leading to the internal jugular vein. It is important to note that emissary veins also connect the intracranial cavernous sinus with the extracranial pterygoid plexus. Since cerebral veins and sinuses are valveless, this means blood may potentially move in either direction—both intracranially or extracranially. Due to this anatomy, extracranial infections may move intracranially via this venous system.

Ref: Waxman SG. *Clinical Neuroanatomy.* 27th ed. New York, NY: McGraw Hill; 2013.

11. In the adult, the inferior end of the spinal cord, or conus medullaris, is typically at what level of the vertebral column?

(A) **L2**
(B) L3
(C) L4
(D) L5
(E) S1

In the adult, the conus medullaris ends at the L1 or L2 level of the vertebral column. The spinal cord extends from the medulla to the conus medullaris. There is a cervical enlargement, which is the origin of the nerves of the upper extremity, and a lumbosacral enlargement, which is the origin of the nerves of the lower extremity. The dura mater of the spinal cord extends from the foramen magnum (where it is contiguous with the cranial dura mater) to approximately the second **sacral** vertebra. The cauda equina is made up of the spinal roots from the lumbar and sacral spinal cord. These roots descend below the conus medullaris within the dural sac. Their appearance is like a horse's tail, hence the name cauda equina.

Ref: Waxman SG. *Clinical Neuroanatomy.* 27th ed. New York, NY: McGraw Hill; 2013.

12. A medial branch block is often performed in the diagnosis of facet joint pain in the spine. The "medial branch" is the mainly sensory component of which branch of a spinal nerve?

(A) **dorsal ramus**
(B) ventral ramus
(C) rami communicantes
(D) dorsal root ganglion
(E) ventral root

There are 31 paired spinal nerves: 8 cervical, 12 thoracic, 5 lumbar, 5 sacral, and 1 coccygeal. Each spinal nerve is composed of a dorsal root and a ventral root. Each dorsal and ventral root is formed from rootlets that connect with the spinal cord. The dorsal (posterior) root contains the dorsal root ganglion, which is the cell body of the sensory axons. The ventral (anterior) root contains the descending motor tracts from the spinal cord. At the thoracic and lumbosacral levels, the ventral root also contains preganglionic autonomic fibers. Outside the intervertebral foramen, the spinal nerve divides into the:

- primary dorsal (posterior) ramus,
- primary ventral (anterior) ramus, and
- rami communicantes (white and gray): join spinal nerves and the sympathetic trunk.

The primary dorsal ramus has a mostly sensory medial branch and a mostly motor lateral branch. A medial branch block is often performed in the diagnosis of facet joint pain in the spine. The primary ventral ramus, which is larger than the dorsal ramus, forms intercostal nerves at the thoracic level, and plexuses at the cervical, brachial, and lumbosacral levels.

Ref: Waxman SG. *Clinical Neuroanatomy.* 27th ed. New York, NY: McGraw Hill; 2013.

13. The T4 dermatome level typically corresponds to which of the following?

(A) **nipple**
(B) umbilicus
(C) anterior aspect of neck
(D) posterior aspect of thumb
(E) anterior aspect of thigh

A dermatome is the sensory component of a corresponding spinal nerve. Clinically, it is important to note there is often overlap from one dermatome to another. Notable dermatomal landmarks include:

- Arm: C5, C6, C7, C8, and T1
- Hand: C6, C7, C8
- Nipple: T4
- Umbilicus: T10
- Groin: L1

C3 and C4 cover the anterior surface of the neck; C6 covers the anterior and posterior surface of the thumb; and L2, L3, and L4 cover the anterior surface of the thigh.

Ref: Waxman SG. *Clinical Neuroanatomy.* 27th ed. New York, NY: McGraw Hill; 2013.

14. A patient undergoes an open abdominal aortic aneurysm repair with supra-renal aortic cross-clamping. Postoperatively, the patient is noted to have paraplegia with preserved proprioceptive sensory function. If the spinal cord injury was due to placement of the aortic cross-clamp, which of the following spinal arteries was likely interrupted?

    (A) anterior sulcal artery
    (B) posterolateral spinal artery
    (C) anterior spinal artery
    (D) anterior medial spinal artery
    (E) **great radicular artery**

The great radicular artery (of Adamkiewicz) usually originates between T5 to T12, although it can originate from the lumbar aorta. Although there can be anatomic variation, the great radicular artery (of Adamkiewicz) is considered the primary supply of the anterior spinal artery in the lower thoracic and lumbar spinal cord. Anterior cord syndrome (ACS) can result from many etiologies including inadequate perfusion of the anterior spinal artery. ACS presents with loss of motor function and loss of pain and temperature sensation below the level of the lesion. Proprioception, vibration, and pressure sensation are preserved. In this situation, inadvertent occlusion of the great radicular artery (of Adamkiewicz) is the cause of ACS. Branches of the vertebral arteries form the anterior spinal artery, which descends along the ventral surface of the spinal cord. Below T4, this artery may be referred to as the anterior medial spinal artery. The anterior sulcal artery is a branch of the anterior spinal artery. The posterolateral arteries also originate from the vertebral arteries.

Ref: Butterworth JF IV, Mackey DC, Wasnick JD. *Morgan and Mikhail's Clinical Anesthesiology.* 5th ed. New York, NY: McGraw Hill; 2013.

15. During the second stage of labor, a patient notes significant perineal pain. Sensory innervation of the perineum originates from which of the following nerves?

    (A) lumbosacral trunk
    (B) superior hypogastric plexus
    (C) hypogastric nerve
    (D) pelvic splanchnic nerves
    (E) **pudendal nerve**

The pudendal nerve (S2, S3, S4) supplies sensory innervation to the perineum. The pelvis receives innervation from the lumbosacral trunk, sacral plexus, coccygeal plexus, the pelvic sympathetic trunk, and parasympathetic nerves. The **sacral plexus** is derived from the ventral rami of L4, L5, S1, S2, S3, and part of S4. (The contribution from L4, L5 is termed the **lumbosacral trunk.**) There are numerous branches from the sacral plexus, including:

- Superior gluteal nerve—L4-S1
- Inferior gluteal nerve—L5-S2
- Pudendal nerve—S2, S3, S4
- Sciatic nerve—L4, L5, S1, S2, S3

Sympathetic fibers for the pelvis originate from T10 to L2 form the superior hypogastric plexus. This plexus then divides into left and right **hypogastric nerves** at the level of the sacral promontory. Parasympathetic and afferent innervation of pelvic viscera is via **pelvic splanchnic nerves** (nervi erigentes) originating from S2-S4. The **hypogastric nerves** and the **pelvic splanchnic nerves** together form the inferior hypogastric plexus (which contains both sympathetic and parasympathetic fibers). The inferior hypogastric plexus further divides into other plexuses, which provide innervation for defecation, urination, ejaculation, and orgasm.

Ref: Morton DA, Albertine K, Foreman KB. *Gross Anatomy: The Big Picture.* 1st ed. New York, NY: McGraw Hill; 2011.

16. At approximately the L3/4 level, an epidural catheter is placed for management of labor pain. The epidural catheter does not function as expected: onset of analgesia is delayed and the analgesia is patchy in distribution. Where is the likely location of the catheter?

    (A) intervertebral foramina
    (B) subarachnoid space
    (C) subdural space
    (D) epidural space
    (E) epidural vein

    Placement of a catheter in the subdural space is suggested by delayed onset of analgesia, a patchy or diffuse block, or a high or total spinal. Relevant anatomy for epidural catheter placement includes knowledge of the various membranes and spaces surrounding the spinal cord. The intrathecal, or subarachnoid space, is filled with cerebrospinal fluid. It is bounded by the pia mater, which is attached to the surface of the spinal cord, and the arachnoid mater. The arachnoid mater and the dura mater are close together, with the subdural space (a potential space) in between. The epidural space, superficial to the dura mater, has no free fluid and is filled with blood vessels, fat, and nerve roots.

    Ref: Hadzic A. *NYSORA Textbook of Regional Anesthesia and Acute Pain Medicine.* 1st ed. New York, NY: McGraw Hill; 2007.

17. Which of the following proposed anatomic boundaries of the posterior epidural space is correct?

    (A) rostral boundary = sacral hiatus
    (B) caudal boundary = base of the skull
    (C) posterior boundary = interspinous ligament
    (D) lateral boundary = pedicle
    (E) anterior boundary = spinal cord

    In the spinal column, an anterior and posterior epidural space surround the dura mater. The boundaries for the posterior epidural space include (Figure 2-3):

    • Rostral—the base of the skull
    • Caudal—the sacral hiatus
    • Posterior—the ligamentum flavum
    • Lateral—the pedicles and intervertebral foramina
    • Anterior—dura mater

    Ref: Hadzic A. *NYSORA Textbook of Regional Anesthesia and Acute Pain Medicine.* 1st ed. New York, NY: McGraw Hill; 2007.

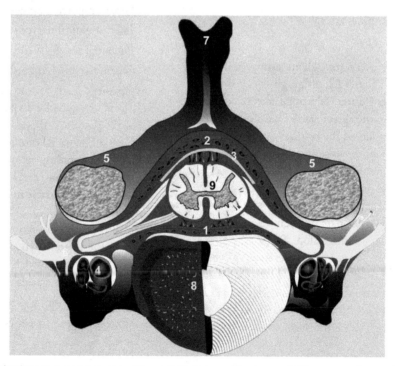

FIG. 2-3. Epidural space: **1.** Anterior epidural space, **2.** Posterior epidural space, **3.** Ligamentum flavum, **4.** Blood vessels in the epidural space, **5.** Pedicles, **6.** Nerve roots, **7.** Spinous process, **8.** Vertebral body, **9.** Spinal cord. (Reproduced with permission from Hadzic A. *NYSORA Textbook of Regional Anesthesia and Acute Pain Medicine.* 1st ed. New York, NY: McGraw Hill; 2007.)

18. The oculomotor nerve (cranial nerve III) provides para-sympathetic innervation of the eye via which of the following ganglia?

(A) geniculate ganglion

(B) sphenopalatine ganglion

(C) otic ganglion

(D) **ciliary ganglion**

(E) Submaxillary ganglion

Cranial nerves III, VII, IX, and X (oculomotor, facial, glossopharyngeal, and vagus nerves) have preganglionic parasympathetic fibers. The parasympathetic innervation of the head is via 4 ganglia (Note: These ganglia also contain sympathetic and sensory fibers):

1. **Ciliary ganglion**—parasympathetic preganglionic fibers from the oculomotor nerve (CN III) travel to the ciliary ganglion. Postganglionic fibers extend to the iris and lens of the eye.

2. **Sphenopalatine (or pterygopalatine) ganglion**—parasympathetic preganglionic fibers from the facial nerve (CN VII) travel via the glossopalatine nerve through the geniculate ganglion and the great petrosal nerve to reach the sphenopalatine ganglion. Postganglionic fibers travel to lacrimal glands and mucous membranes of the nasal cavity and hard and soft palate.

3. **Otic ganglion**—parasympathetic preganglionic fibers from glossopharyngeal nerve (CN IX) travel through the jugular ganglion, the tympanic nerve and small petrosal nerve to reach the otic ganglion. Postganglionic fibers then travel to the parotid gland.

4. **Submaxillary ganglion**—parasympathetic preganglionic fibers from the facial nerve (CN VII) travel through the geniculate ganglion via the glossopalatine nerve, the chorda tympani, and the lingual nerve to the submaxillary ganglion. Postganglionic fibers travel to the submaxillary and sublingual glands.

Ref: Waxman SG. *Clinical Neuroanatomy.* 27th ed. New York, NY: McGraw Hill; 2013.

19. During preoperative anesthetic assessment, a patient feels unwell and "faints." Neurally mediated syncope may be caused by which of the following?

(A) diabetes

(B) volume depletion

(C) supraventricular tachycardia

(D) **ocular pressure**

(E) myocardial ischemia

Causes of syncope (transient loss of consciousness) include:

- Neurally mediated syncope
- Orthostatic hypotension
- Cardiac syncope

Neurally mediated syncope is the result of increased parasympathetic efferent activity (via the vagus nerve) leading to bradycardia, and inhibition of sympathetic efferent activity leading to vasodilation. Triggers for this reflex arc include:

- Vasovagal syncope (provoked by pain, fear, anxiety)
- Airway instrumentation
- Urogenital tract instrumentation
- Gastrointestinal tract instrumentation
- Carotid sinus massage
- **Ocular pressure** and ocular surgery

Orthostatic hypotension is generally due to failure of the autonomic nervous system to provide adequate sympathetically mediated vasoconstriction and increased chronotropy. Causes of ANS dysfunction include:

- Parkinson's disease
- Shy-Drager syndrome
- Diabetes
- Volume depletion
- Hereditary and immune autonomic neuropathies

Cardiac syncope may be caused by arrhythmias (sinus node dysfunction, supraventricular tachycardia, ventricular tachycardias) or structural heart disease (cardiomyopathies, myocardial ischemia, valvular disease).

Ref: Kasper D, Fauci A, Hauser S, Longo D, Jameson J, Loscalzo J. *Harrison's Principles of Internal Medicine.* 19th ed. New York, NY: McGraw Hill; 2015.

20. Various ganglia provide autonomic innervation to the head. Which of the following ganglia contains preganglionic sympathetic fibers?

(A) submaxillary

(B) ciliary

(C) sphenopalatine

(D) otic

(E) **superior cervical**

Sympathetic innervation to the head is via the superior cervical ganglion. Preganglionic sympathetic fibers travel from the spinal cord, via the white rami communicantes, to reach the superior cervical ganglion (The sympathetic chain forms 3 cervical ganglia: inferior cervical, middle cervical, and superior cervical). Postganglionic sympathetic fibers then pass from the superior cervical ganglion, via the carotid plexus, to the head. In the head, there are 4 pairs of autonomic ganglia:

1. Ciliary ganglion
2. Sphenopalatine (or pterygopalatine) ganglion
3. Otic ganglion
4. Submaxillary ganglion

In addition to the postganglionic sympathetic fibers, each of these ganglia also contains parasympathetic and sensory fibers.

Ref: Waxman SG. *Clinical Neuroanatomy.* 27th ed. New York, NY: McGraw Hill; 2013.

21. Activation of receptors in the carotid sinus activates a reflex arc termed the baroreceptor reflex (baroreflex). Which part of this reflex is correctly identified?

(A) Low blood pressure increases the number of baroreceptor action potentials.

(B) Afferent nerve fibers travel from the carotid sinus via the vagus nerve to the medulla.

(C) In the medulla, the nucleus of the tractus solitarius (NTS) releases GABA.

(D) Tonic discharge of sympathetic nerves is inhibited.

(E) Resultant change includes vasoconstriction and tachycardia.

Activation of the baroreceptor reflex results in inhibition of sympathetic outflow. The baroreceptor reflex is a negative feedback loop (Figure 2-4). An **increase** in

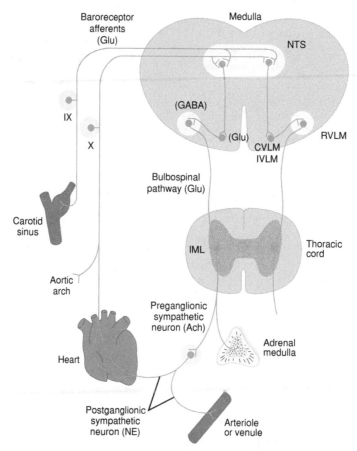

FIG. 2-4. Basic pathways involved in the medullary control of blood pressure. The rostral ventrolateral medulla (RVLM) is one of the major sources of excitatory input to sympathetic nerves controlling the vasculature. These neurons receive inhibitory input from the baroreceptors via an inhibitory neuron in the caudal ventrolateral medulla (CVLM). The nucleus of the tractus solitarius (NTS) is the site of termination of baroreceptor afferent fibers. The putative neurotransmitters in the pathways are indicated in parentheses. Ach, acetylcholine; GABA, γ-aminobutyric acid; Glu, glutamate; IML, intermediolateral gray column; IVLM, intermediate ventrolateral medulla; NE, norepinephrine; NTS, nucleus of the tractus solitarius; IX and X, glossopharyngeal and vagus nerves. (Reproduced with permission from Barrett KE, Boitano S, Barman SM, Brooks HL. *Ganong's Review of Medical Physiology.* 24th ed. New York, NY: McGraw Hill; 2012.)

blood pressure stretches the baroreceptors in the carotid sinus and aortic arch. Stretching increases the number of baroreceptor action potentials. In the carotid sinus, information in the afferent limb of the reflex is relayed to the medulla via the **glossopharyngeal nerve** (the vagus nerve relays information from baroreceptors in the aortic arch). In the medulla, afferent fibers synapse with the nucleus of the tractus solitarius (NTS), which releases an excitatory neurotransmitter, **glutamate**. The NTS interacts with both sympathetic and parasympathetic outflow to the heart and vasculature. In parasympathetic outflow, the NTS releases glutamate and **stimulates** vagal activity in the nucleus ambiguus and dorsal motor nucleus. In sympathetic outflow, the NTS releases glutamate and stimulates inhibitory interneurons in the caudal ventrolateral medulla (CVLM).

Activation of the CVLM releases GABA, which **inhibits** the rostral ventrolateral medulla (RVLM). The RVLM, or vasomotor area, sends excitatory signals to the sympathetic neurons in the spinal cord. In this way, activation of the baroreceptor reflex **stimulates** the parasympathetic nervous system and **inhibits** the sympathetic nervous system, resulting in vasodilation, bradycardia, hypotension, and decreased cardiac output. As an aside, the carotid and aortic **bodies** are chemoreceptors involved in regulation of breathing (they are stimulated by hypoxia and to a lesser degree by altered CO_2 and pH). It should be noted that the carotid and aortic bodies also provide **excitatory** input to the RVLM and the sympathetic nervous system.

Ref: Barrett KE, Boitano S, Barman SM, Brooks HL. *Ganong's Review of Medical Physiology.* 24th ed. New York, NY: McGraw Hill; 2012.

22. In the spinal cord, which of the following components of the sympathetic nervous system forms the white rami communicantes?

(A) **preganglionic neuron**
(B) postganglionic neuron
(C) collateral ganglion
(D) spinal nerve
(E) sympathetic ganglion

Sympathetic nervous system outflow in the spinal cord is from T1 to L2 (thoracolumbar outflow). The

preganglionic cell bodies are found in the intermediolateral cell columns of the spinal cord. The preganglionic fibers follow the ventral roots and spinal nerves out of the intervertebral foramina. The preganglionic fibers connect to the sympathetic ganglia of the paravertebral ganglionic chain via the white rami communicantes (mostly myelinated fibers). The preganglionic fibers may stay at that level or travel up, down, or out of the ganglionic chain, eventually synapsing with postganglionic fibers. Those fibers traveling out of the ganglionic chain without synapsing go on to synapse at collateral (intermediary) sympathetic ganglia such as the celiac and mesenteric ganglia. Gray rami communicantes are the unmyelinated sympathetic postganglionic fibers exiting the paravertebral ganglionic chain and joining the spinal nerves to continue on to their target sites.

Ref: Waxman SG. *Clinical Neuroanatomy.* 27th ed. New York, NY: McGraw Hill; 2013.

23. Afferent nociceptors respond to various harmful stimuli. In order to respond to stimuli, which type of peripheral nociceptor requires activation by inflammatory mediators?

(A) **silent**
(B) polymodal
(C) thermoreceptor
(D) mechanoreceptor
(E) chemoreceptor

A silent nociceptor is not active in uninjured tissue. It requires activation by inflammatory mediators. In general, primary afferent nociceptors may respond to a variety of stimuli including temperature (thermoreceptor), pressure (mechanoreceptor), and chemicals such as prostaglandins, leukotrienes, and bradykinin (chemoreceptor). A polymodal nociceptor responds to multiple stimuli. Aδ fibers include mechano- and thermoreceptors, while the majority of C fibers are polymodal nociceptors.

Ref: Kasper D, Fauci A, Hauser S, Longo D, Jameson J, Loscalzo J. *Harrison's Principles of Internal Medicine.* 19th ed. New York, NY: McGraw Hill; 2015.

24. Pain stimuli, via Aδ fibers, travel to subdivisions of gray matter within the spinal cord. In an uninjured spinal cord, in which lamina of the dorsal horn do Aδ fibers terminate?

(A) lamina I

(B) lamina III

(C) lamina IV

(D) lamina VI

(E) lamina VII

Nociceptive stimuli are transmitted via Aδ and C fibers to the spinal cord (Figure 2-5). Aδ fibers terminate in laminae I and II with collateral branches to laminae V and X. C fibers terminate in laminae I, II, and V. The Rexed subdivisions of the dorsal horn include laminae I-VI (lamina I and II together are also termed the substantia gelatinosa). The ventral horn includes laminae VII-IX, and lamina X surrounds the central canal. Note, after injury, the dorsal horn cytoarchitecture changes, which may explain phenomena such as allodynia and neuropathic pain.

Ref: Butterworth JF IV, Mackey DC, Wasnick JD. *Morgan and Mikhail's Clinical Anesthesiology.* 5th ed. New York, NY: McGraw Hill; 2013.

DIRECTIONS: For each functional description below, select ONE lettered structure that is most closely associated with it. Each lettered structure may be selected once, more than once, or not at all.

(A) amygdala

(B) basal ganglia

(C) cerebral cortex

(D) cerebellum

(E) hippocampus

(F) hypothalamus

(G) internal capsule

(H) medulla

(I) pons

(J) reticular activating system

(K) thalamus

25. This portion of the limbic system is located in the medial aspect of the temporal lobe. It is important for converting short-term memory to long-term memory, and for spatial navigation.

(E) Hippocampus

The hippocampus is one component of the limbic system, along with the thalamus, hypothalamus, and amygdala. Anatomically, these structures are found tucked underneath the edge of the cerebral cortex (Latin *limbus* = border). Each hippocampus is shaped like a small banana or a seahorse (Greek *hippos* meaning "horse" and *kampos* meaning "sea monster").

The hippocampi play an important role in the formation of new memories. Damage to both hippocampi results in difficulty forming new memories, although damage to just one hippocampus generally results in little change in function. Damage to the hippocampus does not appear to affect all types of memory. For example, the learning of a new skill involves memory processing, which is unaffected by hippocampal damage. The hippocampus is one of the very few places in the brain where new neurons are continually formed, and it serves as a source for neural stem cells.

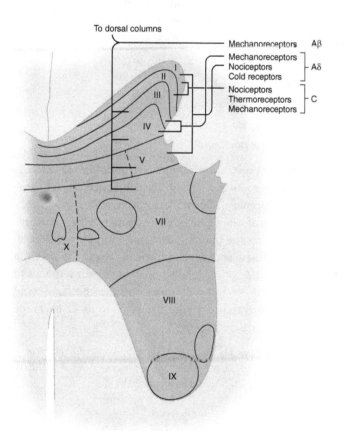

FIG. 2-5. Rexed's spinal cord laminae. Note the termination of the different types of primary afferent neurons. (Reproduced with permission from Butterworth JF IV, Mackey DC, Wasnick JD. *Morgan and Mikhail's Clinical Anesthesiology.* 5th ed. New York, NY: McGraw Hill; 2013.)

It appears that the hippocampus also plays a role in spatial memory—patients with nonfunctioning hippocampi often cannot remember where they have been or where they are going. London taxi drivers, who must pass a rigorous knowledge test of city streets before they are licensed, have been found to have larger-than-average hippocampi. Whether the drivers are predisposed to good navigational skills and are pre-selected for that occupation, or whether navigating the streets exercised the hippocampus and enlarges is, is unclear.

The hippocampus appears to be especially sensitive to stress, and elevations in cortisol cause a reduction in excitability in some neurons, inhibition of new neuronal development, and atrophy of dendrites in hippocampal pyramidal cells. Patients with post-traumatic stress disorder and Cushing's syndrome have been shown to have hippocampal atrophy.

Ref: Ropper AH, Samuels MA, Klein JP. *Adams and Victor's Principles of Neurology.* 10th ed. New York, NY: McGraw Hill; 2014.

26. This diffuse collection of neurons are responsible for regulating arousal behavior.

(J) Reticular activating system

The reticular activating system (RAS) is a set of nuclei in the brainstem that play a role in arousal and sleep-wake transitions, as well as the overall level of CNS activity. It is synonymous with the ascending component of the reticular formation. There are multiple inputs to the RAS including afferent sensory tracts, trigeminal tracts, and auditory and visual input. Neurons from the RAS project to the intralaminar nucleus of the thalamus, as well as a diffuse pathway to the cortex that bypasses the thalamus. Several neurotransmitter systems are present in the RAS, including serotonergic, adrenergic, histaminergic, dopaminergic and cholinergic.

During wakefulness, combined excitatory input from the cortex and the RAS promote the tonic firing of thalamocortical neurons. This promotes a state of vigilance, arousal and attention to detail. On the other hand, during slow-wave deep sleep or general anesthesia, thalamocortical neurons maintain a bursting pattern of firing, which drives a synchronization of the cortex and the slow 1 to 4 Hz delta waves seen on EEG during the deepest stages of non-REM sleep. The principal brainstem nuclei of the RAS that effect ascending excitatory input to the hypothalamus, thalamus and cortex are the locus ceruleus (LC) and dorsal raphe.

Anesthetic drugs may affect components of the RAS and contribute to an unconscious state. Dexmedetomidine exerts its sedative effect by inhibiting the LC a noradrenergic component of the RAS. Similarly, levels of catecholamine in the central nervous system influence MAC. Patients who have ingested cocaine or amphetamines have increased requirements for anesthesia due to activation of the LC. Spinal anesthesia decreases the peripheral input into the RAS and has been shown to render these patients sensitive to sedatives.

Ref: Waxman SG. *Clinical Neuroanatomy.* 27th ed. New York, NY: McGraw Hill; 2013.

27. This is a 2 to 3 mm thick layer of gray matter covering the gyri and sulci, responsible for complex functions such as memory, language, abstraction, and judgment.

(C) Cerebral cortex

The cerebral cortex is the outermost layer of the brain that covers the two cerebral hemispheres. It is a thin layer of 2 to 3 mm, but is deeply folded which vastly increases the surface area. The neocortex, which represents the great majority of the cortex, has six distinct layers, labeled I through VI. The first three layers (the supragranular layers) are the origin and termination of intracortical connections. Layer IV receives thalamocortical connections. Layers V and VI connect the cortex with subcortical areas such as the basal ganglia, brainstem and spinal cord. The allocortex, a more ancient part of the cortex, has less than six layers and includes the olfactory cortex and the hippocampus.

The functional organization of the neocortex is outlined in Table 2-1.

Ref: Waxman SG. *Clinical Neuroanatomy.* 27th ed. New York, NY: McGraw Hill; 2013.

TABLE 2-1. Organization of the neocortex.

Part of cortex	Location	Function
Primary somatosensory cortex	Post-central gyrus (parietal lobe)	Sensation based on degree of innervation (i.e., lips and fingertips are represented much more than other parts)
Visual cortex	Surrounds calcarine sulcus (occipital lobe)	Interpretation of visual input from optic nerves.
Auditory cortex	Transverse temporal gyri (temporal lobe)	Interpretation of sound. In the dominant hemisphere, the cortex surrounding the auditory cortex (Wernicke's area) is required for understanding verbal and written language.
Primary motor cortex	Precentral gyrus (frontal lobe)	Origin of the corticospinal tract. Also some cortical bulbar fibers and projections to thalamus and basal ganglia.
Prefrontal cortex	Frontal lobe	Executive functions such as working memory, judgment, planning, abstract reasoning and dividing attention. Also impulse control, personality, reactivity to surroundings and mood.

28. A group of nuclei situated at the base of the forebrain that are associated with voluntary motor control.

(B) Basal ganglia

The basal ganglia are composed of the striatum (caudate nucleus and putamen), the globus pallidus (substantia nigra and nucleus accumbens), and the subthalamic nucleus. These structures play a role in voluntary motor control as well as reward. The neurotransmitter that subserves both of these functions is dopamine. Parkinson's disease is a degenerative disorder of the CNS resulting from the loss of dopamine-generating cells in the substantia nigra. The result is rigidity, bradykinesia, resting tremor, and gait disturbances. Huntington's chorea, characterized by uncontrollable movements, loss of coordination, and neuropsychiatric symptoms, affects many brain structures, but the most sensitive appears to be the striatum.

Ref: Waxman SG. *Clinical Neuroanatomy.* 27th ed. New York, NY: McGraw Hill; 2013.

29. A large band of white matter providing a thoroughfare for axons leaving and entering the cerebral cortex.

(G) Internal capsule

The internal capsule is a mass of myelinated axons that transmit signals from the cortex to the subcortical areas, as well as sensory information upward from subcortical areas to the sensory cortex. It contains the pyramidal tracts, which are the pathways for voluntary motor signals to travel from the cortex to the pyramids of the medulla, and eventually to the spinal cord.

The internal capsule runs from the corona radiata (just below the gray matter of the cortex) and separates the basal ganglia (laterally) from the thalamus (medially). It is here that the fibers tend to "bottleneck" before entering the brainstem. The

internal capsule is the most common location for lacunar strokes.

Ref: Waxman SG. *Clinical Neuroanatomy.* 27th ed. New York, NY: McGraw Hill; 2013.

30. A healthy 30 year-old man is receiving general anesthesia for a sinus procedure. During the case, he becomes light and bucks on the endotracheal tube. His next blood pressure reading from the cuff is 175/90 mm Hg (baseline 120/80 mm Hg). What is the effect of this increase in systemic blood pressure on his cerebral blood flow (assuming no change in intracranial pressure)?

(A) cerebral vasodilation with increased cerebral blood flow

(B) cerebral vasodilation with decreased cerebral blood flow

(C) cerebral vasoconstriction with increased cerebral blood flow

(D) cerebral vasoconstriction with decreased cerebral blood flow

(E) cerebral vasoconstriction with no change in cerebral blood flow

Cerebral perfusion pressure (CPP) is the pressure gradient causing blood flow to the brain. It is calculated by subtracting the intracranial pressure (ICP) from the mean arterial pressure (MAP). If jugular venous pressure is higher than the ICP, then this is subtracted from MAP instead. Cerebral perfusion pressure is normally between 70 and 90 mm Hg in adults. A patient with a CPP below 70 mm Hg will begin to show signs of cerebral ischemia.

Cerebral autoregulation is the ability of the cerebral vasculature to vasodilate and vasoconstrict in response to changes in the MAP to maintain constant cerebral

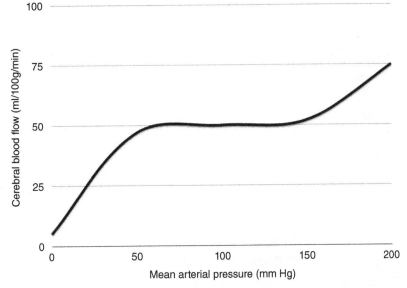

FIG. 2-6. Normal cerebral autoregulation curve.

blood flow (CBF). As the pressure gradient to the brain falls, vessels dilate to keep CBF constant; conversely, as pressure increases, the vessels constrict to keep flow constant by way of increased resistance. Autoregulation *normally* occurs within the MAP range of 50 to 150 mm Hg. Below this, vessels are already maximally vasodilated and further reductions in pressure result in a linear decrease in CBF (Figure 2-6).

At the other end of the spectrum, increases in MAP beyond 150 mm Hg cannot be constrained by further vasoconstriction and flow begins to increase linearly. This autoregulation is often dysfunctional or abolished in the presence of pathology (e.g., trauma, tumor), so increases in MAP are more likely to result in an increased CBF, with a concomitant rise in the volume of the blood compartment in the skull. This leads to increased ICP and the beginning of a vicious cycle that ends in cerebral ischemia.

Ref: Longnecker DE, Brown DL, Newman MF, Zapol WM. *Anesthesiology.* 2nd ed. New York, NY: McGraw Hill; 2012.

31. Which of the following statements about cerebral blood flow (CBF) is TRUE?

(A) CBF averages 150 mL/100 g/min of brain tissue.

(B) White matter has a higher CBF compared to gray matter.

(C) CBF increases logarithmically with increases in PaCO$_2$.

(D) CBF is unresponsive to changes in PaO$_2$ above 60 mm Hg.

(E) Volatile anesthetics produce a dose-dependent decrease in CBF.

CBF represents approximately 750 mL/min, or about 15% of cardiac output (although it is only 2% of the total mass of the body). Put another way, this is about 50 mL/100 g/min of brain tissue. Flow is not constant to all areas, and those with metabolically active cell constituents (i.e., cell bodies) require more perfusion. For this reason, gray matter receives about 4 times the CBF as neighboring white matter, which is just composed of axons and supporting cells. All of the volatile anesthetics increase CBF in a dose-dependent manner. This effect is most potent for halothane, but still occurs with isoflurane, sevoflurane and desflurane, especially at levels >1.5 MAC. However, while the CBF increases with the volatile agents, cerebral metabolism decreases, a phenomenon known as "uncoupling," since the decrease in metabolic demand is not proportionally met with a decrease in CBF.

Cerebral vascular resistance, one of the two determinants of CBF along with cerebral perfusion pressure, is influenced chemically by changes in PaCO$_2$ and PaO$_2$. In the normal brain, as PaCO$_2$ increases, there is a linear increase in CBF (Figure 2-7). Normoxia and hyperoxia have little influence on CBF, while a drop in the cerebral PaO$_2$ below a critical threshold of 60 mm Hg results in a significant vasodilatory response and increase in CBF in an attempt to maintain oxygen delivery to the cells.

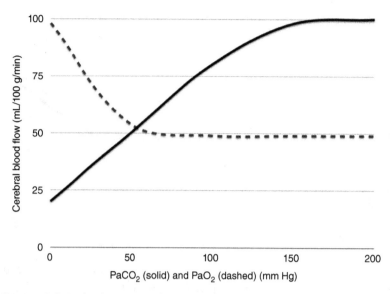

FIG. 2-7. Relationship between cerebral blood flow and oxygen/carbon dioxide tension.

Ref: Longnecker DE, Brown DL, Newman MF, Zapol WM. *Anesthesiology.* 2nd ed. New York, NY: McGraw Hill; 2012.

32. Regarding cerebral blood flow (CBF), "inverse steal" refers to which of the following?

    (A) decreased relative CBF to pathologic areas during hypocapnia

    (B) increased relative CBF to pathologic areas during hypercapnia

    (C) increased relative CBF to pathologic areas during hypocapnia

    (D) decreased relative CBF to normal areas during hypocapnia

    (E) increased relative CBF to normal areas during hypercapnia

The response of the cerebral vasculature to hypercapnia is ordinarily linear and consistent (i.e., the higher the $PaCO_2$, the higher the CBF). However, in areas surrounding tumors, traumatically injured areas, or areas of infarct, vasodilation may already be maximal, presumably due to accumulation of acidic metabolic products. If hypercapnia then occurs, normal cerebral vasculature in other parts of the brain will dilate, accommodating an increase in flow and producing a shunt away from the injured portion of the brain. This is termed "intracerebral steal syndrome."

The reverse is true with hypocapnia. As the $PaCO_2$ decreases, normal vessels will constrict, increasing the resistance to those areas and creating favorable conditions for increased flow to the diseased areas. This

is known as the "inverse steal syndrome" or "Robin Hood effect."

Ref: Longnecker DE, Brown DL, Newman MF, Zapol WM. *Anesthesiology.* 2nd ed. New York, NY: McGraw Hill; 2012.

33. Which of the following statements best reflects the relationship between cerebral metabolic rate for oxygen ($CMRO_2$) and cerebral blood flow (CBF)?

    (A) CBF remains constant until a threshold minimum level of is $CMRO_2$ is reached.

    (B) CBF increases proportionally as $CMRO_2$ decreases.

    (C) CBF decreases proportionally as $CMRO_2$ increases.

    (D) CBF decreases proportionally as $CMRO_2$ decreases.

    (E) CBF is independent of $CMRO_2$.

Cerebral metabolic rate is one of the principal determinants of CBF. Normally, the cells in the adult brain use 3 to 3.8 mL/100 g of brain tissue/min of oxygen. This is not equally distributed, as gray matter has a metabolic rate approximately 4 times that of white matter. This oxygen utilization is normally coupled with oxygen delivery in a ratio of 15:1 (since CBF is typically 50 mL/100 g/min). The mechanisms by which this coupling occur are not fully clear but may include local production of nitric oxide, adenosine, cyclooxygenases, astrocytic cytochrome p450, and potassium. The $CMRO_2$ can be manipulated clinically to decrease the requirement for oxygen during times when blood flow is substantially reduced or absent (i.e., deep hypothermic cardiac arrest).

Factors increasing the $CMRO_2$ include arousal and alertness, seizures, and an increase in brain temperature up to 42°C. Most anesthetics (except ketamine) decrease the $CMRO_2$, and barbiturates in particular have been used to induce electrical silence on the EEG, which corresponds to a reduction in $CMRO_2$ of approximately 60% (40% of metabolism is required for cellular homeostasis). Hypothermia decreases the metabolic rate by 6% to 7% for every degree celcius, and is the only means of further reducing the constitutive portion (the 40% for cellular homeostasis) of $CMRO_2$.

Ref: Longnecker DE, Brown DL, Newman MF, Zapol WM. *Anesthesiology.* 2nd ed. New York, NY: McGraw Hill; 2012.

34. You are providing anesthesia for a patient with long-standing moderate hypertension that is poorly controlled. Which of the following ranges of mean arterial pressure BEST represents the limits of autoregulation of cerebral blood flow in this patient?

    (A) 50 mm Hg and 100 mm Hg
    (B) 50 mm Hg and 125 mm Hg
    (C) 50 mm Hg and 150 mm Hg
    (D) 75 mm Hg and 150 mm Hg
    (E) 75 mm Hg and 175 mm Hg

The normal cerebral autoregulation curve (see Figure 2-6 from question 30) can be abolished by a number of factors, such as hypercapnia, hypoxia, volatile anesthetics, and cerebral pathology including trauma, tumors, stroke, and ruptured intracranial aneurysms. In these cases, it is important to maintain the mean arterial pressure (and by extension, the cerebral perfusion pressure) in a tightly controlled range to avoid hypo- or hyperperfusion.

The autoregulation curve can also be shifted on its *x*-axis by chronic exposure to elevated arterial pressures (Figure 2-8). This is a protective mechanism by the body to maintain a constant cerebral blood flow. However, the result is that a mean arterial pressure of 70 mm Hg, which might be appropriate for a healthy patient, may in fact sit below the lower limit for autoregulation in a patient who is used to a mean pressure of 125 mm Hg. It is critical for the anesthesiologist to manage the hemodynamics in chronic hypertensives as if they have a right-shifted autoregulation curve to prevent underperfusion of the brain. It can be a clinical challenge to determine which hypertensives are well controlled on medication and therefore have "normalized" autoregulation curves, and which patients are truly shifted. Careful preoperative assessment and notation of clinic and preadmission blood pressures are often valuable clues.

Answer (E) is the only choice in which both values are above the normal range.

Ref: Longnecker DE, Brown DL, Newman MF, Zapol WM. *Anesthesiology.* 2nd ed. New York, NY: McGraw Hill; 2012.

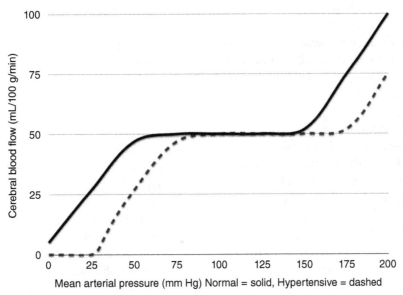

FIG. 2-8. Normal cerebral autoregulation curve (solid line) showing the "right-shift" effect of chronic hypertension (dashed line).

35. Which of the following statements regarding cerebral ischemia is TRUE?

    (A) The penumbra area of an ischemic insult is the area most affected by the lack of oxygen.

    (B) Global ischemia is defined as interruption of cerebral blood flow to one entire cerebral hemisphere.

    (C) Ischemic depolarization occurs when cerebral blood flow is diminished to 30 mL/100 g/min.

    (D) Cell death in ischemia involves activation of the AMPA receptor by glutamate and the influx of calcium into the cell.

    (E) Autoregulation of cerebral blood flow is maintained at the affected area during focal but not global ischemia.

Cerebral ischemia is classified as either global or focal. Global ischemia is seen during a severe reduction in cerebral blood flow (CBF) to the entire brain, as is seen following cardiac arrest. Focal ischemia is limited to a specific vascular territory and is usually due to thromboembolic or atherosclerotic stroke.

Normal CBF is 50 mL/100 g/min. When CBF is diminished to approximately 18 mL/100 g/min, depletion of ATP causes ion pumps to fail (ischemic depolarization), and calcium enters the cells, triggering the release of glutamate. This accelerates the entry of calcium by binding to AMPA and NMDA receptors, leading to the generation of free radical and reactive oxygen species, as well as harmful phospholipases and caspase. Water enters the cell following an osmotic gradient and results in localized swelling of the affected area (cytotoxic edema). These processes culminate in apoptosis and cell death; the release of byproducts from cellular damage and necrotic cells activates components of the inflammatory pathway. Generally this process is irreversible if CBF falls to below 10 mL/100 g/min.

In focal ischemia, there are two areas of pathology. The first area receives no blood flow (the "ischemic core") and responds in a similar manner as globally ischemic tissue; the second area, surrounding the core, is termed the "penumbra" and is comprised of tissue that is marginally perfused. Penumbra regions are often served by collateral vessels. The outcome following focal ischemia depends on ischemic severity and duration; if the insult is maintained for a prolonged period, the neurons in the penumbra die. More neurons in the penumbra region survive if collateral blood flow can be recruited or if reperfusion is reestablished quickly by opening of the culprit vessel.

Autoregulation of CBF is not effective during early ischemia and flow becomes pressure dependent.

Ref: Longnecker DE, Brown DL, Newman MF, Zapol WM. *Anesthesiology.* 2nd ed. New York, NY: McGraw Hill; 2012.

36. Which of the following statements regarding glucose and cerebral ischemia are TRUE?

    (A) Hyperglycemia has been demonstrated to be harmful for both focal and global ischemia.

    (B) Hyperglycemia has been demonstrated to be harmful in focal but not global ischemia.

    (C) Hyperglycemia has been demonstrated to be harmful in global but not focal ischemia.

    (D) Dextrose-containing solutions are safe to use in brain-injured patients due to the small amount of sugar present.

    (E) Patients with brain injury, stroke or brain tumor should be managed with intensive insulin therapy to ensure tight glycemic control.

A number of studies have demonstrated that glycemic control is an important predictor of outcome following ischemia, whether global or focal. The mechanism for the harmful effect of hyperglycemia (generally defined as blood glucose >126 mg/dL) has not been fully elucidated, but proposed mechanisms include accentuation of the release of excitatory amino acids (e.g., glutamate), reduction in levels of inhibitory neurotransmitters, recruitment of neutrophils, and mitochondrial damage. Glucose reduction has been shown to decrease ischemic damage in experimental models, strengthening the argument for avoiding marked elevation of blood sugar in these patients.

Dextrose-containing solutions should be avoided in patients with suspected or confirmed brain injury. However, the optimal blood glucose range is unclear. The AHA/ASA guidelines for acute ischemic stroke recommend that blood glucose be maintained between 140 and 180 mg/dL. Intensive insulin therapy (blood glucose goal of approximately 80 to 110 mg/dL) has been the subject of many investigations, with conflicting results. Intensive control of blood sugar in critical care patients has been shown to increase the risk of severe hypoglycemia (and in some cases the risk of mortality), which can mimic focal neurologic deficits, and if severe enough, result in neuronal injury. In summary, both hyper- and hypoglycemia are associated with worsened outcome in neurologic injury, and careful monitoring and management of the glycemic status is warranted.

Ref: Longnecker DE, Brown DL, Newman MF, Zapol WM. *Anesthesiology.* 2nd ed. New York, NY: McGraw Hill; 2012.

37. Which of the following cerebral autoregulation curves shown in Figure 2-9 best describes the traumatically injured brain?

(C)

The injured brain (from trauma, stroke, tumor, vascular malformation, etc.) exhibits a disturbed autoregulation curve for those affected portions. Because of local inflammatory and/or ischemic mediators, local blood flow is often maximized through vasodilation and is fairly resistant to the usual influences to cerebral vascular resistance such as $PaCO_2$ and cerebral perfusion pressure (CPP). For example, if the patient becomes hypercapnic, healthy vessels in noninjured parts of the brain will vasodilate appropriately, whereas there is no more room to vasodilate at the site of injury. This can create a steal phenomenon, where healthy tissue accommodates more flow and diverts it from the injured areas.

Similarly, the relationship between pressure and flow in these areas is linear (i.e., as CPP increases, so does the flow). There is a real danger in allowing the mean arterial pressure to become elevated in these patients, as there will be a increase in blood volume as well as a rise in the hydrostatic pressure gradient that will further worsen edema at the injured site.

Ref: Longnecker DE, Brown DL, Newman MF, Zapol WM. *Anesthesiology.* 2nd ed. New York, NY: McGraw Hill; 2012.

38. Where in the central nervous system is cerebrospinal fluid (CSF) produced?

(A) cerebral aqueduct
(B) cisterna magna
(C) fourth ventricle
(D) choroid plexus
(E) Interpeduncular cistern

CSF is produced by the choroid plexus, which is located in the lateral, third, and fourth ventricles. The choroid plexus is formed by invagination of the vascular pia mater into the ventricular lumen, where it becomes a highly folded, cauliflower-like mass.

CSF production is both an active secretory process and a passive filtration process. There is a well-defined circulation pattern to CSF, starting from the lateral ventricle (where most of the CSF is produced) and flowing through the interventricular foramen into the third ventricle. After passing through the cerebral aqueduct into the fourth ventricle, CSF leaves the ventricular system through the median aperture and two lateral apertures, thereby entering the subarachnoid

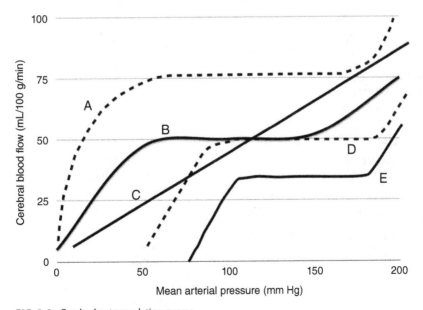

FIG. 2-9. Cerebral autoregulation curves.

space of the brain stem. From here, CSF flows through foramen magnum to bathe the spinal cord, as well as superiorly around the cerebral hemispheres to be reabsorbed. CSF is reabsorbed into the venous system by passing through numerous arachnoid villi, which consist of invaginations of arachnoid mater through the wall of the dural sinuses. The driving force for reabsorption is hydrostatic pressure.

Ref: Waxman SG. *Clinical Neuroanatomy.* 27th ed. New York, NY: McGraw Hill; 2013.

39. Which of the following statements regarding cerebral spinal fluid (CSF) is TRUE?

    (A) The total volume of CSF is approximately 250 mL,

    (B) CSF is produced by the arachnoid granulations of the lateral ventricles.

    (C) The pressure in the CSF with the patient sitting is approximately 20 to 30 cm H₂O.

    (D) CSF is formed at a rate of approximately 60 mL/hr.

    (E) CSF circulation exhibits nonpulsatile flow.

CSF is largely produced by the choroid plexuses of the cerebral ventricles, at a rate of roughly 500 mL/day (or 30 mL/hr). Much of this is resorbed by the arachnoid granulations and lymphatic channels along nerve roots, so the constant volume of CSF in the central nervous system is only between 100 and 150 mL. Its role is to serve is a physical cushion to the brain and spinal cord, increase the buoyancy of the brain, and remove metabolic and neuroendocrine substances from the brain by absorption into the blood.

CSF circulates throughout the lateral ventricles, the third and fourth ventricle, and the subarachnoid space of the brain and spinal cord. This circulation is driven by bulk flow from the new production of CSF by the choroid plexus as well as by pulsations transmitted from intracerebral vasculature.

CSF pressure varies depending on the position of the patient. When lying on their side, the pressure is approximately 10 to 20 cm H₂O, and can be thought of as equal to intracranial pressure. When sitting, measurement of the CSF pressure via lumbar puncture will be elevated to approximately 20 to 30 cm H₂O, due to the column of CSF between the needle orifice and the brain.

Ref: Waxman SG. *Clinical Neuroanatomy.* 27th ed. New York, NY: McGraw Hill; 2013.

40. Which of the following regarding the blood-brain barrier (BBB) is TRUE?

    (A) The BBB regulates the CSF and brain interstitial potassium level.

    (B) The BBB is readily permeable to plasma glutamate.

    (C) The main barrier structure in the BBB is the basement membrane of the capillaries.

    (D) The BBB is immature at birth and takes 3 to 4 months to fully develop.

    (E) The only cells capable of crossing the BBB in the healthy brain are neutrophils.

The barrier function of the BBB prevents the unrestricted movement of ions, neurotransmitters, macromolecules, and ingested neurotoxins from the plasma to the delicate environment of the CNS. For example, plasma levels of the excitatory amino acid glutamate may spike after ingestion of food, but the BBB prevents its passage into the CNS, where it has been shown to cause neurotoxic damage if released in an uncontrolled fashion. The ionic environment in the brain must be kept ideal for synaptic signaling. Ion transporters and channels ensure that while the plasma potassium concentration may vary widely, the brain interstitial and CSF concentration is maintained at about 2.9 mEq/L. The BBB also permits active transport of nutrients and metabolites required by neural tissue.

The BBB to macromolecules and most ionized solutes is created by the presence of tight junctions between cerebral endothelial cells. These are formed by proteins called claudins and occludin that span the distance between two adjacent cells. These are connected to an interior cellular scaffolding. Alterations in both intracellular and extracellular calcium concentration can modulate tight junction structure and alter the electrical resistance across the cell layer.

The BBB develops during fetal life and is fully formed at birth, especially to proteins and macromolecules. While cells from the monocyte lineage enter the brain during embryonic development and become immunologically competent microglia. In inflammation (i.e. with tumors or trauma), the BBB is incompetent and neutrophils may elude the barrier and reside in the perivascular space around small vessels; however, this is abnormal, and in the absence of pathology the central nervous system is an immunologically privileged site.

Ref: Waxman SG. *Clinical Neuroanatomy.* 27th ed. New York, NY: McGraw Hill; 2013.

41. Which one of the statements regarding transport across the blood-brain barrier (BBB) is TRUE?

    (A) CO_2 must dissociate into HCO_3^- and H^+ before crossing the BBB.

    (B) Hydrogen ions readily diffuse across the BBB.

    (C) Glucose is transported by the GLUT-5 transporter.

    (D) **Lipid soluble drugs with a molecular weight <400 Da can cross the BBB by diffusion.**

    (E) Drugs with a high (>8) number of hydrogen bonds in aqueous solution cross the BBB readily.

Few substances pass through the BBB easily. The blood gases oxygen and carbon dioxide are freely diffusible through the BBB. Substances that are charged are generally unable or very slow to cross without specific transporters due to the large electrical resistance of the BBB. This explains why hydrogen ions are unable to freely pass into the CSF. Glucose transport across the BBB is facilitated by the GLUT-1 transporter.

Water moves easily across the BBB, but charged ions are restricted. Marked changes in the concentration of plasma solutes can create a large osmotic gradient between the CNS and plasma that results in water moving in or out. The immediate effect of this is offset by equilibration, but if it occurs rapidly enough, cerebral edema can occur, as in severe hyponatremia.

Some drugs can cross the BBB by lipid-mediated free diffusion. In general, these substances have a low molecular weight (<400 Da) and are lipid soluble (e.g., propofol has a molecular weight of 178 Da). The degree of hydrogen bonding is inversely proportional to the degree of lipid solubility.

Ref: Waxman SG. *Clinical Neuroanatomy.* 27th ed. New York, NY: McGraw Hill; 2013.

42. In traumatic brain injury, which of the following mechanisms best describes the mechanism for breakdown of the blood-brain barrier (BBB)?

    (A) Astrocytes secrete transforming growth factor-β.

    (B) Lipopolysaccharide promotes disruption of the tight junctions via free radicals and interleukins.

    (C) **Production of bradykinin releases IL-6 from astrocytes, leading to opening of the BBB.**

    (D) Accumulation of amyloid-β.

    (E) Reduction in the efficacy of P-glycoprotein.

There are multiple mechanisms for disruption of the BBB, and many are present in the same disease process. BBB breakdown has been shown to be partly attributable in trauma to the release of the inflammatory mediator bradykinin. This stimulates the production and release of interleukin-6 from astrocytes, which results in a leaky BBB.

BBB disruption in stroke is a complex pathologic process, and involves the secretion of transforming growth factor-β, which downregulates endothelial expression of tPA and thrombomodulin; induction of aquaporin proteins; and proteolysis of basement membrane.

Lipopolysaccharide-based disruption is characteristic of bacterial meningitis or encephalitis. Amyloid-β is a key pathologic feature in Alzheimer's disease, and accumulation of this substance has a deleterious effect on the integrity of the basal lamina of the BBB. Altered levels of P-glycoprotein is implicated in many disease processes. Decreased efficacy of this protein is one hallmark of Parkinson's disease.

Ref: Waxman SG. *Clinical Neuroanatomy.* 27th ed. New York, NY: McGraw Hill; 2013.

43. A patient is admitted to the critical care unit with a closed head injury. The admitting resident leaves orders to hyperventilate the patient with a goal $PaCO_2$ of 25 mm Hg. Which of the following is the likely consequence to this therapeutic decision?

    (A) a rise in CSF bicarbonate levels

    (B) **a reduction in CSF bicarbonate levels**

    (C) an elevation in CSF potassium levels

    (D) a reduction in CSF sodium levels

    (E) a reduction in CSF pH

Hyperventilation is one known method of rapidly lowering intracranial pressure, since cerebral blood flow (and therefore cerebral blood volume) is directly linked to $PaCO_2$ through cerebral vasoconstriction. For every 1 mm Hg decrease in $PaCO_2$, there is roughly a 2% decrease in CBF. This can be useful in the short term as bridging therapy to a more definitive interventional or surgical solution, if there is evidence of increased intracranial pressure (ICP).

It is important to note that carbon dioxide diffuses freely across the blood-brain barrier (BBB), while charged ions such as bicarbonate do not. As such, hyperventilation produces a local alkalosis and vasoconstriction by causing an imbalance in the acid-base status across the BBB. This effect is attenuated within 6 to 24 hours by a reduction of CSF bicarbonate ions, which brings the pH between CSF and blood back into balance. At this point, the cerebral arteriole diameters have returned to baseline. However, when the clinical decision is made to discontinue hyperventilation and return to normocapnia, the increased CO_2 load serves to dilate the vessels and increases cerebral blood flow (up to >120% of baseline), which may worsen ICP and lead to edema in the injured area where the BBB is incompetent.

Current guidelines for treatment of head-injured patients advocate for careful consideration of hyperventilation, and using it only in those patients who have an acute rise in ICP. In addition, $PaCO_2$ should be maintained above 30 mm Hg.

Ref: Longnecker DE, Brown DL, Newman MF, Zapol WM. *Anesthesiology*. 2nd ed. New York, NY: McGraw Hill; 2012.

44. Blood and CSF are sampled at the same time from a patient. Which of the following solute values would you expect to be equal for both CSF and plasma?

    (A) $PaCO_2$
    (B) K^+
    (C) Ca^{2+}
    (D) glucose
    (E) **osmolality**

The composition of CSF is in many ways similar to plasma, a finding that led some in the past to believe that it was simply an ultrafiltrate. However, there are certain characteristics that demonstrate that this is unlikely, and in fact CSF is actively secreted. For example, most ionic concentrations in the CSF remain static despite wide fluctuations in the plasma. Moreover, choroid plexus cells cultured in vitro can produce CSF in the absence of a blood supply.

The principal differences between the two fluids are that the potassium, calcium, and glucose levels are lower in CSF; magnesium and chloride levels are higher in CSF. The pH is lower in CSF, due to the higher PCO_2 content and the diminished buffering capacity compared to plasma. CSF protein levels are markedly reduced compared to plasma. Osmolality is the one value that is consistently identical between the two fluids (Table 2-2).

TABLE 2-2. Comparison of CSF and plasma solutes.

	CSF	Plasma
Na^+ (mEq/L)	141	142
K^+ (mEq/L)	2.9	4.6
Ca^{2+} (mEq/L)	2.5	5.0
Mg^{2+} (mEq/L)	2.2	1.7
Cl^- (mEq/L)	124	101
HCO_3^- (mEq/L)	21	23
Glucose (mg/dL)	61	95
Protein (mg/dL)	30	7000
pCO_2 (mm Hg)	50.5	41.1
pH	7.33	7.41
Osmolality (mosm/L)	289	289

Ref: Waxman SG. *Clinical Neuroanatomy*. 27th ed. New York, NY: McGraw Hill; 2013.

45. Assuming a normothermic brain can tolerate 4 minutes of ischemia, what is the approximate expected duration of ischemia that can be tolerated at 27°C?

    (A) 5 minutes
    (B) 6 minutes
    (C) **9 minutes**
    (D) 12 minutes
    (E) 15 minutes

Hypothermia decreases both the metabolic and functional activities of the brain, decreasing the $CMRO_2$ by approximately 7% for each degree Celsius. However, this relationship is not linear throughout the range of temperatures used clinically. The relationship can be expressed using the temperature coefficient (Q_{10}), the amount that cerebral metabolism decreases globally for a each 10°C reduction in temperature. The Q_{10} is approximately 2.3 between 37°C and 27°C. In other words, there is 57% reduction in $CMRO_2$ when a patient's brain is cooled to 27°C. In our example, if the normothermic brain (37°C) can tolerate 4 minutes of complete ischemia, at 27°C the brain should tolerate 9 minutes of ischemia ($4 \times 2.3 = 9.2$).

Below 27°C the Q_{10} doubles to 4.5. This correlates with the gradual loss of neuronal function, as demonstrated by an isoelectric EEG (which occurs between 18°C and 21°C) and the ability of the brain to tolerate more prolonged ischemia than would be predicted based on a linear model. Even mild hypothermia (1−2°C) can provide benefit in reducing the damage from cerebral ischemia. Possible mechanisms include decreased calcium influx, decreased glutamate release, preserved integrity of the blood-brain barrier, and prevention of lipid peroxidation.

Avoidance of hyperthermia in neurologically injured patients is critical as above-normal temperatures markedly increase $CMRO_2$ and further worsen ischemic damage.

Ref: Longnecker DE, Brown DL, Newman MF, Zapol WM. *Anesthesiology.* 2nd ed. New York, NY: McGraw Hill; 2012.

46. Which of the following is LEAST likely to promote cerebral protection during anesthesia for patients with ischemic brain injury?

 (A) propofol

 (B) etomidate

 (C) dexmedetomidine

 (D) lidocaine

 (E) xenon

Many anesthetic agents have been investigated as potential neuroprotective agents, particularly since many of them reduce the functional component of $CMRO_2$.

Propofol has demonstrated neuroprotective effects in animal models of both global and focal ischemia. One proposed mechanism is its antioxidant effect, mediated by the phenolic hydroxyl group. Other theories include reductions in glutamate uptake, activation of GABA receptors, and reduced dopamine release.

Dexmedetomidine likely confers neuroprotection in multiple ways. It has been shown to lower plasma catecholamine levels and improve neurologic outcome in rodent models of ischemia. It also maintains the integrity of the mitochondrial membrane and promotes the uptake and metabolism of glutamate by astrocytes.

Lidocaine, a sodium channel blocker, has been shown to reduce the extent of cerebral infarction following focal ischemia. Xenon, an inert gas that acts as an antagonist of NMDA receptors, has also been shown to improve outcome in hypoxic-ischemic brain injury.

Etomidate has a history of use as a neuroprotective agent during aneurysm clipping. However, more recent data show that this drug increases infarct size by reducing nitric oxide levels (and hence blood flow) in ischemic tissue.

Ref: Longnecker DE, Brown DL, Newman MF, Zapol WM. *Anesthesiology.* 2nd ed. New York, NY: McGraw Hill; 2012.

47. You are administering anesthesia for a patient undergoing coronary artery bypass. Which of the following is the BEST agent to use to induce preconditioning of the brain against ischemia?

 (A) propofol

 (B) thiopental

 (C) fentanyl

 (D) isoflurane

 (E) ketamine

Preconditioning of the brain using volatile anesthetics has been well documented, and improves neurologic outcomes. Administration of these agents either immediately prior or up to 4 days before commencement of the ischemic insult reduces the amount of neuronal loss. This effect has been documented for both isoflurane and sevoflurane. The mechanisms of preconditioning appear to be related primarily to activation of potassium-ATP channels and signaling pathways but may also relate to a demonstrated increase in the expression of anti-apoptotic factors such as Bcl-2 that reduce the mitochondrial membrane permeability and hence the release of cytochrome c into the cytoplasm.

Intravenous anesthetic agents lack this preconditioning effect. Ketamine has mixed actions in this setting: on one hand, it is an NMDA receptor antagonist and blocks calcium entry into the cell; on the other hand, it has been shown to cause vacuolation of some subtypes of neurons, and its role as a neuroprotective agent is unclear. The noble gases (e.g., xenon) also appear to be efficacious as preconditioning agents.

Ref: Longnecker DE, Brown DL, Newman MF, Zapol WM. *Anesthesiology.* 2nd ed. New York, NY: McGraw Hill; 2012.

48. Which of the following anatomic segments forms the inferior (distal) end of the spinal cord?

 (A) cervical enlargement

 (B) lumbosacral enlargement

 (C) conus medullaris

 (D) cauda equina

 (E) filum terminale

The spinal cord is continuous with the medulla and extends inferiorly to the conus medullaris, which typically ends at the L1 or L2 level (adults) or L2 or L3 level (infants). The filum terminale is a fibrous filament of glial cells enclosed in pia that travels from the conus medullaris and extends to the coccyx where it anchors the spinal cord. The cauda equina ("horse's tail") is a collection of lumbar and sacral nerves that originate from the conus medullaris and travel in the dural sac within the spinal column before exiting. The dural sac within the spinal column ends at ~S1 (adults) and ~S3 (infants). A spinal anesthetic or lumbar puncture typically accesses the cerebrospinal fluid below the level of the conus medullaris at ~L3-L4 interspace or L4-L5 interspace.

The cervical and lumbosacral enlargements are the origins of the nerves to the upper extremities and brachial plexus; and the lower extremities and lumbosacral plexus, respectively.

Ref: Waxman SG. *Clinical Neuroanatomy.* 27th ed. New York, NY: McGraw Hill; 2013.

49. A cross-section of the spinal cord shows an "H" of gray matter surrounded by white matter. Which portion of the spinal cord gives rise to preganglionic fibers of the autonomic nervous system?

    (A) anterior horn

    (B) **intermediolateral horn**

    (C) posterior horn

    (D) dorsal column

    (E) ventral column

The "H" of gray matter in the spinal cord extends the length of the spinal cord in columns. The anterior horn (or anterior column, or ventral column) is the origin of the lower motor neurons of the spinal cord, which pass to the spinal nerves via the ventral roots. The dorsal horn (or dorsal column or posterior column) receives sensory information for pain, temperature, pressure, and proprioception. The intermediolateral horn (or intermediolateral column), which separates the anterior and dorsal horns, gives rise to preganglionic fibers of the autonomic nervous system in the thoracic, upper lumbar, and sacral regions of the spinal cord.

Ref: Waxman SG. *Clinical Neuroanatomy.* 27th ed. New York, NY: McGraw Hill; 2013.

50. The gray matter of the spinal can be divided into a number of different layers or laminae (Rexed's laminae). Which of the following laminae gives rise to the lower motor neurons that innervate the arms and legs?

    (A) I

    (B) II

    (C) V

    (D) VI

    (E) **IX**

Laminas I to VI form the dorsal horn:

- Laminas I and II (substantia gelatinosa) respond to painful stimuli.
- Laminas III and IV, which form the nucleus proprius, receive sensory information regarding light touch and position.
- Lamina V receives sensory information for both pain and visceral sensation.
- Lamina VI receives sensory information from muscle spindles and participates in spinal reflexes.

Lamina VII contains Clarke's column (interneurons involved in proprioception) and also the origins of the intermediolateral column, which gives rise to preganglionic fibers of the autonomic nervous system. **Laminas VIII and IX contain the lower motor neurons that innervate axial musculature, the arms, and the legs.** Lamina X contains the neurons around the central canal of the spinal cord. Function is not fully elucidated.

Ref: Waxman SG. *Clinical Neuroanatomy.* 27th ed. New York, NY: McGraw Hill; 2013.

51. A deep tendon reflex (an example of a spinal reflex) involves which of the following components?

    (A) stretch of extrafusal muscle fibers in muscle spindles.

    (B) **activation of afferent Ia fibers.**

    (C) activation of alpha motor neurons by interneurons.

    (D) activation of gamma motor neurons by interneurons.

    (E) contraction of intrafusal muscle fibers.

A deep tendon reflex (or stretch reflex) is a type of monosynaptic spinal reflex with the following components (or reflex arc):

- Muscle receptor
- Sensory axons
- Lower motor neuron
- Muscle

A deep tendon reflex is initiated with activation of muscle spindles within the muscle. A muscle spindle is a mechanoreceptor with **intrafusal** muscle fibers responding to changes in muscle length, and rate of change of muscle length. Muscle spindles in turn activate afferent nerve fibers, mainly **Ia fibers,** which then directly synapse with motor neurons in the spinal cord. Activation of alpha motor neurons leads to contraction of **extrafusal** muscle fibers.

Gamma motor neurons innervate the **intrafusal** muscle fibers of the muscle spindles. Activated by higher centers in the brain, gamma motor neuron activation does not lead to discernible muscle contraction, but rather regulates the set point for deep tendon reflex activation.

Interneurons (Renshaw cells) are **inhibitory** and involved in either inhibitory reflex arcs to prevent overactivity of alpha motor neurons or polysynaptic reflexes to cause contralateral muscle relaxation.

Ref: Waxman SG. *Clinical Neuroanatomy.* 27th ed. New York, NY: McGraw Hill; 2013.

52. The afferent limb of the oculocardiac reflex is which of the following nerves?

(A) III
(B) **V**
(C) X
(D) VII
(E) II

The oculocardiac reflex, a type of visceral reflex, involves cranial nerve V as the afferent limb and cranial nerve X as the efferent limb.

In general, spinal reflexes may be classified into 4 groups:

1. Superficial reflexes (e.g., corneal reflex with cranial nerve V as afferent limb and cranial nerve VII as efferent limb, or light reflex with cranial nerve II as afferent limb and cranial nerve III as efferent limb).
2. Deep tendon reflexes (e.g., patellar reflex with femoral nerve as both afferent and efferent limb).
3. Visceral reflexes (e.g., carotid sinus reflex with cranial nerve IX as the afferent limb and cranial nerve X as the efferent limb).
4. Abnormal reflexes (e.g., Babinski's sign [plantar reflex] with tibial nerve as afferent and limb and peroneal nerve as efferent limb).

Ref: Butterworth JF IV, Mackey DC, Wasnick JD. *Morgan and Mikhail's Clinical Anesthesiology.* 5th ed. New York, NY: McGraw Hill; 2013.

53. Ascending fibers of the spinothalamic tract travel in which of the following areas of the spinal cord?

(A) central canal
(B) **ventral column**
(C) lateral column
(D) dorsal column
(E) dorsal gray column

Sensory information for pain and temperature enters the spinal cord via the dorsal horn, crosses over to the opposite side of the spinal and cord, and ascends within the spinothalamic tracts in **the ventral (anterior) column.**

A cross-section of the spinal cord shows an "H" of gray matter surrounded by white matter. The "H" of gray matter is divided into an anterior horn (or anterior gray column, or ventral column), a dorsal horn (or dorsal gray column or posterior column) and an intermediolateral horn (or intermediolateral gray column), which separates the anterior and dorsal horns. The surrounding white matter of the spinal cord is divided into dorsal (posterior) columns, ventral (anterior columns), and lateral columns. The central canal is filled with cerebrospinal fluid and runs through the middle of the spinal cord. The spinal cord is divided into two symmetric halves with the midline anterior (ventral) medial fissure and posterior (dorsal) median fissure serving as the dividing point.

Ref: Waxman SG. *Clinical Neuroanatomy.* 27th ed. New York, NY: McGraw Hill; 2013.

54. Descending fibers of the corticospinal tract travel mainly in which of the following areas of the spinal cord?

(A) central canal
(B) ventral column
(C) **lateral column**
(D) dorsal column
(E) dorsal gray column

The descending fibers of the corticospinal tract decussate at the medullary pyramids and continue down through the spinal cord via the lateral corticospinal tract in the **lateral column.** Some of the fibers do not cross over and continue down the spinal cord via the anterior corticospinal tract in the anterior (ventral) column.

A cross section of the spinal cord shows an "H" of gray matter surrounded by white matter. The "H" of gray matter is divided into an anterior horn (or anterior gray column, or ventral column), a dorsal horn (or dorsal gray column or posterior column) and an intermediolateral horn (or intermediolateral gray column), which separates the anterior and dorsal horns. The surrounding white matter of the spinal cord is divided into dorsal (posterior) columns, ventral (anterior columns), and lateral columns. The central canal is filled with cerebrospinal fluid and runs through the middle of the spinal cord. The spinal cord is divided into two symmetric halves with the midline anterior (ventral) medial fissure and posterior (dorsal) median fissure serving as the dividing point.

Ref: Waxman SG. *Clinical Neuroanatomy.* 27th ed. New York, NY: McGraw Hill; 2013.

55. A patient is undergoing a complex scoliosis repair. Which of the following monitors may potentially indicate ventral (anterior) spinal cord ischemia?

(A) SSEP
(B) MEP
(C) BAEP
(D) EEG
(E) VEP

Motor evoked potentials (MEPs) deliver a stimulus to the motor cortex and elicit evoked potentials at the muscle. This provides insight into the integrity of the ventral (anterior) spinal cord.

Somatosensory evoked potentials (SSEPs) deliver a stimulus to sensory peripheral nerves and elicit evoked potentials at the scalp (sensory cortex). This provides insight into the integrity of the dorsal (posterior) spinal cord.

Brain stem auditory evoked potentials (BAEPs) deliver an auditory stimulus and elicit evoked potentials at the cerebral cortex. This provides insight into the integrity of the auditory pathway including brain stem.

Electroencephalography (EEG) records electric potential differences in the cerebral cortex. A multichannel EEG may be used to detect cerebral ischemia.

Visual evoked potentials (VEPs) deliver a visual stimulus and elicit evoked potentials at the visual cortex. This provides insight into the integrity of the visual pathway including optic nerve and visual cortex.

Ref: Butterworth JF IV, Mackey DC, Wasnick JD. *Morgan and Mikhail's Clinical Anesthesiology.* 5th ed. New York, NY: McGraw Hill; 2013.

56. Which of the following correctly identifies the number of subunits in a nicotinic acetylcholine-gated ion channel?

(A) 2
(B) 3
(C) 4
(D) 5
(E) 7

Nicotinic cholinergic receptors are found in the neuromuscular junction of skeletal muscle as well as autonomic ganglia, and are similar in structure to both $GABA_A$ and glycine receptors. Each nicotinic receptor is made up of five subunits that form a central channel through which sodium and potassium flow when opened (although these channels are nonselective, and other cations such as calcium can also pass through). The subunits are classified as α, β, δ, γ, and ε and are each structurally different. Nicotinic receptors that are specific to the neuromuscular junction are comprised of two α, one β, one δ, and either a γ or a ε subunit, for a total of five (Figure 2-10). The α subunits contain binding sites for acetylcholine, which promotes a configurational change that opens the central channel.

Ref: Barrett KE, Boitano S, Barman SM, Brooks HL. *Ganong's Review of Medical Physiology.* 24th ed. New York, NY: McGraw Hill; 2012.

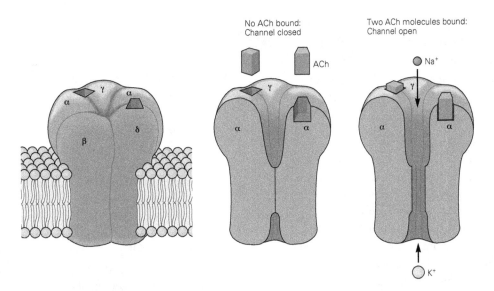

No ACh bound:
Channel closed

Two ACh molecules bound:
Channel open

ACh

Na⁺

K⁺

FIG. 2-10. Three-dimensional model of the nicotinic acetylcholine-gated ion channel. The receptor–channel complex consists of five subunits, all of which contribute to forming the pore. When two molecules of acetylcholine bind to portions of the α-subunits exposed to the membrane surface, the receptor–channel changes conformation. This opens the pore in the portion of the channel embedded in the lipid bilayer, and both K⁺ and Na⁺ flow through the open channel down their electrochemical gradient. (Reproduced with permission from Barrett KE, Boitano S, Barman SM, Brooks HL. *Ganong's Review of Medical Physiology.* 24th ed. New York, NY: McGraw Hill; 2012.)

57. The mature type of nicotinic receptor is characterized by which ONE of the following?

 (A) **They are densely concentrated in the folds of the synaptic clefts.**

 (B) They are expressed at extrajunctional sites in response to burn injury.

 (C) They contain a γ subunit in place of an ε subunit.

 (D) They have a relatively long open time compared with immature nicotinic receptors.

 (E) They are upregulated in myasthenia gravis.

During embryonic development, muscle cells produce immature (fetal) nicotinic receptors that are distributed evenly throughout the cell membrane. These receptors differ structurally from the adult type in that they contain a γ subunit (along with the usual two ∝ subunits and one β subunit) rather than an ε subunit. As the muscle becomes innervated in late fetal development and early infancy, the cell begins to produce mature adult receptors, which are densely concentrated at the neuromuscular junction, especially at the crests of the junctional folds. The fetal isoform of the receptor is inhibited by any neuromuscular activity, and therefore disappears within several weeks after birth.

Extrajunctional receptors (i.e., located in areas of the muscle cell membrane apart from the synaptic cleft) are normally not present in large numbers but are expressed in response to upper or lower motor neuron injury, burns or sepsis. The receptor that is upregulated in these cases is the immature isoform, and is associated with a long open time compared with mature isoform by a factor of 2- to 10-fold. These factors together represent a danger when succinylcholine is used in these patients, as overwhelming leakage of intracellular potassium can result in lethal hyperkalemia from activation of the upregulated, dysfunctional receptors.

Myasthenia gravis is caused by circulating antibodies to the muscular nicotinic cholinergic receptors. This results in sparse, shallow and abnormally wide or absent synaptic clefts in the motor end plate, and a decreased response to acetylcholine.

Ref: Barrett KE, Boitano S, Barman SM, Brooks HL. *Ganong's Review of Medical Physiology.* 24th ed. New York, NY: McGraw Hill; 2012.

58. Which of the following statements regarding the resting potential of neurons is TRUE?

 (A) A high external concentration of K⁺ ions maintains a resting potential of −90 mV.

 (B) **A high internal concentration of K⁺ ions maintains a resting potential of −70 mV.**

(C) A high external concentration of Ca_2^+ ions maintains a resting potential of -90 mV.

(D) A high internal concentration of K^+ ions maintains a resting potential of -55 mV.

(E) A high internal concentration of Na^+ ions maintains a resting potential of -90 mV.

Excitable tissue such as neurons maintain an electrochemical differential across their membrane by the establishment of ion gradients. In neurons, the Na^+/K^+-ATPase pump uses ATP to move three sodium ions outside the cell and two potassium ions inside, both against their concentration gradients. The result is that the extracellular sodium concentration (140 mmol/L) is much higher than intracellular (10 mmol/L); the reverse is true for potassium (140 mmol/L vs. 4 mmol/L). The membrane has ion-selective channels that allow for the passive diffusion of K^+ ions out and Na^+ ions in along their respective concentration gradients. If left unchecked, this would return the electrochemical gradient to zero. However, this is prevented by the Na^+/K^+-ATPase. Since there are substantially more K^+ channels open at rest, it is the relative difference in the intra- and extracellular potassium concentration that primarily determines the resting potential. This transmembrane potential is -70 mV. Note that -90 mV is the resting membrane potential for cardiac muscle, another type of excitable tissue.

Ref: Barrett KE, Boitano S, Barman SM, Brooks HL. *Ganong's Review of Medical Physiology.* 24th ed. New York, NY: McGraw Hill; 2012.

59. Which of the following statements regarding the electrochemistry of action potentials in neurons is TRUE?

(A) The threshold potential is -90 mV.

(B) Potassium efflux is the initiating event in the action potential.

(C) Voltage-gated potassium channels are slower to open than sodium channels.

(D) Hyperpolarization (or "undershoot") is the result of sodium channels remaining in an open state.

(E) Hyperkalemia decreases the excitability of neurons.

At rest, voltage-gated sodium and potassium channels are both closed. In response to depolarizing stimulus (i.e., stimulation of a sensory receptor in the skin), a series of ion channel events occur that change the electrical potential across the neuron cell membrane (Figure 2-11). First, sodium channels open in the membrane, allowing sodium to enter the cell and making the interior less negative. If the stimulus is brief or of insufficient intensity, a critical threshold potential (-55 mV) is not reached, and an action potential does not occur. However, if the threshold potential is reached, this triggers a significantly increased rate of sodium channel opening, resulting in depolarization. The transmembrane potential becomes briefly positive ($+30$ mV), a phenomenon known as overshoot, before starting to fall again. The downstroke in the action potential curve is the result of depolarization-induced inactivation (closure) of sodium channels but more importantly the opening of potassium channels that allow efflux of K^+ ions and the return of the potential down to its resting state. Sodium channels are open for only 0.7 ms, but potassium channels are both slower to open and are open for a longer duration. This contributes to "undershoot," where the potential is more negative briefly due to a relative increase in the concentration of intracellular K^+ ions before the Na^+/K^+-ATPase can return the gradient to its resting potential.

Hyperkalemia increases the resting potential (typically by about 10–15 mV) so that less of a stimulus is required to reach the threshold potential—this makes the nerve hyperexcitable. This is true for other excitable tissue such as cardiac muscle. The reason that calcium is administered as part of the treatment for hyperkalemia is that it raises the **threshold current** of myocardial muscle by approximately the same amount that the potassium excess raises the resting potential. This re-establishes the difference between the two potentials, decreasing the excitability of cardiac muscle, buying some time for you to get rid of the potassium by other means. Now you have a better answer to why we give calcium in this scenario than just to say, "calcium stabilizes the membrane."

Ref: Barrett KE, Boitano S, Barman SM, Brooks HL. *Ganong's Review of Medical Physiology.* 24th ed. New York, NY: McGraw Hill; 2012.

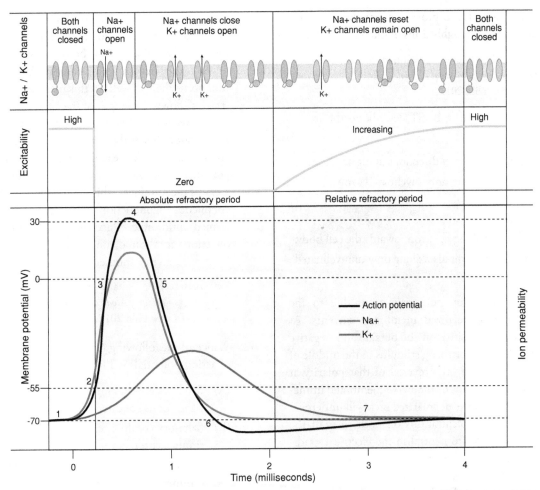

FIG. 2-11. Changes in membrane potential and relative membrane permeability to Na⁺ and K⁺ during an action potential. These changes in threshold for activation (excitability) are correlated with the phases of the action potential. (Adapted with permission from Silverman, *Human Physiology: An Integrated Approach*, 5th edition, Pearson 2010.)

60. Which of the following is TRUE regarding the refractory period of action potentials?

(A) During the absolute refractory period, only electrical stimuli can produce another action potential.

(B) It is impossible to produce another action potential during the relative refractory period in humans.

(C) The relative refractory period is twice as long as the absolute refractory period.

(D) **Voltage-gated potassium channels are open during both refractory periods.**

(E) The absolute refractory period follows the relative refractory period.

The refractory period refers to that portion of the action potential where neuronal excitability is decreased, and action potentials are more difficult to generate. Upon depolarization, the nerve tissue enters an "absolute refractory" period, where no stimulus, regardless of the intensity, is possible of generating a subsequent action potential (see Figure 2-11 from previous question). During this time, sodium channels are in their inactive state (note: this is different than their **closed**, resting state). As long as the majority of sodium channels are inactivated, the neuronal membrane will remain in the absolute refractory period. During repolarization, potassium channels gradually close, returning the hyperpolarized membrane potential to −70 mV. At the same time, sodium channels gradually return to their closed position (from the **inactive** state), making the membrane more permeable to sodium and increasing the excitability of the cell. This period is known as the relative refractory period—while generation of an action potential is possible during this time, it requires a larger than normal stimulus to provoke depolarization. Each refractory period is roughly 2 ms in duration.

Ref: Barrett KE, Boitano S, Barman SM, Brooks HL. *Ganong's Review of Medical Physiology.* 24th ed. New York, NY: McGraw Hill; 2012.

61. Which of the following BEST describes orthodromic conduction?

(A) conduction in both directions along an axon.

(B) conduction along only myelinated axons.

(C) **conduction from the cell body of a nerve to its axonal terminals.**

(D) conduction along the axon towards the cell body.

(E) conduction of impulses along only unmyelinated axons.

Conduction of action potentials occur due to the propagation of depolarized membrane currents. At rest, neurons are positive on the outside and negative on the inside. A depolarizing stimulus in the middle of an axon will cause a brief reversal of that polarity at that point. The regions of the nerve membrane immediately adjacent to the depolarized area will undergo a shift in the ion concentrations on both sides of the membrane in order to neutralize the electrical gradient. In other words, positively charged ions will flow toward the depolarized area, while remaining on the outside of the cell, so that the depolarized area becomes

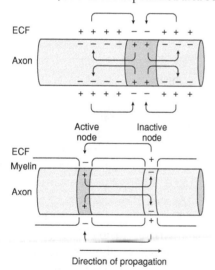

FIG. 2-12. Local current flow (movement of positive charges) around an impulse in an axon. **Top:** Unmyelinated axon. **Bottom:** Myelinated axon. Positive charges from the membrane ahead of and behind the action potential flow into the area of negativity represented by the action potential ("current sink"). In myelinated axons, depolarization appears to "jump" from one node of Ranvier to the next (saltatory conduction). (Reproduced with permission from Barrett KE, Boitano S, Barman SM, Brooks HL. *Ganong's Review of Medical Physiology.* 24th ed. New York, NY: McGraw Hill; 2012.)

less negative on the outside (Figure 2-12). A similar event occurs on the inside of the cell. The net result is that the adjacent areas now become less negative themselves; if they become sufficiently negative, depolarization occurs here as well. In this manner, depolarization "travels" down the length of the axon.

Normally, impulses do not originate in the middle of axons, but rather at the dendrites of the cell, where synapses occur with upstream neurons. Therefore the action potentials will usually only travel in one direction, towards the terminals. This is referred to as orthodromic conduction. Conduction in the opposite direction is termed antidromic. Since synapses only occur in one direction, antidromic conduction is unable to synapse from one nerve to another, and dies out at that point.

Ref: Barrett KE, Boitano S, Barman SM, Brooks HL. *Ganong's Review of Medical Physiology.* 24th ed. New York, NY: McGraw Hill; 2012.

62. Which of the following regarding saltatory conduction of action potentials is TRUE?

(A) Saltatory conduction requires more energy than continuous conduction.

(B) Saltatory conduction is twice as faster than continuous conduction.

(C) The distance between nodes of Ranvier is up to 4 mm.

(D) **The concentration of voltage-gated sodium channels at a Node of Ranvier exceed that of unmyelinated axon by a factor of up to 100 times.**

(E) Saltatory conduction is so-named because of the sodium (e.g., salt ~ saltatory) channels that facilitates its propagation.

Saltatory conduction is a property of neuronal transmission along myelinated nerves only. Myelin is rich in lipid and is an effective electrical insulator. However, the myelin is not continuous along the axon, but is intermittent, with small gaps of unmyelinated axon present in between. These are the so-called Nodes of Ranvier (Figure 2-13). Rather than propagate the transmission continuously along the axon, as is the case in unmyelinated neurons, the current sink is forced to "jump" to the next node in order to continue traveling down the nerve axon. "Saltatory" comes from the Latin *saltere* (to jump). This jumping action dramatically increases the speed of conduction. Myelinated nerves conduct impulses at rates of 60 to 100 m/sec, compared to the 1 m/sec observed in small, unmyelinated C fibers.

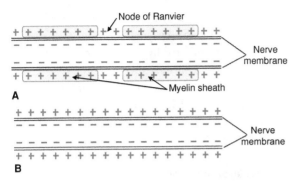

FIG. 2-13. A. Schematic anatomic and electrophysiologic structure of nerve fibers of myelinated and **(B)** unmyelinated nerve fibers. (Reproduced with permission from Hadzic A. *NYSORA Textbook of Regional Anesthesia and Acute Pain Medicine.* 1st ed. New York, NY: McGraw Hill; 2007.)

Nodes are very small in length (approximately 1–2 micrometers). The distance between nodes (termed the "internodal distance") is much greater than the nodes themselves, and can be up to 1.5 mm in some nerves. The concentration of sodium channels is very high at the nodes, in the range of 2000 to 12,000 per square micrometer; in contrast, unmyelinated axons have a concentration of approximately 100 sodium channels per square micrometer. This is the means by which a sufficiently large depolarizing current can be formed in order to "jump" to the next node. Despite this high concentration, saltatory conduction is more efficient than continuous conduction, since less overall sodium and potassium ions are pumped in and out of the neuron.

Ref: Barrett KE, Boitano S, Barman SM, Brooks HL. *Ganong's Review of Medical Physiology.* 24th ed. New York, NY: McGraw Hill; 2012.

63. Which of the following is a neurotransmitter that takes part in presynaptic inhibition?

(A) **gamma-aminobutyric acid (GABA)**
(B) glutamate
(C) norepinephrine
(D) glycine
(E) aspartate

Presynaptic inhibition occurs when inhibitory neurons terminate on the terminal endings of excitatory neurons (this synapse is therefore ***axo-axonal***, rather than axo-dendritic or axosomatic). Stimulation of the presynaptic neuron results in increased Cl^- conductance, reducing the size of the action potentials reaching the axon terminal of the excitatory neuron. As a result, less excitatory neurotransmitter is released by the postsynaptic neuron. A reduced influx of calcium ions into the excitatory neuron also play a role in this inhibition.

GABA, the neurotransmitter most implicated in this synaptic event, stimulates both $GABA_A$ and $GABA_B$ receptors, which increases permeability to Cl^- and K^+ ions respectively. Baclofen is a GABA-agonist and an anti spasticity medication that works to inhibit motor neurons in both spinal cord injury and multiple sclerosis.

Ref: Barrett KE, Boitano S, Barman SM, Brooks HL. *Ganong's Review of Medical Physiology.* 24th ed. New York, NY: McGraw Hill; 2012.

64. Which of the following neurotransmitters binds to N-methyl-D-aspartate (NMDA) receptors in the central nervous system?

(A) acetylcholine
(B) norepinephrine
(C) GABA
(D) **glutamate**
(E) substance P

Glutamate is the most prevalent excitatory neurotransmitter in the brain and spinal cord. Roughly 75% of excitatory transmission involves glutamate as the transmitter. As you might expect with such a widespread molecule, there are a variety of different receptors that glutamate acts upon. They can be subdivided functionally into two groups:

• **The ligand-gated receptors:** AMPA, NMDA, and kainate receptors. When glutamate binds to these, the channel opens and permits the influx of Na^+ (AMPA and kainate) or calcium (NMDA), as well as the efflux of K^+. Interestingly, glycine, an inhibitory neurotransmitter, is a required cofactor in the activation of the NMDA receptor by glutamate.

• **The G protein-coupled receptors:** There are a number of different varieties, all of which decrease intracellular cAMP.

Acetylcholine acts on nicotinic and muscarinic cholinergic receptors. Norepinephrine acts on the adrenergic alpha and beta receptors. GABA, the predominant inhibitory neurotransmitter in the brain, activates $GABA_A$ and $GABA_B$ receptors. Substance P acts on neurokinin receptors.

Ref: Barrett KE, Boitano S, Barman SM, Brooks HL. *Ganong's Review of Medical Physiology.* 24th ed. New York, NY: McGraw Hill; 2012.

65. Which of the following is a biochemical precursor to epinephrine?

(A) isoproterenol

(B) dihydroxy-phenylalanine

(C) glutamine

(D) tryptophan

(E) acetyl-CoA

Catecholamines such as norepinephrine, epinephrine and dopamine are synthesized by the body through the hydroxylation and decarboxylation of the amino acid tyrosine (Figure 2-14). Most tyrosine present in the body is obtained through dietary intake, although some can be synthesized from phenylalanine. The rate limiting step in the production of catecholamines is the conversion of tyrosine to dihydroxy-phenylalanine (DOPA) by the enzyme tyrosine hydroxylase. This enzyme is inhibited by the presence of both dopamine and norepinephrine, thereby providing a negative feedback loop for the production of catecholamines.

Isoproterenol is a synthetic drug that acts on the adrenergic system (as a nonselective beta agonist). Other synthetic adrenergic medications include phenylephrine, dobutamine and salbutamol. Glutamine is a precursor in the production of glutamate, just as tryptophan and acetyl-CoA are substrates for the synthesis of serotonin and acetylcholine, respectively.

Ref: Barrett KE, Boitano S, Barman SM, Brooks HL. *Ganong's Review of Medical Physiology.* 24th ed. New York, NY: McGraw Hill; 2012.

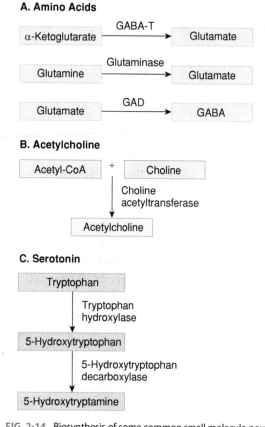

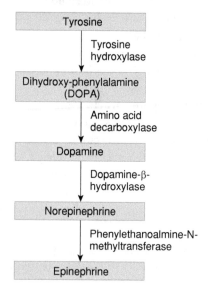

FIG. 2-14. Biosynthesis of some common small molecule neurotransmitters. **A.** Glutamate is synthesized in the Krebs cycle by the conversion of α-ketoglutarate to the amino acid via the enzyme γ-aminobutyric acid transferase (GABA-T) or in nerve terminals by the hydrolysis of glutamine by the enzyme glutaminase. GABA is synthesized by the conversion of glutamate by the enzyme glutamic acid decarboxylase (GAD). **B.** Acetylcholine is synthesized in the cytoplasm of a nerve terminal from acetyl-Co-A and choline by the enzyme choline acetyltransferase. **C.** Serotonin is synthesized from the amino acid tryptophan in a two-step process: the enzymatic hydroxylation of tryptophan to 5-hydroxytryptophan and the enzymatic decarboxylation of this intermediate to form 5-hydroxytryptamine (also called serotonin). **D.** Catecholamines are synthesized from the amino acid tyrosine by a multi-step process. Tyrosine is oxidized to dihydroxy-phenylalanine (DOPA) by the enzyme tyrosine hydroxylase in the cytoplasm of the neuron; DOPA is then decarboxylated to dopamine. In dopaminergic neurons the process stops there. In noradrenergic neurons, the dopamine is transported into synaptic vesicles where it is converted to norepinephrine by dopamine-β-hydroxylase. In neurons that also contain the enzyme phenylethanolamine-N-methyltransferase, norepinephrine is converted to epinephrine. (Reprinted with permission from Barrett KE, Boitano S, Barman SM, Brooks HL. *Ganong's Review of Medical Physiology.* 24th ed. New York, NY: McGraw Hill; 2012.)

66. Which of the following sequences correctly identifies the steps in muscle fiber excitation-contraction coupling?

(A) **motor neuron discharge ▸ binding of acetylcholine to nicotinic receptors ▸ increased Na$^+$ and K$^+$ conductance in motor end-plate membrane ▸ generation of action potential in muscle fibers ▸ binding of calcium to troponin C ▸ formation of cross-linkages between actin and myosin.**

(B) inward spread of depolarization along T tubules ▸ binding of acetylcholine to nicotinic receptors ▸ release of Ca^{2+} from sarcoplasmic reticulum ▸ generation of action potential in muscle fibers ▸ binding of calcium to troponin C ▸ formation of cross-linkages between actin and myosin.

(C) motor neuron discharge ▸ inward spread of depolarization along T tubules ▸ increased Na$^+$ and K$^+$ conductance in end-plate membrane ▸ generation of action potential in muscle fibers ▸ binding of calcium to troponin C ▸ formation of cross-linkages between actin and myosin.

(D) motor neuron discharge ▸ binding of acetylcholine to nicotinic receptors ▸ increased Na$^+$ and K$^+$ conductance in end-plate membrane ▸ generation of action potential in muscle fibers ▸ release of Ca^{2+} from troponin ▸ formation of cross-linkages between actin and myosin.

(E) generation of action potential in muscle fibers ▸ generation of end-plate potential ▸ increased Na$^+$ and K$^+$ conductance in end-plate membrane ▸ generation of action potential in muscle fibers ▸ binding of calcium to troponin C ▸ formation of cross-linkages between actin and myosin.

Excitation-contraction coupling is the term for muscle fiber depolarization and subsequent contraction. The correct order of events is:

- Motor neuron discharge.
- Release of acetylcholine at motor-end plate
- Binding of acetylcholine to nicotinic receptors
- Increased Na and K conductance in end-plate membrane
- Generation of end-plate potential
- Generation of action potential in muscle fibers
- Inward spread of depolarization along T tubules
- Release of Ca^{2+} from sarcoplasmic reticulum
- Binding of Ca to troponin C; myosin binding sites uncovered
- Formation of cross-linkages between actin and myosin

Ref: Barrett KE, Boitano S, Barman SM, Brooks HL. *Ganong's Review of Medical Physiology.* 24th ed. New York, NY: McGraw Hill; 2012.

67. The molecular mechanism of muscle contraction involves "thin filaments" sliding over "thick filaments." Known as the sliding filament theory, the "thin filament" refers to:

(A) **actin**
(B) myosin
(C) tropomyosin
(D) troponin C
(E) sarcoplasmic reticulum

The "thin filament" of the sliding filament theory is actin. Muscle contraction occurs when thin filaments (actin) slide over thick filaments (myosin):

- Depolarization of the muscle cell causes release of calcium from the sarcoplasmic reticulum.
- Calcium binds to troponin C which alters the configuration of troponin I, actin, and tropomyosin.
- This change exposes an actin binding site for myosin.
- Myosin heads and actin form cross-bridges and ADP is released.
- Myosin heads move the actin filaments with a "power stroke".
- Binding of ATP to the myosin head results in detachment from actin.
- Intracellular calcium and ATP levels influence how many cycles are completed.

Ref: Barrett KE, Boitano S, Barman SM, Brooks HL. *Ganong's Review of Medical Physiology.* 24th ed. New York, NY: McGraw Hill; 2012.

68. Which of the following statements regarding nociception is TRUE?

(A) Most nociceptors are either Meissner corpuscles or Pacinian corpuscles.

(B) Nociceptive afferent fibers are comprised primarily of Aβ and C-fibers.

(C) **Polymodal nociceptors can respond to both pressure and extremes of temperature.**

(D) C fibers conduct at a rate of 12 to 35 m/s.

(E) Eating a Carolina Reaper pepper will activate TRPM8 receptors.

The sensation of pain begins with the conversion of the painful stimulus into an action potential. Nociceptors are nerve cell endings that transduce noxious mechanical, chemical and thermal stimuli into electrical action potentials that are then conducted centrally along afferent neurons to the spinal cord. The majority of nociceptors are relatively unspecialized free nerve endings. In contrast, specialized cutaneous mechanoreceptors such as Meissner and Pacinian corpuscles respond to light touch and vibration, respectively. The most prevalent type of free nerve ending is the polymodal (mechanothermal) nociceptor–these respond to both pressure and extremes of cold and heat, as well as a variety of chemical stimuli.

Pain is conducted from nociceptors by two types of nerve fibers. Thinly myelinated Aδ fibers are 2 to 5 μm in diameter and conduct quickly, at a rate of 12 to 35 m/s. Activation of these fibers is what causes "first pain," a rapid response that allows you to discriminate precisely where the pain is coming from and how intense it is. In contrast, unmyelinated C fibers (0.4–1.2 μm in diameter) conduct slowly at 0.5 to 2 m/s and are responsible for the delayed "second pain." This is a dull, achy, poorly localized pain. Aα fibers are motor fibers, whereas Aβ and Aγ fibers subserve muscle spindles.

Chili peppers contain the chemical capsaicin, which is an irritant that causes a sensation of burning in any tissue that comes into contact with it. Capsaicin binds to the transient receptor potential cation channel subfamily V member 1 (TRPV1) receptor, also known as the vanilloid receptor 1. Activators of this receptor include temperatures higher than 43°C, acidic conditions, allyl isothiocyanate (the pungent compound in wasabi), and of course, capsaicin. TRPV1 antagonists have been investigated as a possible analgesic; while some success has been achieved in reducing experimental pain, blockade of TRPV1 also causes hyperthermia, which so far limits its applicability. The Carolina Reaper pepper is (since 2013 and at the time of writing) the hottest chili pepper in the world, registering a whopping 2.2 million units on the Scoville heat scale; by comparison, jalapeño peppers score between 1000 and 4000 units.

TRPM8 receptors are activated by cold and by menthol in mint.

Ref: Butterworth JF IV, Mackey DC, Wasnick JD. *Morgan and Mikhail's Clinical Anesthesiology.* 5th ed. New York, NY: McGraw Hill; 2013.

69. Substance P acts on which receptor type?

(A) NMDA

(B) AMPA

(C) cholinergic

(D) serotonergic

(E) neurokinin-1

Substance P is a peptide neurotransmitter that is synthesized and released by 1st order neurons both at the peripheral site of tissue damage and in the dorsal horn of the spinal cord. Substance P is also found in various other locations in the central nervous system as well as the gut. Activation of substance P neurons by a noxious stimulus in the periphery results in generation of impulses down collaterals that end at blood vessels, mast cells, and sweat glands in the skin. This causes vasodilation, histamine release and sweating. It also sensitizes nearby neurons to be activated at a lower threshold, releases serotonin from platelets, and acts as a chemoattractant for white blood cells. Substance P acts on the neurokinin-1 (NK1) receptor. NK1 receptors are highly concentrated in the substantia gelatinosa of the dorsal horn of the spinal cord, where primary nociceptive afferent fibers terminate.

Ref: Butterworth JF IV, Mackey DC, Wasnick JD. *Morgan and Mikhail's Clinical Anesthesiology.* 5th ed. New York, NY: McGraw Hill; 2013.

70. Which of the following statements regarding wide dynamic range neurons is TRUE?

(A) They serve only noxious stimuli.

(B) They are primarily responsible for the windup phenomenon.

(C) They are a third-order neuron.

(D) They are most abundant in lamina II.

(E) They are efferent neurons.

Second order neurons are the next step after pain stimuli have been transduced and transmitted via first order nociceptive neurons to the spinal cord. These have cell bodies in the gray matter of the dorsal horn and for the most part project upwards on the contralateral side of the cord as the spinothalamic tract. There are two types of second order neurons. Nociceptive specific neurons serve only noxious stimuli, are arranged in lamina I, and have a discrete receptive field. They are usually quiescent, and only fire in response to a high-threshold noxious stimulus. In contrast, wide dynamic range (WDR) neurons receive both noxious input via Aδ and C fibers as well as non-noxious input via Aβ fibers that usually code for somatic mechanoreception. When a painful stimulus happens, the incoming nociceptive barrage from the C-fibers causes the WDR neuron to steadily increase its firing rate, until it becomes hyperexcited. At this stage, normally non-noxious stimuli (e.g., stroking the skin) that occurs in the same receptive field is perceived as painful. This phenomenon of central sensitization is also known as "windup."

WDR neurons are the most prevalent cell type in the dorsal horn and are most abundant in lamina V.

Ref: Butterworth JF IV, Mackey DC, Wasnick JD. *Morgan and Mikhail's Clinical Anesthesiology.* 5th ed. New York, NY: McGraw Hill; 2013.

71. Which of the following regarding the substantia gelatinosa is TRUE?

(A) It is the most ventral of all the Rexed laminae.

(B) It is also known as lamina V.

(C) It receives primarily Aδ afferents from the periphery.

(D) **It is the site of opioid induced modulation of pain transmission.**

(E) It contains cell bodies of the preganglionic sympathetic neurons.

Spinal cord gray matter has been functionally divided into 10 different laminae by Rexed, with laminae I as the most dorsal (Figure 2-15). The first six laminae form the dorsal horn and receive almost all of the afferent input. Nociceptive C fibers terminate or send collaterals to second-order neurons in laminae I and II, as well a some to lamina V. Aδ fibers terminate primarily in laminae I and V. Lamina VII is the intermediolateral column and contains the cell bodies of preganglionic sympathetic neurons.

Laminae II, also known as the substantia gelatinosa, is chock full of interneurons and plays a large role in the spinal modulation of the primary afferent impulses. The substantia gelatinosa doesn't so much send fibres up the spinothalamic or spinoreticular tracts to the brain, but principally connect with other laminae within the gray matter of the cord, including the contralateral lamina II. It is also a target for descending inhibitory fibers. The substantia gelatinosa contains a high concentration of mu- and kappa-type opioids receptors, which respond to endogenous or exogenous opioids and are believed to help in the modulation of pain perception.

Ref: Butterworth JF IV, Mackey DC, Wasnick JD. *Morgan and Mikhail's Clinical Anesthesiology.* 5th ed. New York, NY: McGraw Hill; 2013.

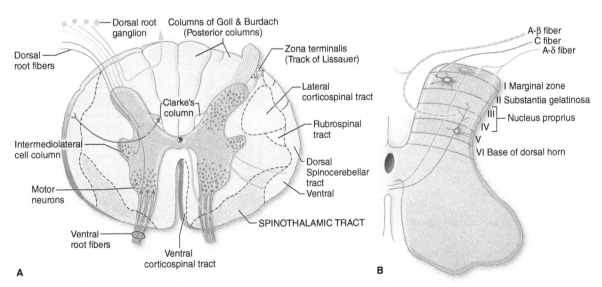

FIG. 2-15. **A.** Spinal cord in transverse section illustrating the course of the afferent fibers and the major ascending pathways. Fast conducting pain fibers are not confined to the spinothalamic tract but are scattered diffusely in the anterolateral funiculus. (Reprinted with permission from Ropper AH, Samuels MA, Klein JP: *Adams and Victor's Principles of Neurology,* 10th Ed. New York, NY: McGraw Hill; 2014. After Martin JH: Neuroanatomy: Text and Atlas. New York, McGraw-Hill, 2003.) **B.** Transverse secton through a cervical segment of the spinal cord illustrating the subdivision of the gray matter into laminae according to Rexed and the entry and termination of the main sensory fibers. (Reprinted with permission from Ropper AH, Samuels MA, Klein JP. *Adams and Victor's Principles of Neurology,* 10th ed. New York, NY: McGraw Hill; 2014. After Fields HL: Pain. New York, McGraw-Hill, 1987.)

72. Which of the following neural structures is involved in the transmission of pain impulses to higher levels of the central nervous system?

(A) fasciculus gracilis

(B) **ventral posterior lateral nucleus**

(C) fasciculus cuneatus

(D) medial lemniscal tract

(E) lateral corticospinal tract

Pain impulses are transduced at the periphery or in the viscera before synapsing with second order neurons in the dorsal horn. Most of these second order neurons cross the midline (that's "*decussate*" to you fancy pants out there.) and ascend the cord via the spinothalamic tract. Some second order neurons ascend one to two levels in Lissauer's Tract before crossing over and ascending via the same route.

The spinothalamic tract has two pathways that run side by side. The anterior spinothalamic tract carries information about crude touch; the lateral spinotha- lamic tract is the one that carries info about pain and temperature. The spinothalamic tract exhibits somato- tropic organization, meaning that the most medial fibers correspond to cervical layers, while the most lat- eral fibers originate in the sacral levels.

As the name implies, these second-order spinotha- lamic fibers synapse in the thalamus, specifically the medial dorsal, ventral posterior lateral and ventral pos- terior medial nuclei. Third-order neurons then project to the somatosensory cortex, cingulate cortex and insular cortex.

The cuneate and gracilis nuclei, as well as the medial lemniscal tract are part of the dorsal column system, for transmission of touch, vibration and proprioception. As the name implies, the corticospinal tract is a descending pathway involved in motor function.

Figure 2-16 shows ascending tracts from both the dorsal column and spinothalamic pathway.

Ref: Barrett KE, Boitano S, Barman SM, Brooks HL. *Ganong's Review of Medical Physiology.* 24th ed. New York, NY: McGraw Hill; 2012.

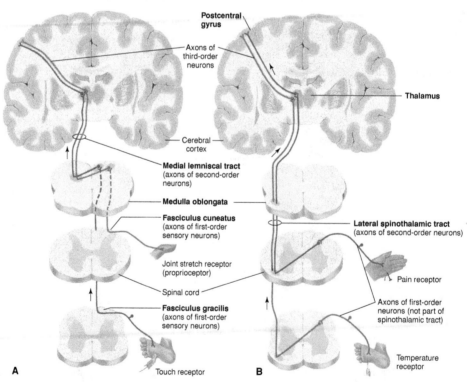

FIG. 2-16. Ascending tracts carrying sensory information from peripheral receptors to the cerebral cortex. **A.** Dorsal column pathway mediates touch, vibratory sense, and proprioception. Sensory fibers ascend ipsilaterally via the spinal dorsal columns to medullary gracilis and cuneate nuclei; from there the fibers cross the midline and ascend in the medial lemniscus to the contralateral thalamic ventral posterior lateral (VPL) and then to the primary somatosensory cortex. **B.** Ventrolateral spinothalamic tract mediates pain and temperature. These sensory fibers terminate in the dorsal horn and projections from there cross the midline and ascend in the ventrolateral quadrant of the spinal cord to the VPL and then to the primary somatosensory cortex. (Reproduced with permission from Barrett KE, Boitano S, Barman SM, Brooks HL. *Ganong's Review of Medical Physiology.* 24th ed. New York, NY: McGraw Hill; 2012.)

73. Which one of the following pain treatment modalities is best explained by Melzack and Wall's gate control theory of pain modulation?

(A) **dorsal column stimulation**

(B) amitriptyline

(C) carbamazepine

(D) transcutaneous lidocaine patches

(E) pregabalin

For many years, the predominant theory of pain processing was the so-called Cartesian view—an impulse in the periphery traveled to the spinal cord and to the brain in much the same way an electrical current is conducted. In other words, nerves were seen as static highways that were not influenced to a great degree in their task of shunting pain messages.

The gate control theory of Melzack and Wall changed that thinking. It was put forward as an attempt to explain the apparent way in which pain intensity could be modulated by other factors, particularly by spinal input from non-noxious sources. In Figure 2-17

panel A, small, unmyelinated C fibers activate the wide dynamic range (WDR) second-order neuron in the dorsal horn of the spinal cord. This results in the experience of pain. WDR neurons also receive input from non-noxious A-beta fibers which contribute to the firing rate of the second order neuron and cause allodynia, hyperalgesia and windup (panel B). However, Melzack and Wall postulated the existence of interneurons located in the substantia gelatinosa that could be activated by branches of the A-beta fibers (panel C). These in turn would inhibit the WDR neuron, effectively "closing the gate" so that the nociceptive input from the C fibers was prevented from increasing the firing rate. Transcutaneous electrical nerve stimulation uses this as its basis for decreasing pain by producing low amplitude electrical signal that stimulated A-beta fibers and held the gate "closed." Implantable dorsal column stimulators also do the same thing presumably, albeit in an antidromic fashion.

Finally, small nociceptive fibers also modulate the interneurons in the substantia gelatinosa, but by

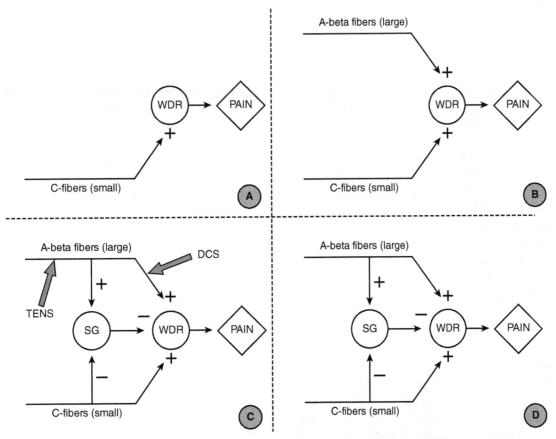

FIG. 2-17. Schematic of the gate control theory. **A.** C fibers activate wide dynamic range (WDR) neurons in the dorsal horn. **B.** Non-noxious A-beta fibers also synapse on the WDR neuron, contributing to its firing rate. **C.** An inhibitory mechanism located in the substantia gelatinosa (SG) is activated by A-beta stimulation, thereby shutting down the WDR neuron or "gate". **D.** C fibers release the inhibition of WDR neurons, opening the gate.

inhibiting them and therefore keeping the gate open (panel D). When no pain is present, the A-beta fibers are thought to tonically keep the gate closed; upon initiation of the painful stimulus, the C fibers work in two ways to open it. Clearly, the experience of pain depends on the relative balance between these two opposing forces. We all make use of the gate theory intuitively. When you hit your thumb with a hammer, you instinctively grab and rub the injured digit, not just at the particular site of injury, but the whole thing; this aids in sending a cascade of non-noxious stimuli originating from the same receptive field to the dorsal column in the hopes of slamming that gate shut.

Ref: Cousins MJ, Carr DB, Horlocker TT, Bridenbaugh PO. *Cousins and Bridenbaugh's Neural Blockade in Clinical Anesthesia and Pain Medicine.* 4th ed. Philadelphia, PA: Lippincott Williams and Wilkins; 2009.

74. Supraspinal descending inhibitory pathways that modulate pain transmission are mediated primarily through:

    (A) substance P
    (B) calcitonin gene-related peptide (CGRP)
    (C) glycine
    (D) glutamate
    (E) **norepinephrine**

Transmission of a pain impulse may be modulated in the spinal cord. Examples of excitatory modulation include windup and central sensitization, receptor field expansion, and hyperexcitability of flexion reflexes.

Inhibitory modulation also occurs at both the segmental level and from higher centers in the CNS. Activation of large non-noxious afferent fibers inhibits wide dynamic range (WDR) neurons as per the gate theory (see previous question). Both glycine and GABA are inhibitory amino acids that facilitate segmental inhibition. Antagonism of either of these increases WDR activity and results in hyperesthesia and allodynia.

Several supraspinal structures project inhibitory neurons down to the spinal cord to inhibit pain in the dorsal horn. These include the periaqueductal gray area, reticular formation, and nucleus raphe magnus. Norepinephrine mediates this action through activation of spinal alpha-2 receptors (this explains why spinal clonidine increases the quality and duration of a spinal block). Some descending neurons use serotonin as a neurotransmitter. The other class of neurotransmitters that are important in descending modulation are the opioids. Endogenous opioids such as endorphins

and enkephalins hyperpolarize primary afferent neurons and inhibit the release of substance P. Exogenous opioids work on second-order neurons or interneurons in the substantia gelatinosa.

Ref: Butterworth JF IV, Mackey DC, Wasnick JD. *Morgan and Mikhail's Clinical Anesthesiology.* 5th ed. New York, NY: McGraw Hill; 2013.

75. Which of the following regarding visceral pain is TRUE?

    (A) Visceral nociceptive afferents are primarily B fibers.
    (B) **Viscera contain "silent" nociceptors that are minimally responsive at baseline.**
    (C) Visceral afferent input makes up >40% of total spinal cord afferent input.
    (D) Vagal afferents project to the cuneate nucleus.
    (E) Afferent first-order neurons enter the spinal cord at a specific level and synapse immediately with a single second order neuron at that same level.

Visceral pain, which arises from the internal organs in the body, is different in several ways to somatic pain. While it is still subserved by Aδ and C fibers, the quality of pain is described as poorly localized, dull, achy, or crampy. It is also frequently associated with referred cutaneous somatic pain and autonomic responses such as sweating and vomiting. These differences can be explained by the structure of visceral pain pathways.

Primary afferents from the viscera project to the CNS by three separate pathways: (1) via the vagus nerve; (2) within and alongside sympathetic efferent fibers; and (3) in the parasympathetic pelvic splanchnic nerves in the sacral region. Primary afferents within the vagus project to the nucleus tractus solitarius in the brainstem with cell bodies in the nodose ganglion. The other two types enter the dorsal horn of T2-L2 (sympathetic) and S2-4 (pelvic splanchnic nerves).

Once in the dorsal horn, these fibers arborize quickly and extensively, including within Lissauer's tract, to enter multiple spinal segments above and below the entry segment. This is partly why visceral pain is diffuse and so poorly localized. Moreover, synaptic contact is made with both superficial and deep dorsal horn neurons on both the ipsilateral and contralateral side, which explains why many visceral pain processes are experienced in the midline and not

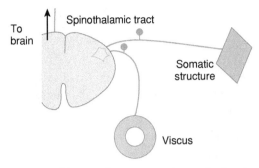

FIG. 2-18. Diagram of convergence theory of referred pain. (Reproduced with permission from Waxman SG. *Clinical Neuroanatomy.* 27th ed. New York, NY: McGraw Hill; 2013.)

exclusively to one side or the other in the abdomen or thorax. Unlike discrete somatic pain processing, visceral pain can be thought of as diffuse central nervous system activation. Despite this extensive branching, visceral afferent fibers are relatively underrepresented in the spinal cord, and account for less than 10% of all incoming first order neurons.

Referred pain from a visceral process is probably caused by the convergence of visceral and somatic afferent fibers on the same wide dynamic range second order neuron in the dorsal horn, which then projects to the thalamus and somatosensory cortex (Figure 2-18). Typically the referred cutaneous or muscular pain is felt in the dermatome or myotome corresponding to the visceral afferent fiber's level of entry.

"Silent" nociceptors are a subtype of free nerve ending, which do not respond to mechanical stimuli like typical cutaneous nociceptors but do become activated in the presence of inflammation. The viscera have the highest concentration of silent nociceptors. Silent nociceptors are also known as mechanically insensitive afferents (MIAs), which is probably a more appropriate name.

Ref: Butterworth JF IV, Mackey DC, Wasnick JD. *Morgan and Mikhail's Clinical Anesthesiology.* 5th ed. New York, NY: McGraw Hill; 2013.

76. Which of the following statements regarding pain and affective disorders is TRUE?

   (A) Pain severity is more predictive of functional limitation than fear of movement or re-injury.

   (B) Approximately 10% of chronic pain patients suffer from depression.

   (C) Chronic pain patients are more likely to express anger than nonchronic pain patients.

   (D) **Internalization of anger is associated with pain intensity.**

   (E) Anxiety is not prevalent in patients with fibromyalgia.

The International Association for the Study of Pain recognizes that pain is not only a subjective sensory feeling, but also an unpleasant emotional experience. Patients with pain frequently have emotional distress. While much of this is no doubt a consequence of the pain experience (reactive depression), the converse can be true as well. Anxiety and depression, for example, have been shown to influence pain severity, the incidence of complications following surgery and the hospital length of stay. Depression and pain appear to be mutually reinforcing factors. Depression is prevalent in patients with chronic pain (approximately 40% to 50%) and has been shown to lead to premature termination from pain rehabilitation programs.

Pain related fear appears to be one of the best predictors of behavioral performance and functional recovery, even more than pain severity or duration. Patients with low back pain tend to avoid back straining activities because of fear of re-injury, and lead to increased amount of time away from work. Avoidance behaviors are natural and serve to reduce re-injury, but can become maladaptive. Anxiety is highly prevalent in chronic pain patients. Up to 40% to 50% of patients with fibromyalgia report feeling chronically anxious.

There appears to be an association between pain and anger as well, as up to 90% of patients surveyed in pain clinics acknowledge feelings of anger. However, several studies have shown that chronic pain patients are less likely to express their anger than nonchronic pain patients, for reasons that are unclear. Anger can be focused toward many different targets—healthcare providers, loved ones, employers, insurance companies, lawyers, and so on. The most common target is often the patient themselves. Over half of patients with anger identify that they were angry primarily with themselves. Internalization of angry feelings is strongly related to increased pain intensity.

Ref: Fishman SM, Ballantyne JC, Rathmell JP. *Bonica's Management of Pain.* 4th ed. Philadelphia, PA: Lippincott Williams and Wilkins; 2010.

77. Which of the following statements regarding the influence of gender on pain perception is TRUE?

    (A) Men are more likely to be diagnosed with temporomandibular disorders and migraine headaches.

    (B) Women report overall increased pain severity than men.

    (C) Estrogen functions to decrease analgesic requirements.

    (D) Red hair and fair skin in women are a marker for increased sensitivity to pain.

    (E) Sociocultural elements likely play a role in any perceived differences.

Population-based research consistently demonstrates that women are at substantially higher risk for pain than men. The population prevalence for several common pain conditions is increased for women than for men, including fibromyalgia, migraine and tension-type headache, irritable bowel syndrome, temporomandibular disorders, and interstitial cystitis. However, studies looking at gender differences in reported pain severity have shown mixed results.

In attempting to explain these differences in pain perception between women and men, many researchers have turned to sex hormones as a mechanism. However, associations between pain or analgesic requirements and plasma levels of estrogen have been all over the board, with some studies showing that estrogen decreased the response to pain, while others drew the opposite conclusion. There does appear to be some difference in gender-related response to some opioids in redheaded females. The melanocortin-1 receptor (MC1R) codes for melanin, the brown pigment in skin and hair. Women carrying two non-functional alleles for the gene demonstrated a greater analgesic response to the kappa-opioid agonist pentazocine (they got better analgesia from the same dose) compared to men with two nonfunctional alleles. In other words, lack of the functioning MC1R gene makes you tougher. Interestingly, about 75% of individuals with red hair and fair skin carry two or more inactive variants of MC1R. The same may not be true with anesthesia requirements, where redheads have been shown to require more anesthesia.

Sociocultural beliefs are thought to play a role in pain responses. For example, in many cultures it is macho to not complain about pain, whereas it is much more acceptable for women to express their pain.

Ref: Longnecker DE, Brown DL, Newman MF, Zapol WM. *Anesthesiology.* 2nd ed. New York, NY: McGraw Hill; 2012.

78. In the autonomic nervous system (ANS), all preganglionic neurons release which of the following neurotransmitters?

    (A) acetylcholine

    (B) norepinephrine

    (C) adenosine triphosphate (ATP)

    (D) substance P

    (E) neuropeptide Y (NPY)

All preganglionic neurons in the ANS release acetylcholine. Acetylcholine is also released by all parasympathetic postganglionic neurons and certain sympathetic postganglionic neurons that innervate sweat glands and those that cause vasodilation in skeletal muscle. Other sympathetic postganglionic neurons release norepinephrine. ATP, substance P, and NPY are nonadrenergic, noncholinergic transmitters released by postganglionic sympathetic neurons.

Ref: Barrett KE, Boitano S, Barman SM, Brooks HL. *Ganong's Review of Medical Physiology.* 24th ed. New York, NY: McGraw Hill; 2012.

79. Classically, which of the following adrenergic receptors is considered an "autoreceptor," thereby playing a role in ANS negative feedback?

    (A) α_1

    (B) α_2

    (C) β_1

    (D) β_2

    (E) β_3

Sympathetic adrenergic receptors are examples of G protein-coupled receptors. Postganglionic sympathetic fibers act on several different adrenergic receptors: α_1 effects include venoconstriction, arteriolar constriction, contraction of intestinal and bladder sphincters, mydriasis (dilatation of pupil), and uterine contraction. Mediates effects via G_q protein stimulation, activation of phospholipase C, and increased levels of inositol triphosphate (IP_3) and calcium.

α_2 classically viewed as an autoreceptor on presynaptic nerve terminals, α_2 activation acts to inhibit norepinephrine release. CNS effects include sedation and analgesia. Mediates effects via G_i protein stimulation, which inhibits adenylyl cyclase and decreases cAMP levels.

β_1 effects include increased heart rate, increased myocardial contractility, and increased cardiac output. Mediates effects via G_s protein stimulation, which activates adenylyl cyclase and increases cAMP levels.

β_2 effects include smooth muscle relaxation in bronchi, GI tract, and uterus; dilation of coronary arteries and blood vessels in skeletal muscle; also increases heart rate and myocardial contractility (to a lesser extent than β_1 activation). Mediates effects via G_s protein stimulation, which activates adenylyl cyclase and increases cAMP levels.

β_3 effects include increased lipolysis in adipose tissue and bladder relaxation. Mediates effects via G_s protein stimulation, which activates adenylyl cyclase and increases cAMP levels.

Ref: Barrett KE, Boitano S, Barman SM, Brooks HL. *Ganong's Review of Medical Physiology.* 24th ed. New York, NY: McGraw Hill; 2012.

80. At postganglionic sympathetic nerve endings the termination of action of norepinephrine is due mainly to:

(A) metabolism by monoamine oxidase (MOA).

(B) metabolism by catechol-O-methyltransferase (COMT).

(C) metabolism by DOPA decarboxylase.

(D) reuptake by uptake-1 mechanism.

(E) reuptake by uptake-2 mechanism.

The termination of action of norepinephrine at postganglionic sympathetic nerve endings is due mainly to reuptake by uptake-1 mechanism. Uptake-2 mechanism refers to non-neuronal tissue. Norepinephrine is also metabolized by MAO and COMT.

DOPA decarboxylase is an enzyme involved in the formation of dopamine.

Ref: Barrett KE, Boitano S, Barman SM, Brooks HL. *Ganong's Review of Medical Physiology.* 24th ed. New York, NY: McGraw Hill; 2012.

81. At a noradrenergic synapse, which of the following enzymes is the rate-limiting step in the production of norepinephrine?

(A) phenylalanine hydroxylase

(B) tyrosine hydroxylase

(C) L-DOPA decarboxylase

(D) dopamine-β-hydroxylase

(E) phenylethanolamine-N-methyltransferase

Tyrosine hydroxylase is the rate-limiting steps in the production of norepinephrine at noradrenergic synapses. Both norepinephrine and dopamine act to inhibit tyrosine hydroxylase activity via negative feedback mechanisms.

Norepinephrine synthesis requires several steps:

- In the liver, dietary phenylalanine can be converted into tyrosine by the enzyme phenylalanine hydroxylase.

- Dietary tyrosine and tyrosine derived from phenylalanine metabolism is taken up into the cytoplasm of the noradrenergic nerve terminal.

- Tyrosine is converted into DOPA by tyrosine hydroxylase.

- DOPA is converted into dopamine by L-DOPA decarboxylase.

- Dopamine is transported into vesicles and subsequently converted into norepinephrine by dopamine-β-hydroxylase.

Note, the enzyme phenylethanolamine-N-methyltransferase is required to convert norepinephrine into epinephrine. This enzyme is found mainly in the adrenal medulla (and to a lesser extend in the CNS). It is not required for norepinephrine synthesis.

Ref: Barrett KE, Boitano S, Barman SM, Brooks HL. *Ganong's Review of Medical Physiology.* 24th ed. New York, NY: McGraw Hill; 2012.

82. Botulinum toxin ("Botox") has a number of medical indications and side effects related to muscle weakness. How does botulinum toxin affect cholinergic transmission?

(A) blocks the transport of choline from the extracellular space into the nerve terminal.

(B) blocks the synthesis of acetylcholine in the nerve terminal.

(C) blocks transport of acetylcholine into vesicles at the nerve terminal.

(D) blocks the influx of Ca^{2+} into the nerve terminal.

(E) blocks exocytosis of acetylcholine into the synaptic cleft.

Botulinum toxin blocks exocytosis of acetylcholine into the synaptic cleft (Note: there are a variety of different botulinum toxins and each blocks a different aspect of the exocytosis process.)

Cholinergic transmission in autonomic ganglia, postganglionic parasympathetic nerve fibers, and at the neuromuscular junction relies on acetylcholine. Acetylcholine synthesis occurs in the nerve terminal. Synthesis and release of acetylcholine involves the following steps:

- Choline is transported into the nerve terminal via a choline transporter.
- Choline acetyltransferase catalyzes the reaction of choline and acetyl-CoA to form acetylcholine.
- Acetylcholine is then packaged into vesicles via a vesicle-associated transporter.
- Nerve impulses open voltage-sensitive Ca^{2+} channels leading to Ca^{2+} influx into the nerve terminal.
- Exocytosis occurs as vesicles fuse with the surface membrane and release acetylcholine.

Ref: Barrett KE, Boitano S, Barman SM, Brooks HL. *Ganong's Review of Medical Physiology.* 24th ed. New York, NY: McGraw Hill; 2012.

83. Which of the following autonomic nervous system neurons principally release norepinephrine?

(A) preganglionic neurons
(B) parasympathetic postganglionic neurons
(C) sympathetic postganglionic neurons innervating sweat glands
(D) sympathetic postganglionic neurons innervating skeletal muscle blood vessels
(E) sympathetic postganglionic neurons innervating systemic veins

The principal neurotransmitters of the autonomic nervous system (ANS) are acetylcholine and norepinephrine. The release of acetylcholine (cholinergic transmission) occurs at:

- All preganglionic neurons,
- All parasympathetic postganglionic neurons,
- Sympathetic postganglionic neurons innervating sweat glands, and
- Sympathetic postganglionic neurons innervating skeletal muscle blood vessels.

The release of norepinephrine (noradrenergic transmission) occurs at all remaining sympathetic postganglionic neurons including those innervating systemic veins.

Ref: Barrett KE, Boitano S, Barman SM, Brooks HL. *Ganong's Review of Medical Physiology.* 24th ed. New York, NY: McGraw Hill; 2012.

84. Acetylcholine's actions on parasympathetic postsynaptic receptors are terminated mainly by:

(A) pseudocholinesterase
(B) butyrylcholinesterase
(C) acetylcholinesterase
(D) reuptake of acetylcholine by autoreceptors on the presynaptic membrane
(E) downregulation of muscarinic receptors on the postsynaptic membrane

Acetylcholine's actions on parasympathetic postsynaptic receptors are terminated mainly by acetylcholinesterase. Acetylcholinesterase, found at the neuromuscular junction and the synaptic cleft of other sites of cholinergic transmission, catalyzes the enzymatic breakdown of acetylcholine into choline and acetate.

Pseudocholinesterase, or butyrylcholinesterase, is a nonspecific cholinesterase produced in the liver and found in blood plasma.

Deficiency of pseudocholinesterase will delay metabolism and prolong the action of medications including succinylcholine, mivacurium, and ester local anesthetics.

Acetylcholine autoreceptors exist on the presynaptic membrane. Their role is somewhat unclear in that studies have found they can either inhibit or augment acetylcholine release. They do not have a role in the metabolism of acetylcholine. Examples of neurotransmitters which rely on reuptake to terminate synaptic transmission include glutamate, norepinephrine, and dopamine.

Receptor downregulation is a negative feedback mechanism whereby the number of postsynaptic receptors decreases in response to a receptor agonist. Receptor downregulation should not be confused with receptor desensitization. Desensitization occurs when a receptor becomes unresponsive due to prolonged exposure to a neurotransmitter.

Ref: Barrett KE, Boitano S, Barman SM, Brooks HL. *Ganong's Review of Medical Physiology.* 25th ed, Ch 7. New York, NY: McGraw Hill; 2012.

85. At parasympathetic ganglia, acetylcholine acting on nicotinic receptors will lead to the activation or influx of which of the following second messengers or ions?

(A) Na^+
(B) Cl^-
(C) cAMP
(D) IP_3
(E) DAG

At parasympathetic ganglia, acetylcholine acting on nicotinic receptors will lead to influx of Na^+. Nicotinic receptors are ligand-gated ion channels and may be classified as those found at either the neuromuscular junction (N_M) or autonomic ganglia and CNS (N_N or "neuronal"). The nicotinic receptor requires two acetylcholine molecules to bind to two α-subunits. This activation results in pore opening and influx of Na^+ and K^+ down their electrochemical gradients (N_N receptors are also highly permeable to Ca^{2+}).

Acetylcholine may also act on a variety of muscarinic receptors (M_1-M_5). M_1, M_3, M_5 receptor activation increases levels of IP3 and DAG and Ca^{2+} conductance. M_2 and M_4 receptor activation decreases levels of cAMP and increases K^+ conductance. In general, M_1 receptors are located in the CNS and autonomic ganglia, M_2 receptors are located in the heart, and M_3 receptors are located on smooth muscle.

Increased chloride permeability occurs when $GABA_A$ receptors are activated.

Ref: Barrett KE, Boitano S, Barman SM, Brooks HL. *Ganong's Review of Medical Physiology*. 24th ed. New York, NY: McGraw Hill; 2012.

86. Which of the following provides sympathetic nervous system innervation to the head and neck?

(A) cranial nerve III

(B) cranial nerve X

(C) splanchnic nerve

(D) **inferior cervical ganglion**

(E) celiac ganglion

The three-paired ganglia of the cervical sympathetic chain, which includes the superior, middle, and inferior cervical ganglia, provide sympathetic nervous system innervation to the head and neck. Cranial nerves III, VII, IX, and X are part of the parasympathetic nervous system. The splanchnic nerve provides sympathetic innervation to a variety of abdominal organs via the celiac ganglion.

Ref: Waxman SG. *Clinical Neuroanatomy*. 27th ed. New York, NY: McGraw Hill; 2013.

87. The autonomic nervous system is influenced by many higher CNS centers. The rostral ventrolateral medulla (RVLM) plays a role in regulation of peripheral vascular tone. Descending neurons from the RVLM

modulate preganglionic sympathetic neurons by releasing which one of the following neurotransmitters?

(A) **glutamate**

(B) GABA

(C) acetylcholine

(D) norepinephrine

(E) dopamine

Descending neurons from the RVLM modulate preganglionic sympathetic neurons via release of glutamate, an excitatory neurotransmitter.

The autonomic nervous system is regulated by a number of higher centers including the limbic system, hypothalamus, and medulla.

The RVLM is influenced by the peripheral baroreceptors, which synapse in the nucleus of the tractus solitarius (NTS). Activation of baroreceptors results in transmission of glutamate. This activates an inhibitory interneuron which in turn decreases descending activation of preganglionic sympathetic neurons (and causes vasodilation).

Ref: Barrett KE, Boitano S, Barman SM, Brooks HL. *Ganong's Review of Medical Physiology*. 24th ed. New York, NY: McGraw Hill; 2012.

88. A patient with a spinal cord injury (SCI) suffers from autonomic dysreflexia. Which of following statements best explains why the patient is potentially at risk of hypertensive crises?

(A) SCI interrupts peripheral baroreceptor activation.

(B) SCI interrupts ascending sensory input to sympathetic nerves.

(C) **SCI interrupts descending inhibitory input to sympathetic nerves.**

(D) SCI interrupts descending activation of parasympathetic nerves.

(E) SCI interrupts ascending sensory input to parasympathetic nerves.

Autonomic dysreflexia may result in hypertensive crises due to activation of the sympathetic nervous system below the level of the spinal cord injury (SCI). SCI interrupts descending inhibitory input to thoracolumbar sympathetic nerves.

Autonomic dysreflexia often occurs in patients with SCIs above the T6 level. Sensory stimuli originating below the level of the injury, such as bladder of bowel distention, may lead to significant sympathetic outflow and intense vasoconstriction. Baroreceptors are intact and sense the change in blood pressure. Descending inhibition of sympathetic nerves is not possible due to the SCI. However, descending parasympathetic pathways (via the vagus nerve) are intact and lead to reflex bradycardia. In this way, sympathetic nervous system clinical features predominate below the level of the lesion (pallor, pilomotor erection, and increased spasticity), and parasympathetic nervous system clinical features predominate above the level of the lesion (facial flushing, nasal congestion, and diaphoresis).

Ref: Hall JB, Schmidt GA, Kress JP. *Principles of Critical Care.* 4th ed. New York, NY: McGraw Hill; 2015.

89. Which type of nerve fibers are responsible for the transmission of afferent input regarding cold tissue temperature throughout the body?

(A) Aα fibers

(B) Aβ fibers

(C) **Aδ fibers**

(D) B fibers

(E) C fibers

Afferent input is transmitted to the central nervous system from a variety of sources, including the skin, spinal cord, brain, and deep abdominal and thoracic tissues. Independent of the anatomical source of the input, temperature transmission occurs via specific sensory neuron fibers for both cold and heat. Cold signals travel via Aδ fibers, whereas heat signals are carried by unmyelinated C fibers (*Quick memory aid: Think A for arctic and C for Caribbean*).

Both of these thermoreceptors increase their firing rates when the respective thermal event occurs (e.g., Aδ fibers increase firing rates in response to cold and slow down when heated; the reverse is true for C fibers). The thermoreceptor itself, which is the free end of the sensory neuron, is a nonspecialized ending that carries one or more types of Transient Receptor Potential (TRP) receptors. The vanilloid (V) subtype (e.g., TRPV1 and TRPV3) respond to heat, while the menthol (M) receptor subtypes (e.g., TRPM8) respond to cold. This latter fact is what gives mints their "cool" feeling in the mouth and airways.

Ref: Longnecker DE, Brown DL, Newman MF, Zapol WM. *Anesthesiology.* 2nd ed. New York, NY: McGraw Hill; 2012.

90. The primary thermoregulatory control center is located in the:

(A) spinothalamic tract.

(B) pons.

(C) reticular activating system.

(D) **hypothalamus.**

(E) anterior pituitary gland.

The hypothalamus is a component of the forebrain that coordinates and regulates many of the autonomic and neuroendocrine activities, such as thermoregulation, hunger, thirst, sex drive, sleep/wake cycles, and aggressiveness. Input from thermoreceptors located in the skin, visceral organs and spinal cord is fed to the anterior hypothalamus where it is integrated and processed, and if necessary, a response generated. In addition, there are thermoreceptors in the hypothalamus itself that contribute approximately 20% of the integrative input. Cooling or heating, the hypothalamus with thermodes in animals drives an appropriate thermoregulatory response in the absence of skin or core temperature change.

Ref: Sessler DI. Mild perioperative hypothermia. *N Engl J Med.* 1997; 336:1730-7.

91. The "set point" is best described by which of the following concepts:

(A) **the temperature of the input to the hypothalamus where the output is zero.**

(B) the point at which sweating begins during heating.

(C) the point at which further vasodilation cannot occur.

(D) the point below which shivering begins.

(E) an exciting moment in a tennis match.

The set point in a negative feedback system such as the thermoregulation system in mammals refers to the point that is being defended by the responses (i.e. the output). For example, the normal set point for temperature in the hypothalamus in humans is 36.9°C. Deviations in core temperature outside a very narrow range (0.2°C) result in thermoregulatory responses including vasoconstriction and shivering for cold or vasodilation and sweating for warmth. The further the deviation from the set point, the higher the degree of thermoregulatory response—this is the concept of "gain." The set point is not fixed; for example, the hypothalamus is subject to the influence of circulating cytokines (e.g., IL-1, TNF, IFN, IL-6) and other pyrogens present during inflammation and infection, which leads to hyperthermia or fever. When the cytokine levels diminish, the set point returns to normal.

Heat stroke is a failure of the set point mechanism that occurs in the setting of prolonged exposure or overexertion in hot environments. Extreme hypovolemia and hypotension brought on by sweating and failure to replenish fluids leads to a decrease in cutaneous blood flow, which prevents the sweating response. The core temperature subsequently rises to the point where the hypothalamic neuronal circuitry is thermally disrupted. Core temperature then continues to rise until irreversible neurologic injury and death occurs.

Ref: Sessler DI. Mild perioperative hypothermia. *N Engl J Med.* 1997; 336: 1730-7.

92. Which of the following mechanisms of heat production most accurately describes the EARLIEST thermoregulatory response to cold?

(A) neuroendocrine release of dopamine

(B) shunting of blood away from visceral organs

(C) **vasoconstriction**

(D) shivering

(E) neuroendocrine release of thyroxine

A normal, healthy, nonanesthetized adult will undergo a number of physiologic responses in response to a 0.1 to 0.2°C drop in core temperature. The first is the cessation of any sweating that had been occurring along with cutaneous vasoconstriction of the skin to prevent radiant, convective and evaporative heat loss from occurring. Vasoconstriction is mediated both by the release of norepinephrine and epinephrine, and to a larger degree by local sympathetic activation of alpha-adrenergic receptors. Vasoconstriction also takes place in the arteriovenous shunts in the fingers, toes, and nose, which increases resistance to flow into the cool extremities. If this does not return the core temperature back to set point, the skeletal muscles of the body begin shivering, an involuntary activity that can increase the metabolic rate up to three times that of

normal. If exposed to a cold environment for a prolonged period of time, the hypothalamus signals the thyroid gland to secrete thyroxine, thereby increasing the metabolic rate in an attempt to generate heat.

Shunting of blood during hypothermia occurs in the direction of the visceral organs in the core compartment, not away from them.

Ref: Longnecker DE, Brown DL, Newman MF, Zapol WM. *Anesthesiology.* 2nd ed. New York, NY: McGraw Hill; 2012.

93. Which of the following is NOT a factor in the increased risk for hypothermia in neonates?

(A) a large skin-to-surface-area ratio.

(B) increased thermal conductance of the skin.

(C) higher evaporative losses.

(D) immature thermoregulatory responses.

(E) **nonfunctional shunts in the fingers and toes.**

The term neonate has a 2.5 times higher skin-surface to body mass ratio compared with an adult, meaning that radiant and convective losses occur at a substantially faster rate. Neonates (and especially preterm infants) have a relatively thin layer of subcutaneous fat, making it easier to conduct heat to the environment (i.e., less "insulation"). Newborns also have less keratin in their skin, increasing the tendency to lose water through evaporation compared to the tougher, keratinized skin of an adult. Whereas an unclothed adult can maintain thermoregulation down to approximately 0°C, infants can only maintain a lower limit of their thermoregulatory responses of about 20 to 22°C. After this point, core body temperature begins to drop rapidly. Infants do in fact have functional shunts in their fingers and toes, and this is not a contributory factor to their increased risk for hypothermia.

One mechanism that infants have to combat hypothermia that adults lack is nonshivering thermogenesis. This refers principally to the generation of heat through metabolically active brown fat, although it has also been detected in skeletal muscle, liver tissue and white fat. Brown fat comprises about 5% of a newborn's body weight, and is primarily located in the chest, neck, axillae and between the scapulae. It is a richly innervated and vascularized tissue that responds to beta-adrenergic activation by the uncoupling of oxidative phosphorylation; this results in heat production instead of the usual generation of ATP. Up to 25% of cardiac output can be diverted to the brown fat deposits, increasing the temperature of the blood. Non-shivering thermogenesis can double the production of heat compared to baseline metabolic activity.

Ref: Butterworth JF IV, Mackey DC, Wasnick JD. *Morgan and Mikhail's Clinical Anesthesiology.* 5th ed. New York, NY: McGraw Hill; 2013.

94. The synthesis of acetylcholine is catalyzed in the terminal of cholinergic nerves by which of the following enzymes?

    (A) choline acetyltransferase
    (B) choline methyltransferase
    (C) acetylcholinesterase
    (D) pseudocholinesterase
    (E) specific cholinesterase

Acetylcholine is synthesized in cytoplasm of the terminal from acetyl CoA and choline by the enzyme choline acetyltransferase. Acetylcholine is then transported from the cytoplasm into vesicles by a vesicle-associated transporter (VAT). These are arranged at the distal terminal near the surface membrane where they await the stimulus to fuse and discharge their payload of acetylcholine.

Acetylcholinesterase is also called specific cholinesterase or true cholinesterase and is responsible for the breakdown of acetylcholine. Pseudocholinesterase (also called plasma cholinesterase or butyrylcholinesterase) is found in the plasma and hydrolyses a number of choline esters such as succinylcholine, mivacurium, heroin and the ester-type local anesthetics such as procaine, chloroprocaine, tetracaine and cocaine.

Ref: Barrett KE, Boitano S, Barman SM, Brooks HL. *Ganong's Review of Medical Physiology.* 24th ed. New York, NY: McGraw Hill; 2012.

95. Release of acetylcholine from synaptic vesicles into the synaptic cleft is dependent on the influx of which ion?

    (A) sodium
    (B) potassium
    (C) calcium
    (D) magnesium
    (E) hydrogen

Action potentials arriving at the terminal of a cholinergic neuron result in the opening of membrane bound calcium ion channels. The influx of calcium causes vesicles that are docked at the surface membrane to fuse and release their load of acetylcholine. This is a complicated process and requires the activation and interaction of a variety of membrane bound proteins. These proteins, known as synaptosome-associated proteins (SNAPs) and vesicle-associated membrane proteins (VAMPs) regulate the fusion of the vesicle membrane with the surface membrane. There are two types of fusion events: The first type is complete absorption and incorporation of the spherical vesicle into the surface plasma membrane. The other type involves the discharge of the vesicular contents through a shared membrane pore, followed by the separation of the vesicle inside the terminal to be recycled (the so-called "kiss-and-run"). Both fusion events are known to occur, but it is unclear why and under which specific circumstances the latter event occurs.

Fun fact: Latrotoxin, the active ingredient in the venom of black widow spiders, is thought to exert its effects by stimulating a G-protein coupled receptor that promotes the presynaptic fusion of vesicles from several types of neurons, most notably cholinergic neurons. While black widow bites are in fact rarely fatal, they may cause severe muscle cramping and abdominal cramping due to the unregulated release of acetylcholine.

Ref: Barrett KE, Boitano S, Barman SM, Brooks HL. *Ganong's Review of Medical Physiology.* 24th ed. New York, NY: McGraw Hill; 2012.

96. Spontaneous, small-amplitude depolarizing potentials at the neuromuscular junction are typically seen:

    (A) with an upper motor neuron lesion.
    (B) with normal quantal release of acetylcholine.
    (C) after fasciculations when using succinylcholine.
    (D) in Lambert-Eaton syndrome.
    (E) in hypercalcemia.

Normal skeletal muscle produces small, spontaneous depolarizing potentials at the neuromuscular junction, called *miniature end-plate potentials (MEPPs)*. These are typically of very small amplitude (1/100th of that required to cause muscular contraction), but otherwise behave in the same manner as larger amplitude potentials. Interestingly, there appears to be a base unit value for MEPPs, related to a specific and consistent amount of acetylcholine released. A given MEPP will be equal to or a multiple of this minimum size. MEPPs are thought to be produced by the spontaneous release of uniformly sized vesicles. This has been termed "quantal release," referring to the discharge of these packages (or quanta) of acetylcholine.

Ref: Miller RD. *Miller's Anesthesia.* 8th ed. Philadelphia, PA: Elsevier; 2015.

97. Which of the following statements regarding the neuromuscular junction is TRUE?

   (A) Acetylcholine binds to one specific subtype of muscarinic cholinergic receptor.
   (B) Cholinergic receptor activation results in the influx of potassium ions in the muscle cell.
   (C) Calcium efflux through the acetylcholine receptor channel is necessary for the generation of end-plate potentials.
   (D) Cholinergic receptors in the neuromuscular junction have two acetylcholine binding sites.
   (E) Junctional folds in the motor end plate serve to reduce the exposure of cholinergic receptors to acetylcholine.

The acetylcholine receptor found in the neuromuscular junction is of the nicotinic variety. Nicotinic receptors that are specific to the neuromuscular junction are comprised of five subunits: two α, one β, one δ, and either a γ or a ϵ subunit. The two α subunits each contain a binding site for acetylcholine, which promotes a configurational change that opens the central channel. When this occurs, calcium and sodium enter the muscle cell, while potassium moves outward. The muscle cell membrane directly across from the nerve terminal contains many junctional folds, which serve to increase the surface area and the number of acetylcholine receptors available. Each neuromuscular junction contains approximately 5 million receptors, although only 10% of these need to be occupied in order to cause muscle cell contraction.

Ref: Butterworth JF IV, Mackey DC, Wasnick JD. *Morgan and Mikhail's Clinical Anesthesiology.* 5th ed. New York, NY: McGraw Hill; 2013.

98. Prejunctional nicotinic receptors located on motor nerve endings are responsible for:

   (A) decreasing the uptake of choline into the cell.
   (B) increasing the release of acetylcholine via positive feedback mechanism.
   (C) modulating the calcium influx following depolarization.
   (D) decreasing the rate of fusion of vesicles with the plasma membrane.
   (E) hyperpolarizing the membrane to prevent further release of acetylcholine.

Both nicotinic and muscarinic receptors are present on prejunctional motor nerve endings. The role of the nicotinic receptor is to maintain the availability of acetylcholine when the nerve is repeatedly stimulated, as in tetany. This nicotinic receptor is slightly different in structure than either the mature or immature postjunctional forms, having three α subunits and two β subunits. Nondepolarizing neuromuscular blocking agents act on these nicotinic receptors (as well as the postjunctional type). Repeated stimulation (e.g., tetany) in the presence of a partial nondepolarizing neuromuscular block will produce fade, since these receptors are involved in the mobilization of acetylcholine, but not its direct release.

Two types of muscarinic receptors have been described on the prejunctional nerve ending, M1 and M2. These modulate calcium influx to either facilitate or inhibit acetylcholine release, respectively.

Ref: Miller RD. *Miller's Anesthesia.* 8th ed. Philadelphia, PA: Elsevier; 2015.

99. Which of the following statements regarding neuromuscular anatomy and function is TRUE?

   (A) Each muscle fiber is typically innervated by 5 to 10 individual axons.
   (B) Nerve endings on slow-twitch muscles are larger and more complicated than those on fast-twitch muscles.
   (C) The motor unit for the extraocular muscles contains more muscle fibers than the motor unit for the quadriceps muscles.
   (D) The synaptic cleft is approximately 20 to 50 nm wide.
   (E) Acetylcholinesterase is synthesized in the liver and transported to the synaptic cleft.

The motor neuron divides as it approaches the muscle, to terminate on the surface of a number of muscle fibers. Each fiber (muscle cell) has only one neuromuscular junction; however, many fibers may be served by a single, branching motor neuron. Stimulation of that neuron will cause all of the associated muscle fibers to contract at once. The motor neuron and its associated muscle fibers are known as the motor unit. Motor units for muscles that require very precise, rapid action as well as those that require the ability to stay contracted for long periods (e.g., extraocular eye muscles) have motor units with a low ratio of muscle fibers per neuron (in the range of 3–6). In contrast, large muscles involved in posture, and those in the thigh might have several hundred per axon.

The synaptic cleft is very small, allowing acetylcholine to cross the distance rapidly. Acetylcholine is hydrolyzed rapidly by acetylcholinesterase, which is synthesized by muscle cells and attached to the muscle cell by a thin stalk of collagen. Nerve endings on fast-twitch muscles are larger than those associated with slow-twitch, although the reason for this is unclear.

Ref: Miller RD. *Miller's Anesthesia.* 8th ed. Philadelphia, PA: Elsevier; 2015.

CHAPTER 3

Respiratory Anatomy and Physiology

1. A patient requires an awake fiberoptic intubation. The anesthesia team elects to perform the procedure via the nasotracheal route. In order to anesthetize the nasal mucosa, which of the following nerves must be blocked?

   (A) olfactory nerve
   (B) facial nerve
   (C) trigeminal nerve
   (D) glossopharyngeal nerve
   (E) vagus nerve

2. In the emergency department, an unconscious trauma patient is evaluated before transfer to the operating room. Suction to the back of the patient's throat does not elicit a gag reflex. Which of the following nerves innervates the sensory portion of this reflex?

   (A) trigeminal nerve
   (B) glossopharyngeal nerve
   (C) vagus nerve
   (D) facial nerve
   (E) hypoglossal nerve

3. What is the anatomic border between the oropharynx and the laryngopharynx (hypopharynx)?

   (A) sphenoid bone
   (B) oral cavity
   (C) epiglottis
   (D) soft palate
   (E) cricoid cartilage

4. Which of the following laryngeal muscles abduct (open) the vocal cords?

   (A) lateral cricoarytenoid muscle
   (B) transverse arytenoid muscle
   (C) posterior cricoarytenoid muscle
   (D) oblique arytenoid muscle
   (E) thyroarytenoid muscle

5. Which of the following laryngeal muscles is innervated by the *external* branch of the superior laryngeal nerve?

   (A) cricothyroid muscle
   (B) transverse arytenoid muscle
   (C) posterior cricoarytenoid muscle
   (D) lateral cricoarytenoid muscle
   (E) thyroarytenoid muscle

6. In the larynx, the posterior aspect of the vocal ligaments (vocal cords) attach to which of the following cartilages?

   (A) thyroid cartilage
   (B) cricoid cartilage
   (C) cuneiform cartilage
   (D) corniculate cartilage
   (E) arytenoid cartilage

7. In follow-up after surgery and anesthesia, a patient notes significant hoarseness. In order to evaluate the patient's vocal cords, a diagnostic fiberoptic examination is performed. If unilateral injury to the recurrent laryngeal nerve has occurred, what will be the position of the affected vocal cord?

   (A) fixed in adducted position
   (B) fixed in abducted position
   (C) fixed in paramedian position
   (D) able to adduct, but weak abduction
   (E) able to abduct, but weak adduction

8. Following an uneventful general anesthetic for uterine myomectomy, a previously well patient is noted to have complete unilateral vocal cord paralysis in the PACU. Which of the following treatment options is most likely required?

   (A) emergency reintubation
   (B) elective tracheostomy
   (C) biPAP
   (D) eNT referral
   (E) expectant management

9. Compared to an adult larynx, which of the following anatomic features is characteristic of the pediatric larynx?

   (A) epiglottis is firm and broad.
   (B) larynx is cylindrical in shape.
   (C) narrowest portion of larynx is at level of vocal cords.
   (D) larynx is in a more superior (rostral) position.
   (E) anterior vocal cord attachment slants superiorly (rostral).

10. In an emergency "cannot intubate, cannot ventilate" situation, an anesthesia team prepares for a percutaneous surgical airway. In order to secure the airway, which one of the following anatomic sites should be accessed?

    (A) suprasternal notch
    (B) between the second and third tracheal rings
    (C) inferior (caudad) to cricoid cartilage
    (D) thyrohyoid membrane
    (E) cricothyroid membrane

11. At the level of the tracheal bifurcation, or carina, which of the following anatomic relationships is correct?

    (A) Right pulmonary artery is directly posterior to the trachea.
    (B) Xiphoid process is directly anterior to the trachea.
    (C) T9 vertebrae is directly posterior to the trachea.
    (D) Pericardial sac is caudad to the trachea.
    (E) Aortic arch is caudad to the trachea.

12. During active expiration, which of the following muscles is most important?

    (A) rectus abdominis
    (B) trapezius
    (C) diaphragm
    (D) external intercostal muscles
    (E) scalene muscles

13. Which of the following muscles is considered an accessory muscle of inspiration?

    (A) diaphragm
    (B) external intercostal
    (C) internal intercostal
    (D) rectus abdominis
    (E) sternocleidomastoid

14. The sum of the expiratory reserve volume (ERV) plus the tidal volume (V_T) plus the inspiratory reserve volume (IRV) equals which of the following?

    (A) inspiratory capacity
    (B) total lung capacity
    (C) functional residual capacity
    (D) vital capacity
    (E) closing capacity

15. Which of the following BEST approximates the functional residual capacity (FRC) for a healthy, 70-kg adult?

    (A) 1200 mL
    (B) 1600 mL
    (C) 2400 mL
    (D) 3200 mL
    (E) 4000 mL

16. Which of the following factors does NOT influence the functional residual capacity (FRC)?

    (A) advanced age
    (B) body habitus
    (C) sex
    (D) posture
    (E) restrictive pulmonary disease

17. Which of the following is a dynamic lung volume?

    (A) slow vital capacity
    (B) forced expiratory volume in 1 second
    (C) inspiratory capacity
    (D) functional residual capacity
    (E) closing volume

18. A patient presents to preoperative clinic with a 50 pack-year smoking history and severe chronic obstructive pulmonary disease. Which of the following parameters is best measured using spirometry?

    (A) forced vital capacity
    (B) total lung capacity
    (C) residual lung volume
    (D) closing capacity
    (E) functional residual capacity

19. Which of the following best describes the concept of physiologic dead space?

    (A) alveoli that are not perfused
    (B) alveoli and nonrespiratory airways that are not perfused
    (C) alveoli that are perfused but are not ventilated.
    (D) trachea and nonrespiratory airways
    (E) pharynx, endotracheal tube, and y-piece of the circuit

20. Which of the following factors DECREASES dead space?

    (A) upright position
    (B) neck extension
    (C) endotracheal tube
    (D) emphysema
    (E) age

21. At what lung volume is pulmonary vascular resistance the lowest?

    (A) residual volume
    (B) closing volume
    (C) expiratory reserve volume
    (D) functional residual capacity
    (E) total lung capacity

Use the following clinical scenario to answer questions 22 and 23:

A 57-year -old male, weighing 70 kg is scheduled for esophagectomy after a recent diagnosis of carcinoma of the esophagus. He has mild hypertension but is otherwise generally fit. As part of his preoperative workup, he is undergoing cardiopulmonary exercise testing (CPET). At baseline, his VO_2 is measured at 4 mL/kg/min, cardiac output is 5.6 L/min and his arterial oxygen content is 200 ml/L.

22. What is his mixed venous oxygen content?

    (A) 50 mL/L
    (B) 100 mL/L
    (C) 150 mL/L
    (D) 250 mL/L
    (E) 300 mL/L

23. Which of the following factors measured using CPET is the best predictor of postoperative cardiopulmonary complication rate?

    (A) anaerobic threshold
    (B) minute ventilation
    (C) EKG ST analysis
    (D) VCO_2
    (E) stroke volume

24. A spontaneously breathing patient inhales 600 mL of air. During this time, the intrapleural pressure decreases from -4 cm H_2O to -9 cm H_2O. The compliance of this patient's respiratory system under these conditions is:

    (A) 60 mL·cm H_2O^{-1}
    (B) 90 mL·cm H_2O^{-1}
    (C) 100 mL·cm H_2O^{-1}
    (D) 120 mL·cm H_2O^{-1}
    (E) 150 mL·cm H_2O^{-1}

25. The parameters necessary to calculate transmural pressure for thoracic wall compliance (i.e. not lung compliance) are:

    (A) atmospheric pressure and intrapleural pressure
    (B) atmospheric pressure and alveolar pressure
    (C) intrapleural pressure and alveolar pressure
    (D) interstitial pressure and intrapleural pressure
    (E) pericardial pressure and intrapleural pressure

26. A patient is being ventilated in the critical care unit. The change in lung volume observed for a given peak inspiratory pressure BEST describes which of the following concepts?

    (A) static lung compliance.
    (B) inspiratory lung compliance.
    (C) dynamic lung compliance.
    (D) maximal lung compliance.
    (E) effort-independent lung compliance.

27. Hysteresis refers to:

    (A) the tendency of alveoli to collapse at low volumes.
    (B) differing pressure-volume curves for inflation and deflation of the lungs.
    (C) the pleural pressure gradient that exists between the apex and the base of the lung.
    (D) the decrease in airway resistance observed as air moves down the respiratory tree.
    (E) the freak-out observed in the OR when a patient starts to quickly desaturate.

28. Which of the following best explains why alveoli do not collapse when lung volumes become small?

    (A) Surfactant increases the surface tension as spherical volume decreases.
    (B) Surfactant decreases the surface tension as spherical volume decreases.
    (C) Air trapping pneumatically stents open the alveoli.
    (D) Chest wall recoil prevents complete collapse.
    (E) Intrapleural pressure is maintained at -10 cm H_2O at the base.

29. A child experiences bronchospasm shortly after induction of general anesthesia. A decrease in the radius of her mid- to large-caliber airways by 50% will be likely to produce an increase in airway resistance of:

    (A) 2 times baseline
    (B) 4 times baseline
    (C) 8 times baseline
    (D) 16 times baseline
    (E) 32 times baseline

30. Which of the following descriptions best matches the flow-volume loop shown below in Figure 3-9?

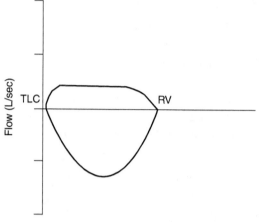

FIG. 3-9. A flow-volume loop.

    (A) extrathoracic variable obstruction
    (B) intrathoracic variable obstruction
    (C) fixed obstruction
    (D) chronic obstructive pulmonary disease
    (E) restrictive pulmonary disease

31. Total lung capacity (TLC) may be measured by all of the following methods EXCEPT:

    (A) helium dilution
    (B) nitrogen washout
    (C) spirometry
    (D) body plethysmography
    (E) chest radiograph measurements

32. At what age will a healthy individual experience some closure of their small airways in the supine position?

    (A) 20 years of age
    (B) 40 years of age
    (C) 50 years of age
    (D) 60 years of age
    (E) 80 years of age

33. A 24-year-old woman is experiencing an acute asthma exacerbation. What alteration in her respiratory mechanics will decrease the work of breathing?

    (A) recruitment of additional muscles of respiration
    (B) taking shallow breaths near total lung capacity
    (C) breath holding
    (D) increasing her respiratory rate
    (E) decreasing her respiratory rate

34. During quiet breathing, the portion of the respiratory system that offers the greatest resistance to airflow is the:

    (A) mouth
    (B) trachea
    (C) large bronchi
    (D) mid-sized bronchi
    (E) small bronchi

35. Which of the following acts to constrict the bronchial smooth muscle?

    (A) parasympathetic stimulation
    (B) beta-2 (β2) agonists
    (C) nitric oxide
    (D) local hypercarbia
    (E) local hypoxemia

36. Which of the following is NOT an example of V/Q mismatch leading to pulmonary shunt?

    (A) mucus plugging of a lobar bronchus
    (B) pulmonary thromboembolism
    (C) a bronchial blocker placed in the left mainstem bronchus
    (D) atelectasis
    (E) pneumonia

37. During normal tidal inspiration, what percentage of ventilation will dependent (lowermost) alveoli receive compared to alveoli in the nondependent (i.e. uppermost aspect) of the lung?

    (A) No ventilation
    (B) 50%
    (C) 100%
    (D) 150%
    (E) 500%

38. According to the zone theory of lung perfusion as described by West, alveoli in zone 3 are characterized by:

    (A) alveolar pressure > pulmonary arterial pressure
    (B) alveolar pressure > pulmonary venous pressure
    (C) pulmonary arterial pressure > alveolar pressure
    (D) pulmonary venous pressure = alveolar pressure
    (E) pulmonary venous pressure > pulmonary arterial pressure

39. Following administration of an antibiotic during a general anesthetic, a patient's end-tidal carbon dioxide decreases from 38 mm Hg to 30 mm Hg. No changes in the ventilatory settings were made during this time. The noninvasive blood pressure cuff is set to cycle again in 2 minutes. Which of the following statements is most accurate regarding this clinical situation?

    (A) Dead space has decreased.
    (B) Dead space has increased.
    (C) Shunt fraction has decreased.
    (D) Shunt fraction has increased.
    (E) The patient requires more PEEP.

40. A pulmonary artery catheter is placed to monitor pulmonary artery occlusion pressure (PAOP). In which West zone(s) must the catheter lie in order to be accurate?

    (A) West zone 1
    (B) West zone 2
    (C) West zone 3
    (D) West zones 1 or 2
    (E) West zone 2 or 3

41. Which of the following factors interferes with effective hypoxic pulmonary vasoconstriction (HPV)?

    (A) propofol
    (B) fentanyl
    (C) thoracic epidural analgesia
    (D) 6% desflurane
    (E) nitroprusside

42. Which of the following is NOT required to calculate the diffusion rate of a gas across the alveolar membrane?

    (A) combined surface area of the alveoli
    (B) diffusion coefficient for the particular gas
    (C) viscosity of the gas
    (D) partial pressure of the gas in the blood
    (E) thickness of alveolar/capillary interface

DIRECTIONS: Use the following scenario to answer questions 43 and 44:

A healthy 30-year-old weighing 70 kg undergoes induction of general anesthesia with paralysis after breathing room air. The patient is neither ventilated nor oxygenated following induction. The patient has a VO_2 of 3.5 mL/kg/min and an FRC of 2400 mL.

43. From the time that apnea is initiated, how long will the patient's oxygen stores last until he begins to desaturate?

    (A) 30 seconds
    (B) 60 seconds
    (C) 2 minutes
    (D) 4 minutes
    (E) 6 minutes

44. The medical student accompanying the anesthesiologist decides to show off and ask about "apneic oxygenation." This backfires when he is then asked to explain what he knows about it. A good answer would be:

    (A) It's a myth—it doesn't really exist.
    (B) There are conflicting data about how it works.
    (C) It's only been shown to work in experimental situations, not in humans.
    (D) It works via the creation of a low pressure zone in the alveoli, which draws in oxygen from the upper airway.
    (E) Hypoxic pulmonary vasoconstriction gradually shunts flow away from underperfused lung, preserving V/Q matching.

45. Diffusion hypoxia is a phenomenon most likely seen in which of the following settings?

    (A) upon induction of anesthesia with air/oxygen and fentanyl
    (B) upon induction of anesthesia with nitrous oxide/oxygen and fentanyl
    (C) upon induction of anesthesia with nitrous oxide/oxygen and morphine
    (D) upon emergence from anesthesia with air/oxygen and morphine
    (E) upon emergence from anesthesia with nitrous oxide/oxygen and fentanyl

46. An intubated patient is breathing 30% oxygen in a critical care unit in Miami. Arterial blood gas analysis reveals her PaO_2 is 140 mm Hg and her $PaCO_2$ is 40 mm Hg. Which of the following best represents her alveolar-arterial (A-a) gradient:

    (A) 6
    (B) 10
    (C) 12
    (D) 18
    (E) 24

47. Assuming the solubility coefficient of oxygen in blood is 0.003 mL/mm Hg/dL, which of the following best estimates the amount of dissolved oxygen in a 70-kg man breathing room air?

    (A) 5 mL
    (B) 15 mL
    (C) 150 mL
    (D) 1500 mL
    (E) 2100 mL

48. Which of the following statements regarding normal adult hemoglobin is correct?

    (A) Hemoglobin is made up of four protein subunits surrounding a single heme group.
    (B) Hemoglobin is made up of two alpha chains and two gamma chains.
    (C) Each gram of hemoglobin can carry 1.34 mL of oxygen.
    (D) Only the ferric form of iron (Fe^{3+}) can bind oxygen.
    (E) As each binding site becomes occupied with oxygen, conformational changes occur that make it more difficult to bind more oxygen.

49. Which of the following factors is most likely to shift the oxyhemoglobin dissociation curve to a position that favors unloading of oxygen?

    (A) hyperthermia
    (B) alkalosis
    (C) decreased 2,3-diphosphoglycerate (2,3-DPG) levels
    (D) carboxyhemoglobin
    (E) fetal hemoglobin

50. Hemoglobin from which one of the following would be expected to have the highest levels of 2,3-DPG?

    (A) an 80-year-old man
    (B) a 45-year-old woman from Florida enjoying a ski holiday in Breckenridge, Colorado
    (C) a healthy 6-month-old child
    (D) a healthy 25-year-old woman 2 weeks postpartum
    (E) a unit of red blood cells stored in a blood bank for 40 days

51. Which of the following best represents the oxygen partial pressure where normal adult hemoglobin will be 50% saturated?

    (A) 19 mm Hg
    (B) 27 mm Hg
    (C) 40 mm Hg
    (D) 50 mm Hg
    (E) 75 mm Hg

52. A patient under general anesthesia has an arterial blood gas drawn, which reveals $PaO_2 = 85$ mm Hg, $PaCO_2 = 42$ mm Hg, Hb = 13 g/dL, and $SpO_2 = 96\%$. Which of the following best approximates his oxygen content?

    (A) 10 mL/dL
    (B) 12 mL/dL
    (C) 14 mL/dL
    (D) 17 mL/dL
    (E) 19 mL/dL

53. Which of the following statements regarding methemoglobin is FALSE?

    (A) Methemoglobin contains the oxidized (ferric or 3^+) form of the iron ion.
    (B) Agents that cause methemoglobinemia include nitrates, nitrites, and prilocaine.
    (C) The remaining binding sites in the hemoglobin tetramer exhibit increased affinity for oxygen.
    (D) Significant amounts of methemoglobin cause the pulse oximeter to display a value of 100% no matter what the oxygen carrying capacity.
    (E) Methemoglobin is converted back to oxyhemoglobin by the enzyme methemoglobin reductase.

54. Carbon dioxide is carried in blood in multiple ways. Which of the following best describes the relative importance of the method of transport?

    (A) dissolved in solution > bound to blood proteins > as bicarbonate ions
    (B) bound to blood proteins > dissolved in solution > as bicarbonate ions
    (C) bound to blood proteins > as bicarbonate ions > dissolved in solution
    (D) as bicarbonate ions > dissolved in solution > bound to blood proteins
    (E) as bicarbonate ions > bound to blood proteins > dissolved in solution

55. Carbonic anhydrase catalyzes which of the following reactions?

    (A) the conversion of CO_2 and H_2O into carbonic acid within the erythrocyte
    (B) the conversion of CO_2 and H_2O into carbonic acid within the plasma
    (C) the splitting of carbonic acid into protons and bicarbonate within the erythrocyte
    (D) the splitting of carbonic acid into protons and bicarbonate within the plasma
    (E) the splitting of carbonic acid into protons and bicarbonate within the interstitial fluid

56. The mechanism by which red blood cells maintain electrical neutrality while generating bicarbonate ions is termed the:

    (A) sodium shift.
    (B) potassium shift.
    (C) calcium shift.
    (D) phosphate shift.
    (E) chloride shift.

57. Compared to the oxyhemoglobin dissociation curve, the carbon dioxide dissociation curve is:

    (A) more sigmoidal shaped.
    (B) logarithmic.
    (C) steeper in slope.
    (D) inversely related.
    (E) left-shifted.

58. The Haldane effect explains why:

    (A) the oxyhemoglobin dissociation curve is sigmoidal.
    (B) fetal hemoglobin has a greater affinity for oxygen that adult hemoglobin.
    (C) carbon dioxide has a greater solubility than oxygen.
    (D) the carbon dioxide dissociation curve is sigmoidal.
    (E) deoxygenated blood can carry more carbon dioxide than oxygenated blood.

59. A healthy 30-year-old patient has an arterial pCO_2 of 60 mm Hg. Which of the following would you expect to DECREASE in association with this lab value?

    (A) heart rate
    (B) pulmonary arterial pressure
    (C) myocardial contractility
    (D) cerebral vascular resistance
    (E) plasma norepinephrine level

60. Due to an error in ventilator settings, a patient's PCO_2 is 25 mm Hg. Which of the following is most likely to occur as a result?

    (A) reduced coronary flow
    (B) decreased coronary vascular resistance
    (C) decreased oxygen extraction
    (D) decreased systemic vascular resistance
    (E) decreased myocardial contractility

61. Administering high concentrations of oxygen (hyperoxia) is most likely to have which of the following effects?

    (A) decreased systemic vascular resistance
    (B) increased heart rate
    (C) increased coronary flow
    (D) increased risk of acute lung injury
    (E) increased cerebral blood flow

62. A 59-year old patient with pneumonia has a room air arterial PaO_2 of 50 mm Hg. Which of the following physiologic findings would most likely be observed in this patient?

    (A) decreased cerebral blood flow
    (B) decreased coronary blood flow
    (C) a respiratory rate of 11/min
    (D) decreased pulmonary vascular resistance
    (E) increased cardiac output

63. The group of neurons responsible for the initiation of each breath are known as the:

    (A) ventral respiratory group.
    (B) dorsal respiratory group.
    (C) medial respiratory group.
    (D) lateral respiratory group.
    (E) central respiratory group.

64. Central respiratory chemoreceptors in the brainstem are stimulated by which of the following?

    (A) plasma hydrogen ion concentration
    (B) plasma bicarbonate ion concentration
    (C) CSF stays capped hydrogen ion concentration
    (D) CSF bicarbonate ion concentration
    (E) CSF oxygen concentration

65. A reduction in plasma PO_2 will result in the increase in firing rate of neurons from which of the following locations?

    (A) carotid body
    (B) carotid sinus
    (C) pulmonary trunk
    (D) right atrium
    (E) bronchioles

66. Which of the following best describes the Hering-Breuer reflex?

    (A) rapid shallow breathing in response to pulmonary vascular congestion
    (B) the slowing of breathing with activation of pulmonary stretch receptors
    (C) apnea in response to immersion of the face in water
    (D) hyperpnea in response to low PaO_2
    (E) hyperpnea in response to pain in an extremity

67. Which of the following would be expected to cause a left shift in the carbon dioxide response curve?

    (A) normal physiologic sleep
    (B) opioids
    (C) chronic obstruction
    (D) metabolic acidosis
    (E) sevoflurane anesthesia with a MAC of 1.0

68. Which of the following vasoactive substances is largely inactivated by the lung?

    (A) dopamine
    (B) epinephrine
    (C) histamine
    (D) oxytocin
    (E) serotonin

69. Which of the following is NOT a physiologic consequence of cigarette smoking?

    (A) decreased FEV_1
    (B) small airway narrowing
    (C) left shift of the oxyhemoglobin dissociation curve
    (D) arterial hypertension
    (E) decreased platelet aggregation and primary clot failure

70. Which of the following is INCREASED for patients who have quit smoking prior to anesthesia, compared to current smokers?

    (A) the risk of ICU admission postoperatively
    (B) the P50 of the oxyhemoglobin dissociation curve
    (C) the risk of pneumonia
    (D) the risk of laryngospasm
    (E) the sputum volume

Answers and Explanations: Respiratory Anatomy and Physiology

1. A patient requires an awake fiberoptic intubation. The anesthesia team elects to perform the procedure via the nasotracheal route. In order to anesthetize the nasal mucosa, which of the following nerves must be blocked?

   (A) olfactory nerve
   (B) facial nerve
   (C) **trigeminal nerve**
   (D) glossopharyngeal nerve
   (E) vagus nerve

   Sensation to the nasal cavity is supplied by the V_1 and V_2 branches of the trigeminal nerve (cranial nerve V). The V_1 branch of the trigeminal nerve, the ophthalmic nerve, branches into the anterior ethmoidal nerve which provides sensation to the anterior portion of the nasal septum. The V_2 branch of the trigeminal nerve, the maxillary nerve, branches into the greater and lesser palatine nerves which provide sensation to the nasal turbinates and majority of the nasal septum. The glossopharyngeal nerve (cranial nerve IX) provides sensation to the pharynx, posterior third of the tongue, anterior surface of epiglottis, and tonsils. The vagus nerve (cranial nerve X), via the internal branch of the superior laryngeal nerve, provides sensation to the root of the tongue, posterior epiglottis, arytenoids, and aryepiglottic folds. The vagus nerve, via the recurrent laryngeal nerve, provides sensation to the vocal folds and trachea. The olfactory nerve (cranial nerve I) is responsible for sense of smell. A branch of the facial nerve (cranial nerve VII) is responsible for sense of taste on the anterior two thirds of the tongue, while the glossopharyngeal nerve is responsible for sense of taste on the posterior third of the tongue.

   Ref: Hadzic A. *NYSORA Textbook of Regional Anesthesia and Acute Pain Medicine.* 1st ed. New York, NY: McGraw Hill; 2007.

2. In the emergency department, an unconscious trauma patient is evaluated before transfer to the operating room. Suction to the back of the patient's throat does not elicit a gag reflex. Which of the following nerves innervates the sensory portion of this reflex?

   (A) trigeminal nerve
   (B) **glossopharyngeal nerve**
   (C) vagus nerve
   (D) facial nerve
   (E) hypoglossal nerve

   The sensory (afferent) portion of the gag reflex is mediated by the glossopharyngeal nerve (cranial nerve IX). The motor (efferent) portion of the gag reflex is mediated by the vagus nerve (cranial nerve X). Overall, touching the posterior pharyngeal wall elicits elevation of the soft palate and pharyngeal muscle contraction. The V_2 (maxillary) branch of the trigeminal nerve (cranial nerve V) innervates the nasopharynx. The facial nerve (cranial nerve VII) via the chorda tympani provides taste sensation to the anterior two thirds of the tongue. The hypoglossal nerve (cranial nerve XII) provides motor innervation to the tongue.

   Ref: Morton DA, Albertine K, Foreman KB. *Gross Anatomy: The Big Picture.* 1st ed. New York, NY: McGraw Hill; 2011.

3. What is the anatomic border between the oropharynx and the laryngopharynx (hypopharynx)?

   (A) sphenoid bone
   (B) oral cavity
   (C) **epiglottis**
   (D) soft palate
   (E) cricoid cartilage

   The epiglottis is the anatomic border separating the oropharynx from the laryngopharynx (Figure 3-1).

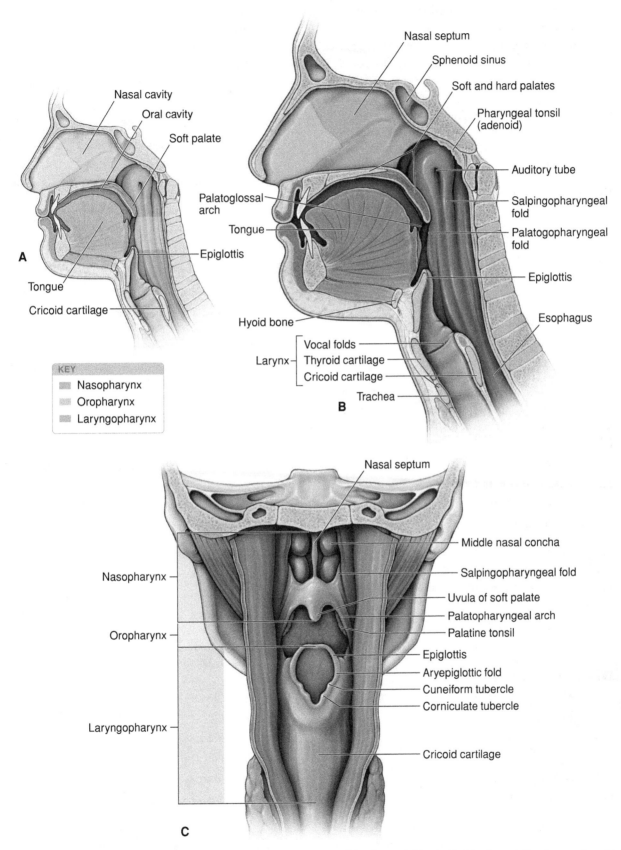

FIG. 3-1. A. Regions of the pharynx. **B.** Sagittal section of the head. **C.** Posterior view of the pharynx (midsagittal incision through the pharyngeal constrictor muscles). (Reproduced with permission from Morton DA, Albertine K, Foreman KB. *The Big Picture: Gross Anatomy*. 1st ed. New York, NY: McGraw Hill; 2011.)

The pharynx (or throat) is divided into three subdivisions: nasopharynx, oropharynx, and laryngopharynx (hypopharynx). The pharynx serves as the common pathway for the aerodigestive tracts. The nasopharynx is the area above the soft palate, below the sphenoid bone, and behind the nasal cavity. The oropharynx is located between the soft palate and epiglottis, posterior to the oral cavity. The laryngopharynx (or hypopharynx) is located between the epiglottis and cricoid cartilage, posterior to the larynx.

Ref: Morton DA, Albertine K, Foreman KB. *Gross Anatomy: The Big Picture.* 1st ed. New York, NY: McGraw Hill; 2011.

4. Which of the following laryngeal muscles abduct (open) the vocal cords?

   (A) lateral cricoarytenoid muscle

   (B) transverse arytenoid muscle

   (C) posterior cricoarytenoid muscle

   (D) oblique arytenoid muscle

   (E) thyroarytenoid muscle

The posterior cricoarytenoid muscles abduct (open) the vocal cords. They are innervated by the recurrent laryngeal nerve (cranial nerve X). Muscles that adduct (close) the vocal cords include:

• lateral cricoarytenoid muscles

• transverse arytenoid muscles

• oblique arytenoid muscles

• aryepiglottic muscles

The thyroarytenoid muscles decrease the length and tension of the vocal cords, while the cricothyroid muscles increase the length and tension of the vocal cords.

Ref: Morton DA, Albertine K, Foreman KB. *Gross Anatomy: The Big Picture.* 1st ed. New York, NY: McGraw Hill; 2011.

5. Which of the following laryngeal muscles is innervated by the *external* branch of the superior laryngeal nerve?

   (A) cricothyroid muscle

   (B) transverse arytenoid muscle

   (C) posterior cricoarytenoid muscle

   (D) lateral cricoarytenoid muscle

   (E) thyroarytenoid muscle

Sensation to the upper airway is innervated by branches of the cranial nerves. The anterior two-thirds of the tongue is innervated by the mandibular branch (V3)

of the trigeminal nerve. Moving deeper into the oropharynx, the glossopnaryhgeal nerve innervates the posterior third of the tongue down to the vallecula and the superior aspect of the epiglottis, as well as the roof of the pharynx, the tonsils and the undersurface of the soft palate. The posterior aspect of the epiglottis, the hypopharynx and the larynx are all innervated by branches that originate from the vagus (cranial nerve X) nerve.

TABLE 3-1. **Sensory and motor innervation of the airway.**

	Superior laryngeal nerve	Recurrent laryngeal nerve
Sensory	Posterior epiglottis, hypopharynx, larynx above vocal cords	Larynx below vocal cords, trachea
Motor	Cricothyroid muscle (external branch of superior laryngeal nerve)	Remainder of the muscles of the larynx

The cricothyroid muscle is innervated by the external branch of superior laryngeal nerve (cranial nerve X). This muscle increases the length and tension of the vocal cords (i.e., "stretches them"), when you're trying to hit that high C note.

The airway is bilaterally innervated, which protects against acute airway obstruction in the event of injury to one of these nerves. The most dangerous situation is bilateral acute injury (i.e., transection) of the recurrent laryngeal nerves. This results in unopposed tension by the cricothyroid muscle, bringing the cords to the midline and resulting in stridor and respiratory distress. Chronic recurrent laryngeal nerve injuries are less dangerous because atrophy of the musculature prevents excessive tension.

Ref: Morton DA, Albertine K, Foreman KB. *Gross Anatomy: The Big Picture.* 1st ed. New York, NY: McGraw Hill; 2011.
Butterworth JF IV, Mackey DC, Wasnick JD. *Morgan and Mikhail's Clinical Anesthesiology.* 5th ed. New York, NY: McGraw Hill; 2013.

6. In the larynx, the posterior aspect of the vocal ligaments (vocal cords) attach to which of the following cartilages?

   (A) thyroid cartilage

   (B) cricoid cartilage

   (C) cuneiform cartilage

   (D) corniculate cartilage

   (E) arytenoid cartilage

In the larynx, the vocal ligaments (vocal cords) attach **posteriorly to the arytenoid cartilages** and anteriorly to the thyroid cartilage. The larynx is formed by nine cartilages, three paired and three unpaired:

- Cuneiform and corniculate cartilages: Small, paired cartilages that, on direct laryngoscopy, lie posterior to the glottis.
- Arytenoid cartilages: Paired cartilages, pyramidal in shape. Posterior attachment for vocal ligaments (vocal cords).
- Epiglottis: Single cartilage, attached to posterior surface of thyroid cartilage. Acts to cover laryngeal opening during swallowing.
- Thyroid cartilage: "Adam's apple," inferior to hyoid bone. Anterior attachment for vocal ligaments. Posterior surface of thyroid cartilage also acts as attachment for epiglottis.
- Cricoid cartilage: Complete ring of cartilage that forms the inferior border of the larynx. Given its circumferential shape, cricoid pressure may be applied during rapid sequence induction in an attempt to occlude the esophagus, which lies posteriorly to the cricoid cartilage.

Ref: Morton DA, Albertine K, Foreman KB. *Gross Anatomy: The Big Picture.* 1st ed. New York, NY: McGraw Hill; 2011.

7. In follow-up after surgery and anesthesia, a patient notes significant hoarseness. In order to evaluate the patient's vocal cords, a diagnostic fiberoptic examination is performed. If unilateral injury to the recurrent laryngeal nerve has occurred, what will be the position of the affected vocal cord?

(A) fixed in adducted position
(B) fixed in abducted position
(C) fixed in paramedian position
(D) able to adduct, but weak abduction
(E) able to abduct, but weak adduction

A unilateral injury to the recurrent laryngeal nerve will result in unilateral vocal cord paralysis with the cord fixed in a paramedian position. All intrinsic muscles of the larynx are innervated by the vagus nerve (cranial nerve X). It's important to note that only the cricothyroid muscle is innervated by the external branch of superior laryngeal nerve. All other intrinsic muscles of the larynx are innervated by the recurrent laryngeal nerves. The fixed paramedian position results from unopposed action of the cricothyroid muscle which increases the length and tension of the vocal cords.

Refs: Longnecker DE, Brown DL, Newman MF, Zapol WM. *Anesthesiology.* 2nd ed. New York, NY: McGraw Hill; 2012.
Morton DA, Albertine K, Foreman KB. *Gross Anatomy: The Big Picture.* 1st ed. New York, NY: McGraw Hill; 2011.

8. Following an uneventful general anesthetic for uterine myomectomy, a previously well patient is noted to have complete unilateral vocal cord paralysis in the PACU. Which of the following treatment options is most likely required?

(A) emergency reintubation
(B) elective tracheostomy
(C) BiPAP
(D) ENT referral
(E) expectant management

Unilateral vocal cord paralysis is not typically an emergency in healthy patients. Presenting symptoms include significant hoarseness. ENT referral is required for workup and treatment. Bilateral vocal cord paralysis may require emergency treatment as both vocal cords are fixed in the paramedian position. Resulting stridor and respiratory distress may necessitate emergency reintubation or tracheostomy. Bilevel positive airway pressure (BiPAP) is a form of noninvasive pressure support ventilation that may be considered as a temporizing measure for patients with bilateral vocal cord paralysis until more definitive treatment can be instituted.

Ref: Longnecker DE, Brown DL, Newman MF, Zapol WM. *Anesthesiology.* 2nd ed. New York, NY: McGraw Hill; 2012.

9. Compared to an adult larynx, which of the following anatomic features is characteristic of the pediatric larynx?

(A) epiglottis is firm and broad.
(B) larynx is cylindrical in shape.
(C) narrowest portion of larynx is at level of vocal cords.
(D) larynx is in a more superior (rostral) position.
(E) anterior vocal cord attachment slants superiorly (rostral).

Compared to an adult larynx, a pediatric larynx is in a more superior (rostral) position in the neck (C3-C4 level) compared to adults (C4-C5 level). This makes the angle for endotracheal tube insertion into the trachea more acute in infants than in adults. There are multiple differences in airway and laryngeal anatomy between adults and infants.

In general, airway differences include:

- Infants have a relatively larger tongue and larger occiput compared to adults. For this reason, a straight laryngoscope blade may be preferred for infants and a shoulder roll may be required to facilitate visualization of laryngeal structures.

- Infants have a floppy, narrower, omega-shaped epiglottis, which angles over the trachea to a greater degree and covers the glottic opening more than in adults. The adult epiglottis is firm and broad.

- Infants have a funnel-shaped larynx with the narrowest portion at the level of the cricoid cartilage. Adults have a cylindrical-shaped larynx with the narrowest portion at the level of the vocal cords.

- In infants, the anterior attachment of the vocal cords slants inferiorly (caudad) relative to the posterior attachment. Hence, during direct laryngoscopy, they slant "away," and blind passage of an endotracheal tube is more prone to lodging in the anterior commissure. The anterior and posterior attachments of vocal cords in adults are perpendicular to each other.

- Infants have a relatively smaller cricothyroid membrane than adults, which makes identification and performance of a surgical airway impractical.

Ref: Hung O, Murphy MF. *Management of the Difficult and Failed Airway.* 2nd ed. New York, NY: McGraw Hill; 2012.

10. In an emergency "cannot intubate, cannot ventilate" situation, an anesthesia team prepares for a percutaneous surgical airway. In order to secure the airway, which one of the following anatomic sites should be accessed?

(A) suprasternal notch

(B) between the second and third tracheal rings

(C) inferior (caudad) to cricoid cartilage

(D) thyrohyoid membrane

(E) **cricothyroid membrane**

In an emergency "cannot intubate, cannot ventilate" situation, a percutaneous cricothyrotomy can be utilized to secure the airway. This technique accesses the trachea via puncture and dilation of the cricothyroid membrane. The cricothyroid membrane lies between the inferior (caudad) aspect of the thyroid cartilage and the cricoid cartilage. A patient should be positioned with neck extended and other landmarks may be noted including:

- suprasternal notch, located at the base of cervical trachea, at superior border of manubrium between the heads of the clavicles;

- hyoid bone, located between the mandible and thyroid cartilage, and

- thyrohyoid membrane, which connects hyoid bone to thyroid cartilage is located above the level of the vocal cords.

Note, a percutaneous **tracheotomy** is usually performed at the level of the second and third tracheal rings (or one space higher or lower). This technique is usually done in an elective setting (although it may be performed by experienced surgeons in the emergency situation). Anesthesiology teams tend not to have experience with this technique and a percutaneous cricothyrotomy is preferred.

Ref: Hung O, Murphy MF. *Management of the Difficult and Failed Airway.* 2nd ed. New York, NY: McGraw Hill; 2012.

11. At the level of the tracheal bifurcation, or carina, which of the following anatomic relationships is correct?

(A) Right pulmonary artery is directly posterior to the trachea.

(B) Xiphoid process is directly anterior to the trachea.

(C) T9 vertebrae is directly posterior to the trachea.

(D) **Pericardial sac is caudad to the trachea.**

(E) Aortic arch is caudad to the trachea.

At the level of the tracheal bifurcation, or carina, the superior (rostral) aspect of the pericardial sac is caudad to the trachea. This relationship is important when assessing the position of a central venous catheter (CVC). If accessed from the internal jugular vein, the tip of a CVC should be within the superior vena cava and outside the pericardial sac. A CVC within the pericardial sac may lead to cardiac effusion or tamponade. Therefore, on chest X-ray, a correctly positioned CVC should be within the superior vena cava **above** the level of the carina, as this is typically above the level of the pericardium. Other anatomic relationships of the tracheal bifurcation, or carina, include anterior (right pulmonary artery, sternal angle) and posterior (T5 vertebrae, bronchial arteries). The aortic arch wraps over the anterior surface of the left mainstem bronchi and then descends inferiorly (caudad).

Ref: Morton DA, Albertine K, Foreman KB. *Gross Anatomy: The Big Picture.* 1st ed. New York, NY: McGraw Hill; 2011.

12. During active expiration, which of the following muscles is most important?

(A) **rectus abdominis**

(B) trapezius

(C) diaphragm

(D) external intercostal muscles

(E) scalene muscles

During active expiration, the abdominal wall muscles (rectus abdominis, internal and external oblique muscles, transversus abdominis) and the internal intercostal muscles are most important. Note, usually expiration is passive, as the elastic recoil of alveoli allows for emptying. Active expiration takes places during coughing, speaking, or exercise. The diaphragm, external intercostals, scalene, and parasternal intercostal muscles are the main muscles of inspiration. (Other accessory muscles are involved in more active inspiration.)

Ref: Levitzky MG. *Pulmonary Physiology.* 8th ed. New York, NY: McGraw Hill; 2013.

13. Which of the following muscles is considered an accessory muscle of inspiration?

(A) diaphragm

(B) external intercostal

(C) internal intercostal

(D) rectus abdominis

(E) **sternocleidomastoid**

The accessory muscles of inspiration include the sternocleidomastoid, trapezius, and muscles of the vertebral column. They are not active during quiet inspiration but become more important for active inspiration during activities such as exercise or during an asthma exacerbation. Quiet inspiration relies on the diaphragm, external intercostals, scalene, and parasternal intercostal muscles. Expiration is usually passive; although during active expiration, the abdominal muscles (including rectus abdominis) and internal intercostal muscles become more important.

Ref: Levitzky MG. *Pulmonary Physiology.* 8th ed. New York, NY: McGraw Hill; 2013.

14. The sum of the expiratory reserve volume (ERV) plus the tidal volume (V_T) plus the inspiratory reserve volume (IRV) equals which of the following?

(A) inspiratory capacity

(B) total lung capacity

(C) functional residual capacity

(D) **vital capacity**

(E) closing capacity

The lungs can be thought of as being made up of four "static" lung volumes, which cannot be further divided (Figure 3-2). The tidal volume (V_T) is the volume exchanged during normal, quiet breathing. *Expiratory reserve volume* (ERV) is the volume of gas expelled from the lungs if a subject is asked to exhale as much as he/she can when starting from resting volume. The volume left

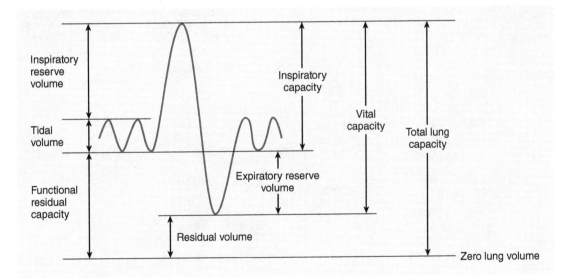

FIG. 3-2. Spirogram showing static lung volumes. (Reproduced with permission from Nunn JF. *Nunn's Applied Physiology,* 4th edition. Butterworth, 2000.)

over in the lungs after maximal exhalation is termed *residual volume* (RV). Finally, the maximum possible volume inhaled starting at the end of normal tidal inspiration is the *inspiratory reserve volume* (IRV).

A capacity is formed by the combination of two or more static lung volumes. For example, the FRC is formed by the combination of RV and ERV. Vital capacity (VC) is ERV plus V_T plus IRV. Total lung capacity (TLC) is the sum of all four static lung volumes.

Ref: Butterworth JF IV, Mackey DC, Wasnick JD. *Morgan and Mikhail's Clinical Anesthesiology*. 5th ed. New York, NY: McGraw Hill; 2013.

15. Which of the following BEST approximates the functional residual capacity (FRC) for a healthy, 70-kg adult?

    (A) 1200 mL
    (B) 1600 mL
    (C) 2400 mL
    (D) 3200 mL
    (E) 4000 mL

The average total lung capacity for a 70-kg adult is approximately 5600 mL, of which about 2100 to 2400 mL is FRC (Figure 3-3).

Ref: Barrett KE, Boitano S, Barman SM, Brooks HL. *Ganong's Review of Medical Physiology*. 24th ed. New York, NY: McGraw Hill; 2012.

16. Which of the following factors does NOT influence the functional residual capacity (FRC)?

    (A) advanced age
    (B) body habitus
    (C) sex
    (D) posture
    (E) restrictive pulmonary disease

Body morphology has an impact on the FRC. It is decreased in obesity and increases proportionally with height. Females have a slightly (10%) decreased FRC compared to males. FRC decreases when changing from an upright to supine or prone position. This is primarily due the pressure of the abdominal contents against the diaphragm resulting in decreased chest compliance. Restrictive lung or chest wall disease also decreases the compliance and results in a diminished FRC. In contrast, FRC is largely independent of age and is a constant 30 mL/kg in both children and adults of all ages.

Ref: Butterworth JF IV, Mackey DC, Wasnick JD. *Morgan and Mikhail's Clinical Anesthesiology*. 5th ed. New York, NY: McGraw Hill; 2013.

17. Which of the following is a dynamic lung volume?

    (A) slow vital capacity
    (B) forced expiratory volume in 1 second
    (C) inspiratory capacity
    (D) functional residual capacity
    (E) closing volume

The dynamic lung volumes are those which are dependent on flow (i.e., have a time limitation) and include forced vital capacity and forced expiratory volume in 1 second (or 0.5, 3, 6 seconds, etc.). Static spirometric measures reflect dimensional volumes and are independent of flow. They are therefore not limited by time and include slow vital capacity, inspiratory capacity, tidal volume, expiratory reserve volume, functional reserve volume, and closing volume.

Ref: Butterworth JF IV, Mackey DC, Wasnick JD. *Morgan and Mikhail's Clinical Anesthesiology*. 5th ed. New York, NY: McGraw Hill; 2013.

Inspiratory reserve volume (40–45 mL/kg)	Inspiratory capacity (50 mL/kg)	Vital capacity (65 mL/kg)	Total lung capacity (80 mL/kg)
Tidal volume (7 mL/kg)			
Expiratory reserve volume (15 mL/kg)	Functional residual capacity (30 mL/kg)		
Residual volume (15–20 mL/kg)			

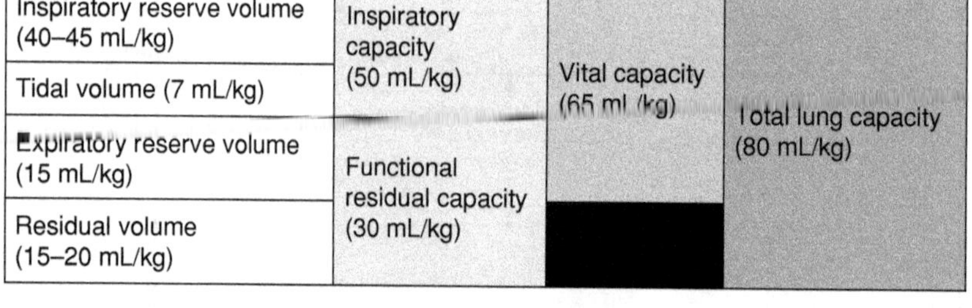

FIG. 3-3. Approximate lung volumes and capacities for a healthy adult.

18. A patient presents to preoperative clinic with a 50 pack-year smoking history and severe chronic obstructive pulmonary disease. Which of the following parameters is best measured using spirometry?

(A) forced vital capacity

(B) total lung capacity

(C) residual lung volume

(D) closing capacity

(E) functional residual capacity

Spirometry, where the patient blows forcefully or slowly (depending on the test) through a mouthpiece attached to a flow meter, is useful for calculating the static lung volumes such as inspiratory and expiratory reserve volume, and slow vital capacity. It is also very useful to quantify the dynamic lung volumes such as forced vital capacity and FEV_1. Spirometry cannot be used to estimate residual volume or any capacity that relies on the quantification of it, such as FRC or TLC.

Ref: Butterworth JF IV, Mackey DC, Wasnick JD. *Morgan and Mikhail's Clinical Anesthesiology.* 5th ed. New York, NY: McGraw Hill; 2013.

19. Which of the following best describes the concept of physiologic dead space?

(A) alveoli that are not perfused

(B) alveoli and nonrespiratory airways that are not perfused

(C) alveoli that are perfused but are not ventilated

(D) trachea and non-respiratory airways

(E) pharynx, endotracheal tube, and y-piece of the circuit

Dead space is defined as the part of the tidal volume that does not participate in gas exchange. The ratio of tidal volume that is wasted to dead space (VD/V_T) is approximately 33% in an average adult breathing spontaneously. This includes those alveoli that are ventilated but not perfused (termed alveolar dead space), and parts of the pharynx and tracheobronchial tree that do not participate in gas exchange (anatomic dead space). The sum of these two dead spaces together is termed physiologic dead space. Apparatus dead space is the set of ventilatory equipment that receives a portion of the tidal volume; this includes the endotracheal tube, extraglottic airway, facemask, and any additional tubing (e.g., accordion tubing, heat/moisture exchangers) that are inserted into the breathing system on the *patient* side of the y-piece. Any gas on the *machine* side of the y-piece of the circle circuit is not considered dead space because the presence of one-way valves in each limb ensure that gas only travels in one direction around the circle.

Dead space is approximately 2 mL/kg and can be calculated using the Bohr equation:

$$VD/V_T = (P_ACO_2 - P_ECO_2)/P_ACO_2$$

Where P_ACO_2 is the alveolar carbon dioxide tension and P_ECO_2 is the mixed (not end tidal) expired gas tension of carbon dioxide.

Ref: Butterworth JF IV, Mackey DC, Wasnick JD. *Morgan and Mikhail's Clinical Anesthesiology.* 5th ed. New York, NY: McGraw Hill; 2013.

20. Which of the following factors DECREASES dead space?

(A) upright position

(B) neck extension

(C) endotracheal tube

(D) emphysema

(E) age

Multiple factors affect dead space (Table 3-2). Compared to the volume of the airway and proximal trachea that normally contributes to the 2 mL/kg of VD/V_T, the volume that gas within an endotracheal tube displaces is less.

TABLE 3-2. **Factors affecting dead space.**

Factor	Effect
Posture	
Upright	↑
Supine	↓
Position of airway	
Neck extension	↑
Neck flexion	↓
Age	↑
Artificial airway	↓
Positive-pressure ventilation	↑
Drugs—anticholinergic	↑
Pulmonary perfusion	
Pulmonary emboli	↑
Hypotension	↑
Pulmonary vascular disease	
Emphysema	↑

From: Butterworth JF IV, Mackey DC, Wasnick JD. *Morgan and Mikhail's Clinical Anesthesiology.* 5th ed. New York, NY: McGraw Hill; 2013.

Ref: Butterworth JF IV, Mackey DC, Wasnick JD. *Morgan and Mikhail's Clinical Anesthesiology.* 5th ed. New York, NY: McGraw Hill; 2013.

21. At what lung volume is pulmonary vascular resistance the lowest?

(A) residual volume

(B) closing volume

(C) expiratory reserve volume

(D) functional residual capacity

(E) total lung capacity

The pulmonary vasculature has two sets of vessels that can be considered to influence the overall pulmonary vascular resistance (PVR). As the lung increases in volume from FRC, the alveoli expand, and with them the small capillaries that surround the alveoli. This traction on the capillaries stretches these tiny vessels so that the luminal diameter is diminished, increasing resistance to flow, and elevating PVR. On the other hand, as lung volumes shrink, the larger extra-alveolar arterioles and venules are exposed to increased transmural pressure due to the elevation in intrathoracic pressure, and the lumens of these become both compressed and kinked, increasing resistance. As such, the "sweet spot" for PVR is right at FRC, with changes in lung volume on either side leading to increases in resistance (Figure 3-4).

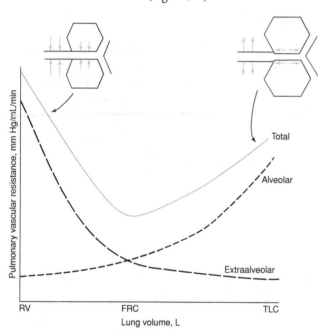

FIG. 3-4. The effects of lung volume on pulmonary vascular resistance (PVR). PVR is lowest near the functional residual capacity (FRC) and increases at both high and low lung volumes because of the combined effects on the alveolar and extraalveolar vessels. To achieve low lung volumes, one must generate positive intrapleural pressures so that the extraalveolar vessels are compressed, as seen at left in the figure. RV = residual volume; TLC = total lung capacity. (Reprinted from Graph after Murray *The Normal Lung*, 1st and 2nd editions (1976, 1986).)

Ref: Levitzky MG. *Pulmonary Physiology.* 8th ed. New York, NY: McGraw Hill; 2013.

Use the following clinical scenario to answer questions 22 and 23:

A 57-year-old male, weighing 70 kg is scheduled for esophagectomy after a recent diagnosis of carcinoma of the esophagus. He has mild hypertension but is otherwise generally fit. As part of his preoperative workup, he is undergoing cardiopulmonary exercise testing (CPET). At baseline, his VO_2 is measured at 4 mL/kg/min, cardiac output is 5.6 L/min, and his arterial oxygen content is 200 mL/L.

22. What is his mixed venous oxygen content?

(A) 50 mL/L

(B) 100 mL/L

(C) **150 mL/L**

(D) 250 mL/L

(E) 300 mL/L

The relationship between cardiac output and oxygen consumption is described by the Fick equation, which states that:

$$VO_2 = CO \times (CaO_2 - CvO_2)$$

Where VO_2 is oxygen consumption, CO is cardiac output, CaO_2 is arterial oxygen content and CvO_2 is mixed venous oxygen content. Filling in the Fick equation with the numbers above, we get:

$$4\ mL/kg/min \times 70\ kg = 5.6\ L/min \times (200\ mL/min - CvO_2)$$

Rearranging, we get:

$$280\ mL/min/5.6\ L/min = 200\ mL/min - CvO_2$$
$$50 + CvO_2 = 200\ mL/min$$
$$CvO_2 = 150\ mL/min$$

Ref: Longnecker DE, Brown DL, Newman MF, Zapol WM. *Anesthesiology.* 2nd ed. New York, NY: McGraw Hill; 2012.

23. Which of the following factors measured using CPET is the best predictor of postoperative cardiopulmonary complication rate?

(A) **anaerobic threshold**

(B) minute ventilation

(C) EKG ST analysis

(D) VCO_2

(E) stroke volume

CPET is used increasingly as a means to quantify the combined pulmonary, cardiac and circulatory system. It is safe, reliable, objective, and noninvasive. Subjects are exercised on a stationary cycle, and physiologic parameters including continuous EKG, blood pressure, and SpO_2 are monitored. The subject breathes through a mouthpiece or a tight-fitting mask, and gases can be measured for quantification of VO$_2$ and VCO$_2$, respiratory exchange ratio (ratio of molecules of O$_2$ breathed in versus molecules of CO$_2$ breathed out), oxygen pulse (VO$_2$/HR, an approximation of stroke volume) and anaerobic threshold. This last value can be used to note at which point in the VO$_2$ curve the oxygen demand begins to exceed supply, and muscle cells begin to respire anaerobically. The anaerobic threshold is usually achieved about halfway through the test, well before VO$_2$ max is reached and the test is terminated; for this reason, it is felt to be independent of motivation and therefore a reliable marker of functional capacity.

Indeed, it appears that anaerobic threshold is a valid predictor of postoperative outcome, with a value of 11 mL/kg/min required to safely undergo significant surgery in several studies. Ever noticed how nearly every patient preop note contains a phrase to the effect of, "exercise tolerance >4 mets"? One MET (or "metabolic equivalent" on the Duke Activity Status Index) is the oxygen consumption of an adult at rest, or approximately 3.5 mL/kg/min. Four METs is therefore about 13 to 14 mL/kg/min, which is roughly the same as the anaerobic threshold validated in the CPET studies.

Ref: Agnew N. Preoperative cardiopulmonary exercise testing. *CEACCP.* 2010;10:33–37.

24. A spontaneously-breathing patient inhales 600 mL of air. During this time, the intrapleural pressure decreases from −4 cm H$_2$O to −9 cm H$_2$O. The compliance of this patient's respiratory system under these conditions is:

(A)   60 mL·cm H$_2$O^{-1}
(B)   90 mL·cm H$_2$O^{-1}
(C)   100 mL·cm H$_2$O^{-1}
(D)   **120 mL·cm H$_2$O^{-1}**
(E)   150 mL·cm H$_2$O^{-1}

Compliance is defined as the change in lung volume per unit change in airway pressure ($\Delta V/\Delta P$), and is a measure of the distensibility of the lungs. Compliance can also be thought of as the slope of the pressure-volume curve (Figure 3-5). The lungs and the chest wall each have a distinct compliance curve, and the sum of the two provides the overall compliance of the respiratory system. At FRC, the inward recoil of

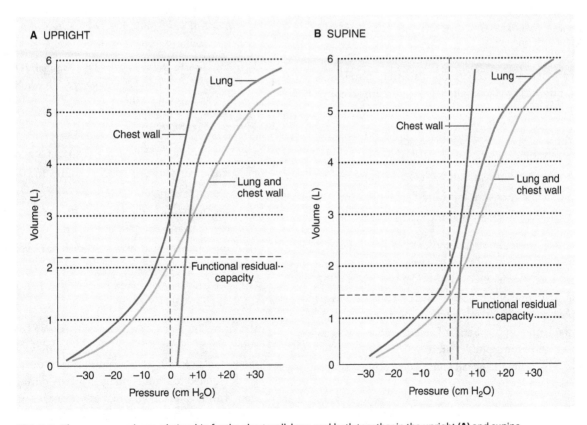

FIG. 3-5. The pressure–volume relationship for the chest wall, lung, and both together in the upright **(A)** and supine **(B)** positions. (Modified and reproduced with permission from Scurr C, Feldman S. *Scientific Foundations of Anesthesia*, 2nd edition. Butterworth-Heinemann, 1982.)

the lungs is balanced by the outward recoil of the chest wall, and there is no net transmural pressure. Compliance is highest around FRC (i.e., the slope is steepest), whereas at very low and very high lung volumes, additional changes in pressure result in minimal changes in volume (i.e. compliance is low). Normal compliance at FRC is approximately 0.2 L/cm H_2O in a healthy adult male.

Compliance is reduced in pulmonary fibrosis, pulmonary edema, decreased surfactant levels as in prematurity and when guys puff their chest out for the benefit of females while walking around on the beach. Compliance is increased in the course of normal aging, and also when elasticity of the lungs is reduced (e.g., emphysema).

In the above example, the change in pressure is 5 cm H_2O (the intrapleural pressure, which is normally negative, became 5 cm H_2O **more** negative with inspiration), divided into 600 mL gives 120 mL·cm H_2O^{-1}. Normal adult pulmonary compliance is approximately 100 to 200 mL·cm H_2O^{-1}.

Refs: Butterworth JF IV, Mackey DC, Wasnick JD. *Morgan and Mikhail's Clinical Anesthesiology.* 5th ed. New York, NY: McGraw Hill; 2013.

Barrett KE, Boitano S, Barman SM, Brooks HL. *Ganong's Review of Medical Physiology.* 24th ed. New York, NY: McGraw Hill; 2012.

25. The parameters necessary to calculate transmural pressure for thoracic wall compliance (i.e., not lung compliance) are:

(A) **atmospheric pressure and intrapleural pressure**
(B) atmospheric pressure and alveolar pressure
(C) intrapleural pressure and alveolar pressure
(D) interstitial pressure and intrapleural pressure
(E) pericardial pressure and intrapleural pressure

For any given lung volume, there are three distinct compliance curves and three corresponding transmural pressure gradients used to calculate them. The transmural pressure gradient used to calculate lung compliance is alveolar-intrapleural; for thoracic wall, it is intrapleural-atmospheric. The difference between alveolar and atmospheric pressures is the gradient required to calculate overall compliance of the respiratory system.

Ref: Butterworth JF IV, Mackey DC, Wasnick JD. *Morgan and Mikhail's Clinical Anesthesiology.* 5th ed. New York, NY: McGraw Hill; 2013.

26. A patient is being ventilated in the critical care unit. The change in lung volume observed for a given peak inspiratory pressure BEST describes which of the following concepts?

(A) static lung compliance
(B) inspiratory lung compliance
(C) **dynamic lung compliance**
(D) maximal lung compliance
(E) effort-independent lung compliance

Pulmonary compliance is measured in two different ways. The static lung compliance is defined as compliance in the absence of gas flow. In a patient receiving positive pressure ventilation, the static compliance can be calculated by creating an inspiratory pause of 1 to 2 seconds at a known lung volume, and measuring the resulting *plateau* pressure. In contrast, dynamic compliance is the distensibility of the respiratory system during inspiratory and expiratory tidal ventilation. The *peak* inspiratory pressure (PIP) is used to calculate the dynamic compliance using the following equation:

$$C_{dynamic} = \text{tidal volume}/(PIP - PEEP)$$

As a memory aid, imagine you're climbing a mountain. If your leg muscles become **static**, you pause and reach a **plateau**; if your body becomes a **dynamic** piece of athletic machinery, you'll reach the **peak**.

Ref: Butterworth JF IV, Mackey DC, Wasnick JD. *Morgan and Mikhail's Clinical Anesthesiology.* 5th ed. New York, NY: McGraw Hill; 2013.

27. Hysteresis refers to:

(A) the tendency of alveoli to collapse at low volumes.
(B) **differing pressure-volume curves for inflation and deflation of the lungs.**
(C) the pleural pressure gradient that exists between the apex and the base of the lung.
(D) the decrease in airway resistance observed as air moves down the respiratory tree.
(E) the freak-out observed in the OR when a patient starts to quickly desaturate.

If a set of lungs are inflated and deflated slowly, the pressure-volume curves will not be identical for the two phases (Figure 3-6). This is largely due to the additional work required to recruit and open alveoli during inspiration. This phenomenon, which is present in most elastic structures, is termed elastic hysteresis. The practical result is that, for any given pressure, lung volume during inhalation will be less than the lung volume during exhalation.

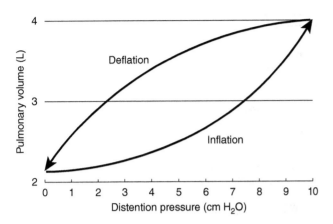

FIG. 3-6. Hysteresis during lung inflation and deflation.

Ref: Levitzky MG. *Pulmonary Physiology.* 8th ed. New York, NY: McGraw Hill; 2013.

28. Which of the following best explains why alveoli do not collapse when lung volumes become small?

   (A) Surfactant increases the surface tension as spherical volume decreases.

   (B) Surfactant decreases the surface tension as spherical volume decreases.

   (C) Air trapping pneumatically stents open the alveoli.

   (D) Chest wall recoil prevents complete collapse.

   (E) Intrapleural pressure is maintained at −10 cm H$_2$O at the base.

The alveoli are lined with a layer of fluid, which results in an air-fluid interface. This interface creates surface tension forces that tends to reduce the volume of the alveolus. The pressure inside the alveolus can be calculated using LaPlace's Law:

$$P = 2T/R$$

where P = pressure within the alveolus, T = surface tension of the liquid, and R = the radius of the alveolus. As the radius decreases, the molecules of the surface film become closer together (and have a stronger mutual attraction), increasing the pressure within the alveolus. On the other hand, if the radius increases, the molecules move apart, and the pressure within the alveolus decreases.

If we imagine two interconnected alveoli (Figure 3-7) and assume equal surface tension, the increased pressure in the smaller alveolus will tend to create flow into the larger alveolus, eventually collapsing the smaller one. However, the presence of pulmonary surfactant, a phospholipid secreted by type II alveolar cells, serves to reduce the surface tension *in proportion to the concentration at the air-fluid interface* by acting as a detergent. During expiration, the alveolar volume decreases and surfactant molecules are packed more tightly on the alveolar film surface, exerting a greater reduction in surface tension.

Ref: Levitzky MG. *Pulmonary Physiology.* 8th ed. New York, NY: McGraw Hill; 2013.

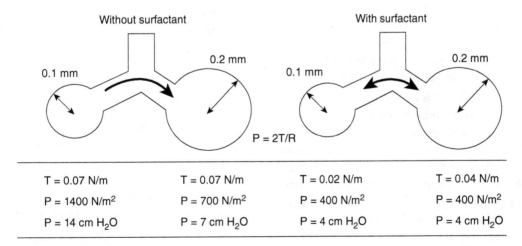

FIG. 3-7. The effect of pulmonary surfactant on surface tension and gas flow between two interdependent alveoli of different sizes.

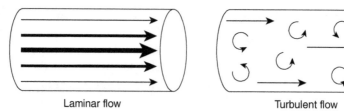

FIG. 3-8. Laminar and turbulent flow within tubes.

29. A child experiences bronchospasm shortly after induction of general anesthesia. A decrease in the radius of her mid- to large-caliber airways by 50% will be likely to produce an increase in airway resistance of:

(A)   2 times baseline

(B)   4 times baseline

(C)   8 times baseline

(D)   16 times baseline

(E)   **32 times baseline**

The flow of gas within the pulmonary system is dependent of several factors. It is important to realize that there are two distinct flow patterns. Laminar flow describes an ordered pattern where all the molecules are moving in layers (or "laminae") of straight lines down the tube. Flow rates in laminar flow are fastest in the center, and slowest at the periphery (Figure 3-8). In the pulmonary system, laminar flow occurs primarily in small (<1 mm) airways. Turbulent flow, a disorganized movement associated with the presence of eddy currents within the lumen, is present in large and medium airways, at branching points, points of obstruction, and when the lumen diameter abruptly decreases. These eddy currents interfere with forward movement of molecules and increase the energy input required to achieve a given flow rate.

In laminar flow, resistance is calculated by:

$$\text{Resistance} = (8 \times \text{length} \times \text{viscosity})/(\pi \times \text{radius}^4)$$

The radius of the lumen is clearly the most important factor in this equation because it affects the resistance inversely by the fourth power; in other words, a halving of the radius will increase the resistance by a factor of 16 during laminar flow. In contrast, resistance during turbulent flow depends on the gas flow rate, increasing proportionally as flow rate increases. Additionally, the resistance during turbulent flow is inversely proportional to the radius to the *fifth* power (or 32 times), as described below:

$$\text{Pressure gradient} \approx \text{flow}^2 \times (\text{density}/\text{radius}^5)$$

As such, during turbulent flow, resistance is exquisitely dependent on airway caliber.

Ref: Levitzky MG. *Pulmonary Physiology.* 8th ed. New York, NY: McGraw Hill; 2013.

30. Which of the following descriptions best matches the flow-volume loop shown below in Figure 3-9?

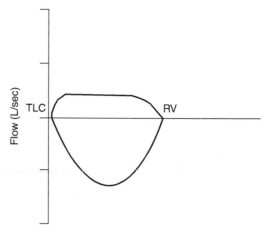

FIG. 3-9. A flow-volume loop.

(A)   extrathoracic variable obstruction

(B)   **intrathoracic variable obstruction**

(C)   fixed obstruction

(D)   chronic obstructive pulmonary disease

(E)   restrictive pulmonary disease

While there are various spirometric tests that pulmonary labs can perform, the flow-volume loop is often a useful one to characterize overall patterns of airflow resistance. Volume is charted on the x-axis and flow on the y-axis. The test is commenced at residual volume (RV) and the patient is instructed to take a forced vital capacity breath. By convention, this flow is assigned a negative value, and a normal inspiratory curve appears as a bowl or semi-circular shape. At total lung capacity (TLC), the patient immediately expires forcefully back to RV, and flow is represented as a positive value. Normally, flow is high at the beginning of expiration but diminishes near the end (linearly) due to reduced lung volumes.

There are several characteristic patterns of flow-volume loops that can aid in the diagnosis of obstructive or

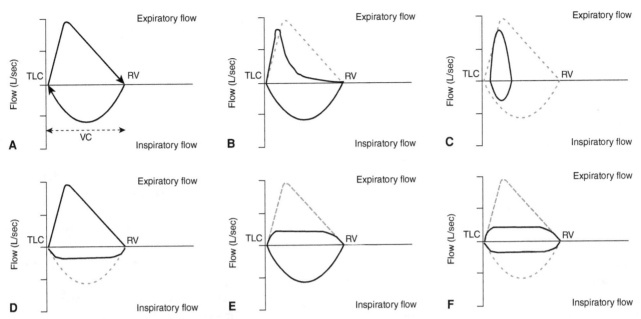

FIG. 3-10. Flow-volume loops. **A.** Normal. **B.** Small airways disease (e.g., COPD). **C.** Restrictive lung disease. **D.** Variable extrathoracic obstruction. **E.** Variable intrathoracic obstruction. **F.** Fixed airway obstruction.

restrictive conditions (Figure 3-10). Small airways obstruction, as seen in chronic obstructive airways disease, is typically characterized by a "scooped-out" pattern in the latter half of the expiratory curve, caused by delayed emptying. Flow-volume loops in restrictive lung disease (e.g., pulmonary fibrosis) have decreased overall volumes and flows, but the shape is more or less preserved.

Dynamic obstruction can occur in the airways either inside or outside the thoracic cage. This differs from fixed obstruction in that the obstruction is somewhat mobile and limitations to airflow will change depending on the phase of respiration. Extrathoracic variable obstruction (e.g., a mass just below the glottis) is one in which negative pressure in the extrathoracic trachea during inspiration as airflow increases in speed past the narrowed lumen (the Bernoulli principle) causes a pulling together of the tracheal walls, thereby reducing flow during this phase. During expiration, the positive pressure pushes open the extrathoracic airway, allowing for normal flow patterns again. Conversely, with an intrathoracic variable obstruction, the negative transmural pressure during inspiration "pulls open" the airway, keeping flow normal during this phase; during expiration (especially forced expiration), the more positive intrathoracic pressure tends to further worsen the obstruction. These dynamic changes can be seen as flattening of the respective portions of the flow-volume loops.

A fixed obstruction, one that does not change position in phase of respiration (e.g., tracheal stenosis), will produce airflow limitation in both phases of respiration and a flattening of both portions of the curve.

Ref: Butterworth JF IV, Mackey DC, Wasnick JD. *Morgan and Mikhail's Clinical Anesthesiology.* 5th ed. New York, NY: McGraw Hill; 2013.

31. Total lung capacity (TLC) may be measured by all of the following methods EXCEPT:

(A) helium dilution

(B) nitrogen washout

(C) spirometry

(D) body plethysmography

(E) chest radiograph measurements

The gold standard for measuring TLC is body plethysmography. This device, also called a "body-box," is a phone booth–type instrument that is capable of measuring the volume and pressure of air surrounding a subject who is sealed within and breathing through a mouthpiece. Boyle's law is used to determine the relationship between pressure and volume at FRC, TLC, and RV. In the helium dilution method, a known *amount* of helium (which is not absorbed by the alveolar capillaries), is inhaled and diluted by the gas already present in the lungs. The exhaled *concentration* is then used to calculate FRC and TLC. The nitrogen washout method is somewhat similar, during which a subject breathes 100% oxygen and expired gas collected via a one-way valve. The nitrogen concentration is measured until it reaches zero, at which point the total volume of gas expired is determined, along with the total mixed nitrogen concentration. Assuming 79% of the initial lung volume was nitrogen, the lung volume can then be calculated by cross-multiplying. Chest X-rays can be used to estimate TLC within with a 10% to 15% margin of error. Spirometry, which can be used to measure tidal volume, inspiratory volume and expiratory volume, cannot be used to calculate or measure RV, FRC or TLC because it cannot measure the gas left in the lungs at maximal exhalation (RV), a component of all of those capacities.

Ref: Levitzky MG. *Pulmonary Physiology.* 8th ed. New York, NY: McGraw Hill; 2013.

32. At what age will a healthy individual experience some closure of their small airways in the supine position?

   (A) 20 years of age
   (B) **40 years of age**
   (C) 50 years of age
   (D) 60 years of age
   (E) 80 years of age

As air is exhaled from end inspiration, a point is reached where the positive pleural pressure causes dynamic collapse of the very small airways in the most dependent portions of the lung. This volume is termed the closing volume. Note that technically speaking, the closing **capacity** is the total volume remaining in the lungs at this collapse point and is estimated by closing volume plus residual volume; closing volume is closing

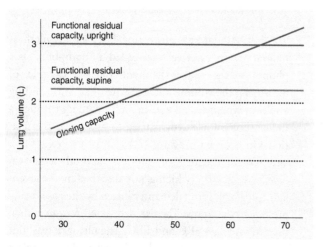

FIG. 3-11. Closing volume. (Reproduced with permission from Nunn JF. *Nunn's Applied Physiology,* 4th edition. Butterworth, 2000.)

capacity minus residual volume. These terms are sometimes used interchangeably, although they technically are distinct.

Closing volume increases with age, as the elastic recoil of the lung decreases and there is less radial tension keeping airways open as the volumes decrease (Figure 3-11). In childhood and early adulthood, closing volume is below functional residual capacity (FRC). However, closing volume equals FRC while in the supine position at approximately 40 years of age, and in the seated position at approximately 60 years of age. The implication here is that, at the end of every breath, some alveoli are collapsed, leading to small areas of shunt and decreased arterial oxygen tension. The reduced FRC seen during anesthesia in the spontaneously breathing patient leads to an earlier reduction in FRC below closing volume, so that otherwise unaffected younger patients may experience V/Q mismatch.

Ref: Butterworth JF IV, Mackey DC, Wasnick JD. *Morgan and Mikhail's Clinical Anesthesiology.* 5th ed. New York, NY: McGraw Hill; 2013.

33. A 24-year-old woman is experiencing an acute asthma exacerbation. What alteration in her respiratory mechanics will decrease the work of breathing?

   (A) recruitment of additional muscles of respiration
   (B) taking shallow breaths near total lung capacity
   (C) breath holding
   (D) increasing her respiratory rate
   (E) **decreasing her respiratory rate**

There are two principal components to the work of breathing: That related to overcoming elastic recoil of the chest wall and pulmonary parenchyma as well as the surface tension of the alveoli, and that related to airflow resistance. These are additive and the summed total gives the overall work of breathing. Normally, the work of breathing is low and represents 3% to 5% of total VO_2.

The effect of elastic recoil and airway resistance are respiratory rate dependent (Figure 3-12). Under normal circumstances, the balance between these two resistances results in a nadir of the total work of breathing curve at about 12 to 15 breaths per minute. As the elastic resistance curve increases (as in restrictive lung disease), it becomes more difficult to take deep breaths without substantially increasing work. To maintain minute ventilation with minimal work, the respiratory rate increases. The reverse occurs with an isolated increase in airway resistance, where slower breathing is easiest. This

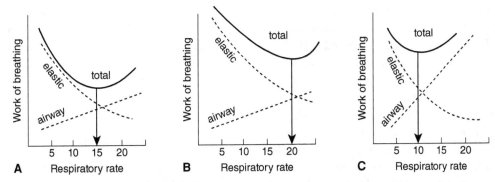

FIG. 3-12. Work of breathing related to respiratory rate for **(A)** normal circumstances; **(B)** increased elastic resistance (e.g., restrictive lung disease); and **(C)** increased airway resistance (e.g., asthma, COPD).

is because a slower rate allows for more complete exhalation to FRC with minimal breath stacking or dynamic compression of the airways.

Ref: Levitzky MG. *Pulmonary Physiology.* 8th ed. New York, NY: McGraw Hill; 2013.

34. During quiet breathing, the portion of the respiratory system that offers the greatest resistance to airflow is the:

    (A) mouth
    (B) trachea
    (C) large bronchi
    (D) mid-sized bronchi
    (E) small bronchi

Resistance is highest in the individual lumen with the smallest radius. For this reason, it may be concluded that the small bronchi in the terminal portion of the conducting airways offer the greatest resistance to airflow. However, because these small bronchi are so numerous and are arranged in parallel, the total cross-sectional area is very large. Accordingly, the combined resistance is very low in these small airways. It is the mid-sized airways where the highest resistance occurs during normal breathing.

Ref: Levitzky MG. *Pulmonary Physiology.* 8th ed. New York, NY: McGraw Hill; 2013.

35. Which of the following acts to constrict the bronchial smooth muscle?

    (A) parasympathetic stimulation
    (B) beta-2 (β2) agonists
    (C) nitric oxide
    (D) local hypercarbia
    (E) local hypoxemia

Increased cholinergic parasympathetic activity via the vagus nerve results in constriction of the smooth muscle in the bronchial wall as well as increased production of mucus by respiratory epithelial goblet cells. Other substances that provoke bronchoconstriction include systemic acetylcholine, histamine, leukotrienes, serotonin, alpha-adrenergic agonists, and direct exposure to noxious agents such as smoke, dust, or other irritants.

In contrast, bronchodilation is mediated primarily by the stimulation of beta-2 (β2) receptors located widely throughout the bronchial muscle. This usually occurs following an increase in circulating catecholamines through activation of the sympathetic system, or by direct activation by sympathetic fibers. Nitric oxide is commonly used as a pulmonary vasodilator but also acts on the bronchial smooth muscle to dilate it as well. Any process produces hypercarbia or hypoxemia in the small airways will also result in bronchodilation.

Ref: Levitzky MG. *Pulmonary Physiology.* 8th ed. New York, NY: McGraw Hill; 2013.

36. Which of the following is NOT an example of V/Q mismatch leading to pulmonary shunt?

    (A) mucus plugging of a lobar bronchus
    (B) pulmonary thromboembolism
    (C) a bronchial blocker placed in the left mainstem bronchus
    (D) atelectasis
    (E) pneumonia

Ideally, ventilation and perfusion (V and Q) are matched so that parts of the lung receiving the greatest proportion of gas during a breath also enjoy the most perfusion. In normal healthy lungs, this is generally true, but V and Q are never 100% matched due to regional differences in both ventilation and perfusion. There are some circumstances or disease processes where substantial V/Q mismatch occurs. Shunt refers to a situation where there is perfusion but no ventilation. This may occur in instances where larger airways are blocked by mucus, the use of lung separation such as double-lumen tubes and bronchial blockers, or in alveolar processes such as pneumonia, atelectasis, pulmonary hemorrhage or severe pulmonary edema. The degree of shunting as a proportion of total cardiac output is termed the shunt fraction (Q_s/Q_t). This can be calculated by:

$$Q_s/Q_t = (C_{CO2} - C_AO_2)/(C_{CO2} - C_VO_2),$$

where Q_s = amount of shunted cardiac output; Q_t = total cardiac output; C_{CO2} = end-capillary O_2 content; C_AO_2 = arterial O_2 content; C_VO_2 = mixed venous O_2 content.

Shunt can occur via nonpulmonary causes such as intracardiac shunts (e.g., Thebesian veins) and that portion of bronchial circulation that empties into the pulmonary veins rather than bronchial veins. This fraction of deoxygenated blood that enters the left heart is relatively fixed, and is largely responsible for the normal shunt fraction of <5%. The increased shunt fraction (and subsequent reduction in arterial oxygen tension)

observed in pulmonary processes is never truly as bad as it seems—this is due to hypoxic pulmonary vasoconstriction which diverts flow away from poorly ventilated areas and improves V/Q matching (discussed further in question 41).

Ref: Butterworth JF IV, Mackey DC, Wasnick JD. *Morgan and Mikhail's Clinical Anesthesiology.* 5th ed. New York, NY: McGraw Hill; 2013.

37. During normal tidal inspiration, what percentage of ventilation will dependent (lowermost) alveoli receive compared to alveoli in the non-dependent (i.e., uppermost aspect) of the lung?

   (A) no ventilation
   (B) 50%
   (C) 100%
   (D) 150%
   (E) 500%

Alveolar ventilation is not uniform throughout the lungs. This is primarily because of gravitational effects on the lung tissue and the resulting compression of dependent alveoli (Figure 3-13). Alveoli in the uppermost aspect of the lung are exposed to a more negative intrapleural pressure and are therefore larger at FRC. Imagine the lungs as two soaking wet sponges set on a table. The weight of the sponge will tend to compress

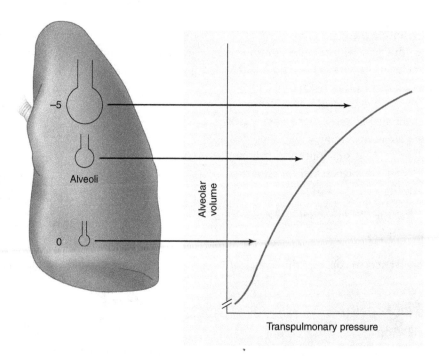

FIG. 3-13. The effect of gravity on alveolar compliance in the upright position. (Reproduced with permission from Butterworth JF IV, Mackey DC, Wasnick JD. *Morgan and Mikhail's Clinical Anesthesiology.* 5th ed. New York, NY: McGraw Hill; 2013.)

the bottom section, whereas the top of the sponge is fully expanded; an imperfect analogy technically speaking, but you get the picture. The volume and transpulmonary (alveolar; pleural) pressure both start small near the dependent aspect and increase toward the uppermost areas. The curve is steep at first but flattens out near the top. The shape of this compliance curve explains the distribution of ventilation: as the breath is initiated, the steepest (i.e., most compliant) portion is the most dependent alveoli, and they draw in gas first. The uppermost alveoli that are already almost fully filled do not receive ventilation until the end of inspiration, if at all. During normal tidal breathing, the ratio of basal to apical ventilation is 1.5 to 1.

Note that the terms lowermost and uppermost are used here, not base and apex. This is because this relationship is preserved no matter what the patient position, although the amount of difference in pleural pressure between the top and bottom will be less when a patient is supine or prone than when he/she is upright.

Ref: Butterworth JF IV, Mackey DC, Wasnick JD. *Morgan and Mikhail's Clinical Anesthesiology.* 5th ed. New York, NY: McGraw Hill; 2013.

38. According to the zone theory of lung perfusion as described by West, alveoli in zone 3 are characterized by:

(A) alveolar pressure > pulmonary arterial pressure

(B) alveolar pressure > pulmonary venous pressure

(C) **pulmonary arterial pressure > alveolar pressure**

(D) pulmonary venous pressure = alveolar pressure

(E) pulmonary venous pressure > pulmonary arterial pressure

The relationship between pulmonary ventilation and perfusion has been simplified by West such that the lung can be considered to be composed of four zones (Figure 3-14). The relationships between pulmonary arterial and venous pressures, alveolar pressures, and interstitial pressures follow the observation that the vascular pressures are higher at the most dependent and lowest at the least dependent aspects of the lung; at the same time, alveolar pressure is relatively constant throughout the lung.

In zone 1, the alveolar pressure exceeds even the pulmonary arterial pressure (and certainly the venous pressure). Therefore, although this zone is ventilated, no blood flow occurs here (i.e., dead space). In zone 2, arterial pressure is now higher than alveolar pressure, and so flow occurs. However, venous pressure is lower than alveolar pressure in most of zone 2 (they are equal at the zone 2/3 interface), meaning that flow in this zone is dependent on the difference between arterial and alveolar pressures, and venous pressure has no bearing on flow.

West zone 3 is where both arterial and venous pressures exceed alveolar, and flow is dependent on the gradient between the two (and not alveolar pressure).

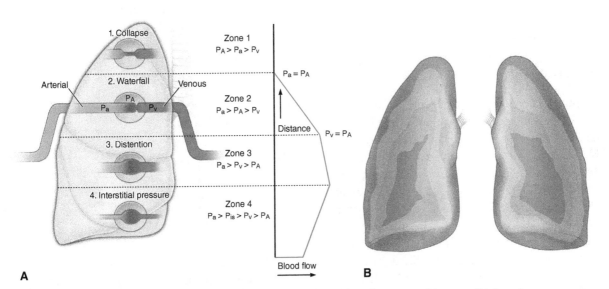

FIG. 3-14. Pulmonary blood flow distribution relative to the alveolar pressure (P_A), the pulmonary arterial pressure (P_a), the pulmonary venous pressure (P_V), and the interstitial pressure (P_{is}) at various gravitation levels. **A.** Classic West Zones of blood flow distribution in the upright position. (Redrawn from West JB. *Respiratory Physiology: The Essentials,* 6th edition. William and Wilkins, 2000.) **B.** In vivo perfusion scanning illustrating central-to-peripheral, in addition to gravitational blood flow distribution, in the upright position. (Reproduced with permission from Lohser J. Evidence based management of one lung ventilation. *Anesthesiol Clin* 2008;26:241.)

Flow still increases in moving down zone 3 because the overall volume of vessels increases (the pressure gradient remains the same). Zone 4 arises in aspects of the lung where reduced lung volumes (and resultant increased interstitial pressures) decrease the size of extra-alveolar vessels, thereby increasing their resistance and reducing flow.

These zones are dynamic; for example, during times of decreased cardiac output, there will be a relative increase in zone 1 and a shrinking of zones 2 and 3. Conversely, during exercise, the increased cardiac output "pushes" blood up to the top of the column, effectively eliminating zone 1 and increasing zone 3 substantially.

This is a simplified conceptual description of the distribution of perfusion within the lungs. For example, it is known that perfusion also exists in a central-to-peripheral gradient, with the hilar areas receiving more flow and the periphery receiving less blood flow.

Ref: Butterworth JF IV, Mackey DC, Wasnick JD. *Morgan and Mikhail's Clinical Anesthesiology.* 5th ed. New York, NY: McGraw Hill; 2013.

39. Following administration of an antibiotic during a general anesthetic, a patient's end-tidal carbon dioxide decreases from 38 mm Hg to 30 mm Hg. No changes in the ventilatory settings were made during this time. The noninvasive blood pressure cuff is set to cycle again in 2 minutes. Which of the following statements is most accurate regarding this clinical situation?

(A) Dead space has decreased.

(B) Dead space has increased.

(C) Shunt fraction has decreased.

(D) Shunt fraction has increased.

(E) The patient requires more PEEP.

End-tidal carbon dioxide represents the partial pressure of CO_2 in the exhaled gas just before inspiration occurs. Under conditions where cardiac output is stable and V/Q matching is ideal, there is minimal gradient between the partial pressure of CO_2 present in the alveoli ($PACO_2 = 40$ mm Hg) and at end-expiration ($EtCO_2 = 38$ mm Hg). The small difference that does exist is due to alveoli at the apices of the lung that are ventilated but not well-perfused (i.e., dead space).

As such, the composition of exhaled gas returning from this zone (West zone 1) reflects inhaled gas and has no CO_2 in it. When it mixes with alveolar gas from well-perfused zones of the lung (i.e., West zone 3), the unchanged gas lowers the overall CO_2 concentration.

The higher the proportion of dead space alveoli, the lower the $EtCO_2$.

An increase in dead space can be caused by a number of mechanisms but is commonly seen when pulmonary perfusion drops, as in pulmonary thrombo- or gas-embolism, cardiac arrest, or (less dramatically) vasodilation and decreases in right-sided preload that decrease pulmonary artery pressures and increase the proportion of West zone 1 in the lungs. This can be a useful clinical monitor. In our example, the antibiotic likely caused vasodilation that resulted in a drop in preload and cardiac output. Before the next cycle of the blood pressure cuff could detect the arterial hypotension that would surely accompany this pulmonary preload reduction, the end-tidal CO_2 alerts the clinician to a potentially serious change in cardiopulmonary function that warrants attention.

Shunting has little effect on end-tidal CO_2 because transfer of CO_2 across the intact capillary/alveolar interface is very efficient. Therefore, endobronchial intubation (resulting in a large initial shunt fraction due to no ventilation on one lung) will typically not be detected with a decrease in end-tidal CO_2. The addition of positive end-expiratory pressure (PEEP) is a maneuver well-suited to patients suffering from impaired oxygenation. However, the increased alveolar pressure tends to be transferred to the capillaries, reducing perfusion and **increasing** dead space.

Ref: Butterworth JF IV, Mackey DC, Wasnick JD. *Morgan and Mikhail's Clinical Anesthesiology.* 5th ed. New York, NY: McGraw Hill; 2013.

40. A pulmonary artery catheter is placed to monitor pulmonary artery occlusion pressure (PAOP). In which West zone(s) must the catheter lie in order to be accurate?

(A) West zone 1

(B) West zone 2

(C) West zone 3

(D) West zones 1 or 2

(E) West zone 2 or 3

Pulmonary arterial catheters estimate left ventricular end diastolic pressure by occluding a segment of the pulmonary artery with a balloon (a "wedged" position). Pressure measured at the catheter tip should theoretically be reflective of an uninterrupted column of fluid that continues through the pulmonary capillary bed, to the pulmonary venules and veins, the left atrium and finally the left ventricle. However, if the

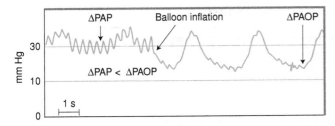

FIG. 3-15. Pressure trace recorded during positive pressure mechanical ventilation from a pulmonary artery catheter located in West's lung zone 1. Pressure swings in the pulmonary artery occlusion pressure (ΔPAOP) reflect changes in airway pressure and are significantly higher than swings in pulmonary artery pressure (ΔPAP), which result from changes in pleural pressure. (Reprinted from Longnecker DE, Brown DL, Newman MF, Zapol WM. *Anesthesiology.* 2nd edition. New York, NY: McGraw-Hill, 2012. After Teboul JL, Pinsky MR, Mercat A, et al. Estimating cardiac filling pressure in mechanically ventilated patients with hyperinflation. *Crit Care Med.* 2000;28(11):3631–3636.)

alveolar pressure is greater than the pulmonary venous pressure (as is the case in West zones 1 and 2), the column of fluid will be interrupted and the pressure transduced will be reflective of airway pressure (Figure 3-15).

Catheters are normally directed into West zone 3 because they are balloon tipped and probably follow the arterial path with the greatest flow. However, if the same patient then becomes hypovolemic or is exposed to positive pressure ventilation (especially with a large amount of PEEP), a portion of zone 3 may be converted to zone 2 or even 1. This may be detected on the monitor when the PAOP tracing develops large swings corresponding to the respiratory rate.

Ref: Longnecker DE, Brown DL, Newman MF, Zapol WM. *Anesthesiology.* 2nd ed. New York, NY: McGraw Hill; 2012.

41. Which of the following factors interferes with effective hypoxic pulmonary vasoconstriction (HPV)?

(A) propofol

(B) fentanyl

(C) thoracic epidural analgesia

(D) 6% desflurane

(E) **nitroprusside**

HPV is a physiologic mechanism that serves to reduce the shunt fraction caused by poor V/Q mismatching in areas of the lung where ventilation is poor. Because it is a local response, only those areas that are hypoxic undergo vasoconstriction, a smooth muscle response that is likely mediated by oxygen-sensitive potassium channels. In response to hypoxia, these channels are blocked, leading to depolarization and an increase in intracellular calcium concentration, thereby causing contraction of the smooth muscle. HPV can reduce the shunt fraction during one lung ventilation by about half, markedly increasing the arterial oxygen tension (Figure 3-16).

HPV is a relatively weak response, and can be overcome by a number of factors including mechanical (elevated pulmonary arterial pressure), pharmacologic (vasodilators) and metabolic (alkalosis) (Table 3-3). Many common anesthetic drugs have little to no effect, including propofol, volatile anesthetics at concentrations of 1 MAC, opioids, and thoracic epidural analgesia.

Ref: Levitzky MG. *Pulmonary Physiology.* 8th ed. New York, NY: McGraw Hill; 2013.

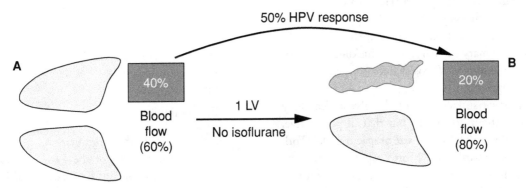

FIG. 3-16. **A.** Schematic diagram showing that the 2-lung ventilation nondependent-to-dependent lung blood flow ratio is 40% to 60%. **B.** When 2-lung ventilation is converted to 1-lung ventilation (as indicated by atelectasis of the nondependent lung), the HPV response decreases the blood flow to the nondependent lung by 50% so that the nondependent-to-dependent lung blood flow ratio is now 20% to 80%. (Reproduced with permission from Wernly JA, et al. Clinical value of quantitative ventilation-perfusion lung scans in the surgical management of bronchogenic carcinoma. *J Thorac Cardiovasc Surg.* 1980;80:535.)

TABLE 3-3. Common factors influencing hypoxic pulmonary vasoconstriction.

Factor	Effect on hypoxic pulmonary vasoconstriction
Alkalosis	Inhibits
Hypothermia	Inhibits
Increased cardiac output; increased pulmonary artery pressures	Inhibits
Hypocapnia	Inhibits
Positive end expiratory pressure (PEEP)	Inhibits (increased pressure in aerated lung shunts blood to nonaerated lung)
Vasodilators (nitroglycerin, nitroprusside)	Inhibits
Vasoconstrictors (phenylephrine, norepinephrine)	Inhibits (overcome HPV by increasing PAP)
Volatile anesthetics	Minimal or no change at 1.0 MAC; desflurane >1.5 MAC inhibits HPV
Lateral decubitus position (vs supine)	Enhances
Propofol	Either no change (high dose: 6–12 mcg/kg/hr), or enhances (clinically used doses)
Thoracic epidural analgesia	Enhances
Fentanyl	No change
Labetalol	No change
Nicardipine	No change

42. Which of the following is NOT required to calculate the diffusion rate of a gas across the alveolar membrane?

    (A) combined surface area of the alveoli

    (B) diffusion coefficient for the particular gas

    (C) viscosity of the gas

    (D) partial pressure of the gas in the blood

    (E) thickness of alveolar/capillary interface

Diffusion rate of a gas through a barrier can be calculated using Fick's law for diffusion (How many laws did this guy invent? Enough already!). This law states that:

$$\dot{v}gas = [A \times D \times (P_1 - P_2)]/T$$

Where $\dot{v}$ = volume of gas diffusing through the membrane per unit of time; A = surface area of the membrane; D = diffusion coefficient of the particular gas; $P_1 - P_2$ = difference in partial pressure between alveolus and pulmonary capillary; T = thickness of alveolar/capillary interface. Viscosity does not play a role in diffusion capacity.

The average surface area of the alveolar/capillary interface is about 70 m². To put that in perspective, that is roughly 750 ft², or the size of spacious New York City studio apartment. More capillaries can be recruited during exercise to increase this (effectively decreasing the West zone 1 volume); conversely, hypotension or excessive PEEP may decrease the surface area by derecruiting capillaries. Diffusion coefficient for a gas is related to molecular weight and solubility. The lighter the gas and the higher the solubility, the easier it passes through the membrane. The thickness of this interface is between 0.2 to 0.5 mm, but this can increase with pulmonary edema or interstitial fibrosis.

Ref: Levitzky MG. *Pulmonary Physiology.* 8th ed. New York, NY: McGraw Hill; 2013.

DIRECTIONS: Use the following scenario to answer questions 43 and 44:

A healthy 30-year-old weighing 70 kg undergoes induction of general anesthesia with paralysis after breathing room air. The patient is neither ventilated nor oxygenated following induction. The patient has a VO_2 of 3.5 mL/kg/min and an FRC of 2400 mL.

43. From the time that apnea is initiated, how long will the patient's oxygen stores last until he begins to desaturate?

    (A) 30 seconds

    (B) 60 seconds

    (C) 2 minutes

    (D) 4 minutes

    (E) 6 minutes

In this scenario, the pulmonary oxygen stores at time zero are the volume of the FRC multiplied by the FiO_2. Since the patient has been breathing room air, the oxygen stores are 2400 mL × 0.21, or 504 mL. The oxygen consumption is 3.5 mL/kg/min × 70 kg, or 245 mL/min. Therefore, the pulmonary oxygen stores will be used up in about 2 minutes, and desaturation will begin to commence.

The time to desaturation can be markedly extended by pre-oxygenating the patient prior to the apnea period. If the patient had been completely de-nitrogenated by breathing 100% oxygen for several minutes, the oxygen stores would effectively equal the volume at FRC, which is 2400 mL in this example. Given an uptake of 245 mL/min, this would provide almost 10 minutes of apneic time before desaturation occurred. This calculation is an oversimplification, and in reality the effects of atelectasis and V/Q mismatching would likely reduce that number by some amount.

Ref: Levitzky MG. *Pulmonary Physiology.* 8th ed. New York, NY: McGraw Hill; 2013.

44. The medical student accompanying the anesthesiologist decides to show off and ask about "apneic oxygenation." This backfires when he is then asked to explain what he knows about it. A good answer would be:

(A) It's a myth—it doesn't really exist.

(B) There are conflicting data about how it works.

(C) It's only been shown to work in experimental situations, not in humans.

(D) **It works via the creation of a low pressure zone in the alveoli, which draws in oxygen from the upper airway.**

(E) Hypoxic pulmonary vasoconstriction gradually shunts flow away from underperfused lung, preserving V/Q matching.

In the 1940s, researchers began to investigate the idea of providing a continuous source of oxygen to the upper airway while the patient was apneic as a means of extending this apneic time further. During apnea, it is estimated that CO_2 enters the alveoli at a rate of approximately 10 mL/min. As stated above, oxygen is removed at a rate of approximately 200 to 250 mL/min. This discrepancy results in a reduction in barometric pressure in the alveoli. Assuming a patent airway, gas from the pharynx, tracheal and conducting airways will move via bulk flow down the pressure gradient to replace the oxygen that has diffused into the capillaries.

Practically speaking, providing the patient is pre-oxygenated, has a patent airway, and there is a source of oxygen flowing (e.g., nasal, pharyngeal or tracheal cannula), apneic oxygenation can allow patients to maintain a PaO_2 in the 200 to 400 mm Hg range for beyond 15 minutes. With an endotracheal tube and insufflation with 100% oxygen, patients can theoretically tolerate up to 100 minutes of apnea. Apneic oxygenation can be extremely useful in short cases where surgical access to the airway is required (e.g., laryngoscopy and/or bronchoscopy) or where immobility of the chest wall is desired (e.g., high-resolution imaging of the chest). Clearly, a consideration when performing apneic oxygenation is the hypercarbia that develops due to hypoventilation, and the effects on the cerebral, systemic, and pulmonary vasculature.

Ref: Lumb AB. *Nunn's Applied Respiratory Physiology.* 7th ed. Philadelphia, PA: Elsevier; 2010.

45. Diffusion hypoxia is a phenomenon most likely seen in which of the following settings?

(A) upon induction of anesthesia with air/oxygen and fentanyl

(B) upon induction of anesthesia with nitrous oxide/oxygen and fentanyl

(C) upon induction of anesthesia with nitrous oxide/oxygen and morphine

(D) upon emergence from anesthesia with air/oxygen and morphine

(E) **upon emergence from anesthesia with nitrous oxide/oxygen and fentanyl**

Diffusion hypoxia is a phenomenon observed upon emergence from an anesthetic where nitrous oxide was used extensively. Because of its relative insolubility, nitrous oxide is eliminated from the bloodstream rapidly. If large amounts of this gas diffuse into the alveoli in a short period of time, these can displace or dilute the oxygen already present, provoking hypoxia. This is particularly dangerous during emergence, as this is a time where the patient is at increased risk for obstruction and hypoventilation, further worsening the oxygenation. However, if supplemental oxygen is provided to these patients and a patent airway ensured, diffusion hypoxia is unlikely.

The risk is greatest during the first 5 to 10 minutes following emergence, since nitrous oxide is rapidly eliminated into the room air. A technique known as "nitrous-narcotic anesthesia," which is not practiced often these days, relies heavily on both nitrous oxide and opioids—this tended to worsen the risk for diffusion hypoxia because of the opioid-induced respiratory depression on emergence.

Ref: Butterworth JF IV, Mackey DC, Wasnick JD. *Morgan and Mikhail's Clinical Anesthesiology.* 5th ed. New York, NY: McGraw Hill; 2013.

46. An intubated patient is breathing 30% oxygen in a critical care unit in Miami. Arterial blood gas analysis reveals her PaO_2 is 140 mm Hg and her $PaCO_2$ is 40 mm Hg. Which of the following best represents her alveolar-arterial (A-a) gradient:

(A) 6
(B) 10
(C) 12
(D) 18
(E) 24

The alveolar-arterial (A-a) gradient quantifies the difference between the calculated alveolar oxygen tension and the measured arterial oxygen tension. It is an important value, used to estimate the degree of impairment of gas exchange and the health of the alveolar-capillary interface:

$$Alveolar\ oxygen\ tension\ (PAO_2)$$
$$= FiO_2\ (P_{atm} - P_{H_2O}) - PaCO_2/0.8$$

Where FiO_2 is fraction of inspired oxygen, P_{atm} is atmospheric pressure, P_{H_2O} is water vapor pressure, and $PaCO_2$ is arterial carbon dioxide tension. Atmospheric pressure at sea level (e.g., Miami) is 760 mm Hg. Water vapor pressure, assuming 100% humidity in the alveoli, is 47 mm Hg. Substituting in our example, we get:

$PAO_2 = 0.3 \times (760 - 47\ mm\ Hg) - 40\ mm\ Hg/0.8$

$PAO_2 = 214 - 50\ mm\ Hg$

$PAO_2 = 164\ mm\ Hg$

Subtracting the measured PaO_2 gives:

A-a gradient $= 164 - 140\ mm\ Hg = 24\ mm\ Hg$

A rough guideline for the normal range is a gradient less than [age/4] + 4. Normal A-a gradients increase with both age and FiO_2. Therefore, while a healthy, nonsmoking 18-year-old breathing room air would be expected to have a gradient between 5 and 10 mm Hg, an elderly person breathing room air would likely have a gradient of 14 to 15 mm Hg. Similarly, breathing 100% oxygen would result in a gradient of approximately 30 mm Hg in a young person and 55 mm Hg in an elderly person.

The A-a gradient can be helpful in refining the differential diagnosis for hypoxemia. For example, hypoxemia in the presence of a normal A-a gradient suggests either alveolar hypoventilation or a low FiO_2.

In contrast, hypoxemia with an elevated gradient suggests one of the following:

1. V/Q mismatch
2. Left-to-right shunt (cardiac or pulmonary)
3. Diffusion impairment
4. Decreased venous admixture (e.g., increased extraction from sepsis, fever, thyrotoxicosis, etc.)

Ref: Lumb AB. *Nunn's Applied Respiratory Physiology.* 7th ed. Philadelphia, PA: Elsevier; 2010.

47. Assuming the solubility coefficient of oxygen in blood is 0.003 mL/mm Hg/dL, which of the following best estimates the amount of dissolved oxygen in a 70-kg man breathing room air?

(A) 5 mL
(B) 15 mL
(C) 150 mL
(D) 1500 mL
(E) 2100 mL

According to Henry's Law, the concentration of dissolved gas in a liquid is in direct proportion to its partial pressure and solubility. In other words:

$$CO_{2dissolved} = solubility\ coefficient \times PaO_2$$

Substituting the above solubility coefficient and assuming a room air PaO_2 of 100 mm Hg, we get:

$CO_{2dissolved} = 0.003\ mL/mm\ Hg/dL \times 100\ mm\ Hg$, or

$CO_{2dissolved} = 0.3\ mL/dL$

The average 70-kg male has 75 mL of blood/kg, or about 5 L (50 dL) of blood volume. Multiplying 50 dL $\times$ 0.3 mL/dL gives us 15 mL of dissolved oxygen in the body.

This is a pitifully small amount of dissolved oxygen, especially when considering the average oxygen consumption is 250 mL/min. The cardiac output required to deliver that much dissolved oxygen to meet the metabolic needs would be physiologically impossible. This is precisely why the ability of hemoglobin to bind and transport oxygen to the tissues is critical for the development and survival of complicated heme-based organisms.

Ref: Butterworth JF IV, Mackey DC, Wasnick JD. *Morgan and Mikhail's Clinical Anesthesiology.* 5th ed. New York, NY: McGraw Hill; 2013.

48. Which of the following statements regarding normal adult hemoglobin is correct?

(A) Hemoglobin is made up of four protein subunits surrounding a single heme group.

(B) Hemoglobin is made up of two alpha chains and two gamma chains.

(C) **Each gram of hemoglobin can carry 1.34 mL of oxygen.**

(D) Only the ferric form of iron (Fe^{3+}) can bind oxygen.

(E) As each binding site becomes occupied with oxygen, conformational changes occur that make it more difficult to bind more oxygen.

Hemoglobin, the principal means of oxygen carrying capacity, is a metalloprotein that consists of four protein subunits and four heme groups. In normal adult hemoglobin, there are two alpha subunits and two beta subunits, each of which is attached by a histidine amino acid residue to the heme group. Heme itself consists of a porphyrin ring surrounding an iron ion. Oxygen can only binds to the ferrous form of the iron ion (Fe^{2+}); heme containing the oxidized, ferric form (Fe^{3+}) is known as methemoglobin and cannot bind oxygen. There is normally a very small amount of methemoglobin in healthy individuals, which is converted back to hemoglobin by the enzyme methemoglobin reductase. Each gram of adult hemoglobin can carry 1.34 mL of oxygen, which (assuming a hemoglobin concentration of 14 g/dL) increases the oxygen carrying capacity by over 60-fold compared to dissolved oxygen.

Other hemoglobin species exist. For example, fetal hemoglobin is composed of a similar structure but has two gamma subunits instead of two beta subunits. This changes the shape of the oxyhemoglobin dissociation curve for fetal hemoglobin, increasing its affinity for oxygen and making it easier to bind to oxygen at low tensions present in placenta.

The four binding sites demonstrate "cooperativity," which describes the conformational changes that occur as oxygen occupies each site in turn. Rather than obey the law of mass action (in which the fourth heme-O_2 binding reaction should be slowest due to a decreased amount of oxygen and heme available), the kinetics of the fourth reaction are actually fastest, and the overall result is that all four binding reactions occur at the same rate.

Refs: Butterworth JF IV, Mackey DC, Wasnick JD. *Morgan and Mikhail's Clinical Anesthesiology.* 5th ed. New York, NY: McGraw Hill; 2013.

Lumb AB. *Nunn's Applied Respiratory Physiology.* 7th ed. Philadelphia, PA: Elsevier; 2010.

49. Which of the following factors is most likely to shift the oxyhemoglobin dissociation curve to a position that favors unloading of oxygen?

(A) **hyperthermia**

(B) alkalosis

(C) decreased 2,3-diphosphoglycerate (2,3-DPG) levels

(D) carboxyhemoglobin

(E) fetal hemoglobin

The oxyhemoglobin dissociation curve is a representation of the effect of tissue PO_2 on the loading and unloading characteristics of hemoglobin. The loading status is characterized as the percent saturation on the y-axis. As can be seen in Figure 3-17, the relationship is a sigmoidal one—the slope of the curve is steep at low oxygen tensions, and begins to flatten out as the PO_2 approaches 70 mm Hg. This is very important for the physiology of oxygen transport and delivery. Hemoglobin has a high affinity for oxygen at high oxygen tensions, such as those found in the alveoli.

This allows the rapid loading of the four binding sites to a fully saturated state. Even if the alveolar PO_2 is reduced from normal conditions (e.g., 70 mm Hg down from ~100 mm Hg), the curve demonstrates that the SpO_2 is still 94%. On the other hand, the steep portion of the curve at low oxygen tensions encourages the offloading of oxygen. A small reduction in PO_2 results in a large decrease in saturation as oxygen becomes unbound and therefore available to the relatively hypoxic tissues.

Certain factors can cause the oxyhemoglobin dissociation curve to shift its position on the x-axis (Table 3-4 and Figure 3-18). The most common factors are

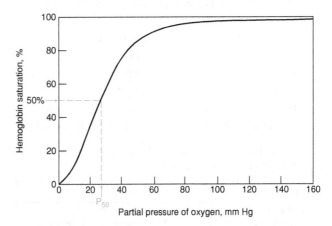

FIG. 3-17. A typical "normal" adult oxyhemoglobin dissociation curve for blood at 37°C with a pH of 7.40 and a PCO_2 of 40 mm Hg. The P_{50} is the partial pressure of oxygen at which hemoglobin is 50% saturated with oxygen. (Reproduced with permission from Levitzky MG. *Pulmonary Physiology.* 8th ed. New York, NY: McGraw Hill; 2013.)

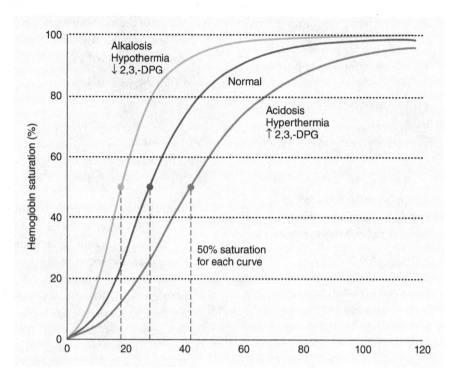

FIGURE 3-18. The effects of changes in acid–base status, body temperature, and 2,3-DPG concentration on the hemoglobin–oxygen dissociation curve. (Reproduced with permission from Butterworth JF IV, Mackey DC, Wasnick JD. *Morgan and Mikhail's Clinical Anesthesiology.* 5th ed. New York, NY: McGraw Hill; 2013.)

temperature, hydrogen ion concentration, and the concentration of 2,3-DPG (a by-product of glycolysis that accumulates during anaerobic metabolism). An increase in any of these factors will shift the curve to the right, which will reduce the affinity of hemoglobin for oxygen. In other words, a right shift of the curve will tend to promote unloading. A decrease in any of these three factors will result in a left shift, and an increased affinity for oxygen. This increased tendency for hemoglobin to "hold on" to oxygen is undesirable when oxygen delivery to the tissues is critical.

The oxyhemoglobin dissociation curve can be shifted by abnormal hemoglobin forms as well as substances that displace oxygen. For example, hemoglobin has a vastly higher (200–300×) affinity for carbon monoxide than oxygen; exposure to carbon monoxide displaces oxygen from the binding sites and makes it unavailable

TABLE 3-4. Factors promoting a left or right shift of the oxyhemoglobin dissociation curve.

Left shift	Right shift
↓ temperature	↑ temperature
↓ hydrogen ions (alkalosis)	↑ hydrogen ions (acidosis)
↓ 2,3-DPG concentration	↑ 2,3-DPG concentration
Carboxyhemoglobin, methemoglobin	
Fetal hemoglobin	

to the tissues. Carbon monoxide also shifts the curve to the left, making what oxygen that *is* bound even less available to the tissues. Methemoglobinemia (commonly caused by nitrates, nitrites, sulfonamides, and some local anesthetics) also displaces oxygen and left-shifts the curve. Fetal hemoglobin is naturally displaced to the left compared with adult hemoglobin; this is adaptive for the fetus so that loading can proceed efficiently at low oxygen tensions present in the placenta.

Ref: Butterworth JF IV, Mackey DC, Wasnick JD. *Morgan and Mikhail's Clinical Anesthesiology.* 5th ed. New York, NY: McGraw Hill; 2013.

50. Hemoglobin from which one of the following would be expected to have the highest levels of 2,3-DPG?

(A) an 80-year-old man

(B) a 45-year-old woman from Florida enjoying a ski holiday in Breckenridge, Colorado

(C) a healthy 6-month-old child

(D) a healthy 25-year-old woman 2 weeks postpartum

(E) a unit of red blood cells stored in a blood bank for 40 days

2,3-diphosphoglycerate (2,3-DPG) is produced by red blood cells during normal cellular respiration. Within the erythrocyte, it binds to hemoglobin, reducing the molecule's affinity for oxygen. As such, increased levels of 2,3-DPG result in a right-shift of the oxyhemoglobin dissociation curve. This normally occurs during chronic hypoxic conditions, such as exposure to high altitudes. An individual accustomed to partial pressures of oxygen present at sea level would be expected to generate up to 20% higher levels of 2,3-DPG when exposed to high altitudes (e.g., Breckenridge, CO, which is located at 9600 ft above sea level). Elevated levels of 2,3-DPG are found during normal pregnancy, with concentrations returning to normal within days of delivery. Newborns have elevated levels of 2,3-DPG, but these drop quickly and reach adult concentrations by age 2 months. Increased 2,3-DPG concentrations are also seen in iron deficiency anemia. Blood stored in blood banks is quickly depleted of 2,3-DPG. This has the undesirable effect of causing a left shift in the oxyhemoglobin dissociation curve, reducing the ability of hemoglobin to off-load oxygen in the relatively hypoxic tissue.

Ref: Levitzky MG. *Pulmonary Physiology.* 8th ed. New York, NY: McGraw Hill; 2013.

51. Which of the following best represents the oxygen partial pressure where normal adult hemoglobin will be 50% saturated?

   (A) 19 mm Hg
   (B) 27 mm Hg
   (C) 40 mm Hg
   (D) 50 mm Hg
   (E) 75 mm Hg

The P50 is the partial pressure of oxygen at which the hemoglobin is 50% saturated. Under normal conditions in an adult, this number is 26.6 mm Hg. This is a useful concept for understanding changes in hemoglobin physiology. Since the P50 exists at the steepest part of the sigmoidal oxyhemoglobin dissociation curve, it is a sensitive point on the *x*-axis to compare curves that have been shifted left or right. For example, the P50 of fetal hemoglobin is approximately 19 mm Hg. The curve for fetal hemoglobin is therefore left-shifted, allowing fetal hemoglobin to load oxygen more efficiently at relatively lower partial pressures (such as at the placenta).

The four key points on the oxyhemoglobin dissociation curve that are worth remembering are:

- Arterial point: pO_2 100 mm Hg with SaO_2 98%
- Saturation "fall-off" point: pO_2 60 mm Hg with SpO_2 90%

- Mixed venous point: pO_2 40 mm Hg with SaO_2 75%
- P50: pO_2 26.6 mm Hg with SaO_2 50%

Ref: Levitzky MG. *Pulmonary Physiology.* 8th ed. New York, NY: McGraw Hill; 2013.

52. A patient under general anesthesia has an arterial blood gas drawn, which reveals PaO_2 = 85 mm Hg, $PaCO_2$ = 42 mm Hg, Hb = 13 g/dL, and SpO_2 = 96%. Which of the following best approximates his oxygen content?

   (A) 10 mL/dL
   (B) 12 mL/dL
   (C) 14 mL/dL
   (D) 17 mL/dL
   (E) 19 mL/dL

Oxygen content (CaO_2) is defined as the sum total of the dissolved oxygen and that oxygen bound to hemoglobin. The equation is as follows:

$$CaO_2 = (0.003 \times PaO_2) + (1.34 \times Hb \times SpO_2)$$

The constant 1.34 reflects that amount of oxygen that 1 g of hemoglobin can bind under standard conditions. Some sources cite a constant of 1.39, which is an experimental and theoretical maximum, but in reality the presence of a small amount of other species of hemoglobins (e.g., methemoglobin, carboxyhemoglobin) brings that number down by a small amount. Note that the first term is very small since PaO_2 is multiplied by 0.003. This is the dissolved fraction, which is negligible compared to the amount carried by hemoglobin.

Substituting in our example, we get:

$$CaO_2 = (0.003 \times 85) + (1.34 \times 13 \times 0.96)$$
$$= 0.255 + 16.72$$
$$= 17 \text{ mL/dL}$$

Ref: Butterworth JF IV, Mackey DC, Wasnick JD. *Morgan and Mikhail's Clinical Anesthesiology.* 5th ed. New York, NY: McGraw Hill; 2013.

53. Which of the following statements regarding methemoglobin is FALSE?

   (A) Methemoglobin contains the oxidized (ferric or 3^+) form of the iron ion.
   (B) Agents that cause methemoglobinemia include nitrates, nitrites and prilocaine.
   (C) The remaining binding sites in the hemoglobin tetramer exhibit increased affinity for oxygen.

(D) **Significant amounts of methemoglobin cause the pulse oximeter to display a value of 100% no matter what the oxygen carrying capacity.**

(E) Methemoglobin is converted back to oxyhemoglobin by the enzyme methemoglobin reductase.

Methemoglobin is the form of hemoglobin that occurs when the normal ferrous ion (2^+) is oxidized to its ferric form (3^+). There are a variety of oxidizing agents that may provoke this reaction; important examples in anesthesiology practice include nitroglycerin, nitric oxide, sulfonamides, metoclopramide, benzocaine, and prilocaine. When oxidized, the iron ion is no longer able to serve as a binding site; however, the presence of methemoglobin on one of the four tetramers increases the affinity for oxygen on the part of the remaining reduced hemoglobin molecules.

In normal day-to-day living, auto-oxidation results in approximately 1% of circulating hemoglobin present as methemoglobin. This is normally not a problem, since the enzyme methemoglobin reductase converts this back to its ferrous state. In clinically significant methemoglobinemia, the volume of methemoglobin outstrips the ability of the enzyme to keep up, and methemoglobin begins to accumulate. Symptoms are nonspecific and relate to inadequate oxygen delivery, typically beginning when methemoglobin represents 8% to 12% of total hemoglobin. Pulse oximetry is inaccurate, and with significant ($>20\%$) concentrations tends to read as 85%, independent of the actual oxygen saturation.

Bonus fun fact: Unlike in carboxyhemoglobinemia, where blood typically has a bright red appearance, blood with a significant amount of methemoglobin appears "chocolate brown." Mmmmmmm, chocolate …

Ref: Levitzky MG. *Pulmonary Physiology.* 8th ed. New York, NY: McGraw Hill; 2013.

54. Carbon dioxide is carried in blood in multiple ways. Which of the following best describes the relative importance of the method of transport?

(A) dissolved in solution > bound to blood proteins > as bicarbonate ions

(B) bound to blood proteins > dissolved in solution > as bicarbonate ions

(C) bound to blood proteins > as bicarbonate ions > dissolved in solution

(D) as bicarbonate ions > dissolved in solution > bound to blood proteins

(E) **as bicarbonate ions > bound to blood proteins > dissolved in solution**

Like oxygen, a small fraction of CO_2 is carried in blood dissolved in solution. The solubility of CO_2 is higher than oxygen, but the overall contribution is still roughly 5%. Another 6% to 23% of total CO_2 is transported bound to histidine residues on the hemoglobin chain, forming carbaminohemoglobin (n.b. NOT the same as carboxyhemoglobin. This is hemoglobin bound to carbon monoxide instead of oxygen). The vast majority (70%–90%) of CO_2 is transported as bicarbonate ions. The wide ranges on these percentages reflect the differences between arterial and venous carriage of carbon dioxide.

Ref: Butterworth JF IV, Mackey DC, Wasnick JD. *Morgan and Mikhail's Clinical Anesthesiology.* 5th ed. New York, NY: McGraw Hill; 2013.

55. Carbonic anhydrase catalyzes which of the following reactions?

(A) **the conversion of CO_2 and H_2O into carbonic acid within the erythrocyte**

(B) the conversion of CO_2 and H_2O into carbonic acid within the plasma

(C) the splitting of carbonic acid into protons and bicarbonate within the erythrocyte

(D) the splitting of carbonic acid into protons and bicarbonate within the plasma

(E) the splitting of carbonic acid into protons and bicarbonate within the interstitial fluid

At the tissue level, CO_2 diffuses out of the cells, into the interstitial fluid, and into the capillaries along a concentration gradient. Once in the blood, CO_2 is able to combine with water to form H_2CO_3 (carbonic acid), which then dissociates into hydrogen ions and bicarbonate ions. This reaction is very slow on its own. However, erythrocytes contain a high concentration of carbonic anhydrase, an enzyme that catalyzes the combination of CO_2 with water to form carbonic acid at a rate 13,000 times faster (Figure 3-19):

$$CO_2 + H_2O \xrightleftharpoons[\text{anhydrase}]{\text{carbonic}} H_2CO_3 \rightleftharpoons H^+ + HCO_3^-$$

FIG. 3-19. The conversion of CO_2 and water to carbonic acid to protons and bicarbonate.

Ref: Levitzky MG. *Pulmonary Physiology.* 8th ed. New York, NY: McGraw Hill; 2013.

56. The mechanism by which red blood cells maintain electrical neutrality while generating bicarbonate ions is termed the:

(A) sodium shift.

(B) potassium shift.

(C) calcium shift.

(D) phosphate shift.

(E) **chloride shift.**

CO_2 freely diffuses into red blood cells, whereupon it combines with water (in the presence of carbonic anhydrase) to form carbonic acid. The carbonic acid spontaneously dissociates into protons and bicarbonate ions. In response to the falling intracellular CO_2 levels, additional CO_2 diffuses into the cell from the plasma. The erythrocyte cell membrane is impermeable to protons but does allow bicarbonate ions to pass out of the cell. However, in order to maintain electrical neutrality, extracellular chloride ions are exchanged for intracellular bicarbonate ions via an anion exchanger protein. The intracellular chloride concentration is higher in venous blood than arterial blood as a result, due to increased partial pressures of CO_2 in venous blood.

As a historical side-note, this mechanism is also known as the "Hamburger" shift, after the Dutch physiologist Hartog Jacob Hamburger. He also developed a drug that we use for almost every case in some form or another: normal saline.

Ref: Levitzky MG. *Pulmonary Physiology.* 8th ed. New York, NY: McGraw Hill; 2013.

57. Compared to the oxyhemoglobin dissociation curve, the carbon dioxide dissociation curve is:

(A) more sigmoidal shaped.

(B) logarithmic.

(C) **steeper in slope.**

(D) inversely related.

(E) left-shifted.

The carbon dioxide dissociation curve describes the relationship between the PCO_2 and the whole blood CO_2 content (in all three forms: dissolved, as carbamino compounds, and as bicarbonate). In general, the curve is straighter (less "S-shaped"), and while it appears to be fairly flat in the normal physiologic range (Figure 3-20), it is in fact steeper than the oxygen dissociation curve for whole blood. In other words, for each 1 mm Hg change in PCO_2, there is a larger corresponding change in carbon dioxide content.

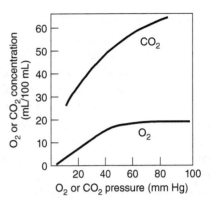

FIG. 3-20. Whole blood CO_2 and O_2 concentration plotted against partial pressure.

Ref: Levitzky MG. *Pulmonary Physiology.* 8th ed. New York, NY: McGraw Hill; 2013.

58. The Haldane effect explains why:

(A) the oxyhemoglobin dissociation curve is sigmoidal.

(B) fetal hemoglobin has a greater affinity for oxygen that adult hemoglobin.

(C) carbon dioxide has a greater solubility than oxygen.

(D) the carbon dioxide dissociation curve is sigmoidal.

(E) **deoxygenated blood can carry more carbon dioxide than oxygenated blood.**

Carbon dioxide is carried in the blood in three forms (in order of importance):

• as bicarbonate ions,

• as carbamino compounds (bound to proteins in the blood), and

• dissolved in solution.

When carbon dioxide diffuses out of tissues and into the blood at the capillary level, much of it will diffuse into red blood cells, where some will combine with water in the presence of carbonic anhydrase to form carbonic acid and subsequently hydrogen ions and bicarbonate in the following reaction:

$$CO_2 + H_2O \rightarrow H_2CO_3 \rightarrow H^+ + HCO_3^-$$

Within the red blood cell, some CO_2 is dissolved. However, most CO_2 is converted into bicarbonate by the above reaction or is combined with the amino acids of hemoglobin to form carbamino compounds. The end result is a decrease in the concentration of dissolved CO_2 in the cell, which favors increase diffusion into the red blood cells from the plasma. The decrease in red blood cell CO_2 concentration also favors the right shift of the equation, and the generation of more hydrogen ions and bicarbonate.

The Haldane effect refers to the relationship between the degree of oxygenation of hemoglobin and manner in which carbon dioxide is carried in the blood. Specifically, *deoxygenated* hemoglobin has a much greater affinity for hydrogen ions than oxyhemoglobin. This means that at the tissue level, when oxygen is being released, more CO_2 can be carried as bicarbonate and carbamino compounds, hastening the elimination of CO_2 from the tissues. In other words, venous blood has a greater capacity for carbon dioxide (in all forms) than oxygenated arterial blood. The equation below represents the Haldane effect. At the tissue level, it is shifted to the left.

$$H^+ + HbO_2 \longleftrightarrow H^+Hb + O_2$$

In the oxygen-rich environment of the lungs, the equation is reversed, and protons dissociate readily from hemoglobin. These then combine with bicarbonate, forming carbon dioxide which is eliminated via the alveoli.

Ref: Levitzky MG. *Pulmonary Physiology.* 8th ed. New York, NY: McGraw Hill; 2013.

59. A healthy 30-year-old patient has an arterial pCO_2 of 60 mm Hg. Which of the following would you expect to DECREASE in association with this lab value?

(A) heart rate
(B) pulmonary arterial pressure
(C) myocardial contractility
(D) cerebral vascular resistance
(E) plasma norepinephrine level

Hypercarbia produces a spectrum of physiologic effects. Many of these are related to the increase in plasma levels of catecholamines that occurs in response to an elevated PCO_2. These effects include:

- **Neurologic**
  - increased cerebral blood flow
  - cerebral vasodilation (decreased cerebral vascular resistance)
  - increased intracranial pressure
  - narcosis and obtundation (PCO_2 >90 mm Hg)
- **Endocrine/metabolic**
  - increased plasma levels of epinephrine and norepinephrine
  - respiratory acidosis with compensatory metabolic alkalosis
  - decreased affinity of hemoglobin for oxygen
  - hyperkalemia

- **Cardiovascular**
  - increased contractility (indirect effect via sympathetic system)
  - tachycardia (indirect effect via sympathetic system)
  - increased cardiac output
  - increased systemic and pulmonary blood pressures
  - increased incidence of cardiac arrhythmias
- **Pulmonary**
  - increased respiratory rate (mild hypercarbia)
  - respiratory depression (PCO_2 >90 mm Hg)

Note that at high carbon dioxide tensions (>90–120 mm Hg), the direct action of hypercarbia results in a depressant effect on many of these variables, including cardiac output, contractility, blood pressure, level of consciousness, and respiratory drive. Hypercarbia also has the potential to alter pharmacokinetics, by multiple mechanisms including the altered perfusion of organs, and changes in ionization and protein binding.

Ref: Lumb AB. *Nunn's Applied Respiratory Physiology.* 7th ed. Philadelphia, PA: Elsevier; 2010.

60. Due to an error in ventilator settings, a patient's PCO_2 is 25 mm Hg. Which of the following is most likely to occur as a result?

(A) reduced coronary flow
(B) decreased coronary vascular resistance
(C) decreased oxygen extraction
(D) decreased systemic vascular resistance
(E) decreased myocardial contractility

Hypocarbia (PCO_2 <35 mm Hg) has a number of potentially deleterious effects, primarily in the neurologic and cardiovascular systems. These include:

- **Neurologic**
  - Increased cerebral vascular resistance
  - Decreased cerebral blood flow
  - Decreased cerebral blood volume
  - Decreased intracranial pressure
  - Psychomotor and higher intellectual functional impairment
  - Neonatal brain injury (multicystic encephalomalacia, cystic periventricular leukomalacia, pontosubicular necrosis, cerebral infarction, reactive hyperemia and hemorrhage)
- **Cardiovascular**
  - Decrease in myocardial oxygen supply via:
    - reduced coronary flow

- reduced collateral flow
- increased coronary vascular resistance
- increased risk of coronary vasospasm
- increased platelet aggregation; thrombocytosis
  - Increase in myocardial oxygen demand via:
    - Increased oxygen extraction
    - Increased intracellular calcium concentration; increased contractility
    - Increased systemic vascular resistance
  - Increased incidence of arrhythmias

Ref: Laffey and Kavanaugh. Hypocapnia. *N Engl J Med.* 2002; 347:43.

61. Administering high concentrations of oxygen (hyperoxia) is most likely to have which of the following effects?

(A) decreased systemic vascular resistance

(B) increased heart rate

(C) increased coronary flow

(D) increased risk of acute lung injury

(E) increased cerebral blood flow

Abnormally high oxygen tensions are known to have several effects on the cardiovascular system. In general, hyperoxia causes vasoconstriction and decreased blood flow in most vascular beds including the brain, retina, skeletal muscle, and the coronary circulation. Coronary vascular resistance increases up to 20% to 40% from baseline, reducing coronary flow significantly. Systemic vascular resistance is elevated, which leads to a reflex decrease in heart rate and cardiac output of approximately 10% each. The retina is especially susceptible to hyperoxia-mediated vasoconstriction in the premature neonate; oxygen therapy should be avoided in newborns unless hypoxia is present to avoid retinopathy. The mechanism for vasoconstriction may be related to alternations in the bioavailability of vasoactive substances prostaglandins, adenosine and nitric oxide.

Respiratory rate is initially decreased but quickly increases to above normal, for reasons that are unclear, but may involve a reverse Haldane effect (where oxygenated blood has a reduced affinity for carbon dioxide, leading to stimulation of the respiratory center from hypercarbia). Oxygen toxicity of pulmonary tissues is a serious problem, and can develop in only a few hours after exposure to 100% oxygen (i.e., during anesthesia). Reactive oxygen species readily react with cell constituents such as lipids, proteins, and nucleic

acids. The onset of hyperoxia and the resulting high levels of reactive oxygen species can lead to overwhelming of the hemoglobin-O_2 buffering system, oxidative stress, cell damage, apoptosis, and necrosis. This results in an acute lung injury similar to acute respiratory distress syndrome, with alveolar injury, edema.

On the other hand, high oxygen tensions are used to treat infections such as necrotizing fasciitis, improve wound healing in certain settings, and to treat carbon monoxide poisoning. The evidence base for efficacy in these (and other) scenarios is limited however.

Ref: Sjöberg F, Singer M. The medical use of oxygen: A time for critical reappraisal. *J Int Med.* 2013; 274:505–28.

62. A 59-year-old patient with pneumonia has a room air arterial PaO_2 of 50 mm Hg. Which of the following physiologic findings would most likely be observed in this patient?

(A) decreased cerebral blood flow

(B) decreased coronary blood flow

(C) a respiratory rate of 11/min

(D) decreased pulmonary vascular resistance

(E) increased cardiac output

Hypoxia is a state of inadequate oxygen supply to tissues and can be either global or localized. Hypoxemia is defined as an arterial PaO_2 of less than 60 mm Hg (SpO_2 of 90%). Hypoxia is a critical event, and the body responds with a variety of compensatory mechanisms in an effort to maintain cellular homeostasis and integrity. These include:

- **Hyperventilation.** This response is nonlinear and little effect is noticed until the PaO_2 falls below 55 mm Hg (Figure 3-21). Maximal hyperventilation (of about 40 L/min) occurs at a PaO_2 of approximately 30 mm Hg. This response depends to a degree on the $PaCO_2$ as well, with hypercapnia shifting the curve to the right.

- **Increased pulmonary arterial pressure.** This improves the distribution of pulmonary blood flow and reduces V/Q mismatch when areas of hypoxia are localized. However, when all regions of the lung are relatively hypoxic (e.g., when at high altitudes), this effect is deleterious and counterproductive.

- **Increased cardiac output,** with increased regional blood flow to critical organs such as the heart and brain. This is principally mediated by an increase in sympathetic tone affected via chemoreceptors in the carotid and aortic bodies.

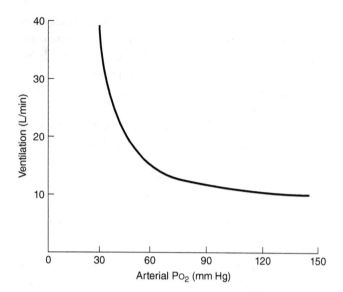

FIG. 3-21. The ventilatory response to arterial oxygenation.

- Over hours to days, the oxyhemoglobin dissociation curve is shifted to the right due to an increase in erythrocyte 2,3-DPG. If hypoxia is chronic, hematopoiesis is stimulated and circulating hemoglobin concentration is increased.

Ref: Lumb AB. *Nunn's Applied Respiratory Physiology.* 7th ed. Philadelphia, PA: Elsevier; 2010.

63. The group of neurons responsible for the initiation of each breath are known as the:

(A) ventral respiratory group.

(B) dorsal respiratory group.

(C) medial respiratory group.

(D) lateral respiratory group.

(E) central respiratory group.

Breathing is an automatic activity that is primarily controlled by the respiratory center in the reticular formation of the medulla beneath the floor of the fourth ventricle. This area of the brainstem contains two groups of neurons that influence breathing: the dorsal respiratory group (DRG) and the ventral respiratory group (VRG). While there is a degree of intermingling of the fibers and hence function of these two groups, it is believed that the DRG serves as the initiator, or pacemaker, of the diaphragm. The DRG is closely associated with the nucleus tractus solitarius, which receives projections from the glossopharyngeal nerve, among others; this is the pathway by which information about PO_2, PCO_2 and pH from carotid and aortic chemoreceptors are carried to the respiratory center. The neurons of the

VRG innervate intercostal and abdominal muscles, and aid in both inspiration and expiration.

Neurons located in the pons also exert some control over the respiratory center. These include the apneustic center and the pneumotaxic center, which are excitatory and inhibitory, respectively. These pontine centers probably serve to fine tune respiration.

Ref: Butterworth JF IV, Mackey DC, Wasnick JD. *Morgan and Mikhail's Clinical Anesthesiology.* 5th ed. New York, NY: McGraw Hill; 2013.

64. Central respiratory chemoreceptors in the brain stem are stimulated by which of the following?

(A) plasma hydrogen ion concentration

(B) plasma bicarbonate ion concentration

(C) CSF hydrogen ion concentration

(D) CSF bicarbonate ion concentration

(E) CSF oxygen concentration

The blood brain barrier is freely permeable to carbon dioxide. Increases in PCO_2 are very quickly reflected in the CSF (in about 60 seconds); this causes the CSF hydrogen ion concentration to increase, as seen by the equation:

$$CO_2 + H_2O \rightarrow H_2CO_3 \rightarrow H^+ + HCO_3^-$$

This increase in hydrogen ions stimulates the central chemoreceptors, which in turn stimulates the firing of respiratory neurons in the nearby respiratory center. The central chemoreceptors are much slower to respond to a reduction in arterial pH caused by a metabolic acidosis, since the blood-brain barrier is impermeable to both hydrogen and bicarbonate ions. Hypoxia does not trigger the central chemoreceptors.

Ref: Butterworth JF IV, Mackey DC, Wasnick JD. *Morgan and Mikhail's Clinical Anesthesiology.* 5th ed. New York, NY: McGraw Hill; 2013.

65. A reduction in plasma PO_2 will result in the increase in firing rate of neurons from which of the following locations?

(A) carotid body

(B) carotid sinus

(C) pulmonary trunk

(D) right atrium

(E) bronchioles

Peripheral chemoreceptors include the carotid bodies, located at the bifurcation of the common carotid artery, and the aortic bodies which are scattered throughout the aortic arch. These neurons have a baseline firing rate, which increases in response to arterial hypercarbia, hypoxemia, or acidemia. The carotid bodies appear to be much more important for driving ventilatory changes, whereas the aortic bodies are more important for regulation of cardiovascular reflexes.

Ref: Butterworth JF IV, Mackey DC, Wasnick JD. *Morgan and Mikhail's Clinical Anesthesiology.* 5th ed. New York, NY: McGraw Hill; 2013.

66. Which of the following best describes the Hering-Breuer reflex?

    (A) rapid shallow breathing in response to pulmonary vascular congestion.

    (B) the slowing of breathing with activation of pulmonary stretch receptors.

    (C) apnea in response to immersion of the face in water.

    (D) hyperpnea in response to low PaO_2.

    (E) hyperpnea in response to pain in an extremity.

There are two pulmonary reflexes that have been described by Hering and Breuer. Both are mediated by pulmonary smooth muscle stretch receptors. The first, the inflation reflex, describes the decreased respiratory effort in response to sustained inflation of the lungs. The afferent pathway is via the vagus nerve. The response is slowing of the respiratory rate as well as bronchodilation. It is thought that this inflation reflex may aid in reducing the work of breathing by inhibiting large tidal volumes.

The Hering-Breuer deflation reflex refers to an increase in respiratory rate that is thought to be mediated by a decrease in tonic stretch receptors in the lung. While the adaptive benefit of this is not entirely clear, it may be that this reflex serves to produce periodic "sighs" that help prevent atelectasis.

Ref: Butterworth JF IV, Mackey DC, Wasnick JD. *Morgan and Mikhail's Clinical Anesthesiology.* 5th ed. New York, NY: McGraw Hill; 2013.

67. Which of the following would be expected to cause a left shift in the carbon dioxide response curve?

    (A) normal physiologic sleep

    (B) opioids

    (C) chronic obstruction

    (D) metabolic acidosis

    (E) sevoflurane anesthesia with a MAC of 1.0

The normal carbon dioxide response curve is shown in Figure 3-22. The slope of the curve in an awake, normal individual is linear and quite steep. In other words, small increases in $PaCO_2$ will serve to rapidly increase alveolar ventilation to correct the hypercarbic state.

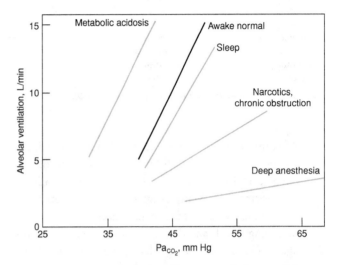

FIG. 3-22. The effects of sleep, narcotics, chronic obstructive pulmonary disease, deep anesthesia, and metabolic acidosis on the ventilatory response to carbon dioxide. (Reproduced with permission from Levitzky MG. *Pulmonary Physiology.* 8th ed. New York, NY: McGraw Hill; 2013.)

Sleep normally increases the PCO_2 by approximately 5 mm Hg, which shifts the curve to the right. This means that for a given PCO_2, the respiratory rate will be lower than the awake individual. This may play a role in central sleep apnea. Both anesthetics and opioid drugs are powerful depressants of the CO_2 response curve. Chronic obstruction is known to have a decreased response to CO_2, probably due to chronic hypercarbia as well as the increased work of breathing required to normalize the PCO_2.

Metabolic acidosis shifts the curve to the left, so that for a given PCO_2, the minute ventilation will be greater. Hypoxia (see question 49) is also a potent stimulant of the CO_2 response curve.

Ref: Levitzky MG. *Pulmonary Physiology.* 8th ed. New York, NY: McGraw Hill; 2013.

68. Which of the following vasoactive substances is largely inactivated by the lung?

    (A) dopamine

    (B) epinephrine

    (C) histamine

    (D) oxytocin

    (E) serotonin

TABLE 3-5. Drugs that undergo first-pass pulmonary extraction.

Drug	Approximate degree of first-pass extraction
Lidocaine	30%–40%
Bupivacaine	5%–10%
Morphine	30%
Meperidine	>90%
Fentanyl	>90%
Sufentanil	60%
Alfentanil	10%–60%
Thiopental	15%
Propofol	30%

Ref: Boer F. Drug handling by the lungs. *Br J Anaesth*. 2003;91:50–60.

After injection into the venous circulation, many drugs are taken up by the cells in the pulmonary parenchyma, a phenomenon known as "first-pass pulmonary extraction." Many drugs used in common anesthetic practice exhibit first pass uptake into the lungs, including local anesthetics, opioids and induction agents (Table 3-5). By and large, these are not eliminated from the circulation by the lungs, but rather are a temporary depot for eventual reuptake by the blood when the concentration gradient reverses to favor redistribution. An exception to this is methadone, which is metabolized to a certain degree in the lung. Neuromuscular blocking agents such as rocuronium and vecuronium are not taken up in any appreciable quantity by the pulmonary tissues.

Metabolism of circulating vasoactive substances by the lungs is common. A number of vasoactive substances are inactivated or removed from the circulation by the endothelium of the pulmonary blood vessels. Since the surface area of this vascular bed is so large, these processes are very efficient—some prostaglandins, for example, are almost completely removed from the circulation in one pass through the pulmonary bed. Leukotrienes, serotonin, bradykinin, and angiotensin I are also either largely removed or metabolized in a single pass. Other substances, including histamine, epinephrine, isoproterenol, dopamine, angiotensin II, vasopressin, and oxytocin, are essentially unaffected and are transferred through to the systemic circulation.

Ref: Levitzky MG. *Pulmonary Physiology*. 8th ed. New York, NY: McGraw Hill; 2013.

69. Which of the following is NOT a physiologic consequence of cigarette smoking?

    (A) decreased FEV_1
    (B) small airway narrowing
    (C) left shift of the oxyhemoglobin dissociation curve
    (D) arterial hypertension
    (E) decreased platelet aggregation and primary clot failure

Smoking exerts deleterious effects on multiple organ systems. Chronic obstructive pulmonary disease, cancer, coronary artery, and cerebral and peripheral vascular disease are very common diseases related to long-term use. However, there are also more immediate physiologic effects including:

- increased mucus production and decreased mucociliary transport,
- increased productive cough,
- decrease in FEV_1 and $MEFR_{25}$,
- small airway narrowing and increased airway reactivity,
- increased carbon monoxide levels and left shift of the oxyhemoglobin dissociation curve (limiting oxygen availability to tissues),
- decreased lower esophageal sphincter tone,
- increased platelet aggregation,
- increased sympathetic activation due to nicotine, leading to arterial hypertension, vasoconstriction, tachycardia, and a small but short-lasting increase (10%) in metabolic rate, and
- decreased wound healing and increased rate of wound infection and dehiscence, likely secondary to vasoconstriction.

Ref: Lumb AB. *Nunn's Applied Respiratory Physiology*. 7th ed. Philadelphia, PA: Elsevier; 2010.

70. Which of the following is INCREASED for patients who have quit smoking prior to anesthesia, compared to current smokers?

    (A) the risk of ICU admission postoperatively
    (B) the P50 of the oxyhemoglobin dissociation curve
    (C) the risk of pneumonia
    (D) the risk of laryngospasm
    (E) the sputum volume

Smoking cessation prior to anesthesia has been shown to confer a reduced risk of respiratory failure, postoperative ICU admission, pneumonia, and laryngospasm. It is clear that compared to nonsmokers, current smokers are at significantly higher risk for postoperative pulmonary complications. What is less clear is the best timing to stop smoking: older evidence suggested that quitting less than 8 weeks prior to cardiac surgery resulted in increased mucociliary transport, sputum production, and a fourfold risk of increased pulmonary complications. This has since been refuted by more recent studies and it seems as if smoking cessation at ANY time prior to surgery does not increase the risk of pulmonary complications compared to patients who continue to smoke. Quitting 2 weeks ahead of time appears to decrease the amount of mucus produced, and even quitting 24 to 48 hours in advance decreases carbon monoxide levels significantly and shifts the oxyhemoglobin dissociation curve to the right, increasing the ability of hemoglobin to deliver oxygen to the tissues.

Ref: Longnecker DE, Brown DL, Newman MF, Zapol WM. *Anesthesiology.* 2nd ed. New York, NY: McGraw Hill; 2012.

CHAPTER 4

Cardiovascular Anatomy and Physiology

1. Which of the following statements regarding normal cardiac anatomy is TRUE?

   (A) The pulmonic valve is attached by chordae tendinae to the right ventricle.
   (B) The coronary sinus empties into the left atrium.
   (C) A patent foramen ovale is found in 25% to 30% of adults.
   (D) The ligamentum arteriosum connects the aorta to the pulmonary vein.
   (E) The root of the aorta is positioned between the left auricle and the pulmonary trunk.

2. Which of the following coronary vessels supplies the majority of the interventricular septum?

   (A) left coronary artery
   (B) left circumflex artery
   (C) left anterior descending artery
   (D) right coronary artery
   (E) posterior descending artery

3. The left recurrent laryngeal nerve loops around which major vessel in the mediastinum?

   (A) aorta
   (B) superior vena cava
   (C) left brachiocephalic vein
   (D) left subclavian artery
   (E) left pulmonary artery

4. Which of the following statements BEST describes the function of the cardiac skeleton?

   (A) It provides an anchor for the chordae tendinae to attach.
   (B) It is the same structure as the fibrous pericardium.
   (C) It provides a framework for the coronary arteries and veins.
   (D) It electrically insulates the atria from the ventricles.
   (E) It prevents excessive torsion of the heart during systole.

5. The cardiomyocytes of the apex of the heart are MOST likely innervated by which branch of the conducting system?

   (A) the bundle of His
   (B) the right bundle branch
   (C) the left septal fascicle
   (D) the left anterior fascicle
   (E) the left posterior fascicle

6. Which of the following organs receives the MOST cardiac output at rest?

   (A) heart
   (B) lungs
   (C) brain
   (D) kidneys
   (E) liver

7. An anesthesiology resident, on a hiking vacation in the Pacific Northwest, comes face to face with a large grizzly bear. A "fight-or-flight" response ensues. How does sympathetic activation alter the intrinsic heart rate of the sinoatrial (SA) node?

   (A) It increases permeability of resting membrane to K^+.
   (B) It causes hyperpolarization of resting membrane potential.
   (C) It releases acetylcholine.
   (D) It decreases threshold potential of SA nodal cells.
   (E) It increases permeability of resting membrane to Na^+ and Ca^{2+}.

8. During a cardiac cycle, the beginning of isovolumetric contraction corresponds to which of the following events?

   (A) closure of atrioventricular valves
   (B) V wave on venous pulse
   (C) opening of aortic valve
   (D) P wave on ECG
   (E) peak aortic blood flow

9. The sinoatrial (SA) node rhythmically discharges. In phase 4 of the action potential, the "pacemaker potential" declines until the depolarization threshold is reached and the next impulse is triggered. During the late stages of phase 4, which of the following currents (I) is most predominant?

   (A) I_f
   (B) I_{CaL}
   (C) I_{CaT}
   (D) I_K
   (E) I_{Na}

10. Which of the following cardiac events does the PR interval of the ECG correspond to?

    (A) atrial depolarization
    (B) ventricular depolarization
    (C) plateau phase of ventricular depolarization
    (D) atrial depolarization and AV nodal conduction
    (E) ventricular repolarization

11. Which of the following cardiac tissues has the slowest rate of conduction?

    (A) tract of Wenckebach
    (B) AV node
    (C) bundle of His
    (D) Purkinje system
    (E) ventricular muscle

12. A curve of left ventricular pressure vs. time is depicted in Figure 4-4 below. Which part of the left ventricular pressure-time curve represents the maximal rate of force development by the ventricle?

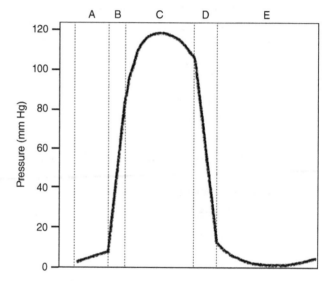

FIG. 4-4. Left ventricular pressure-time curve.

    (A) A
    (B) B
    (C) C
    (D) D
    (E) E

13. The Frank-Starling law of the heart describes the relationship between cardiac output and which of the following variables?

    (A) left ventricular contractility
    (B) heart rate
    (C) cardiac rhythm
    (D) left ventricular end-diastolic volume
    (E) left ventricular compliance

14. How does an increase in afterload affect the Frank-Starling curve?

    (A) Shifts curve down and to the left.
    (B) Shifts curve down and to the right.
    (C) Shifts curve up and to the left.
    (D) Shifts curve up and to the right.
    (E) No change.

15. Which phase of the cardiac cycle is associated with the greatest proportion of myocardial oxygen consumption?

    (A) rapid ventricular ejection
    (B) atrial systole
    (C) isovolumetric contraction
    (D) rapid ventricular filling
    (E) isovolumetric relaxation

16. Left ventricular wall stress or tension is a determinant of myocardial oxygen utilization. Which of the following changes will reduce myocardial oxygen demand the most?

    (A) increasing left ventricular radius
    (B) increasing left ventricular pressure
    (C) increasing left ventricular wall thickness
    (D) increasing left ventricular stroke volume
    (E) increasing heart rate

17. Which of the following assessments of left ventricular function is independent of preload and afterload?

    (A) cardiac output
    (B) ejection fraction
    (C) wall stress
    (D) maximum dP/dt
    (E) end-systolic elastance

18. An increase in which of the following parameters will cause a decrease in cardiac output?

    (A) heart rate
    (B) contractility
    (C) afterload
    (D) preload
    (E) stroke volume

19. Left ventricular diastolic dysfunction is most likely indicated by which of the following findings?

    (A) Doppler echocardiography showing increased flow velocities across the aortic valve during diastole
    (B) Doppler echocardiography of mitral inflow with increased E wave and reduced A wave
    (C) tissue Doppler echocardiography of mitral annular velocities with e' wave greater than a' wave
    (D) ECG with widened QRS in V1
    (E) radionuclide study showing ejection fraction of 35%

20. Venous return may be augmented by:

    (A) increasing central venous pressure.
    (B) increasing intrathoracic pressure.
    (C) decreasing peripheral venous pressure.
    (D) decreasing venous resistance.
    (E) decreasing peripheral venous volume.

21. In comparison to control of arteriolar tone, which of the following factors is a major determinant of only venous tone?

    (A) basal tone
    (B) sympathetic mediated vasoconstriction
    (C) external compression
    (D) vasodilating metabolites
    (E) active myogenic response

22. Positive pressure ventilation (PPV) and PEEP can affect venous return. Which of the following mechanisms explains how PPV and PEEP may *increase* venous return?

    (A) increasing intra-abdominal pressure
    (B) increasing intra-abdominal vascular capacitance
    (C) increasing right atrial pressure
    (D) increasing intra-thoracic pressure
    (E) decreasing RV filling

23. Approximately what percentage of total circulating blood volume is contained in venules and veins?

    (A) 2%
    (B) 5%
    (C) 12%
    (D) 20%
    (E) 60%

24. Pulse pressure is indirectly proportional to which of the following variables?

    (A) heart rate
    (B) stroke volume
    (C) total peripheral resistance
    (D) arterial compliance
    (E) cardiac output

25. Mean arterial pressure (MAP) can be calculated by which of the following formulas?

    (A) MAP = cardiac output × total peripheral resistance
    (B) MAP = systolic pressure − diastolic pressure
    (C) MAP = diastolic pressure + 2/3(systolic pressure − diastolic pressure)
    (D) MAP = stroke volume × heart rate
    (E) MAP = 80 × (systolic pressure − central venous pressure)/cardiac output

26. A pulmonary artery catheter is placed in a surgical patient for intraoperative monitoring. For a normal patient, which of the following values is typically indicative of correct placement in the pulmonary artery?

    (A) mean <5 mm Hg
    (B) 25/5 mm Hg
    (C) 25/10 mm Hg
    (D) 130/8 mm Hg
    (E) 135/80 mm Hg

27. Which of the following changes will result in a decrease in pulmonary vascular resistance (PVR)?

    (A) increased lung volume above FRC
    (B) increased pulmonary blood volume
    (C) increased blood viscosity
    (D) increased alveolar pressure
    (E) increased interstitial pressure

28. Which of the following causes of hypotension is the result of decreased systemic vascular resistance (SVR)?

    (A) tension pneumothorax
    (B) cardiac tamponade
    (C) myocardial infarction
    (D) hemorrhage
    (E) liver failure

29. A patient's mean blood pressure remains the same, at approximately 80 mm Hg, while the pulse pressure increases. This increase in pulse pressure will affect baroreceptors in the carotid sinus and aortic arch resulting in which of the following changes?

    (A) increase in rate of discharge from the baroreceptors
    (B) profound bradycardia and hypotension (Bezold-Jarisch reflex)
    (C) excitation of sympathetic nerves facilitating long-term control of blood pressure
    (D) baroreceptor activity will only be elicited if mean blood pressure <50 mm Hg
    (E) no change in baroreceptor firing, as baroreceptors are more sensitive to changes in mean blood pressure rather than pulse pressure

30. Tissue edema due to heart failure is a result of:

    (A) decreased Starling forces.
    (B) increased capillary hydrostatic pressure.
    (C) increased capillary oncotic pressure.
    (D) increased interstitial oncotic pressure.
    (E) increased interstitial hydrostatic pressure.

31. Laminar blood flow in blood vessels will occur up to a critical velocity, then flow becomes turbulent. The probability of this can be expressed by which of the following?

    (A) Reynolds number
    (B) shear stress
    (C) Poiseuille-Hagen formula
    (D) viscosity
    (E) Law of Laplace

32. Which of the following changes will increase coronary perfusion pressure the most?

    (A) increased left ventricular end diastolic pressure
    (B) increased aortic diastolic pressure
    (C) increased heart rate
    (D) increased time in systole
    (E) increased aortic systolic pressure

33. In zone 1 of the lung, the relative effects of gravity and alveolar pressure on lung perfusion are best expressed as:

(A) $P_A > P_a > P_v$

(B) $P_a > P_A > P_v$

(C) $P_a > P_v > P_A$

(D) $P_v > P_A > P_a$

(E) $P_A > P_v > P_a$

34. Which part of the renal vasculature plays a role in counter-current exchange and regulating water balance?

(A) glomerulus

(B) vasa recta

(C) afferent arteriole

(D) efferent arteriole

(E) arcuate arteries

35. Which organ, at rest, extracts approximately 70% to 75% of the oxygen in the blood that flows through it?

(A) heart

(B) skeletal muscle

(C) liver

(D) kidneys

(E) brain

36. In an otherwise healthy patient, which of the following factors will decrease cerebral blood flow?

(A) decrease in MAP to 65 mm Hg

(B) hyperventilation

(C) hyperthermia

(D) pain

(E) volatile anesthetics

37. Uteroplacental blood flow changes dramatically as pregnancy progresses. Vessels vasodilate and undergo circumferential growth. Which of the following is implicated as the key factor for circumferential enlargement of uterine vessels?

(A) 17β-estradiol

(B) VEGF

(C) angiotensin II

(D) norepinephrine

(E) shear stress

38. Endogenous vasopressin is involved in a variety of homeostatic feedback mechanisms. Which of the following factors will decrease vasopressin secretion?

(A) pain

(B) angiotensin II

(C) increased extracellular fluid (ECF) volume

(D) increased plasma osmolality

(E) carbamazepine

39. Which of the following will cause an increase in renin secretion by the kidneys?

(A) increased afferent arteriole blood pressure

(B) increased Na^+ and Cl^- in the distal renal tubules

(C) norepinephrine

(D) vasopressin

(E) angiotensin II

40. Which of the following hormones will directly increase sodium and water retention by the kidneys?

(A) renin

(B) angiotensin I

(C) aldosterone

(D) bradykinin

(E) ANP

41. A patient is given a large intravenous fluid bolus of isotonic saline and their extracellular fluid (ECF) volume expands. Which of the following hormones is most likely to be released following activation of receptors in the ventricles of the heart?

(A) ANP

(B) BNP

(C) CNP

(D) vasopressin

(E) renin

Answers and Explanations: Cardiovascular Anatomy and Physiology

1. Which of the following statements regarding normal cardiac anatomy is TRUE?

   (A) The pulmonic valve is attached by chordae tendinae to the right ventricle.

   (B) The coronary sinus empties into the left atrium.

   (C) A patent foramen ovale is found in 25% to 30% of adults.

   (D) The ligamentum arteriosum connects the aorta to the pulmonary vein.

   (E) The root of the aorta is positioned between the left auricle and the pulmonary trunk.

The aortic and pulmonic valves are semilunar valves, with three cusps each. They are positioned at the base of the aorta and pulmonary trunk, respectively, and allow blood flow out of the ventricles. Closure of these valves at the end of systole by back pressure in the aorta and pulmonary trunk causes the second heart sound. There are no chordae tendinae attached to the semilunar valves; these structures connect the papillary muscles of the left and right ventricles to the cusps of the mitral and tricuspid valves, respectively.

The coronary sinus, the major drainage vessel of the heart, empties into the right atrium between the inferior vena cava and the tricuspid valve on the inferior aspect of the interatrial septum. Its valve is termed the Thebesian valve.

Both autopsy and transesophageal echocardiographic studies have found a prevalence of patent foramen ovale of approximately 25% to 30%. There appear to be no difference in prevalence rates between males and females. In patients with cryptogenic stroke, PFO prevalence is higher, between 40% and 45%.

The ligamentum arteriosum is the fibrous remains of the embryonic ductus arteriosus, a shunt that allows blood entering the pulmonary trunk to flow to the aorta prior to birth, as resistance to flow within the pulmonary system is high. It becomes fibrosed within three weeks of birth.

The aortic root is positioned in between the *right* auricle and the pulmonary trunk. The right auricle is located on the opposite side of the pulmonary trunk.

Ref: Fuster V, Walsh R, Harrington R. *Hurst's The Heart.* 13th ed. New York, NY: McGraw Hill; 2011.

2. Which of the following coronary vessels supplies the majority of the interventricular septum?

   (A) left coronary artery

   (B) left circumflex artery

   (C) left anterior descending artery

   (D) right coronary artery

   (E) posterior descending artery

The left and right coronary arteries arise from the left and right coronary sinus of the aortic root, respectively. These epicardial arteries traverse the surface of the heart, with the main branches located in the interventricular and atrioventricular sulci (Figure 4-1). The left coronary artery (LCA) gives rise to the left anterior descending (LAD), which travels down the anterior interventricular groove to the apex of the heart before continuing around the apex and up the posterior interventricular groove a variable distance, where it meets the posterior descending artery (PDA). The LAD supplies the anterior walls of both ventricles, the apex, and the anterior two thirds of the intraventricular septum.

The circumflex artery is a branch of the LCA that wraps around the heart between the left atrium and ventricle. The circumflex artery supplies the SA node in about 45% of people by sending a branch to the right atrium.

The right coronary artery (RCA) emerges between the pulmonary trunk and the right auricle, and runs in the coronary sulcus to the posterior aspect of the heart where it anastomoses with the circumflex branch of the LCA. It supplies the right atrium and ventricle, the SA node in 55% of people via the sinoatrial nodal branch, and the posterior one third of the intraventricular septum via the posterior descending artery.

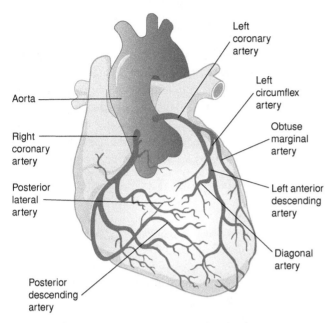

FIG. 4-1. Normal coronary anatomy. (Reproduced with permission from Longnecker DE, Brown DL, Newman MF, Zapol WM. *Anesthesiology*. 2nd ed. New York, NY: McGraw Hill; 2012.)

In roughly 15% of people, the posterior descending artery originates from the left circumflex artery. This is important because it means that the entire left ventricle (including all of the septum) is supplied by the left coronary artery.

Ref: Longnecker DE, Brown DL, Newman MF, Zapol WM. *Anesthesiology*. 2nd ed. New York, NY: McGraw Hill; 2012.

3. The left recurrent laryngeal nerve loops around which major vessel in the mediastinum?

(A) **aorta**

(B) superior vena cava

(C) left brachiocephalic vein

(D) left subclavian artery

(E) left pulmonary artery

The left and right recurrent laryngeal nerves are branches of the vagus nerves. The vagus nerves exit the carotid sheaths and descend into the thorax before giving rise to recurrent branches, which loop back superiorly between the trachea and esophagus. They then ascend to supply all of the intrinsic muscles of the larynx, except the cricothyroid muscles.

The right recurrent laryngeal nerve hooks around the right subclavian artery; the left hooks around the aortic arch, to the left of the ligamentum arteriosum. This difference is due to a quirk of embryology. The

arteries of the fourth pharyngeal arches are the right subclavian and the left-sided aortic arch. During fetal development, the recurrent laryngeal nerves, which originate from the sixth pharyngeal arch, are dragged down into the chest as the great arteries take their position. Because the aortic arch is located further caudad, the left recurrent laryngeal nerve is forced to take a longer course to reach the larynx.

Ref: Fuster V, Walsh R, Harrington R. *Hurst's The Heart*. 13th ed. New York, NY: McGraw Hill; 2011.

4. Which of the following statements BEST describes the function of the cardiac skeleton?

(A) It provides an anchor for the chordae tendinae to attach.

(B) It is the same structure as the fibrous pericardium.

(C) It provides a framework for the coronary arteries and veins.

(D) **It electrically insulates the atria from the ventricles.**

(E) It prevents excessive torsion of the heart during systole.

The cardiac skeleton is a dense fibrous connective tissue structure that surrounds and supports the valves, provides an anchor for cardiomyocytes from both the atria and the ventricles, and importantly, electrically insulates the atria from the ventricles, thereby preventing uncoordinated conduction of atrial impulses to the ventricular muscle. The collagen in the fibrous rings that surround all four valves (Figure 4-2) inhibits the

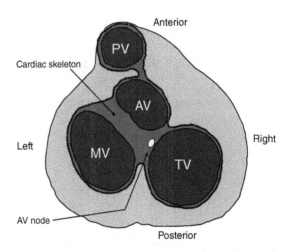

FIG. 4-2. A transverse section through the heart, showing the cardiac skeleton, the four valves, and the atrioventricular (AV) node. AV = aortic valve, MV = mitral valve, PV = pulmonary valve, TV = tricuspid valve.

transmission of electrical signals. The only electrical conduit between atria and ventricles is the AV node.

5. The cardiomyocytes of the apex of the heart are MOST likely innervated by which branch of the conducting system?

(A) the bundle of His
(B) the right bundle branch
(C) the left septal fascicle
(D) the left anterior fascicle
(E) **the left posterior fascicle**

Normal cardiac muscle cells do not depolarize spontaneously but require electrical activation by a cardiac conducting system. Generation of the normal ("sinus") impulse begins in the sinoatrial (SA) node, which is located in the right atrium at the junction of the superior vena cava. The atrioventricular (AV) node is located in the interatrial septum and extends through the cardiac skeleton, transmitting the electrical impulses through to the bundle of His. The SA and AV nodes are connected by three bundles of atrial fibers that are able to conduct action potentials more rapidly than the muscle cells themselves. These internodal pathways are termed the anterior, middle, and posterior tracts.

At the top of the interventricular septum, the bundle of His divides into right and left bundle branches, which run down the subendocardium of each ventricular septal wall and end by giving rise to Purkinje fibers (Figure 4-3). These fibers conduct the action potential to all parts of the ventricular myocardium. The left common bundle splits early into an anterior fascicle, which runs along the anterior aspect of the upper left ventricle, and the posterior fascicle, which continues down the septum to the apex. A third left fascicle, the septal fascicle, is present in approximately two thirds of people, and if present runs down the septum.

Ref: Barrett KE, Boitano S, Barman SM, Brooks HL. *Ganong's Review of Medical Physiology.* 24th ed. New York, NY: McGraw Hill; 2012.

6. Which of the following organs receives the MOST cardiac output at rest?

(A) heart
(B) **lungs**
(C) brain
(D) kidneys
(E) liver

In the absence of an intracardiac shunt, the lungs receive 100% of cardiac output, since the entire stroke volume of the right ventricle passes through the pulmonary system. Cardiac output to other organs is summarized in Table 4-1.

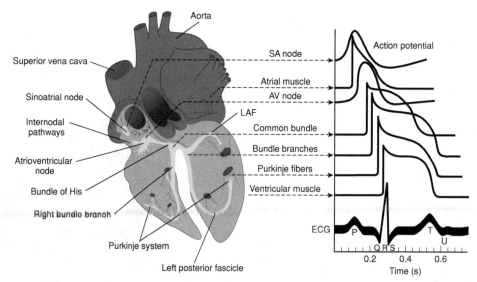

FIG. 4-3. Conducting system of the heart. **Left:** Anatomical depiction of the human heart with additional focus on areas of the conduction system. **Right:** Typical transmembrane action potentials for the SA and AV nodes, other parts of the conduction system, and the atrial and ventricular muscles are shown along with the correlation to the extracellularly recorded electrical activity, that is, the electrocardiogram (ECG). The action potentials and ECG are plotted on the same time axis but with different zero points on the vertical scale for comparison. LAF, left anterior fascicle. (Reproduced with permission from Barrett KE, Boitano S, Barman SM, Brooks HL. *Ganong's Review of Medical Physiology.* 24th ed. New York, NY: McGraw Hill; 2012.)

TABLE 4-1. Proportion of cardiac output delivered to various organ systems at rest.

Organ	Cardiac output
Skeletal muscle	15–20%
Kidneys	20%
Heart	4–5%
Brain	15%
Skin	4–5%
Liver	6%
Gastrointestinal system, spleen	20%

7. An anesthesiology resident, on a hiking vacation in the Pacific Northwest, comes face to face with a large grizzly bear. A "fight-or-flight" response ensues. How does sympathetic activation alter the intrinsic heart rate of the sinoatrial (SA) node?

(A) It increases permeability of resting membrane to K^+.

(B) It causes hyperpolarization of resting membrane potential.

(C) It releases acetylcholine.

(D) It decreases threshold potential of SA nodal cells.

(E) **It increases permeability of resting membrane to Na^+ and Ca^{2+}.**

Sympathetic activation of the sinoatrial node increases permeability of the resting membrane to Na^+ and Ca^{2+}.

The sympathetic and parasympathetic nervous systems are the primary influences on the intrinsic heart rate of the sinoatrial (SA) node.

Sympathetic activation via norepinephrine increases automaticity of the SA node (positive chronotropic effect). At a cellular level, norepinephrine acts via β_1 receptors and G_s proteins to increase intracellular cAMP and ultimately increases permeability of the resting membrane to Na^+ and Ca^{2+} (I_f, "funny current"). This increase in the rate of depolarization, as reflected by increased phase 4 slope of the action potential, causes the heart rate to increase.

Parasympathetic activation via acetylcholine decreases automaticity of the SA node (negative chronotropic effect). The human heart is under tonic parasympathetic control as the intrinsic heart rate of the SA node is approximately 100 beat/minute. At a cellular level, acetylcholine increases permeability of the resting membrane to K^+ and decreases the I_f. Together, this results in hyperpolarization of the resting membrane potential and decreases the rate of depolarization (decreased phase 4 slope of the action potential).

Note, the threshold potential of SA nodal cells (i.e., the membrane potential required for depolarization), is not altered by autonomic activity.

Ref: Mohrman DE, Heller LJ. *Cardiovascular Physiology*. 8th ed. New York, NY: McGraw Hill; 2014.

8. During a cardiac cycle, the beginning of isovolumetric contraction corresponds to which of the following events?

(A) **closure of atrioventricular valves**

(B) V wave on venous pulse

(C) opening of aortic valve

(D) P wave on ECG

(E) peak aortic blood flow

The cardiac cycle describes changes in the ventricles (such as pressure, flow, volume, ECG, and auscultatory events) over time. There are seven specific time periods:

1. Atrial systole
2. Isovolumetric contraction
3. Rapid ejection
4. Reduced ejection
5. Isovolumetric relaxation
6. Rapid ventricular filling
7. Diastasis (reduced ventricular filling)

Isovolumetric contraction refers to the time period when the atrioventricular valves (mitral, tricuspid) close and the aortic valve opens. It signals the initiation of ventricular systole, is associated with the first heart sound (S1), and the R and S waves of the ECG.

Other prominent events of the cardiac cycle include:

1. Atrial systole: P wave of the ECG, and the *a* wave of the venous pulse.

2. Rapid ejection: after opening of the aortic valve, rapid aortic blood flow, rapid increase in ventricular pressure, rapid decrease in ventricular volume, *c* wave of the venous pulse.

3. Reduced ejection: T wave of the ECG, from period of peak ventricular pressure until aortic valve closes, rapid decrease in aortic blood flow.

4. Isovolumetric relaxation: after closure of the aortic valve until the mitral valve opens, signals the initiation of ventricular diastole, rapid decrease in ventricular pressure, associated with lowest ventricular volume, second heart sound (S2), and *v* wave of venous pulse.

5. Rapid ventricular filling: after mitral opens, associated with rapid ventricular filling and reduced ventricular pressure due to continued ventricular relaxation. May be associated with third heart sound (S3).

6. Reduced ventricular filling (diastasis): associated with slow increase in ventricular pressure and volume, ends with onset of atrial systole and P wave of ECG.

Ref: Fuster V, Walsh R, Harrington R. *Hurst's The Heart.* 13th ed. New York, NY: McGraw Hill; 2011.

9. The sinoatrial node (SA node) rhythmically discharges. In phase 4 of the action potential, the "pacemaker potential" declines until the depolarization threshold is reached and the next impulse is triggered. During the late stages of phase 4, which of the following currents (I) is most predominant?

(A) I_f

(B) I_{CaL}

(C) I_{CaT}

(D) I_K

(E) I_{Na}

The I_{CaT} is the principal current responsible for the late stages of phase 4 of the SA node action potential.

The SA node action potential is made up of 3 phases (compared to phases 0–4 for action potentials in ventricular muscle). The principal current responsible for each phase of the SA node action potential is as follows:

- Phase 0: L-type Ca^{2+} channels (long-lasting) open and cause depolarization.

- Phase 3: At the peak of depolarization, outward K^+ current (I_K) initiates depolarization.

- Phase 4: Hyperpolarization activates a channel permeable to both Na^+ and K^+, which produces the "funny current'"(I_f). This initiates the depolarization of the "pacemaker potential." The late stages of this phase involve activation of T-type Ca^{2+} channels (transient-lasting). The I_{CaT} completes phase 4 and ends with the threshold for the next action potential.

Ref: Barrett KE, Boitano S, Barman SM, Brooks HL. *Ganong's Review of Medical Physiology.* 24th ed. New York, NY: McGraw Hill; 2012.

10. Which of the following cardiac events does the PR interval of the ECG correspond to?

(A) atrial depolarization

(B) ventricular depolarization

(C) plateau phase of ventricular depolarization

(D) **atrial depolarization and AV nodal conduction**

(E) ventricular repolarization

The PR interval corresponds to atrial depolarization and AV nodal conduction.

The electrocardiogram (ECG) is a measure of the electrical activity of the heart. The P wave represents atrial depolarization. The QRS complex represents ventricular depolarization, while the T wave represents ventricular repolarization. The ST segment corresponds to the plateau phase of ventricular depolarization. The QT interval corresponds to ventricular systole.

Refs: Fuster V, Walsh R, Harrington R. *Hurst's The Heart.* 13th ed. New York, NY: McGraw Hill; 2011.

Mohrman DE, Heller LJ. *Cardiovascular Physiology.* 8th ed. New York, NY: McGraw Hill; 2014.

11. Which of the following cardiac tissues has the slowest rate of conduction?

(A) tract of Wenckebach

(B) **AV node**

(C) bundle of His

(D) Purkinje system

(E) ventricular muscle

The AV node has the slowest rate of conduction (0.05 m/s) of any of the listed cardiac tissues. Conduction rates for other cardiac tissues are:

- SA node = 0.05 m/s
- Atrial pathways (e.g., tract of Wenckebach) = 1 m/s
- Bundle of His = 1 m/s
- Purkinje system = 4 m/s
- Ventricular muscle = 1 m/s

Atrial depolarization from the SA node to the AV node is fast (~0.1 second). The AV node is relatively slow and delays conduction to the ventricles by an additional 0.1 second. This is important to ensure atrial contraction is complete before ventricular contraction begins and it also prevents rapid atrial rhythms from being transmitted to the ventricles.

Ref: Mohrman DE, Heller LJ. *Cardiovascular Physiology.* 8th ed. New York, NY: McGraw Hill; 2014.

12. A curve of left ventricular pressure vs. time is depicted in Figure 4-4 below. Which part of the left ventricular pressure-time curve represents the maximal rate of force development by the ventricle?

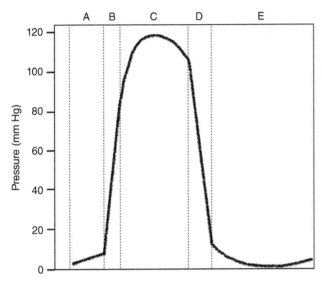

FIG. 4-4. Left ventricular pressure-time curve.

(A) A

(B) **B**

(C) C

(D) D

(E) E

B = slope of ascending limb of the pressure-time curve. This is a measure of change in pressure over time (dP/dt) during isovolumetric contraction. This represents the maximal rate of force (pressure change) development by the ventricle. Doppler echocardiography may be used to make this determination. This reflects contractility at a given set of ventricular loading conditions (preload and afterload).

A = end-diastolic pressure

C = top of curve = ejection phase

D = isovolumetric relaxation (down slope of curve)

E = rapid ventricular filling

Refs: Koeppen BM, Stanton BA. *Berne and Levy Physiology.* 6th ed. Philadelphia, PA: Mosby Elsevier; 2010.

Fuster V, Walsh R, Harrington R. *Hurst's The Heart.* 13th ed. New York, NY: McGraw Hill; 2011.

13. The Frank-Starling law of the heart describes the relationship between cardiac output and which of the following variables?

(A) left ventricular contractility

(B) heart rate

(C) cardiac rhythm

(D) **left ventricular end-diastolic volume**

(E) left ventricular compliance

The Frank-Starling law of the heart describes the relationship between cardiac output (or stroke volume) and left ventricular end-diastolic volume (LVEDV) or preload. If other determinants of cardiac function (contractility, heart rate, and afterload) are held constant, a plot of cardiac output versus LVEDV is relatively linear (for the normal heart); keeping with the adage "the heart pumps what it receives."

An increase in contractility (e.g., exercise) will shift the Frank-Starling curve to the left (increased cardiac output). A decrease in contractility (e.g., heart failure) will shift the curve down and to the right (decreased cardiac output and increased LVEDV).

Ventricular compliance is a plot of end-diastolic pressure vs. end-diastolic volume.

Ref: Butterworth JF IV, Mackey DC, Wasnick JD. *Morgan and Mikhail's Clinical Anesthesiology.* 5th ed. New York, NY: McGraw Hill; 2013.

14. How does an increase in afterload affect the Frank-Starling curve?

(A) Shifts curve down and to the left.

(B) **Shifts curve down and to the right.**

(C) Shifts curve up and to the left.

(D) Shifts curve up and to the right.

(E) No change.

Changes in cardiac determinants such as preload, afterload and contractility can affect the Frank-Starling curve (Figure 4-5). Changes in preload result in changes along the *same* line of the Frank-Starling curve. Changes in afterload or contractility will result in a shift to a *new* Frank-Starling curve:

• Afterload. An increase in afterload shifts the curve down and to the right (as cardiac output/stroke volume is decreased). A decrease in afterload shifts the curve up and to the left (as cardiac output/stroke volume at given preload increases)

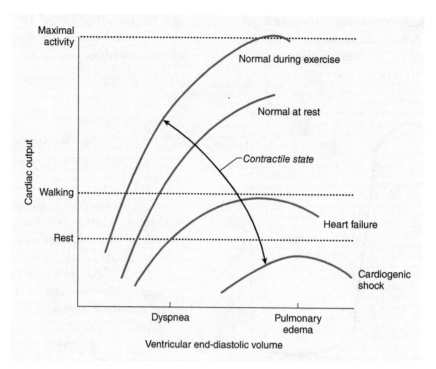

FIG. 4-5. Starling's law of the heart. (Reproduced with permission from Butterworth JF IV, Mackey DC, Wasnick JD. *Morgan and Mikhail's Clinical Anesthesiology.* 5th ed. New York, NY: McGraw Hill; 2013.)

- Contractility. An increase in contractility (e.g., exercise) will shift the Frank-Starling curve up and to the left (increased cardiac output). A decrease in contractility (e.g., heart failure) will shift the curve down and to the right (decreased cardiac output and increased LVEDV).

Ref: Fuster V, Walsh R, Harrington R. *Hurst's The Heart.* 13th ed. New York, NY: McGraw Hill; 2011.

15. Which phase of the cardiac cycle is associated with the greatest proportion of myocardial oxygen consumption?

    (A) rapid ventricular ejection
    (B) atrial systole
    (C) **isovolumetric contraction**
    (D) rapid ventricular filling
    (E) isovolumetric relaxation

The isovolumetric contraction phase of the cardiac cycle is responsible for approximately 50% of myocardial oxygen consumption.

In general, the heart's basal metabolism is responsible for 25% of myocardial energy use, while contraction is responsible for the remaining 75%. The cardiac cycle describes changes in the ventricles (such as pressure,

flow, volume, ECG, and auscultatory events) over time. There are seven specific time periods:

1. Atrial systole
2. Isovolumetric contraction
3. Rapid ejection
4. Reduced ejection
5. Isovolumetric relaxation
6. Rapid ventricular filling
7. Reduced ventricular filling—diastasis

Ref: Mohrman DE, Heller LJ. *Cardiovascular Physiology.* 8th ed. New York, NY: McGraw Hill; 2014.

16. Left ventricular wall stress or tension is a determinant of myocardial oxygen utilization. Which of the following changes will reduce myocardial oxygen demand the most?

    (A) increasing left ventricular radius
    (B) increasing left ventricular pressure
    (C) **increasing left ventricular wall thickness**
    (D) increasing left ventricular stroke volume
    (E) increasing heart rate

Increasing left ventricular wall thickness will reduce left ventricular wall stress and reduce myocardial oxygen demand.

Myocardial oxygen consumption is related to myocardial wall tension, contractility, and heart rate. The Law of Laplace:

$$\text{LV wall stress} = \frac{\text{LV pressure} \times \text{radius}}{2 \times \text{LV wall thickness}}$$

Reductions in left ventricular pressure or left ventricular radius will also reduce LV wall stress and myocardial oxygen demand.

Left ventricular stroke work also correlates with oxygen consumption:

$$\text{LV stroke work} = \text{stroke volume} \times \text{MAP}$$

As from the formula above, stroke work can be viewed as either "volume work" or "pressure work." It is important to note that a greater increase in oxygen consumption occurs due to increases in pressure work compared to similar increases in volume work (mechanism remains unknown).

Ref: Barrett KE, Boitano S, Barman SM, Brooks HL. *Ganong's Review of Medical Physiology.* 24th ed. New York, NY: McGraw Hill; 2012.

17. Which of the following assessments of left ventricular function is independent of preload and afterload?

(A) cardiac output
(B) ejection fraction
(C) wall stress
(D) maximum dP/dt
(E) **end-systolic elastance**

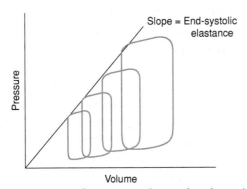

FIG. 4-6. Calculation of time-varying elastance based on variably loaded pressure-volume loops. A family of loops is created by abruptly changing preload, typically with inferior vena caval occlusion. End-systolic elastance is the slope of the line connecting the end-systolic points of each loop and is a load-independent index of contractility. (Reproduced with permission from Mathew JP, Swaminathan M, Ayoub CM. *Clinical Manual and Review of Transesophageal Echocardiography.* 2nd ed. New York, NY: McGraw Hill; 2010.)

End-systolic elastance is an index of contractility, which is independent of preload and afterload. As shown in the Figure 4-6, end-systolic elastance can be calculated as the slope of various pressure-volume loops.

Cardiac output (stroke volume × heart rate) is a measure of ventricular systolic function, diastolic function, pericardial function, and valvular function. Ventricular systolic function is dependent on myocardial contractility, preload, and afterload.

Left ventricular ejection fraction, wall stress, and maximum dP/dt are all load dependent indices (i.e., altered preload and afterload will affect measure of left ventricular performance).

Ref: Mathew JP, Swaminathan M, Ayoub CM. *Clinical Manual and Review of Transesophageal Echocardiography.* 2nd ed. New York, NY: McGraw Hill; 2010.

18. An increase in which of the following parameters will cause a decrease in cardiac output?

(A) heart rate
(B) contractility
(C) **afterload**
(D) preload
(E) stroke volume

An increase in afterload will cause a decrease in cardiac output.

$$\text{Cardiac output} = \text{stroke volume} \times \text{heart rate}$$

Stroke volume is directly proportional to preload and contractility and inversely proportional to afterload. Therefore, increases in heart rate, preload, and contractility will increase cardiac output, while a decrease in afterload will increase cardiac output.

Ref: Barrett KE, Boitano S, Barman SM, Brooks HL. *Ganong's Review of Medical Physiology.* 24th ed. New York, NY: McGraw Hill; 2012.

19. Left ventricular diastolic dysfunction is most likely indicated by which of the following findings?

(A) Doppler echocardiography showing increased flow velocities across the aortic valve during diastole
(B) **Doppler echocardiography of mitral inflow with increased E wave and reduced A wave**
(C) tissue Doppler echocardiography of mitral annular velocities with e' wave greater than a' wave
(D) ECG with widened QRS in V1
(E) radionuclide study showing ejection fraction of 35%

Left ventricular diastolic dysfunction is suggested by Doppler echocardiography of mitral inflow with increased E wave and reduced A wave (restrictive pattern). Pulsed-wave Doppler echocardiography can measure the inflow velocities across the mitral valve. There are two characteristic waves during diastole: E wave = early filling of the ventricle, and A wave = active filling during atrial contraction. The normal E wave is greater than the A wave. Pulsed-wave tissue Doppler echocardiography can measure the velocity of the ventricular wall.

When placed at the lateral wall of the mitral annulus, tissue Doppler shows two characteristic waves during diastole: e' = early myocardial relaxation, and a' = atrial contraction. In the normal ventricle, the, e' wave is larger than the a' wave. As diastolic dysfunction progresses, e' wave gets progressively smaller.

ECG findings of left atrial enlargement include a biphasic P wave in lead V1 with terminal negative portion (P mitrale) and a notched P wave in lead II. The differential diagnosis of left atrial enlargement is broad and includes left ventricular diastolic dysfunction, mitral stenosis, and mitral regurgitation.

Left ventricular ejection fraction, which can be determined via radionuclide imaging, cardiac catheterization, or echocardiography, is a measure of left ventricular systolic function.

Ref: Butterworth JF IV, Mackey DC, Wasnick JD. *Morgan and Mikhail's Clinical Anesthesiology.* 5th ed. New York, NY: McGraw Hill; 2013.

20. Venous return may be augmented by:

(A) increasing central venous pressure.
(B) increasing intrathoracic pressure.
(C) decreasing peripheral venous pressure.
(D) decreasing venous resistance.
(E) decreasing peripheral venous volume.

Venous return may be augmented by decreasing venous resistance.

Venous return is the rate of blood return from the peripheral venous compartment to the central venous compartment. The central venous compartment includes the blood in the right atrium and veins in the thorax, with the more peripheral vessels making up the peripheral venous compartment.

The rate of venous return = Δ pressure/resistance.

$$\Delta \text{ pressure} = \text{peripheral venous pressure} - \text{central venous pressure}$$

resistance = resistance of peripheral veins

Factors that can affect venous return include:

- Peripheral venous pressure. Decreasing peripheral venous pressure will decrease the gradient for venous return.
- Central venous pressure. Increasing central venous pressure will decrease the gradient for venous return.
- Intrathoracic pressure. Increasing intrathoracic pressure will compress the central veins and decrease venous return.
- Peripheral venous volume. Decreasing peripheral venous volume will decrease venous return.

Ref: Mohrman DE, Heller LJ. *Cardiovascular Physiology.* 8th ed. New York, NY: McGraw Hill; 2014.

21. In comparison to control of arteriolar tone, which of the following factors is a major determinant of only venous tone?

(A) basal tone
(B) sympathetic mediated vasoconstriction
(C) external compression
(D) vasodilating metabolites
(E) active myogenic response

A major determinant of venous tone is external compression. External compression does not play a significant role in control of arteriolar tone. In comparison to arterioles, veins are typically in a dilated state without significant basal tone, veins have little response to vasodilating metabolites, and venous diameter is proportional to internal venous pressure.

Vascular tone of arterioles is regulated via a number of different mechanisms:

- Basal tone. Arterioles have a baseline degree of vasoconstriction.
- Metabolites. Decreased oxygen levels cause vasodilation. while increased carbon dioxide levels, acidemia, and hyperkalemia also cause vasodilation (note that local metabolites play the most prominent role in autoregulation of blood flow in arterioles).
- Transmural pressure. Arterioles have both a passive and an active response to changes in transmural pressure. Initially, increased pressure causes passive distension, which is followed by an active myogenic response which causes vasoconstriction to counteract the initial distension.
- Neural influences. Sympathetic-mediated vasoconstriction of arterioles is due to norepinephrine acting via α_1 adrenergic receptors.

- Hormones. Circulating epinephrine, norepinephrine, vasopressin, and angiotensin II all may play a role in regulating vascular tone, albeit to a lesser extent than local metabolites or neural influences.

Ref: Mohrman DE, Heller LJ. *Cardiovascular Physiology.* 8th ed. New York, NY: McGraw Hill; 2014.

22. Positive pressure ventilation (PPV) and PEEP can affect venous return. Which of the following mechanisms explains how PPV and PEEP may *increase* venous return?

(A) **increasing intra-abdominal pressure**
(B) increasing intra-abdominal vascular capacitance
(C) increasing right atrial pressure
(D) increasing intra-thoracic pressure
(E) decreasing RV filling

PPV and PEEP increase intra-thoracic pressure and right atrial pressure. This decreases the gradient for venous return and results in decreased RV filling and RV stroke volume (Note: spontaneous ventilation does the opposite). However, PPV and PEEP can also have a "preload-sparing" effect by causing diaphragmatic descent into the abdomen. The abdomen is a store of venous blood and diaphragmatic descent leads to increased intra-abdominal pressure, decreased intra-abdominal capacitance, and increased venous return.

Ref: Tobin MJ. *Principles and Practice of Mechanical Ventilation.* 3rd ed. New York, NY: McGraw Hill; 2013.

23. Approximately what percentage of total circulating blood volume is contained in venules and veins?

(A) 2%
(B) 5%
(C) 12%
(D) 20%
(E) **60%**

Most of the circulating blood, approximately 60%, is contained in venules and veins. Approximately 12% is in arteries, 2% in arterioles, 5% in capillaries, and 20% in the pulmonary system and heart chambers.

Ref: Mohrman DE, Heller LJ. *Cardiovascular Physiology.* 8th ed. New York, NY: McGraw Hill; 2014.

24. Pulse pressure is indirectly proportional to which of the following variables?

(A) heart rate
(B) stroke volume

(C) total peripheral resistance
(D) **arterial compliance**
(E) cardiac output

Pulse pressure is indirectly proportional to arterial compliance: Pulse pressure ~ stroke volume/arterial compliance. This helps to explain that as you age and arterial compliance decreases, pulse pressure generally increases. Pulse pressure also equals systolic pressure minus diastolic pressure.

Ref: Mohrman DE, Heller LJ. *Cardiovascular Physiology.* 8th ed. New York, NY: McGraw Hill; 2014.

25. Mean arterial pressure (MAP) can be calculated by which of the following formulas?

(A) **MAP = cardiac output × total peripheral resistance**
(B) MAP = systolic pressure − diastolic pressure
(C) MAP = diastolic pressure + 2/3(systolic pressure − diastolic pressure)
(D) MAP = stroke volume × heart rate
(E) MAP = 80 × (systolic pressure − central venous pressure)/cardiac output

Mean arterial pressure (MAP) = cardiac output × total peripheral resistance. MAP can also be approximated by the following equation:

- MAP = diastolic pressure + 1/3 (systolic pressure − diastolic pressure)
- Arterial pulse pressure = systolic pressure − diastolic pressure.
- Cardiac output = stroke volume × heart rate.
- Systemic vascular resistance = 80 × (MAP − CVP)/cardiac output

Ref: Mohrman DE, Heller LJ. *Cardiovascular Physiology.* 8th ed. New York, NY: McGraw Hill; 2014.

26. A pulmonary artery catheter is placed in a surgical patient for intraoperative monitoring. For a normal patient, which of the following values is typically indicative of correct placement in the pulmonary artery?

(A) mean <5 mm Hg
(B) 25/5 mm Hg
(C) **25/10 mm Hg**
(D) 130/8 mm Hg
(E) 135/80 mm Hg

Normal values for hemodynamic parameters measured by a pulmonary artery catheter (PAC) include:

- central venous pressure ~5 mm Hg
- right ventricular pressure 25/5 mm Hg
- pulmonary artery pressure 25/10 mm Hg

When a PAC is floated the pressure waveform tracing shows characteristic changes as it moves from the right atrium, right ventricle, and into the pulmonary artery. Since the pulmonary artery has a higher diastolic pressure than the right ventricle, the PAC waveform shows a characteristic "step-up" change when successfully passed through the pulmonic valve (Figure 4-7).

Other typical pressures (not measured by a pulmonary artery catheter) include:

left ventricular pressure 130/8 mm Hg and aortic pressure 135/80.

Refs: Longnecker DE, Brown DL, Newman MF, Zapol WM. *Anesthesiology.* 2nd ed. New York, NY: McGraw Hill; 2012.

Wasnick JD, Hillel Z, Kramer DC, Littwin S, Nicoara A. *Cardiac Anesthesia and Transesophageal Echocardiography.* New York, NY: McGraw Hill; 2011.

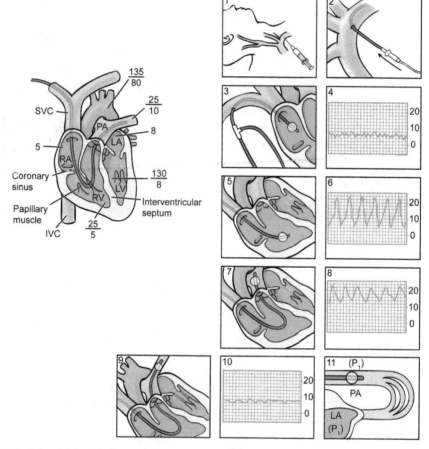

FIG. 4-7. Although its utility is increasingly questioned, pulmonary artery catheters continue to be a part of perioperative management of the cardiac surgery patient. Following placement of a sheath introducer in the central circulation (panels 1 and 2), the pulmonary artery catheter is "floated." Central line placement should always be completed using rigorous sterile technique, full body draping, and only after multiple, redundant confirmations of the correct localization of the venous circulation. Pressure guidance is used to ascertain the localization of the PA catheter in the venous circulation and the heart. Upon entry into the right atrium (panels 3 and 4), the central venous pressure tracing is noted. Passing through the tricuspid valve (panels 5 and 6) right ventricular pressures are detected. At 35 to 50 cm, depending upon patient size, the catheter will pass from the right ventricle through the pulmonic valve into the pulmonary artery (panels 7 and 8). This is noted by the measurement of diastolic pressure once the pulmonic valve is passed.

Lastly, when indicated the balloon-tipped catheter will "wedge" or "occlude" a pulmonary artery branch (panels 9–11). When this occurs, the pulmonary artery pressure equilibrates with that of the left atrium which barring any mitral valve pathology should be a reflection of left ventricular end-diastolic pressure. (Reproduced with permission from Soni N. *Practical Procedures in Anasthesia and Intensive Care.* Boston, MA: Butterworth Heinemann; 1994:43, with permission.)

27. Which of the following changes will result in a decrease in pulmonary vascular resistance (PVR)?

    (A) increased lung volume above FRC
    (B) **increased pulmonary blood volume**
    (C) increased blood viscosity
    (D) increased alveolar pressure
    (E) increased interstitial pressure

A variety of factors may affect pulmonary vascular resistance. These may be classified as neural, humoral, or "passive":

- Neural: Sympathetic activation increases PVR; parasympathetic activation decreases PVR.
- Humoral: α-adrenergic agonists, $PGF_{2\alpha}$, PGE_2, thromboxane, endothelin, angiotensin increase PVR; acetylcholine, β-adrenergic agonists, PGE_1, prostacyclin, nitric oxide, and bradykinin decrease PVR.

"Passive" factors include gravity and body position, lung volume, alveolar pressure/intrapleural pressure, interstitial pressure, blood viscosity, pulmonary artery pressure/blood volume, and cardiac output.

These are considered "passive" factors as pulmonary vasculature has relatively small amounts of smooth muscle. This means PVR is more sensitive to extravascular effects and changes in transmural pressure, in contrast to systemic vasculature and SVR.

Increased pulmonary blood volume causes a decrease in PVR. Recruitment and distention are responsible for this effect. Recruitment occurs as increased pulmonary blood volume opens previously under- or nonperfused capillaries (at normal cardiac output approximately one half of capillaries are not perfused). Distention describes how the radius of a pulmonary vessel will increase in response to increased perfusion pressure, with a resultant decrease in resistance.

Lung volumes above and below FRC increase PVR (above FRC alveolar vessels are compressed, below FRC extra-alveolar vessels are compressed). Increased blood viscosity directly increases PVR and increased alveolar pressure (such as with application of PEEP) can lead to compression of alveolar vessels and increased PVR. Increased interstitial pressure (e.g., congestive heart failure) decreases the transmural pressure gradient for extra-alveolar vessels, leading to compression and increased PVR.

Ref: Levitzky MG. *Pulmonary Physiology.* 8th ed. New York, NY: McGraw Hill; 2013.

28. Which of the following causes of hypotension is the result of decreased systemic vascular resistance (SVR)?

    (A) tension pneumothorax
    (B) cardiac tamponade
    (C) myocardial infarction
    (D) hemorrhage
    (E) **liver failure**

Blood pressure = cardiac output × SVR. Therefore, hypotension is a result of either decreased cardiac output, decreased SVR, or both. Hypovolemia due to hemorrhage, burns, vomiting, and so on is a result of decreased cardiac output with increased SVR.

Cardiogenic causes of hypotension such as myocardial infarction, arrhythmias, or valvular heart disease is a result of decreased cardiac output with increased SVR.

Obstructive causes of hypotension such as tension pneumothorax, cardiac tamponade, or pulmonary embolus is a result of decreased cardiac output with increased SVR.

Distributive causes of hypotension such as sepsis, pancreatitis, thyrotoxicosis, anaphylaxis, spinal cord injury, and liver failure are a result of decreased SVR with increased cardiac output.

Ref: Wasnick JD, Hillel Z, Kramer DC, Littwin S, Nicoara A. *Cardiac Anesthesia and Transesophageal Echocardiography.* New York, NY: McGraw Hill; 2011.

29. A patient's mean blood pressure remains the same, at approximately 80 mm Hg, while the pulse pressure increases. This increase in pulse pressure will affect baroreceptors in the carotid sinus and aortic arch resulting in which of the following changes?

    (A) **increase in rate of discharge from the baroreceptors**
    (B) profound bradycardia and hypotension (Bezold-Jarisch reflex)
    (C) excitation of sympathetic nerves facilitating long-term control of blood pressure
    (D) baroreceptor activity will only be elicited if mean blood pressure <50 mm Hg
    (E) no change in baroreceptor firing, as baroreceptors are more sensitive to changes in mean blood pressure rather than pulse pressure

Baroreceptors in the carotid sinus and aortic arch respond to stretch. An increase in blood pressure and distention leads to increased rate of discharge from the baroreceptors. Activation of the baroreceptor reflex results in inhibition of sympathetic activity and excitation of parasympathetic (vagal) activity. Overall, an increase in blood pressure/stretch is met with reflex vasodilation, hypotension, and bradycardia. This is an important reflex for short-term adjustments in blood pressure such as changes in posture or during exercise.

Although they are more sensitive to changes in pulse pressure, baroreceptors respond both to changes in mean blood pressure and pulse pressure. More baroreceptor activity occurs during systole than diastole; and the threshold for baroreceptor activity is approximately 50 mm Hg to 200 mm Hg.

The Bezold-Jarisch reflex refers to activation of vagal C fibers in the cardiopulmonary region (atria, ventricles, pulmonary vessels) which results in bradycardia, hypotension, and a period of apnea.

Ref: Barrett KE, Boitano S, Barman SM, Brooks HL. *Ganong's Review of Medical Physiology.* 24th ed. New York, NY: McGraw Hill; 2012.

30. Tissue edema due to heart failure is a result of:

    (A) decreased Starling forces.

    (B) **increased capillary hydrostatic pressure.**

    (C) increased capillary oncotic pressure.

    (D) increased interstitial oncotic pressure.

    (E) increased interstitial hydrostatic pressure.

    The Starling equation describes how hydrostatic and oncotic pressures (the Starling forces) determine the movement of fluid between the intravascular space and the interstitial space. Tissue edema due to heart failure is a result of increased capillary hydrostatic pressure, which causes movement of fluid from the intravascular space to the interstitial space. Tissue edema may also occur when there is decreased capillary oncotic pressure (e.g., nephrotic syndrome).

    Ref: Kasper D, Fauci A, Hauser S, Longo D, Jameson J, Loscalzo J. *Harrison's Principles of Internal Medicine.* 19th ed. New York, NY: McGraw Hill; 2015.

31. Laminar blood flow in blood vessels will occur up to a critical velocity, then flow becomes turbulent. The probability of this can be expressed by which of the following?

    (A) **Reynolds number**

    (B) shear stress

    (C) Poiseuille-Hagen formula

    (D) viscosity

    (E) Law of Laplace

Reynolds number (Re) describes the probability at which flow will become turbulent. It relates density of the fluid (ρ), diameter of the tube (D), velocity of flow (V), and viscosity of the fluid (η):

$$Re = \frac{\rho D \dot{V}}{\eta}$$

Law of Laplace describes how tension in the wall of cylinder (T) relates to transmural pressure (P), radius (r), and wall thickness (w):

$$T = Pr/w$$

Viscosity describes a fluid's innate resistance to flow (blood's viscosity is 3–4× greater than water). The Poiseuille-Hagen formula describes flow in a narrow tube (F) as it relates to the pressure difference between the two ends ($P_A - P_B$), viscosity of the fluid (η), radius of the tube (r), length of the tube (L):

$$F = (P_A - P_B) \times \left(\frac{\pi}{8}\right) \times \left(\frac{1}{\eta}\right) \times \left(\frac{r^4}{L}\right)$$

This formula can be reworked to describe resistance (R) in the tube:

$$R = \frac{8\eta L}{\pi r^4}$$

This shows resistance to flow is proportional to the fourth power of the radius of the vessel (and why arterioles are effective at regulating organ blood flow). Shear stress describes the force on the endothelium of the blood vessel as blood flows by. Shear stress (γ) is proportional to viscosity (η) and shear rate (dy/dr):

$$\gamma = \eta(dy/dr)$$

Ref: Barrett KE, Boitano S, Barman SM, Brooks HL. *Ganong's Review of Medical Physiology.* 24th ed. New York, NY: McGraw Hill; 2012.

32. Which of the following changes will increase coronary perfusion pressure the most?

    (A) increased left ventricular end diastolic pressure

    (B) **increased aortic diastolic pressure**

    (C) increased heart rate

    (D) increased time in systole

    (E) increased aortic systolic pressure

Coronary perfusion pressure = arterial diastolic pressure − LVEDP.

The force of left ventricular contraction means that coronary perfusion occurs mostly during diastole. Therefore, increased aortic diastolic pressure will increase coronary perfusion pressure. Anything that increases LVEDP or shortens diastole (e.g., increased heart rate) will decrease coronary perfusion pressure. Arterial diastolic pressure is more important than systolic pressure or mean pressure in determining coronary perfusion pressure.

Ref: Butterworth JF IV, Mackey DC, Wasnick JD. *Morgan and Mikhail's Clinical Anesthesiology.* 5th ed. New York, NY: McGraw Hill; 2013.

33. In zone 1 of the lung, the relative effects of gravity and alveolar pressure on lung perfusion are best expressed as:

(A) $P_A > P_a > P_v$

(B) $P_a > P_A > P_v$

(C) $P_a > P_v > P_A$

(D) $P_v > P_A > P_a$

(E) $P_A > P_v > P_a$

Alveolar dead space (zone 1 of the lung), refers to conditions where alveolar pressure (P_A) is greater than pulmonary artery pressure (P_a) and no blood flow occurs (i.e., the lung is ventilated but not perfused):

$$P_A > P_a > P_v.$$

The middle area of the lung (zone 2) refers to conditions where pulmonary artery pressure (P_a) is greater than alveolar pressure (P_A) which is greater than pulmonary vein pressure (P_v): $P_a > P_A > P_v$. The effective driving pressure for blood flow is $P_a - P_A$.

The bottom area of the lung (zone 3) refers to conditions where pulmonary artery pressure is greater than pulmonary vein pressure which is greater than alveolar pressure: $P_a > P_v > P_A$.

Ref: Levitzky MG. *Pulmonary Physiology.* 8th ed. New York, NY: McGraw Hill; 2013.

34. Which part of the renal vasculature plays a role in counter-current exchange and regulating water balance?

(A) glomerulus

(B) vasa recta

(C) afferent arteriole

(D) efferent arteriole

(E) arcuate arteries

Blood reaches each kidney via a renal artery, which then further divides, eventually leading to arcuate arteries which are at the junction of the renal cortex and renal medulla. Arcuate arteries give rise to interlobular arteries (cortical arteries), which then branch into afferent arterioles. Afferent arterioles supply glom-

eruli and blood is then taken via efferent arterioles to either peritubular capillaries or vasa recta. Peritubular capillaries are found in the renal cortex. Efferent arterioles of juxtamedullary glomeruli branch and descend into the medulla as the vasa recta. A relatively small amount of blood flow reaches the inner medulla. In this way the vasa recta plays a role in counter-current exchange and regulating water balance.

Ref: Eaton DC, Pooler JP. *Vander's Renal Physiology.* 8th ed. New York, NY: McGraw Hill; 2013.

35. Which organ, at rest, extracts ~70–75% of the oxygen in the blood that flows through it?

(A) heart

(B) skeletal muscle

(C) liver

(D) kidneys

(E) brain

In general, the oxygen extraction ratio (oxygen consumption/oxygen delivery) for the body is ~20% to 30%. However, at rest the heart extracts ~70% to 75% of the oxygen delivered via coronary blood flow. This means the myocardium is sensitive to alterations in coronary blood flow and an increase in myocardial oxygen consumption requires an increase in coronary blood flow.

The oxygen extraction ratio for other organs varies:

- brain approximately 30%
- skeletal muscle approximately 25% to 30%
- splanchnic (GI tract, spleen, pancreas, liver) approximately 15% to 20%
- kidneys <15%

Ref: Mohrman DE, Heller LJ. *Cardiovascular Physiology.* 8th ed. New York, NY: McGraw Hill; 2014.

36. In an otherwise healthy patient, which of the following factors will decrease cerebral blood flow?

(A) decrease in MAP to 65 mm Hg

(B) hyperventilation

(C) hyperthermia

(D) pain

(E) volatile anesthetics

Changes in P_aCO_2 alter cerebral vascular resistance. Hyperventilation causes cerebral vasoconstriction, decreased cerebral blood flow, and decreased intracranial pressure. Aggressive hyperventilation (P_aCO_2 <20–25 mm Hg) can potentially cause cerebral ischemia and should be avoided. Cerebral blood flow is autoregulated between cerebral perfusion pressures of approximately 50% and 150 mm Hg. In an otherwise healthy patient, a MAP of 65 mm Hg is within this zone of autoregulation so cerebral blood flow should not change.

Other causes of increased cerebral blood flow (and increased intracranial pressure) include: acidosis, hypoventilation, hyperthermia, hypoxia, pain, seizures, and, volatile anesthetics. The management of elevated intracranial pressure often requires manipulation of these elements.

Ref: Hall JB, Schmidt GA, Kress JP. *Principles of Critical Care.* 4th ed. New York, NY: McGraw Hill; 2015.

37. Uteroplacental blood flow changes dramatically as pregnancy progresses. Vessels vasodilate and undergo circumferential growth. Which of the following is implicated as the key factor for circumferential enlargement of uterine vessels?

   (A) 17β-estradiol
   (B) VEGF
   (C) angiotensin II
   (D) norepinephrine
   (E) **shear stress**

At term pregnancy, uterine blood flow is approximately 500 to 750 mL/min. This increase in blood flow during gestation is due to vasodilation mediated by 17β-estradiol, progesterone, and relaxin. Uterine vessel vasodilation results in increased shear stress, which leads to circumferential vessel growth. Mechanisms for how shear stress causes circumferential vessel growth are not completely understood, but nitric oxide is believed to play an important role. Other factors thought to have a role in uterine vascular remodeling include angiotensin II and VEGF (vascular endothelial growth factor).

Refs: Cunningham FG, Leveno KJ, Bloom SL, Spong CY, Dashe JS, Hoffman BL, et al. *Williams Obstetrics.* 24th ed. New York, NY: McGraw Hill; 2014.
   Osol G, Mandala M. Maternal uterine vascular remodeling during pregnancy. *Physiology.* 2009; 24:58–71.

38. Endogenous vasopressin is involved in a variety of homeostatic feedback mechanisms. Which of the following factors will decrease vasopressin secretion?

   (A) pain
   (B) angiotensin II
   (C) **increased extracellular fluid (ECF) volume**
   (D) increased plasma osmolality
   (E) carbamazepine

Vasopressin (or antidiuretic hormone (ADH)) is secreted from the posterior pituitary when plasma osmolality is greater than 285 mOsm/kg. Vasopressin is also released when extracellular fluid (ECF) volume is decreased. In this way, vasopressin is involved in homeostatic regulation of both tonicity and volume.

Other stimuli for increased vasopressin secretion include: pain or surgical stress Angiotensin II, nausea and vomiting, medications such as opiates, NSAIDs, carbamazepine, and TCAs, and malignancies.

Ref: Barrett KE, Boitano S, Barman SM, Brooks HL. *Ganong's Review of Medical Physiology.* 24th ed. New York, NY: McGraw Hill; 2012.

39. Which of the following will cause an increase in renin secretion by the kidneys?

   (A) increased afferent arteriole blood pressure
   (B) increased Na$^+$ and Cl$^-$ in the distal renal tubules
   (C) **norepinephrine**
   (D) vasopressin
   (E) angiotensin II

Juxtaglomerular cells of the kidney produce renin. As part of the renin-angiotensin system (RAS), renin acts as an enzyme on circulating angiotensinogen leading to the formation of angiotensin I. Angiotensin converting enzyme (ACE) then converts angiotensin I into angiotensin II. Angiotensin II is a potent vasoconstrictor and also has many other effects including: secretion of aldosterone, secretion of vasopressin, increased Na$^+$ reabsorption by the renal tubules.

Renin secretion is stimulated by:
• Decreased blood pressure (afferent arteriole),
• Decreased Na$^+$ and Cl$^-$ in the distal renal tubules,
• Increased sympathetic nervous system activity,
• Increased circulating catecholamines (norepinephrine, epinephrine), and
• Prostaglandins.

Renin secretion is inhibited by:
• Increased blood pressure (afferent arteriole),
• Increased Na$^+$ and Cl$^-$ in the distal renal tubules,
• Angiotensin II, and
• Vasopressin.

Ref: Barrett KE, Boitano S, Barman SM, Brooks HL. *Ganong's Review of Medical Physiology.* 24th ed. New York, NY: McGraw Hill; 2012.

40. Which of the following hormones will directly increase sodium and water retention by the kidneys?

(A) renin

(B) angiotensin I

(C) **aldosterone**

(D) bradykinin

(E) ANP

Aldosterone, a mineralocorticoid hormone, will directly increase Na^+ and water retention by the kidneys. Aldosterone secretion is stimulated by ACTH (adrenocorticotropic hormone), angiotensin II, and hyperkalemia. In the kidney, aldosterone's actions on principal cells in the collecting ducts causes Na^+ absorption in exchange for K^+ and H^+.

As part of the renin-angiotensin system (RAS), renin acts as an enzyme on circulating angiotensinogen leading to the formation of angiotensin I. Angiotensin I, the precursor to angiotensin II, has no known direct action.

Bradykinin is a peptide involved in inflammation. It is important to note that angiotensin converting enzyme (ACE), which converts angiotensin I to angiotensin II, is also involved in the metabolism of bradykinin. The use of ACE inhibitors for hypertension may be associated with a chronic cough, which is attributed to higher levels of tissue bradykinin.

Atrial natriuretic peptide (ANP) secretion is activated by extracellular fluid volume expansion and stretching of the atrial receptors, which leads to increased renal Na^+ and water excretion.

Ref: Barrett KE, Boitano S, Barman SM, Brooks HL. *Ganong's Review of Medical Physiology.* 24th ed. New York, NY: McGraw Hill; 2012.

41. A patient is given a large intravenous fluid bolus of isotonic saline and their extracellular fluid (ECF) volume expands. Which of the following hormones is most likely to be released following activation of receptors in the ventricles of the heart?

(A) ANP

(B) **BNP**

(C) CNP

(D) vasopressin

(E) renin

Brain natriuretic peptide (BNP), although first isolated from the brain is most abundant in the ventricles of the heart. BNP secretion is generated by ECF expansion and stretching of the ventricles. In general, BNP has the opposite actions of the renin-angiotensin system (RAS): BNP will increase renal Na^+ and water excretion, and relax vascular smooth muscle.

Atrial natriuretic peptide (ANP) and C-type natriuretic peptide (CNP) also belong to the same family as BNP and share similar actions. ANP is most abundant in the atria (although small amounts are found in the ventricles). CNP is present in other body tissues, including the brain, pituitary, and kidneys.

Monitoring ANP and BNP levels may play a diagnostic role in congestive heart failure (as volume overload causes a proportional increase in their levels). Both vasopressin and renin secretion are inhibited by an increase in ECF. Vasopressin is released from the posterior pituitary, and renin is released from the kidneys.

Ref: Barrett KE, Boitano S, Barman SM, Brooks HL. *Ganong's Review of Medical Physiology.* 24th ed. New York, NY: McGraw Hill; 2012.

CHAPTER 5

Gastrointestinal/Hepatic/Renal Physiology

1. Which of the following statements regarding hepatic blood supply is CORRECT?

   (A) The portal vein delivers up to 75% of the total blood flow of the liver.

   (B) The liver receives approximately 10% of total cardiac output.

   (C) Seventy-five percent of the oxygen supply to the liver is delivered by the hepatic artery.

   (D) Hepatic capillaries run alongside rows of hepatocytes in each hexagonal lobule.

   (E) Zone 3 cells are most resistant to ischemia in each acinus.

2. Which of the following is NOT a factor in hepatic blood flow regulation?

   (A) hepatic artery myogenic response

   (B) hepatic arterial buffer response

   (C) splanchnic vascular resistance

   (D) intrinsic regulation of portal blood flow

   (E) glucagon levels

3. Which of the following proteins is synthesized in the liver?

   (A) immunoglobulin-G

   (B) acetylcholinesterase

   (C) von Willebrand factor

   (D) pseudocholinesterase

   (E) glucagon

4. Which of the following statements regarding hepatic physiology is CORRECT?

   (A) β-adrenergic agonists stimulate the conversion of glucose to glycogen.

   (B) The liver acts as a reservoir and can add up to 350 mL of blood to the circulation if needed.

   (C) The adult liver can store up to 25 g of glycogen.

   (D) A reduction in serum albumin is the earliest protein marker of reduced hepatic synthetic function.

   (E) Kupffer cells are important for the deamination of proteins in the liver.

5. Which of the following statements regarding the biliary system is CORRECT?

   (A) Bile is only produced on demand, after each meal.

   (B) Bile is composed of approximately 50% bile salts.

   (C) The greenish-yellow color of bile is due to cholesterol and lecithin.

   (D) Inability to synthesize or excrete bile salts may result in a coagulopathy.

   (E) Ammonia is converted to urea in the liver, which is then excreted in bile.

6. Which of the following best describes a Phase II biotransformation reaction?

   (A) oxidation

   (B) hydrolysis

   (C) reduction

   (D) ester cleavage

   (E) conjugation

7. A patient suffers a myocardial infarction. Following her initial recovery, her cardiac output is found to have decreased by 50%. Which of the following drugs is MOST likely to have reduced hepatic elimination as a result?

   (A) thiopental
   (B) midazolam
   (C) fentanyl
   (D) rocuronium
   (E) vecuronium

8. Which portion of the diluting segment of the nephron plays a role in the countercurrent-induced hypertonicity of the renal medulla?

   (A) proximal tubule
   (B) descending thin limb of the loop of Henle
   (C) ascending thin limb of the loop of Henle
   (D) thick ascending limb of the loop of Henle
   (E) distal convoluted tubule

9. Signaling via which of the following areas is directly involved in the non-osmotic release of vasopressin?

   (A) paraventricular nuclei of the hypothalamus
   (B) lateral preoptic area of the hypothalamus
   (C) juxtaglomerular apparatus
   (D) carotid baroreceptors
   (E) zona glomerulosa of the adrenal cortex

10. Angiotensin II plays an important role in the regulation of extracellular fluid volume (ECF). Which of the following actions is due to angiotensin II?

   (A) inhibition of aldosterone secretion
   (B) inhibition of ACTH secretion
   (C) inhibition of vasopressin secretion
   (D) simulation of thirst
   (E) increased renal Na^+ excretion

11. In the proximal convoluted tubule (PCT) of the kidney, what is the predominant mechanism of acid-base regulation?

   (A) HCO_3^- is actively transported and reabsorbed across the apical membrane.
   (B) H^+ is transported into the tubular lumen via a Na-H antiporter.
   (C) H^+ is actively transported into the tubular lumen via a H-ATPase.
   (D) HCO_3^- is transported into the tubular lumen via a Na-3HCO_3 symporter.
   (E) Carbonic anhydrase in the epithelial cells of the PCT catalyzes the formation of CO_2 and H_2O.

12. A patient's renal function, including creatinine concentration, is assessed. A measurement of plasma creatinine concentration is inversely related to:

   (A) renal blood flow
   (B) renal plasma flow
   (C) glomerular filtration rate
   (D) filtration fraction
   (E) urea concentration

13. A patient with gout is prescribed probenecid. The same patient is also prescribed large doses of morphine for chronic pain. Theoretically, how may probenecid alter the renal excretion of morphine and its metabolites?

   (A) decrease glomerular filtration rate (GFR)
   (B) decrease active tubular secretion
   (C) increase passive tubular reabsorption by alkalinizing the urine
   (D) decrease passive tubular reabsorption by acidification of the urine
   (E) increase morphine protein binding

14. In the proximal convoluted tubule, the main driving force for water and other solute reabsorption is generated by which of the following electrolytes?

   (A) Na^+
   (B) K^+
   (C) Cl^-
   (D) Ca^{2+}
   (E) HCO_3^-

Answers and Explanations: Gastrointestinal/Hepatic/Renal Physiology

1. Which of the following statements regarding hepatic blood supply is CORRECT?

(A) **The portal vein delivers up to 75% of the total blood flow of the liver.**

(B) The liver receives approximately 10% of total cardiac output.

(C) Seventy-five percent of the oxygen supply to the liver is delivered by the hepatic artery.

(D) Hepatic capillaries run alongside rows of hepatocytes in each hexagonal lobule.

(E) Zone 3 cells are most resistant to ischemia in each acinus.

The liver receives blood from two distinct supplies: the hepatic artery (25%–35% of total flow), which delivers blood from the general arterial circulation (via the celiac trunk) and the portal vein (65%–75% of total flow), which delivers blood from the gut and associated organs. Total flow to the liver represents approximately 25% to 30% of cardiac output, even though the liver is <3% of body weight. Under normal circumstances, oxygen delivery is shared 50:50 between the two systems, despite this difference in flow, because blood entering via the portal vein is partially deoxygenated.

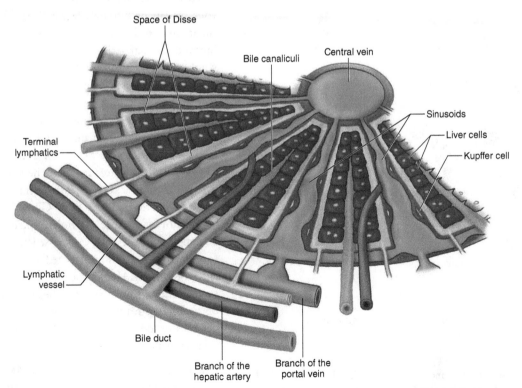

FIG. 5-1. The hepatic lobule. (Reproduced with permission from Butterworth JF IV, Mackey DC, Wasnick JD. *Morgan and Mikhail's Clinical Anesthesiology*. 5th ed. New York, NY: McGraw Hill; 2013.)

Unlike most other organs, the liver lacks capillaries, and blood from the hepatic artery and portal vein mixes together in what are termed the sinusoids of the liver. These are endothelial-lined gaps that run between rows of hepatocytes. Each row converges on a so-called central vein (Figure 5-1) where blood is collected and ultimately fed to the hepatic veins. These large veins empties into the inferior vena cava, which is intimately associated with the posterior aspect of the liver. The hepatocytes, bile canaliculi and sinusoids that surround the central vein in a hexagonal pattern are known as a lobule. Portal triads occupy 4 to 5 of the 6 corners of the lobular hexagon. These triads contain branches from the hepatic artery, the portal vein, and bile ducts that carry bile in the opposite direction.

The functional (metabolic) unit of the liver is called the acinus. It is less clear to imagine histologically than a lobule, but incorporates an elliptical area starting at the portal triad and running along the direction of flow of the hepatic arterioles and portal venules (Figure 5-2). Cells closest to these vessels (zone 1) are well oxygenated and are least at-risk for ischemia; those in zone 3 that are furthest from the nutritive vessels are most susceptible to ischemia if oxygenation and/or perfusion pressure drops.

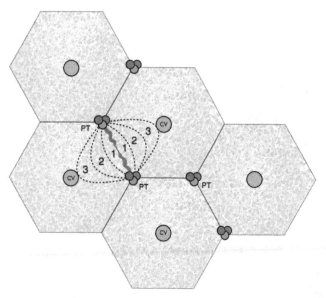

FIG. 5-2. Hepatic acinus with the 3 functional zones, labeled 1, 2 and 3. CV = central vein, PT = portal triad.

Ref: Barrett KE, Boitano S, Barman SM, Brooks HL. *Ganong's Review of Medical Physiology.* 24th ed. New York, NY: McGraw Hill; 2012.

2. Which of the following is NOT a factor in hepatic blood flow regulation?

(A) hepatic artery myogenic response

(B) hepatic arterial buffer response

(C) splanchnic vascular resistance

(D) **intrinsic regulation of portal blood flow**

(E) glucagon levels

Hepatic arterial flow is subject to both intrinsic and extrinsic control. The myogenic response is a reflex constriction of smooth muscle in the walls of the hepatic artery in response to an increase in systemic arterial pressure. The other important intrinsic mechanism is called the hepatic arterial buffer response. Mediated by the vasodilator adenosine, which is produced at a constant rate, this phenomenon serves to balance the flows of the portal and arterial systems. If portal flow is sluggish, adenosine is not washed away quickly, resulting in vasodilation of the hepatic arterioles. With an increase in portal venous flow (e.g., after a meal), adenosine is carried away more rapidly, decreasing its effect on the arterial flow. This counterbalancing effect tends to keep the total blood flow to the liver constant. Note that there is no intrinsic regulation of portal venous flow.

Extrinsic mechanisms relate to the sympathetic nervous system or humoral factors. Increases in sympathetic tone in the arterioles of the splanchnic bed will increase vascular resistance in the splanchnic bed as a whole and decrease portal venous flow. Sympathetic activation increases hepatic arterial resistance and reduces both hepatic arterial flow and liver blood volume. Circulating epinephrine causes constriction of both the hepatic arterial and portal venous systems due to alpha-1 effects. Beta-receptor activation, through low-dose epinephrine, vasodilates hepatic arterioles. In contrast, beta-blockers increase resistance in these vessels and decrease blood flow. Glucagon is a potent vasodilator of hepatic arterioles, whereas vasopressin and angiotensin II both vasoconstrict.

Total liver blood flow is related to the pressure differential between MAP (hepatic artery)/portal venous pressure on the upstream side and hepatic venous pressure on the downstream side. Factors that increase hepatic venous pressure (CHF, volume overload, positive pressure ventilation), will decrease hepatic blood flow.

Ref: Barrett KE, Boitano S, Barman SM, Brooks HL. *Ganong's Review of Medical Physiology.* 24th ed. New York, NY: McGraw Hill; 2012.

3. Which of the following proteins is synthesized in the liver?

    (A) immunoglobulin-G
    (B) acetylcholinesterase
    (C) von Willebrand factor
    (D) **pseudocholinesterase**
    (E) glucagon

One of the most important roles for the liver is the synthesis of a wide variety of proteins (and almost every plasma protein). These include albumin (10–15 g/day), α1-antitrypsin, antithrombin III, complement proteins, C-reactive protein, and α1-acid glycoprotein. It also produces all of the coagulation factors with the exception of von Willebrand factor, which is synthesized in the endothelium and platelets. Factor VIII is also produced in the endothelium as well as in the liver.

Immunoglobulins are synthesized in plasma cells. Acetylcholinesterase (true cholinesterase) is manufactured by neurons in the CNS or by muscle cells at the neuromuscular junction. In contrast, pseudocholinesterase or plasma cholinesterase is synthesized in the liver. This enzyme inactivates many drugs such as the ester-linked local anesthetics, succinylcholine, mivacurium, and heroin. Glucagon is a catabolic peptide hormone that is produced in the alpha cells of the pancreas, acting primarily on the liver to stimulate the release of stored glucose.

Ref: Butterworth JF IV, Mackey DC, Wasnick JD. *Morgan and Mikhail's Clinical Anesthesiology.* 5th ed. New York, NY: McGraw Hill; 2013.

4. Which of the following statements regarding hepatic physiology is CORRECT?

    (A) β-adrenergic agonists stimulate the conversion of glucose to glycogen.
    (B) **The liver acts as a reservoir and can add up to 350 mL of blood to the circulation if needed.**
    (C) The adult liver can store up to 25 g of glycogen.
    (D) A reduction in serum albumin is the earliest protein marker of reduced hepatic synthetic function.
    (E) Kupffer cells are important for the deamination of proteins in the liver.

The liver normally contains approximately 500 mL of blood, although that volume can increase with backpressure associated with caval or hepatic venous congestion. Under circumstances where increased blood volume is required (e.g., hypovolemic shock or exercise), sympathetic mediated vasoconstriction can expel as much as 350 mL of blood into the central circulation. The liver is the most important reservoir organ during hemorrhage.

Epinephrine stimulates β-adrenergic receptors on hepatocytes to increase intracellular cAMP levels. This stimulates glycogenolysis, which results in the release of glucose from stored glycogen. Glucagon also has the same effect, although through a different G protein-coupled receptor. Glycogenolysis is critical for maintenance of a steady plasma glucose concentration. Glycogen is stored by several organs other than the liver, but in only very small amounts. The vast majority of glycogenolysis occurs in the liver. As much as 100 to 120 g of glycogen can be stored after a meal.

In acute liver failure, the synthesis of new proteins is suspended, at least to the degree that hepatocytes are infarcted or impaired. Many plasma proteins have long half-lives; albumin, for example, has a half-life of 22 days. In contrast, factor VII has a half-life of only 4 to 6 hours. Factor VII is used after liver transplantation to assess for acute hepatocellular injury for this reason. Kupffer cells are phagocytic cells that are involved in the immune function of the liver.

Ref: Barrett KE, Boitano S, Barman SM, Brooks HL. *Ganong's Review of Medical Physiology.* 24th ed. New York, NY: McGraw Hill; 2012.

5. Which of the following statements regarding the biliary system is CORRECT?

    (A) Bile is only produced on demand, after each meal.
    (B) Bile is composed of approximately 50% bile salts.
    (C) The greenish-yellow color of bile is due to cholesterol and lecithin.
    (D) **Inability to synthesize or excrete bile salts may result in a coagulopathy.**
    (E) Ammonia is converted to urea in the liver, which is then excreted in bile.

Bile is an aqueous solution of bile salts, bile pigments, and other lipids and salts (Table 5-1) that has two functions: aiding in the absorption of fat in the gut and the excretion of urea, cholesterol, alkaline phosphatase, and many drugs. The pigments bilirubin and biliverdin give bile its characteristic greenish-yellow hue. Bile is produced by hepatocytes continuously, and any excess stored in the gall bladder (i.e., when the sphincter of Oddi is closed). When fatty-rich foods enter the duodenum, the peptide hormone cholecystokinin is released by the mucosa, which stimulates the gallbladder to contract, expelling its contents through the cystic duct to the common bile duct, and into the duodenum via the sphincter of Oddi.

This sphincter is under autonomic control, relaxing with parasympathetic stimulation and contracting with sympathetic discharge. In addition, several drugs have an effect on the sphincter of Oddi. In particular, opioids contract the smooth muscle of the sphincter, causing spasm, which can confound the diagnosis of cholestasis and/or make ERCP difficult. This appears to be a class effect, with little evidence showing that one agent (e.g., meperidine) leading to a decreased incidence or intensity of contraction. Drugs that relax the sphincter include naloxone, atropine, calcium channel blockers, glucagon, prostaglandin E1, and nitroglycerin. Note that in trying to make a diagnosis in atypical chest pain, the administration of nitroglycerin will relax both the coronary arteries and the sphincter of Oddi (which is not so helpful ruling out gallstone cholestasis versus myocardial ischemia). Glucagon is a more useful agent for this indication.

The conversion of ammonia to urea is one of the liver's most important metabolic tasks, as ammonia toxicity is rapidly fatal. Urea is a nontoxic, water-soluble molecule that is taken up by the circulation (not excreted in the bile) and excreted by the kidneys.

Inability to release bile into the duodenum will impact the absorption of fats and fat-soluble vitamins (A, D, E, and K). Untreated, this will manifest as a coagulopathy due to the impaired production of vitamin K–dependent coagulation factors II, VII, IX, and X.

TABLE 5-1. Composition of bile.

97% water
<1% bile salts
Pigments
Inorganic salts
Lipids
Cholesterol
Fatty acids
Lecithin
Alkaline phosphatase

Reproduced with permission from Butterworth JF IV, Mackey DC, Wasnick JD. *Morgan and Mikhail's Clinical Anesthesiology*. 5th ed. New York, NY: McGraw Hill; 2013.

Ref: Butterworth JF IV, Mackey DC, Wasnick JD. *Morgan and Mikhail's Clinical Anesthesiology*. 5th ed. New York, NY: McGraw Hill; 2013.

6. Which of the following best describes a Phase II biotransformation reaction?

(A) oxidation
(B) hydrolysis
(C) reduction
(D) ester cleavage
(E) **conjugation**

A chief responsibility of the liver is the detoxification and removal of xenobiotics from the body. There are generally two steps to the transformation of drugs by the liver. **Phase I** reactions are carried out primarily by the enzymes of the cytochrome P-450 system in the endoplasmic reticulum of hepatocytes. Through oxidation (90%), reduction, and hydrolysis (ester and amide cleavage), drugs are modified by the addition of a reactive and/or polar groups, making them susceptible to further transformation in **Phase II** reactions. In this second step, the activated drugs are conjugated with polar species such as glutathione, sulfate, glycine, or glucuronic acid to render them water-soluble and easily excretable by the kidneys, or less commonly, through the biliary system, lungs, salivary glands, or lacrimal glands.

The cytochrome P-450 system is subject to up- and down-regulation by specific drugs, which may then alter the metabolic rate of other drugs in the body. The classic example is phenytoin, which induces the activity of CYP450. Since the metabolic activity is accelerated, plasma levels of drugs dependent on CYP450 for biotransformation may decrease to subtherapeutic levels. Other inducers include ethanol, barbiturates, and ketamine. Cimetidine, buproprion, and ciprofloxacin are all CYP450 inhibitors and tend to have the opposite effect.

Ref: Butterworth JF IV, Mackey DC, Wasnick JD. *Morgan and Mikhail's Clinical Anesthesiology*. 5th ed. New York, NY: McGraw Hill; 2013.

7. A patient suffers a myocardial infarction. Following her initial recovery, her cardiac output is found to have decreased by 50%. Which of the following drugs is MOST likely to have reduced hepatic elimination as a result?

(A) thiopental
(B) midazolam
(C) **fentanyl**

(D) rocuronium

(E) vecuronium

The hepatic elimination of drugs is dependent on the liver's intrinsic ability to clear the drug, as well as the amount of drug presented to the liver. Hepatic extraction ratio is the fraction of drug flowing into the liver that is extracted by the hepatocytes. Different drugs have varying extraction ratios (Table 5-2). For example, propofol has a very high extraction ratio, meaning that nearly 100% of all propofol flowing through the liver is taken up and metabolized there by the organ. The capacity of the liver to metabolize drugs with high extraction ratios is greater than the the flow of those drugs to the liver; therefore, increases or decreases in hepatic function have little influence over clearance. What does affect clearance for high extraction ratio drugs is liver blood flow, where it assumes a linear relationship: the higher the blood flow, the higher the clearance. Fentanyl also has a high extraction ratio, which is why its clearance will be diminished in the above example.

Drugs with low extraction ratios are not efficiently cleared by the liver, and their clearance is limited by the capacity of the hepatic enzyme systems, rather than blood flow.

TABLE 5-2. Hepatic extraction ratios of commonly used drugs in anesthesia.

Low	Intermediate	High
Diazepam	Alfentanil	Bupivacaine
Lorazepam	Codeine	Diltiazem
Methadone	Etomidate	Fentanyl
Phenytoin	Hydromorphone	Ketamine
Rocuronium	Meperidine	Lidocaine
Thiopental	Methohexital	Metoprolol
	Midazolam	Morphine
	Vecuronium	Naloxone
		Nifedipine
		Propofol
		Sufentanil

Ref: Brunton LL, Chabner BA, Knollman BC. *Goodman and Gilman's The Pharmacological Basis of Therapeutics.* 12th ed. New York, NY: McGraw Hill; 2011.

8. Which portion of the diluting segment of the nephron plays a role in the countercurrent-induced hypertonicity of the renal medulla?

(A) proximal tubule

(B) descending thin limb of the loop of Henle

(C) ascending thin limb of the loop of Henle

(D) **thick ascending limb of the loop of Henle**

(E) distal convoluted tubule

The thick ascending limb of the loop of Henle and the distal convoluted tubule form the diluting segment of the nephron (both segments actively reabsorb NaCl and are impermeable to water, resulting in hypotonic tubular fluid, irrespective of hydration status). The thick ascending limb of the loop of Henle plays a role in the countercurrent-induced hypertonicity of the renal medulla. In general, functions of the various sections of a nephron are as follows:

- Proximal convoluted tubule: ~65% of filtered Na^+ reabsorbed (with water).

- Descending thin limb (DTL) of the loop of Henle: High permeability to water, low permeability to NaCl and urea.

- Ascending thin limb (ATL) of the loop of Henle: Permeable to NaCl and urea, impermeable to water.

- Thick ascending limb (TAL) of the loop of Henle: Actively reabsorbs NaCl, impermeable to water and urea.

- Distal convoluted tubule: Actively reabsorbs NaCl, impermeable to water.

The "passive countercurrent multiplier hypothesis" uses the following model:

- TAL: Active transport of NaCl into outer medullary interstitium. Dilute tubular fluid to collecting ducts.

- Collecting ducts: Water extracted if vasopressin (antidiuretic hormone, ADH) present. Cortical and outer portion of medullary collecting ducts impermeable to urea, meaning urea is concentrated in this area.

- Fluid to inner medullary collecting duct, which is permeable to urea, so it now diffuses into inner medulla.

- This high concentration of urea in the medullary interstitium helps to extract water from the DTL. Low permeability of DTL to NaCl and urea means that NaCl is concentrated.

As fluid enters ATL, NaCl diffuses into medulla and contributes to hypertonicity.

Ref: Brunton LL, Chabner BA, Knollman BC. *Goodman and Gilman's The Pharmacological Basis of Therapeutics.* 12th ed. New York, NY: McGraw Hill; 2011.

9. Signaling via which of the following areas is directly involved in the nonosmotic release of vasopressin?

   (A) paraventricular nuclei of the hypothalamus
   (B) lateral preoptic area of the hypothalamus
   (C) juxtaglomerular apparatus
   (D) **carotid baroreceptors**
   (E) zona glomerulosa of the adrenal cortex

In a response to decreased blood volume, signaling via carotid baroreceptors directly results in the nonosmotic release of vasopressin. Vasopressin secretion may be in response to either changes in plasma osmolality or changes in extracellular fluid volume. Note, when faced with changes to both, vasopressin will defend volume at the expense of plasma osmolality. Changes in plasma osmolality are detected by osmoreceptors in the supraoptic and paraventricular nuclei of the hypothalamus. An increase in plasma osmolality leads to vasopressin secretion from the posterior pituitary and retention of water. An increase in plasma osmolality detected by osmoreceptors in the lateral preoptic area of the hypothalamus activates the thirst mechanism. The juxtaglomerular apparatus (juxtaglomerular cells, macula densa, and lacis cells) in the kidney is involved in regulation of renin secretion. Decreased sodium and chloride delivery to the distal renal tubules and decreased arteriolar pressure both lead to increased renin secretion, which ultimately helps defend extracellular fluid volume via the renin-angiotensin system. Note that activation of angiotensin II causes multiple effects, including increased secretion of vasopressin. The zona glomerulosa of the adrenal cortex is the site where angiotensin II augments the release of aldosterone. Aldosterone increases sodium retention and causes volume expansion.

Refs: Butterworth JF IV, Mackey DC, Wasnick JD. *Morgan and Mikhail's Clinical Anesthesiology.* 5th ed. New York, NY: McGraw Hill; 2013.

Barrett KE, Boitano S, Barman SM, Brooks HL. *Ganong's Review of Medical Physiology.* 24th ed. New York, NY: McGraw Hill; 2012.

10. Angiotensin II plays an important role in the regulation of extracellular fluid volume (ECF). Which of the following actions is due to angiotensin II?

    (A) inhibition of aldosterone secretion
    (B) inhibition of ACTH secretion
    (C) inhibition of vasopressin secretion
    (D) **simulation of thirst**
    (E) increased renal Na^+ excretion

Angiotensin II has multiple effects: increased aldosterone secretion, increased ACTH secretion, increased vasopressin secretion, stimulation of thirst, vasoconstriction, facilitation of norepinephrine release, and direct increase in renal Na^+ absorption. As part of the renin-angiotensin system (RAS), angiotensin II plays a critical role in the regulation of extracellular fluid volume (ECF). In general, angiotensin II causes both vasoconstriction and the retention of Na^+ and water, both of which serve to maintain blood pressure.

Ref: Barrett KE, Boitano S, Barman SM, Brooks HL. *Ganong's Review of Medical Physiology.* 24th ed. New York, NY: McGraw Hill; 2012.

11. In the proximal convoluted tubule (PCT) of the kidney, what is the predominant mechanism of acid-base regulation?

    (A) HCO_3^- is actively transported and reabsorbed across the apical membrane.
    (B) **H^+ is transported into the tubular lumen via a Na-H antiporter.**
    (C) H^+ is actively transported into the tubular lumen via a H-ATPase.
    (D) HCO_3^- is transported into the tubular lumen via a Na-3HCO$_3$ symporter.
    (E) Carbonic anhydrase in the epithelial cells of the PCT catalyzes the formation of CO_2 and H_2O.

The proximal convoluted tubule (PCT) is the main site of HCO_3^- "reabsorption." However, it is interesting to note that no HCO_3^- actually crosses between the tubular lumen and the apical border of the epithelial cells of the PCT. Instead, an acid-base process of H^+ secretion occurs:

- Freely filtered HCO_3^- from the glomerulus and Bowman's capsule enters the lumen of the PCT
- In the lumen, carbonic anhydrase catalyzes a reaction between HCO_3^- and H^+ to form H_2O and CO_2

- The H^+ for this reaction is generated in the epithelial cell of the PCT, with carbonic anhydrase catalyzing the reaction of H_2O and CO_2 to form H^+ and HCO_3^-
- This intracellular H^+ is transported into the tubular lumen via a Na-H antiporter on the apical membrane, generating intracellular HCO_3^-
- This HCO_3^- is then transported across the basolateral membrane into the interstitium via a Na-3HCO₃ symporter.

In this way, freely filtered HCO_3^- is "reabsorbed" in the PCT and returned to the interstitium.

Refs: Eaton DC, Pooler JP. *Vander's Renal Physiology.* 8th ed. New York, NY: McGraw Hill; 2013.

Hammer GD, McPhee SJ. *Pathophysiology of Disease: An Introduction to Clinical Medicine.* 7th ed. New York, NY: McGraw Hill; 2014.

12. A patient's renal function, including creatinine concentration, is assessed. A measurement of plasma creatinine concentration is inversely related to:

(A) renal blood flow

(B) renal plasma flow

(C) **glomerular filtration rate**

(D) filtration fraction

(E) urea concentration

Creatinine concentration in the blood is inversely related to glomerular filtration rate (GFR). GFR is the amount of fluid that the kidney filters per unit time (mL/min). As a rule of thumb, if creatinine concentration doubles then GFR declines by 50%. Renal blood flow (RBF) is the amount of blood passing through the kidneys per unit time (~20% of total cardiac output or ~1 L/min). Renal plasma flow (RPF) is the amount of plasma passing through the kidneys per unit time (plasma is ~55% of blood volume). The filtration fraction is the proportion of renal plasma filtered at the glomeruli (e.g., GFR/RPF). Urea is produced in the liver as a breakdown product of amino acids. A measurement of blood urea nitrogen (BUN) varies depending on hydration status and protein metabolism. Normal BUN/Cr ratio is 10–20:1. A ratio >20:1 suggests prerenal causes, while a ratio <10:1 suggests renal causes.

Ref: Laposata M: *Laboratory Medicine: The Diagnosis of Disease in the Clinical Laboratory.* 2nd ed. New York, NY: McGraw Hill; 2014.

13. A patient with gout is prescribed probenecid. The same patient is also prescribed large doses of morphine for chronic pain. Theoretically, how may probenecid alter the renal excretion of morphine and its metabolites?

(A) decrease glomerular filtration rate (GFR)

(B) **decrease active tubular secretion**

(C) increase passive tubular reabsorption by alkalinizing the urine

(D) decrease passive tubular reabsorption by acidification of the urine

(E) increase morphine protein binding

In general, drug excretion and elimination by the kidney involves a combination of glomerular filtration, tubular secretion, and tubular reabsorption. Amount of drug filtered is proportional to glomerular filtration rate (GFR) and to the amount of free drug in the plasma (morphine is ~35% bound to albumin). In the proximal convoluted tubule, a variety of transporters move anions, cations, and conjugated metabolites into the tubular lumen. Passive reabsorption, which may occur in either the proximal or distal portion of the tubule, depends on the pH of the urine. Alkaline urine favors the excretion of weak acids, while acidification of urine favors excretion of weak bases. Morphine metabolites (morphine-3-glucuronide and morphine-6-glucuronide) are filtered at the glomerulus and also secreted in the tubular lumen by transporters such as OAT (organic anion transporter) and MRP2 (multidrug resistance-associated protein 2). Probenecid is a medication used in the treatment of gout. It also has utility for increasing plasma drug concentrations of certain medications such as penicillin. Probenecid will decrease renal tubular secretion of various drugs (including morphine-3-glucuronide and morphine-6-glucuronide) by inhibiting a variety of transporters including OAT and MRP2.

Refs: Brunton LL, Chabner BA, Knollman BC. *Goodman and Gilman's The Pharmacological Basis of Therapeutics.* 12th ed. New York, NY: McGraw Hill; 2011.

Van Crugten JT, Sallustio BC, Nation RL, et al. Renal tubular transport of morphine, morphine-6-glucuronide, and morphine-3-glucuronide in the isolated perfused rat kidney. *Drug Metab Dispos Biol Fate Chem.* 1991; 19:1087–92.

14. In the proximal convoluted tubule, the main driving force for water and other solute reabsorption is generated by which of the following electrolytes?

   (A) Na^+
   (B) K^+
   (C) Cl^-
   (D) Ca^{2+}
   (E) HCO_3^-

Sodium reabsorption in the proximal convoluted tubule (PCT) plays a key role generating the driving force for transport of water and other solutes. The epithelial cells of the PCT actively extrude sodium into the interstitium via the Na-K-ATPase. This sets up a gradient for passive movement of Na^+ from the tubular lumen into the epithelial cell. In order to maintain electroneutrality, movement of Na^+ into the epithelial cell requires a corresponding movement of anions. Solute movement into the epithelial cells also results in the osmotic movement of water. The majority of potassium is reabsorbed in the PCT and thick ascending limb of the loop of Henle. The distal nephron may either reabsorb or secrete potassium depending on the needs of the body. Calcium is reabsorbed mostly in the PCT and also in the thick ascending limb of the loop of Henle and the distal convoluted tubule.

Ref: Eaton DC, Pooler JP. *Vander's Renal Physiology*. 8th ed. New York, NY: McGraw Hill; 2013.

CHAPTER 6

Intravenous Fluids and Transfusion Medicine

1. What is the daily maintenance fluid requirement for a 80-kg patient?

   (A) 2400 mL
   (B) 2640 mL
   (C) 2880 mL
   (D) 3000 mL
   (E) 4800 mL

2. When transfusing packed red blood cells (PRBCs) it is often recommended to avoid which of the following crystalloids?

   (A) normal saline (0.9% NS)
   (B) lactated Ringer's solution (LR)
   (C) plasmalyte
   (D) 5% Dextrose in water (D_5W)
   (E) D_5W + 1/2 NS (0.45% NS)

3. Glucose is a mandatory fuel source for the brain, adrenal medulla, red blood cells, and wounds. Diabetic patients are often given an infusion of dextrose to meet these basal energy requirements, reduce loss of lean muscle mass, and to prevent hypoglycemia while on insulin infusions. In order to meet these basal glucose requirements, for a 100-kg adult patient, which of the following is the most appropriate infusion of 5% dextrose in water (D_5W)?

   (A) 50 cc/hr
   (B) 140 cc/hr
   (C) 175 cc/hr
   (D) 200 cc/hr
   (E) 280 cc/hr

4. A patient's surgery is postponed due to a scheduling conflict. The adult patient weighs 60 kg and is euvolemic with normal electrolytes. They are to remain NPO until the surgery can be accommodated, which may take up to 24 to 48 hours. While the patient remains NPO, which of the following orders for intravenous fluid is the best for routine maintenance fluids?

   (A) 100 cc/hr 0.9% NS
   (B) 100 cc/hr 0.45% NS + 20 mEq KCl/L
   (C) 100 cc/hr LR
   (D) 100 cc/hr D_5W + 20 mEq KCl/L
   (E) 100 cc/hr D_5W + 0.45% NS + 20 mEq KCl/L

5. There is an ongoing debate about the benefits of intravenous fluid therapy with either crystalloids or colloids. For a critically ill patient, an artificial colloid (e.g., hydroxyethyl starch) is selected for fluid resuscitation. In comparison to the administration of a balanced crystalloid (e.g., lactated ringer's), which of the following is a potential benefit of an artificial colloid?

   (A) decreased tissue edema
   (B) decreased risk of death
   (C) decreased risk of anaphylactic reaction
   (D) decreased risk of coagulopathy
   (E) decreased risk of renal impairment

6. Which of the following is the MOST appropriate indication for transfusion of packed red blood cells?

   (A) a patient with a hemoglobin concentration of 11 g/dL who is about to undergo an extensive orthopedic procedure

   (B) a septic patient in the critical care unit with a hemoglobin concentration of 8.2 g/dL

   (C) an acutely bleeding adult patient with a hemoglobin concentration of 5 g/dL who refuses consent for transfusion

   (D) a hemodynamically stable patient with extensive surgical blood loss, a hemoglobin concentration of 7 g/dL, and a mixed venous oxygen saturation of 72%

   (E) a hemodynamically stable patient with extensive surgical blood loss, a hemoglobin concentration of 8.5 g/dL, and a mixed venous oxygen saturation of 52%

7. In which of the following situations is transfusion of fresh frozen plasma LEAST appropriate?

   (A) an international standardized ratio (INR) of 1.6 prior to urgent surgery for a patient on warfarin

   (B) microvascular bleeding after transfusion of 1 blood volume of packed red blood cells when PT/PTT testing cannot be obtained rapidly

   (C) augmentation of plasma volume in a patient who is bleeding briskly and has already received 1 L of crystalloid

   (D) correction of known factor deficiencies for which specific concentrates are not available

   (E) during massive transfusion of a trauma patient

8. Which of the following regarding the collection and storage of blood components is INCORRECT?

   (A) Blood collection bags contain citrate, adenine and phosphate.

   (B) Frozen red cells may be stored for 10 years or more.

   (C) Red cells have a maximum shelf life of 42 days when refrigerated.

   (D) Plasma can be frozen for up to 1 year before being thawed for use.

   (E) Platelets are stored at a temperature of 1–6°C and are kept for a maximum of 5 days.

9. Which of the following is associated with the red blood cell (RBC) "storage lesion"?

   (A) increased deformability of the RBCs

   (B) increased 2,3-diphosphoglycerate (2,3-DPG)

   (C) increased pH

   (D) vasoconstriction of the microcirculation

   (E) right shift of the oxyhemoglobin dissociation curve

10. Which of the following is the MOST appropriate size of filter to prevent macroaggregate delivery during transfusion?

    (A) 1 micron

    (B) 40 microns

    (C) 110 microns

    (D) 170 microns

    (E) 375 microns

11. An improperly calibrated blood warming device that heats the red blood cells (RBCs) to a temperature >45°C may result in which of the following?

    (A) red cell fragmentation and hemolysis.

    (B) red cell adherence and premature clotting.

    (C) a left shift in the oxyhemoglobin dissociation curve.

    (D) contamination of the blood with plastic polymers from the intravenous tubing.

    (E) disseminated intravascular coagulation (DIC).

12. Cryoprecipitate contains which of the following coagulation factors?

    (A) factor II

    (B) factor VII

    (C) factor VIII

    (D) factor IX

    (E) factor X

13. Which of the following statements regarding albumin solutions for transfusion is NOT true?

    (A) Albumin solutions are available in 5% or 25% concentrations.

    (B) Albumin provides most of the colloid oncotic pressure in the plasma.

    (C) Albumin is heat treated to inactivate viruses.

    (D) Almost all of a 5% albumin solution will remain in the intravascular compartment.

    (E) Patients with an allergy to eggs should not receive an albumin transfusion.

14. When ordering blood from the blood bank, which of the following steps in the type and cross process takes the MOST amount of time?

    (A) testing for ABO type

    (B) testing for Rh (D) type

    (C) antibody screen

    (D) immediate spin crossmatch

    (E) computer crossmatch

15. Which of the following regarding preoperative autologous donation (PAD) is FALSE?

    (A) Aortic stenosis is a contraindication to PAD.

    (B) PAD should be considered when there is a high likelihood of >500–1000 mL blood loss.

    (C) PAD is more expensive than allogeneic blood transfusion.

    (D) By donating their own blood, a patient eliminates the risk of viral transmission associated with transfusion.

    (E) PAD units may be used for other recipients if not used for the intended donor.

16. Which of the following combinations of blood products would MOST likely result in an incompatibility reaction?

    (A) Type O red cells are transfused to a type AB patient.

    (B) Type AB red cells are transfused to a type O patient.

    (C) Type AB plasma is transfused to a type B patient.

    (D) Type B plasma is transfused to a type O patient.

    (E) Type A platelets are transfused to type B patient.

17. Advantages of recombinant hemoglobin-based oxygen carriers over allogeneic blood transfusion may include all EXCEPT:

    (A) longer half-life in the vasculature

    (B) superior shelf-life

    (C) universal compatibility

    (D) may be acceptable to Jehovah's Witnesses

    (E) unlimited availability

18. Features characteristic of febrile non-hemolytic transfusion reactions (FNHTR) include all EXCEPT:

    (A) a rise in temperature >1°C

    (B) a higher incidence with red blood cells (RBCs) than platelets

    (C) rigors

    (D) hypotension

    (E) caused by cytokines typically released by donor leukocytes

19. A 56-year-old woman is receiving a transfusion of RBCs in the operating room for continued bleeding during an abdominal hysterectomy. Over the course of 5 minutes, you notice hives, facial edema and an increase in peak airway pressures from 20 to 35 cmH$_2$O while ventilating her with positive pressure ventilation. Which of the following is the MOST likely cause of this reaction?

    (A) IgA from small amounts of donor plasma

    (B) citrate in the RBC units

    (C) cytokines from leukocytes

    (D) free hemoglobin from lysed RBCs

    (E) a drug error

20. A patient receiving a transfusion of FFP in the PACU complains of pruritus and hives over his chest, neck and face. After stopping the transfusion, which of the following would be MOST appropriate next step?

    (A) Administer epinephrine 0.3 mg SC.

    (B) Administer epinephrine 0.1 mg IV.

    (C) Administer diphenhydramine 50 mg IV.

    (D) Administer hydrocortisone 100 mg IV.

    (E) Administer dexamethasone 8 mg IV.

21. Which of the following clinical features is MOST commonly associated with an acute hemolytic transfusion reaction?

    (A) flank pain
    (B) hypotension
    (C) nausea
    (D) oliguria
    (E) fever

22. Which of the following BEST describes the etiology of a delayed hemolytic transfusion reaction?

    (A) ABO incompatibility
    (B) anamnestic response to an undetected antigen
    (C) lysis of recipient cells by donor complement
    (D) recipient viral illness at time of transfusion
    (E) disseminated intravascular coagulation from fibrin strands

23. Which of the following infectious agents is MOST likely to be transmitted to a patient during allogeneic blood transfusion?

    (A) human immunodeficiency virus (HIV)
    (B) hepatitis B
    (C) hepatitis C
    (D) West Nile virus
    (E) human T-cell lymphotrophic virus (HTLV)

24. In which of the following scenarios is the transfusion of cytomegalovirus-seronegative blood units LEAST likely to offer a safety advantage?

    (A) CMV-seronegative pregnant women
    (B) intrauterine transfusions
    (C) CMV-seronegative allogeneic bone marrow transplant recipients
    (D) a patient infected with HIV
    (E) a patient infected with hepatitis C

25. Which of the following statements regarding citrate intoxication during blood transfusion is CORRECT?

    (A) Citrate is used as an antioxidant in packed red blood cell preparations.
    (B) Citrate is normally metabolized rapidly in the liver to bicarbonate.
    (C) Rapid transfusion of citrated blood can result in hypercalcemia.
    (D) A shortened QT interval is characteristic of citrate toxicity.
    (E) Calcium can be added to blood to prevent citrate toxicity.

26. Which of the following electrolyte disturbances is LEAST likely after transfusion of packed red cells?

    (A) hyponatremia
    (B) hyperkalemia
    (C) hypomagnesemia
    (D) hypocalcemia
    (E) hypokalemia

27. The transfusion of multiple units of cold red blood cells may lead to which of the following complications?

    (A) coronary vasospasm
    (B) hemolysis
    (C) decreased affinity of hemoglobin for oxygen
    (D) dilutional thrombocytopenia
    (E) disseminated intravascular coagulation (DIC)

28. A patient receiving 2 units of fresh frozen plasma on the floor develops hypoxemia and pulmonary failure. Three hours later, auscultation reveals crackles in all lung fields. Her post-intubation chest X-ray is notable for widespread alveolar infiltrates. Which of the following factors best differentiates transfusion-related acute lung injury (TRALI) from transfusion-associated circulatory overload (TACO)?

    (A) blood pressure
    (B) presence of crackles on auscultation
    (C) chest radiograph
    (D) response to diuretics
    (E) TACO is just a way better acronym

29. Transfusion of blood that has not been leukocyte-depleted has been shown to result in which of the following complications?

(A) cerebral edema
(B) postoperative infection
(C) increased rate of renal allograft rejection
(D) snaphylaxis
(E) hypercalcemia

Answers and Explanations:
Intravenous Fluids and Transfusion Medicine

1. What is the daily maintenance fluid requirement for a 80-kg patient?

   (A) 2400 mL
   (B) 2640 mL
   (C) 2880 mL
   (D) 3000 mL
   (E) 4800 mL

   Using the "4/2/1" rule the patient will require: 4 mL/kg/hr for the first 10 kg; 2 mL/kg/hr for the next 10 kg; and 1 mL/kg/hr for the remaining weight greater than 20 kg. Total hourly fluid requirements = 40 mL + 20 mL + 60 mL = 120 mL/hr. Daily requirements = 120 mL/hr × 24 hours = 2880 mL.

   Ref: Miller RD. Miller's *Anesthesia*. 8th ed. Philadelphia, PA: Elsevier; 2015.

2. When transfusing packed red blood cells (PRBCs) it is often recommended to Avoid which of the following crystalloids?

   (A) normal saline (0.9% NS)
   (B) lactated Ringer's solution (LR)
   (C) plasmalyte
   (D) 5% Dextrose in water (D$_5$W)
   (E) D$_5$W + 1/2 NS (0.45% NS)

   Lactated Ringer's (LR) contains 130 mEq/L sodium, 4 mEq/L potassium, 3 mEq/L calcium, and 109 mEq/L chloride. It is recommended to avoid LR with citrated blood products, as theoretically the calcium in the LR can chelate the citrate anticoagulant and lead to clot formation. (However, it should be noted that this common recommendation is in contrast to many research studies that show LR may be used safely in the **rapid** transfusion of PRBCs.) Normal saline, Plasmalyte, and

   D$_5$W do not contain calcium. Another common recommendation is to avoid the use of potassium containing crystalloids (LR or Plasmalyte) in patients with hyperkalemia. This recommendation does not take into account the volume of NS administered. If a large volume of NS is administered (>20 cc/kg), a patient is at risk of developing a hyperchloremic metabolic acidosis which can lead to hyperkalemia (despite the absence of potassium in NS!). With this is mind, large volume fluid resuscitation with isotonic, balanced crystalloids (Lactated Ringer's or Plasmalyte) is recommended.

   Refs: Miller RD. Miller's *Anesthesia*. 8th ed. Philadelphia, PA: Elsevier; 2015.

   Levac B, Parlow JL, van Vlymen J, et al. Ringer's lactate is compatible with saline- adenine-glucose-mannitol preserved packed red blood cells for rapid transfusion. *Can J Anaesth*. 2010; 57(12):1071– 1077.

   O'Malley CM, Frumento RJ, Hardy MA, et al. A randomized, double-blind comparison of lactated Ringer's solution and 0.9% NaCl during renal transplantation. *Anesth Analg*. 2005; 100(5):1518–1524.

3. Glucose is a mandatory fuel source for the brain, adrenal medulla, red blood cells, and wounds. Diabetic patients are often given an infusion of dextrose to meet these basal energy requirements, reduce loss of lean muscle mass, and to prevent hypoglycemia while on insulin infusions. In order to meet these basal glucose requirements, for a 100-kg adult patient, which of the following is the most appropriate infusion of 5% dextrose in water (D$_5$W)?

   (A) 50 cc/hr
   (B) 140 cc/hr
   (C) 175 cc/hr
   (D) 200 cc/hr
   (E) 280 cc/hr

For adults, typical basal glucose requirements are approximately 2 mg/kg/min. (An important note regarding terminology: glucose is also known as D-glucose or dextrose. D_5W is a water soluble form of dextrose, dextrose monohydrate. This slightly alters the energy calculation in that D_5W provides 3.41 kcal/g compared to 4 kcal/g for glucose taken orally. This means that approximately 17% more D_5W than oral glucose is required.)

For a 100-kg patient the basal requirement = (2 mg/kg/min × 100 kg × 60 min/hr)/1000 mg/g = 12 g/hr. D_5W contains 50 g of dextrose per liter. Therefore, the patient requires an infusion of D_5W of 280 cc/hr: (12 g/hr/50 g/L) × 1000 cc/L) × 117%.

Note: Insulin resistance with impaired glucose uptake by muscle is common in surgical and critically ill patients. Therefore, the calculation for basal glucose requirements provides a starting point for glucose infusion and close monitoring of blood glucose is required. For otherwise healthy adults, glucose containing solutions are not routinely administered perioperatively.

Infants and children have different glucose requirements, with recommendations ranging from 5 to 15 mg/kg/min for premature and term infants, and 5 to12 mg/kg/min for children 1 to 3 years old. Risk of intraoperative hypoglycemia is low for children with an appropriate preoperative fasting interval (with clear fluids up to 2 hours before anesthesia). Routine use of glucose-containing solutions is no longer recommended unless a child is at risk of hypoglycemia (preterm, neonate, requiring parenteral nutrition, prolonged preoperative starvation, etc.) Research suggests that lower dextrose concentrations (1% or 2%, D_1W, D_2W) with LR prevent hypoglycemia without the risk of hyperglycemia associated with 5% dextrose (D_5W).

Refs: Miller RD. Miller's *Anesthesia*. 8th ed. Philadelphia, PA: Elsevier; 2015.

Paut O, Lacroix F. Recent developments in the perioperative fluid management for the paediatric patient, *Current Opinion in Anaesthesiology*. 2006; 19:268–277.

Sumpelmann R, Mader T, Eich C, et al. A novel isotonic-balanced electrolyte solution with 1% glucose for intraoperative fluid therapy in children: Results of a prospective multicentre observational post-authorization safety study (PASS), *Pediatric Anesthesia*. 2010; 20:977–981.

Cox JH, Melbardis IM. Parenteral Nutrition. In: Samour PQ, King K, eds. *Handbook of Pediatric Nutrition*. 3rd ed. Burlington, MA: Jones and Bartlett; 2005;533.

4. A patient's surgery is postponed due to a scheduling conflict. The adult patient weighs 60 kg and is euvolemic with normal electrolytes. They are to remain NPO until the surgery can be accommodated, which may take up to 24 to 48 hours. While the patient remains NPO, which of the following orders for intravenous fluid is the best for routine maintenance fluids?

(A) 100 cc/hr 0.9% NS

(B) 100 cc/hr 0.45% NS + 20 mEq KCl/L

(C) 100 cc/hr LR

(D) 100 cc/hr D_5W + 20 mEq KCl/L

(E) 100 cc/hr D_5W + 0.45% NS + 20 mEq KCl/L

For a 60-kg adult patient who is euvolemic without electrolyte abnormalities and NPO, 100 cc/hr D_5W + 0.45% NS + 20 mEq KCl/L is the best choice for routine maintenance fluid. Over the course of 24 hours, this maintenance fluid provides 2400 cc fluid, 120 g dextrose, 48 mEq of K^+, and 185 mEq of Na^+.

The other options provide adequate fluid but in the case of NS and LR, excess sodium and inadequate potassium, and in the case of 0.45% NS + 20 mEq KCl/L, inadequate glucose.

Notes: In general, during the *intraoperative* period isotonic crystalloids (NS or LR) are used for fluid deficits, maintenance, and losses. Surgical patients have a predisposition for hyponatremia due to many intraoperative factors including surgical stress and pain which result in increased secretion of ADH. Hypotonic fluids with excess free water (D_5W or 0.45% NS) are typically avoided.

Twenty mEq KCl/L does not meet the estimated daily needs for potassium replacement. However, intravenous KCl can irritate peripheral veins and the concentration must be limited. If insufficient fluid or energy intake extends for more than 1 or 2 weeks, then enteral or parenteral nutrition should be considered. Maintenance fluids provide a starting point for patient fluid management and ongoing evaluation of the patient (weight, physical exam, electrolytes) is required.

The earlier this was 4/2/1 rule estimates routine maintenance fluids for a 60-kg patient as:

$$4 × 1st\ 10\ kg = 40\ cc/hr$$
$$2 × 2nd\ 10\ kg = 20\ cc/hr$$
$$1 × remaining\ 40\ kg = 40\ cc/hr$$

$$Total = 100\ cc/hr\ or\ 2400\ cc/day$$

Alternatively, daily water loss for the "average" person is approximately 2 L/day:

- urine 1400 cc
- sweat 100 cc
- feces 100 cc
- insensible losses 700 cc

Total = 2300 cc/day

Based on this assumption, a 60-kg patient requires maintenance fluids of approximately 95 cc/hr.

Regarding the composition of the maintenance fluid for adults: sodium requirements = 1.5 to 2 mEq/kg/day; potassium requirements = 1 to 1.5 mEq/kg/day; and glucose requirements = ~2 mg/kg/min. Based on these estimates, a 60 kg patient requires 90 to 120 mEq/day of sodium, 60 to 90 mEq/day of potassium, and approximately 7.2 g of glucose per hour (173 g/day).

Typical intravenous crystalloids have the following composition:

- 0.9% Normal Saline (NS) = Na^+ 154 mEq/L, K^+ 0 mEq/L, glucose 0 mEq/L
- 0.45% NS = Na^+ 77 mEq/L, K^+ 0 mEq/L, glucose 0 mEq/L
- Lactated Ringer's (LR) = Na^+ 130 mEq/L, K^+ 4 mEq/L, glucose 0 mEq/L
- 5% dextrose in water (D_5W) = Na^+ 0 mEq/L, K^+ 0 mEq/L, glucose 50 g/L
- D_5W + 0.45% NS = Na^+ 77 mEq/L, K^+ 0 mEq/L, glucose 50 g/L

Refs: Miller RD. Miller's *Anesthesia*. 8th ed. Philadelphia, PA: Elsevier; 2015.

Sterns RH. Maintenance and replacement fluid therapy in adults. In: UpToDate, Forman JP (Ed), UpToDate, Waltham, MA. (Accessed on September 19, 2014.)

5. There is an ongoing debate about the benefits of intravenous fluid therapy with either crystalloids or colloids. For a critically ill patient, an artificial colloid (e.g., hydroxyethyl starch) is selected for fluid resuscitation. In comparison to the administration of a balanced crystalloid (e.g., lactated ringer's), which of the following is a potential benefit of an artificial colloid?

(A) decreased tissue edema
(B) decreased risk of death
(C) decreased risk of anaphylactic reaction
(D) decreased risk of coagulopathy
(E) decreased risk of renal impairment

Significant controversy exists about the optimal type of fluid for volume replacement perioperatively. Complicating the matter, a significant number of previously published trials involving artificial colloids have been retracted due to academic misconduct.

In comparison to artificial colloids, balanced crystalloids have a reduced risk of anaphylactic reaction, decreased risk of coagulopathy (although crystalloids can still cause a dilutional coagulopathy), and decreased risk of renal impairment.

Meta-analysis of data shows no compelling evidence that one fluid is superior to another with respect to mortality. Given that crystalloids are inexpensive, many authors question the routine use of colloids perioperatively.

A significant proportion of crystalloid volume ends up in extravascular compartments. Peripheral edema and organ edema can result. A potential advantage of colloids is that a relatively smaller volume of fluid is required, as more of it stays in the intravascular space. This reduces tissue edema. As to whether colloids improve tissue microcirculation and oxygenation, again this is controversial. Many studies have been retracted and animal studies do not show improved microcirculation.

Refs: Miller RD. Miller's *Anesthesia*. 8th ed. Philadelphia, PA: Elsevier; 2015.

Reilly C, Retraction. Notice of formal retraction of articles by Dr. Joachim Boldt. *Br J Anaesth*. 2011; 107(1): 116–117.

The SAFE Study Investigators, A Comparison of Albumin and Saline for Fluid Resuscitation in the Intensive Care Unit. *N Engl J Med*. 2004; 350:2247–2256.

Guerci P, Tran N, Menu P, et al. Impact of fluid resuscitation with hypertonic- hydroxyethyl starch versus lactated ringer on hemorheology and microcirculation in hemorrhagic shock. *Clin Hemorheol Microcirc*. 2014; 56(4): 301–317.

6. Which of the following is the MOST appropriate indication for transfusion of packed red blood cells?

(A) a patient with a hemoglobin concentration of 11 g/dL who is about to undergo an extensive orthopedic procedure
(B) a septic patient in the critical care unit with a hemoglobin concentration of 8.2 g/dL
(C) an acutely bleeding adult patient with a hemoglobin concentration of 5 g/dL who refuses consent for transfusion

(D) a hemodynamically stable patient with extensive surgical blood loss, a hemoglobin concentration of 7 g/dL, and a mixed venous oxygen saturation of 72%

(E) **a hemodynamically stable patient with extensive surgical blood loss, a hemoglobin concentration of 8.5 g/dL, and a mixed venous oxygen saturation of 52%**

Traditional teaching dictated that patients should be transfused red cells based on the "10/30 rule" (i.e., a fixed transfusion trigger of a hemoglobin concentration of 10 g/dL or a hematocrit of 30%). However, numerous studies highlighting the adverse effects of unnecessary transfusion, as well as concern over transmission of infectious agents, has led to a more evidence-based restrictive approach. There is essentially only one indication for transfusion: to increase the delivery of oxygen to the cells. This is calculated by the formula:

$$\text{Oxygen delivery (DO}_2) = \text{cardiac output} \times \text{arterial oxygen content}$$

Substituting the factors that produce those terms, we get:

$$DO_2 = [HR \times \text{stroke volume}] \times [(1.34 \times Hb \times SaO_2) + 0.003 \times PaO_2]$$

where HR = heart rate, and Hb is hemoglobin concentration. Stroke volume is influenced by preload, afterload, and contractility. Thus, in order to increase the delivery of oxygen to the tissues, one or more options for therapy exist:

1. Increase the heart rate.
2. Optimize the preload (may require diuresis or volume expansion).
3. Optimize the afterload (usually requires afterload reduction).
4. Increase contractility.
5. Increase the FiO_2 and ventilatory strategies (i.e., PEEP) to improve both SaO_2 and PaO_2.
6. Transfuse red blood cells.

Typically in the healthy, bleeding patient the body automatically compensates by increasing cardiac output. The ASA have published a practice guideline for blood component therapy, stating that red cell transfusion is rarely indicated when hemoglobin concentration is >10 g/dL, and is almost always indicated when hemoglobin concentration is <6 g/dL. These are not hard and fast rules, and other factors must be taken into account, including the rate of bleeding, hemodynamic factors, and institutional speed of blood delivery.

Many anesthesiologists aim to transfuse at a hemoglobin somewhere in between these two values; however, the presence of comorbidities such as coronary disease, pulmonary disease, or those states where metabolic demand is increased (sepsis, fever) should prompt consideration of a more liberal transfusion threshold. Rather than relying on an empiric numerical threshold, transfusion should be guided by clinical signs of inadequate oxygen delivery such as decreased urine output, altered mental status, EKG signs of ischemia and/or hemodynamic instability. The mixed venous oxygen saturation can also aid in decision making. A normal SvO_2 (60%–80%) usually indicates normal delivery and extraction; however, when this begins to fall, one or more of three conditions must be present: inadequate cardiac output (either absolute or relative), inadequate SaO_2, or inadequate hemoglobin concentration.

Critically ill patients (excluding those with acute coronary syndrome) appear to do better with a restrictive transfusion trigger (7 g/dL) compared to a liberal one (9 g/dL). Transfusion of blood products to competent, adult patients who refuse them is ethically unsound and a form of assault. Alternative means of maximizing oxygen delivery should be discussed and implemented.

Ref: Longnecker DE, Brown DL, Newman MF, Zapol WM. *Anesthesiology.* 2nd ed. New York, NY: McGraw Hill; 2012.

7. In which of the following situations is transfusion of fresh frozen plasma LEAST appropriate?

(A) an international standardized ratio (INR) of 1.6 prior to urgent surgery for a patient on warfarin

(B) microvascular bleeding after transfusion of 1 blood volume of packed red blood cells when PT/PTT testing cannot be obtained rapidly

(C) **augmentation of plasma volume in a patient who is bleeding briskly and has already received 1 L of crystalloid**

(D) correction of known factor deficiencies for which specific concentrates are not available

(E) during massive transfusion of a trauma patient

According to the ASA practice guidelines on blood component therapy, plasma therapy should be reserved for specific indications, including:

• urgent reversal of warfarin therapy
• correction of excessive microvascular bleeding with elevated coagulation indices (PT/PTT/INR)

- correction of microvascular bleeding associated with large volume (i.e. >1 blood volume) red cell transfusion and when PT/PTT/INR are not available in a timely manner
- correction of known factor deficiencies when those specific concentrates are not available
- heparin resistance in a patient requiring heparin.

Other indications include severe liver disease or liver transplantation, thrombotic thrombocytopenic purpura, hemolytic uremic syndrome, and HELLP syndrome. Plasma should not ordinarily be administered as a means of increasing volume status. Physiologically balanced crystalloid or synthetic colloid solutions should be used first in these circumstances. An exception to this appears to be in trauma, in which the empiric use of high ratio of plasma to red cell (e.g., 1:1 or 1:2) transfusion early (rather than crystalloid followed by red cells), has been demonstrated in some studies to reduce overall blood loss, transfusion requirements, and mortality.

Dosing of plasma is often prescribed empirically, without thought to the goal. For an increase to a minimum of 30% of plasma factors concentration, a dose of 10 to 15 mL/kg is typical. For reversal of warfarin anticoagulation, a lower dose of 5 to 8 mL/kg is all that is required.

Ref: Longnecker DE, Brown DL, Newman MF, Zapol WM. *Anesthesiology.* 2nd ed. New York, NY: McGraw Hill; 2012.

8. Which of the following regarding the collection and storage of blood components is INCORRECT?

(A) Blood collection bags contain citrate, adenine and phosphate.

(B) Frozen red cells may be stored for 10 years or more.

(C) Red cells have a maximum shelf life of 42 days when refrigerated.

(D) Plasma can be frozen for up to one year before being thawed for use.

(E) Platelets are stored at a temperature of 1–6°C and are kept for a maximum of 5 days.

Whole blood is collected in bags containing citrate-phosphate-dextrose-adenine 1 (CPDA-1). Citrate is an anticoagulant, phosphate is a buffer, dextrose is an energy source for the red cells, and adenine allows RBCs to resynthesize ATP, extending the shelf life from 21 to 35 days (when refrigerated). The shelf life of centrifuged, packed RBCs can be extended to 42 days by adding 100 mL of a nutritive solution containing either dextrose and adenine (NutriCell or AS-3) or dextrose, adenine and mannitol (Adsol or AS-1). Frozen red cells which are suspended in a glycerol solution can be stored for over 10 years. Once thawed, they should be used within 24 hours. Similarly, frozen plasma can be stored for up to 1 year.

In the United States, platelets are typically prepared by centrifuging whole blood using a "soft spin" and separating the platelet rich plasma from red cells. The plasma is then subjected to a "hard spin" to concentrate the platelets. Platelet concentrates from 4 to 6 units are mixed with the plasma from one donor to create one adult dose ("platelet pack"). In Europe, a slightly different method called the buffy-coat method is utilized, but the end product is essentially the same. Both of these products are pooled donor products. In contrast, apheresis platelets are collected from a single donor using special pheresis centrifuge, which removes the platelet component from whole blood and returns the plasma, red cells and leukocytes to the donor using the same intravenous cannula. Platelets must be stored at room temperature on an agitator for no longer than 5 days (7 days in some settings where they are tested for bacterial contamination). Cold temperatures degrade the quality of the platelet, rendering them functionally inactive.

Ref: Longnecker DE, Brown DL, Newman MF, Zapol WM. *Anesthesiology.* 2nd ed. New York, NY: McGraw Hill; 2012.

9. Which of the following is associated with the red blood cell (RBC) "storage lesion"?

(A) increased deformability of the RBCs

(B) increased 2,3-diphosphoglycerate (2,3-DPG)

(C) increased pH

(D) **vasoconstriction of the microcirculation**

(E) right shift of the oxyhemoglobin dissociation curve

ATP levels within stored RBCs fall in a time-dependent manner, which has negative effects on cellular processes such as RBC membrane stability, oxidative stress defense mechanisms, and glucose transport. This leads to increased cell fragility and decreased deformability, which can result in cell rupture, increased free hemoglobin, and blocked capillaries due to the inability of the RBC to "fold" through the tight channel.

One of the most notable changes in stored blood is the fall in 2,3-DPG, an allosteric modifier of hemoglobin that plays a crucial role in the release of oxygen at the tissue level. Levels of 2,3-DPG fall quickly, becoming undetectable within 2 weeks. This leads to a left-shift in the oxyhemoglobin dissociation curve (despite an increase in hydrogen ions, CO_2 and decreased pH). This persists for approximately 6 to 72 hours after transfusion, so that while these donor erythrocytes may be transported to the tissues, oxygen may be less likely to become unbound for a given tissue PO_2. The clinical significance of this is unclear.

When hemoglobin encounters areas of regional hypoxia, it releases the vasodilator S-nitrosothiol (SNO), which is formed when a nitric oxide equivalent binds to hemoglobin. SNO is released in proportion to hemoglobin oxygen desaturation, thereby matching regional tissue perfusion and delivery of oxygen to metabolic demand. During the first few hours of storage, SNO activity is almost obliterated, and this component of the storage lesion is thought to result in altered oxygen delivery within the microcirculation, especially to "at-risk" tissues.

Ref: Longnecker DE, Brown DL, Newman MF, Zapol WM. *Anesthesiology.* 2nd ed. New York, NY: McGraw Hill; 2012.

10. Which of the following is the MOST appropriate size of filter to prevent macroaggregate delivery during transfusion?

(A) 1 micron

(B) 40 microns

(C) 110 microns

(D) **170 microns**

(E) 375 microns

Standard blood administration sets contain 170 micron filters, which are designed to prevent the passage of large clots and aggregates, while ensuring an effective transfusion flow rate. Most standard blood filters of this size are designed to filter 2 to 4 units of blood before changing. Otherwise, these sets should be changed every 12 hours or if flow rates are compromised. The administration set used in most rapid tranfusion devices (e.g., Level 1) also contain a 170-micron filter.

Smaller, 20- to 40-micron micropore filters are used by some to filter out fibrin, leukocytes and red cell components; however, there is insufficient evidence to recommend their routine use. They may be useful in rapid, massive transfusion, although because they may slow down flow rates (especially as they become clogged with debris) they may need to be changed frequently.

Ref: Longnecker DE, Brown DL, Newman MF, Zapol WM. *Anesthesiology.* 2nd ed. New York, NY: McGraw Hill; 2012.

11. A improperly calibrated blood warming device that heats the red blood cells (RBCs) to a temperature >45°C may result in which of the following?

(A) **red cell fragmentation and hemolysis**

(B) red cell adherence and premature clotting

(C) a left shift in the oxyhemoglobin dissociation curve

(D) contamination of the blood with plastic polymers from the intravenous tubing

(E) disseminated intravascular coagulation (DIC)

Heating devices for blood infusion sets must be calibrated properly. Blood that is too cold (below body temperature) will quickly contribute to hypothermia. Prior to the introduction of routine blood warming, the rate of ventricular arrhythmias following cold blood transfusion was alarmingly high. On the other extreme, superheated (>45°C) red cells can exhibit heat denaturation (budding and fragmentation), which leads to hemolysis. Blood should be administered through a warmer that is routinely checked and calibrated. Blood should never be heated in other ways, such as by using a microwave oven. Unless you're a vampire. Then I guess it's okay.

Ref: Longnecker DE, Brown DL, Newman MF, Zapol WM. *Anesthesiology.* 2nd ed. New York, NY: McGraw Hill; 2012.

12. Cryoprecipitate contains which of the following coagulation factors?

(A) factor II

(B) factor VII

(C) **factor VIII**

(D) factor IX

(E) factor X

Cryoprecipitate is prepared by thawing fresh frozen plasma (FFP) between 1°C and 6°C and recovering the precipitate. The FFP may either be derived from a whole blood collection or an apheresis collection. Once obtained by centrifugation, the cold-insoluble precipitate is refrozen, and typically has a volume of 10 to 20 mL.

Cryoprecipitate contains most of the factor VIII, fibrinogen, factor XIII, VWF and fibronectin from the FFP. Fibrinogen is the most important factor, with each bag containing approximately 150 to 250 mg of fibrinogen. In a 70-kg patient, 1 bag of cryoprecipitate should raise the fibrinogen level by about 45 mg/dL. Cryoprecipitate is indicated for the treatment of microvascular or massive bleeding associated with hypofibrinogenemia (<100 mg/dL), or clinical suspicion of hypofibrinogenemia in the setting of massive bleeding where clinical status precludes waiting for laboratory confirmation of fibrinogen concentration. Cryoprecipitate is also used for the treatment of bleeding in patients with von Willebrand's disease or hemophilia A, when specific factor concentrates are unavailable and/or DDAVP is unavailable or ineffective.

Ref: Longnecker DE, Brown DL, Newman MF, Zapol WM. *Anesthesiology.* 2nd ed. New York, NY: McGraw Hill; 2012.

13. Which of the following statements regarding albumin solutions for transfusion is NOT true?

(A) Albumin solutions are available in 5% or 25% concentrations.

(B) Albumin provides most of the colloid oncotic pressure in the plasma.

(C) Albumin is heat treated to inactivate viruses.

(D) Almost all of a 5% albumin solution will remain in the intravascular compartment.

(E) **Patients with an allergy to eggs should not receive an albumin transfusion.**

Albumin is synthesized by the liver and is an abundant protein both in the intravascular compartment and in the interstitial space. Albumin is the primary transport protein in the blood and contributes significantly (approximately 75%) to the oncotic pressure of the plasma.

Albumin solutions are intravenous colloid solutions that are prepared by diluting human-derived albumin protein in isotonic saline. Two concentrations are available, an isotonic 5% solution, and a hyperoncotic 25% solution. While the 5% solution can be used for volume expansion during hypovolemia and blood loss, the 25% solution should only be used to shift fluid from the interstitium into the intravascular space in cases of hypoalbuminemia. Both solutions are heated to 60°C for 10 hours to reduce the risk of transmission of viral diseases.

The vast majority of 5% albumin solution will remain in the intravascular space, expanding the intravascular volume by (approximately) the amount transfused, compared to 25% to 30% of the volume of crystalloid. This makes it an excellent volume expander, as there is little shift to either the interstitial or intracellular compartments.

Allergic reactions to albumin are rare (0.1%), and are generally less common that those seen with the synthetic colloids. Egg allergy is not a contraindication for the use of albumin, as the primary egg protein, ovalbumin (kd), is structurally different than human albumin (67 kd).

Ref: Longnecker DE, Brown DL, Newman MF, Zapol WM. *Anesthesiology.* 2nd ed. New York, NY: McGraw Hill; 2012.

14. When ordering blood from the blood bank, which of the following steps in the type and cross process takes the MOST amount of time?

(A) testing for ABO type

(B) testing for Rh (D) type

(C) **antibody screen**

(D) immediate spin crossmatch

(E) computer crossmatch

Compatibility testing of blood prior to transfusion involves several steps. The first steps are referred to as the "type and screen":

TABLE 6-1. **Type and screen procedures and time required for each step.**

Test	Time (min)	Information
ABO type	5	Recipient RBCs tested for A and B antigen
Rh (D) type	5	Recipient RBCs tested for D antigen
Antibody screen	45	Screens for RBC alloantibodies formed as a result of prior transfusion or pregnancy (using the indirect Coombs test or gel column agglutination)

A type and screen is usually ordered when there is a low risk (<10% chance) of transfusion during a surgical procedure or hospital admission. Most minor surgeries do not require even a type and screen. For procedures in which transfusion is planned or the procedure carries a higher risk (>10%) of transfusion, a serologic cross-match is indicated. Assuming the antibody screen is negative, there are two ways that this can be rapidly performed:

- **Immediate spin crossmatch** (Time required: 5 minutes). Testing involves mixing of donor RBCs and recipient plasma. This is used to verify ABO compatibility only.

- **Computer crossmatch** (Time required: 2 minutes). The computer selects appropriate unit(s) based on ABO status.

However, if the initial antibody screen is positive, an **antiglobulin crossmatch** is mandatory. This involves incubation of donor RBCs with recipient plasma and anti-IgG. Because finding donor units that are compatible with these often rare antibodies present in the recipient blood, patients with a positive antibody screen should have donor red cell units made available before surgery.

Ref: Longnecker DE, Brown DL, Newman MF, Zapol WM. *Anesthesiology.* 2nd ed. New York, NY: McGraw Hill; 2012.

15. Which of the following regarding preoperative autologous donation (PAD) is FALSE?

(A) Aortic stenosis is a contraindication to PAD.

(B) PAD should be considered when there is a high likelihood of >500–1000 mL blood loss.

(C) PAD is more expensive than allogeneic blood transfusion.

(D) **By donating their own blood, a patient eliminates the risk of viral transmission associated with transfusion.**

(E) PAD units may be used for other recipients if not used for the intended donor.

PAD became popular in the 1980s and 1990s during a time of heightened concern about transmission of infectious agents during allogeneic blood transfusion. In recent years, it has experienced a decline, due to a number of factors, including cost, better surgical blood conservation measures, and a lack of evidence supporting its use. Several studies have shown that PAD induces a preoperative anemia and increases the risk for transfusion compared to patients who do not participate in PAD.

Patients who are usually considered for PAD should be in good general health, are able tolerate iron therapy during the collection period, and are undergoing a procedure in which there is a good likelihood of losing 500 to 1000 mL or more of blood. Contraindications relate to the effect of creating acute anemia, and include ischemic heart disease, heart failure, aortic stenosis, ventricular arrhythmias, cerebrovascular disease, and uncontrolled hypertension.

PAD is significantly more expensive (from $70 to >$4000 per unit) compared to allogeneic blood. Contributing to this is the additional time and attention required by autologous donor/patients, the increased clerical requirements, the special handling required (additional labels, special storage, etc.), and the enormous wastage of autologous blood—approximately 50% is not transfused.

PAD units may be designated for "crossover" if not used and are therefore available for use by the blood bank as needed. In these cases, the units must undergo the same infectious testing as allogeneic units, even if transfused to the original donor/patient. One of the purported advantages of PAD, the reduction in infective risk, is not completely eliminated, as clerical error may result in a patient receiving an allogeneic unit.

Ref: Hillyer CD, Silberstein LE, Ness PM, Anderson KC, Roback JD. *Blood Banking and Transfusion Medicine: Basic Principles and Practice.* 2nd ed. Philadelphia, PA: Churchill Livingstone; 2007.

16. Which of the following combinations of blood products would MOST likely result in an incompatibility reaction?

(A) Type O red cells are transfused to a type AB patient.

(B) **Type AB red cells are transfused to a type O patient.**

(C) Type AB plasma is transfused to a type B patient.

(D) Type B plasma is transfused to a type O patient.

(E) Type A platelets are transfused to type B patient.

The ABO blood type is the most important of all the red blood cell antigens. There are four different blood groups, determined by the presence or absence of A and/or B antigens (Table 6-2). Normally, antibodies are produced against the antigen(s) that are NOT present. For example, a patient with type B blood will have anti-A antibodies that attack RBCs donated from both group A and group AB individuals.

TABLE 6-2. Blood groups and compatibility.

Blood group	Red cells express	Plasma contains
O	Neither A nor B antigen	*Both* anti-A and anti-B antibodies
A	A antigen	Anti-B antibody
B	B antigen	Anti-A antibody
AB	*Both* A and B antigen	Neither anti-A nor anti-B antibody

The following principles should be adhered to when managing transfusions:

- Transfused RBCs should be ABO (and Rh-group) specific. In an emergency, group O-negative cells can be used until the group is known. Since group O RBCs lack both antigens, patients with this blood type are considered the universal donor, and these cells can be given to any ABO group. Type AB patients lack antibodies to A and B in their plasma and therefore can *receive* any ABO blood type (universal recipient).

- Plasma and cryoprecipitate should also be ABO compatible with the recipient's red cells. Additional testing beyond ABO and Rh grouping (i.e., antibody screening and crossmatching) are not required for components derived from plasma. Group AB plasma contains no antigens and is therefore considered the universal donor.

- Platelets should ideally be ABO compatible. However, due to supply issues, this is not always possible, and ABO nonidentical platelets may be transfused. Additional testing beyond ABO and Rh grouping (i.e., antibody screening and crossmatching) are not required for platelets.

Ref: Hillyer CD, Silberstein LE, Ness PM, Anderson KC, Roback JD. *Blood Banking and Transfusion Medicine: Basic Principles and Practice.* 2nd ed. Philadelphia, PA: Churchill Livingstone; 2007.

17. Advantages of recombinant hemoglobin-based oxygen carriers over allogeneic blood transfusion may include all EXCEPT:

(A) longer half-life in the vasculature

(B) superior shelf-life

(C) universal compatibility

(D) may be acceptable to Jehovah's Witnesses

(E) unlimited availability

The purpose of hemoglobin-based oxygen carriers is to provide a means for oxygen delivery without the risks and/or reliance on traditional allogeneic donor blood. Several types have been developed, including free acellular human or bovine hemoglobin, polymerized hemoglobin, liposomal encapsulated hemoglobin, and recombinant hemoglobin. However, there are no hemoglobin-based oxygen carriers currently approved for use in the United States (or most other countries), largely because of absence of good effect in animal trials, as well as concern for toxicity related to nitric oxide scavenging, vasoconstriction, reduced oxygen delivery to hypoxic tissues, and systemic and pulmonary hypertension. Nonetheless, research still continues because of a number of theoretical benefits.

One such benefit is a longer shelf life, because these solutions do not contain living, respiring cells. Second, because recombinant hemoglobin is produced by bacteria, the risk of mammalian disease agents is eliminated, and the supply is theoretically very large. Recombinant hemoglobin lacks a cell membrane and its associated antigens, so there are no restrictions with respect to compatibility, and persons of any blood type can receive these products. Modern recombinant hemoglobin molecules have an oxygen affinity that is useful, if not exactly the same as HbA (P_{50} of acellular Hb = 18 mm Hg). However, these molecules are relatively short-lived in the plasma, with an intravascular half-life of less than 1 day. Many Jehovah's Witnesses will consent to receive these solutions (despite their unavailability), as they are not a human-derived blood product.

Ref: Hillyer CD, Silberstein LE, Ness PM, Anderson KC, Roback JD. *Blood Banking and Transfusion Medicine: Basic Principles and Practice.* 2nd ed. Philadelphia, PA: Churchill Livingstone; 2007.

18. Features characteristic of febrile nonhemolytic transfusion reactions (FNHTR) include all EXCEPT:

(A) a rise in temperature >1°C

(B) a higher incidence with red blood cells (RBCs) than platelets

(C) rigors

(D) hypotension

(E) caused by cytokines typically released by donor leukocytes

An FNHTR is classically described as a fever (>1°C) occurring during or shortly after transfusion, associated with chills, rigors, and occasionally hypotension, that is self-limiting. While fever is typical, it is not always present, especially if the patient is taking antipyretic drugs such as acetaminophen.

The cause of FNHTR is thought to be a reaction between recipient antibodies and antigens expressed on the surface of donor cells, usually leukocytes. For that reason, it is substantially more common in platelet transfusion (approximately 1:10 transfusions) than RBC transfusion (1:300 transfusions), since platelet units are typically contaminated by leukocytes. This reaction releases proinflammatory cytokines that produce the fever, chills, and hypotension. The use of leukoreduction filters does not predictably reduce the incidence of FNHTR, because these filters do not prevent the transfusion of prereleased cytokines.

Management of FNHTR centers around ruling out other causes of transfusion reaction (especially acute hemolytic transfusion reaction), followed by symptomatic treatment of the fever with acetaminophen. If the rigors are severe and no contraindications exist, meperidine 25 to 50 mg can be effective.

Ref: Longnecker DE, Brown DL, Newman MF, Zapol WM. *Anesthesiology.* 2nd ed. New York, NY: McGraw Hill; 2012.

19. A 56-year-old woman is receiving a transfusion of RBCs in the operating room for continued bleeding during an abdominal hysterectomy. Over the course of 5 minutes, you notice hives, facial edema and an increase in peak airway pressures from 20 to 35 cmH$_2$O while ventilating her with positive pressure ventilation. Which of the following is the MOST likely cause of this reaction?

(A) IgA from small amounts of donor plasma

(B) citrate in the RBC units

(C) cytokines from leukocytes

(D) free hemoglobin from lysed RBCs

(E) a drug error

Transfusion-associated anaphylactic reactions are rare, with a reported incidence of 1 in 20,000 to 50,000. Reactions usually begin within 1 to 45 minutes of the commencement of transfusion.

There are several causes of transfusion-related anaphylaxis. One of the most well-described is the delivery of plasma containing IgA to patients with selective IgA deficiency who have anti-IgA antibodies. IgA deficiency is not uncommon (1 in 300 to 500 individuals).

Other causes include recipients who lack haptoglobin and have anti-haptoglobin antibodies, and the transfer of food (e.g. peanut) allergens that were ingested by the donor and transfused to a sensitized recipient. If a patient is known to be IgA deficient and requires a transfusion, only washed RBCs should be used. Similarly, if plasma is to be transfused, IgA-deficient plasma from IgA-deficient donors can be specially ordered.

Ref: Longnecker DE, Brown DL, Newman MF, Zapol WM. *Anesthesiology.* 2nd ed. New York, NY: McGraw Hill; 2012.

20. A patient receiving a transfusion of FFP in the PACU complains of pruritus and hives over his chest, neck and face. After stopping the transfusion, which of the following would be the MOST appropriate next step?

(A) Administer epinephrine 0.3 mg SC.

(B) Administer epinephrine 0.1 mg IV.

(C) Administer diphenhydramine 50 mg IV.

(D) Administer hydrocortisone 100 mg IV.

(E) Administer dexamethasone 8 mg IV.

Urticarial transfusion reactions (UTRs) are a minor allergic reaction thought to be caused by soluble allergens in the transfused plasma portion of blood reacting with preexisting IgE recipient antibodies. Degranulation of mast cells and basophils results, with histamine and other vasoactive mediators causing urticaria. Other symptoms may include bronchial reactivity (e.g., coughing, wheezing), abdominal cramps, diarrhea, nausea, and vomiting. These reactions are relatively common, especially with plasma containing components (1 in 100 units transfused).

Immediate management should involve stopping the transfusion followed by the administration of 25 to 50 mg diphenhydramine. If the urticaria resolve and there is an absence of more serious clinical features such as hypotension, dyspnea, or laryngeal edema, the transfusion may be restarted. Epinephrine and corticosteroids should be reserved for anaphylactic and anaphylactoid reactions. Premedication with antihistamines or steroids has not be proven to be effective against these reactions.

Ref: Longnecker DE, Brown DL, Newman MF, Zapol WM. *Anesthesiology.* 2nd ed. New York, NY: McGraw Hill; 2012.

21. Which of the following clinical features is MOST commonly associated with an acute hemolytic transfusion reaction?

    (A) flank pain
    (B) hypotension
    (C) nausea
    (D) oliguria
    (E) fever

Acute hemolytic transfusion reactions (AHTRs) are a medical emergency that typically result from a clerical or procedural error that leads to ABO-incompatibility during transfusion. Half of all errors are due to administering the correctly labeled blood to the incorrect patient. Other errors can occur during the collection of the specimen or during testing of samples in the lab. Anti-A or anti-B antibodies in the recipient serum bind to the donor erythrocytes carrying the respective antigen, fix complement, and lyse the donor cells, releasing free hemoglobin.

Not all AHTRs are ABO-related. Non-ABO incompatibility causes include alloantibodies from a previous transfusion that are not detected by the antibody screen or the transfusion of uncrossmatched blood in an emergency to a patient who is alloimmunized.

The most common presenting features are fever, chills, and hemoglobinuria. Less common features include flank or abdominal pain, hypotension, nausea/vomiting, ooziness/DIC, and renal failure. Fever may be the ONLY presenting sign of an AHTR.

Management priorities should be:
- STOP the transfusion (keep the bag of transfused cells, as repeat crossmatch will likely be required).
- Supportive care (airway, breathing, circulation).
- Begin an infusion of normal saline to induce a brisk diuresis and to prevent/treat hypotension. Ringer's lactate should be avoided as the calcium may clot the remaining blood in the IV line.
- Manage DIC and hemorrhage as indicated.
- Check if there is a clerical error (check identity of patient vs. blood label).
- Notify the blood bank (critical if there has been a switch in blood bags and another patient in the hospital is at risk).

- From another limb, draw a sample for a direct antiglobulin test, plasma free hemoglobin, and repeat type and crossmatch.

Ref: Longnecker DE, Brown DL, Newman MF, Zapol WM. *Anesthesiology.* 2nd ed. New York, NY: McGraw Hill; 2012.

22. Which of the following BEST describes the etiology of a delayed hemolytic transfusion reaction?

    (A) ABO incompatibility
    (B) anamnestic response to an undetected antigen
    (C) lysis of recipient cells by donor complement
    (D) recipient viral illness at time of transfusion
    (E) disseminated intravascular coagulation from fibrin strands

Delayed hemolytic reactions result from the formation of recipient antibodies to previously transfused blood (or from exposure to alloantigens during pregnancy) and the re-exposure to these antigens during subsequent transfusion. These alloantigens are below the level that is detectable on the routine antibody screen (which highlights why compatibility testing is not failsafe), but upon transfusion cause an anamnestic production of antibodies that leads to hemolysis. The usual time lag between transfusion and clinical presentation is between 2 days and 2 weeks. Hemolysis is usually gradual and less severe than acute hemolytic reactions, but it can be rapid and life-threatening. Hemolytic anemia is the main clinical picture, with a low hemoglobin, high bilirubin, reticulocytosis, spherocytosis, and a positive direct antiglobulin test.

Ref: Longnecker DE, Brown DL, Newman MF, Zapol WM. *Anesthesiology.* 2nd ed. New York, NY: McGraw Hill; 2012.

23. Which of the following infectious agents is MOST likely to be transmitted to a patient during allogeneic blood transfusion?

    (A) human immunodeficiency virus (HIV)
    (B) hepatitis B
    (C) hepatitis C
    (D) West Nile virus
    (E) human T-cell lymphotrophic virus (HTLV)

Transfusion-transmitted infection is generally very uncommon. Current estimates of the risk of viral transmission during transfusion are:

Virus	Estimated risk of infection via transfusion
HIV	1 in 1.5–2 million
Hepatitis B virus	1 in 50,000–250,000
Hepatitis C virus	1 in 1–2 million
HTLV	1 in 2 million
West Nile virus	Unknown/very rare

The incidence of transfusion transmitted bacterial infection is higher than viral infection. This risk is highest for platelets, since they are stored at room temperature (risk of contamination is approximately 1 in 1000), whereas the incidence of contamination of red cell units is estimated to be 1 in 50,000. Not every bacterially-contaminated unit leads to a clinical infection, and rates of sepsis with platelets and RBCs are thought to be approximately 1 in 10,000 and 1 in 100,000, respectively.

Ref: Carson JL, Kleinman S. Indications and hemoglobin thresholds for red blood cell transfusion in the adult. In: UpToDate, Silvergleid AJ (Ed), UpToDate, Waltham, MA. Accessed January 12, 2015.

24. In which of the following scenarios is the transfusion of cytomegalovirus-seronegative blood units LEAST likely to offer a safety advantage?

(A) CMV-seronegative pregnant women

(B) intrauterine transfusions

(C) CMV-seronegative allogeneic bone marrow transplant recipients

(D) a patient infected with HIV

(E) a patient infected with hepatitis C

Cytomegalovirus (CMV) is a highly prevalent (40%–60%) community-acquired infection that can be transmitted in a variety of ways through infected body fluids. It primarily infects leukocytes, and in immunocompetent individuals often does nothing more than provoke a mononucleosis syndrome; however, the virus remains latent in the host, and can be reactivated if the patient becomes immunocompromised. In this setting, CMV infection can cause severe and sometimes fatal inflammatory conditions such as pneumonitis, hepatitis, encephalitis, and gastroenteritis that require aggressive treatment with antiviral medications.

The transfusion of blood that is free (or virtually free) of CMV should be considered for certain populations, including seronegative transplant patients (either solid or hematopoietic), severely immunosuppressed patients and HIV-infected patients. In addition, seronegative pregnant patients, fetuses, and low-birthweight infants should also minimize exposure to CMV in order to reduce the risk of congenital CMV infection. One strategy is to use blood units that have been tested for CMV and are CMV-seronegative. Not all units in the United States are tested for this—only enough to maintain an inventory of CMV-seronegative units. However, another approach is simply to use leukoreduction filters, as the virus inhabits the white cells. Most studies have failed to find a difference between the use of specific CMV-seronegative blood and ordinary units that are leukoreduced to below 5 million cells per unit of blood, and so either approach is reasonable.

Ref: Longnecker DE, Brown DL, Newman MF, Zapol WM. *Anesthesiology.* 2nd ed. New York, NY: McGraw Hill; 2012.

25. Which of the following statements regarding citrate intoxication during blood transfusion is CORRECT?

(A) Citrate is used as an antioxidant in packed red blood cell preparations.

(B) Citrate is normally metabolized rapidly in the liver to bicarbonate.

(C) Rapid transfusion of citrated blood can result in hypercalcemia.

(D) A shortened QT interval is characteristic of citrate toxicity.

(E) Calcium can be added to blood to prevent citrate toxicity.

Citrate is an anticoagulant that is added to blood as part of the CPDA solution. It prevents coagulation by chelating ionized calcium, a co-factor in several steps in the coagulation cascade. Normally, citrate is metabolized by the liver into bicarbonate, and circulating ionized calcium levels should not decrease. However, when large volumes of blood are transfused rapidly (i.e., >1 mL/kg/min, or 1 unit every 5 minutes), this may theoretically overwhelm the liver's ability to metabolize the citrate and hypocalcemia may develop. Liver disease may contribute to the rapidity with which this event occurs. Hypocalcemia may be suspected when the QT interval becomes prolonged or when the patient complains of perioral numbness or muscle spasm/tetany. When large volumes of blood are transfused, measurement of arterial blood gases should be routinely performed in order to follow the serum ionized calcium level and to guide intravenous calcium therapy.

Calcium should never be added to blood bags as this will cause clotting. Likewise, calcium-containing intravenous fluids (lactated Ringers solution, Haemaccel 3.5%) should be avoided as carrier solutions.

Ref: Longnecker DE, Brown DL, Newman MF, Zapol WM. *Anesthesiology.* 2nd ed. New York, NY: McGraw Hill; 2012.

26. Which of the following electrolyte disturbances is LEAST likely after transfusion of packed red cells?

    (A) hyponatremia
    (B) hyperkalemia
    (C) hypomagnesemia
    (D) hypocalcemia
    (E) hypokalemia

During storage of blood, metabolism within the red blood cells generates hydrogen ions. In order to maintain electrical neutrality, potassium moves outside the cells. This may be accentuated with "old" blood, where the lysis of cells increases the extracellular potassium content. This is usually not a problem during routine transfusion, but during rapid, massive transfusion, hyperkalemia has been reported. This may be a particular concern for patients with renal impairment or neonates, both of whom are less able to handle potassium loads.

In contrast, upon transfusion, most healthy red cells reverse the storage lesion and reverse the potassium gradient. In addition, the citrate in the CPDA solution is metabolized by the liver to bicarbonate, which induces a metabolic alkalosis, shifting potassium into the cells. For these reasons, hypokalemia has also been seen on occasion after massive transfusion.

Both hypocalcemia and hypomagnesemia can be caused by rapid transfusion by the chelation of these ions by citrate. While stored blood is acidic (pH of 6.6–6.9) due to accumulation of carbon dioxide and lactate, this is rapidly reversed once transfused into a patient with normal tissue perfusion. Citrate and lactate are both metabolized to bicarbonate, provoking a metabolic alkalosis. Prophylactic administration of sodium bicarbonate to counteract the acidic blood is nonsensical, and leads to worsened alkalosis, a left-shift of the oxyhemoglobin dissociation curve, and hypernatremia from the sodium load. Sodium disturbances do not routinely complicate transfusion therapy.

Ref: Longnecker DE, Brown DL, Newman MF, Zapol WM. *Anesthesiology.* 2nd ed. New York, NY: McGraw Hill; 2012.

27. The transfusion of multiple units of cold red blood cells may lead to which of the following complications?

    (A) coronary vasospasm
    (B) hemolysis
    (C) decreased affinity of hemoglobin for oxygen
    (D) dilutional thrombocytopenia
    (E) disseminated intravascular coagulation (DIC)

The administration of multiple units of RBCs without additional platelet or plasma units will eventually result in a clinically significant dilution of both platelets and coagulation factors. Traditionally, RBCs were transfused until evidence of this coagulopathy appeared, or until a certain threshold limit of RBCs was empirically reached. The recognition that dilutional coagulopathies worsen bleeding and outcomes (especially in penetrating trauma) combined with evidence that increased ratios of plasma and platelets to RBCs has led to a rethinking of massive transfusion strategy, with many centers adopting a 1:1 or 1:2 plasma:RBC ratio on the initiation of a massive transfusion protocol.

When massive transfusion is carried out at cold temperatures, the patient is placed at risk for a number of adverse events. First, hypothermia may occur quickly. Six units of RBCs at refrigerator temperature (4°C) will reduce the core body temperature of an average adult male by 1°C. Given that many cases of massive transfusion are being carried out in the trauma population, who may already be hypothermic due to hemorrhage and exposure, the potential for serious hypothermia is substantial. Ventricular arrhythmias begin to occur at about 30°C. Second, significant hypothermic coagulopathy due to clotting cascade dysfunction and platelet sequestration occurs with even mild (<1°C) reductions in core body temperature. This leads to increased bleeding and requirement for allogeneic blood transfusion, with all the attendant potential complications.

Ref: Longnecker DE, Brown DL, Newman MF, Zapol WM. *Anesthesiology.* 2nd ed. New York, NY: McGraw Hill; 2012.

28. A patient receiving 2 units of fresh frozen plasma on the floor develops hypoxemia and pulmonary failure. Three hours later, auscultation reveals crackles in all lung fields. Her post-intubation chest X-ray is notable for widespread alveolar infiltrates. Which of the follow-

ing factors best differentiates transfusion-related acute lung injury (TRALI) from transfusion-associated circulatory overload (TACO)?

(A) blood pressure

(B) presence of crackles on auscultation

(C) chest radiograph

(D) **response to diuretics**

(E) TACO is just a way better acronym

TACO and TRALI may be difficult to distinguish, and in fact may coexist in the same patient, making diagnosis and treatment difficult.

TRALI is an inflammatory condition of the pulmonary microcirculation occurring in approximately 1 in every 5000 units of blood product transfused. The clinical diagnosis is made on the basis of a new acute lung injury/ARDS occurring within 6 hours of blood product administration (documented by room air SpO_2 <90% or P/F ratio <300 and an abnormal CXR). TRALI has occurred following any blood component therapy, and may be particularly prone to occur after transfusion with plasma from female donors. TRALI is thought to occur via a "2-hit" mechanism. The first step is neutrophil sequestration and priming in the lung microvasculature by endothelial injury; this step, which makes the neutrophils more susceptible to activation by a weak stimulus, occurs prior to the transfusion. The second step is neutrophil activation by a factor in the transfused blood, resulting in an inflammatory cascade. Treatment in TRALI is supportive, with ventilatory and hemodynamic support. TRALI is the leading cause of transfusion-related mortality, with rates varying from 5% to 10% to as high as 67% for the critically ill population.

TACO is more common, occurring with every 1500 units transfused. It generally occurs in elderly patients or small children, those with poor ventricular function, and is associated with rapid blood product administration. The clinical picture for TACO appears as simple volume overload: elevated central venous and pulmonary wedge pressures, increased brain natriuretic peptide, and rapid pulmonary improvement with diuretic therapy. There is typically no fever and no elevated white cell count, whereas both of these are usually present in TRALI. Management of TACO is similar to TRALI with the notable exception that

diuresis usually proves very effective at reversing the pulmonary symptoms and clinical picture.

Widespread crackles and alveolar infiltrates on CXR are present in both syndromes; blood pressure can vary and tends to be hypertensive in TACO, but this is not a rule.

Ref: Butterworth JF IV, Mackey DC, Wasnick JD. *Morgan and Mikhail's Clinical Anesthesiology.* 5th ed. New York, NY: McGraw Hill; 2013.

29. Transfusion of blood that has not been leukocyte-depleted has been shown to result in which of the following complications?

(A) cerebral edema

(B) **postoperative infection**

(C) increased rate of renal allograft rejection

(D) anaphylaxis

(E) hypercalcemia

Leukocytes present in the plasma fraction of transfused red cells may cause a number of effects that lead to the suppression of the host immune system. This was first noticed in the 1960s when renal transplant patients who had been transfused blood enjoyed ***reduced*** rejection rates of the transplanted organ, suggesting that an immunosuppressive mechanism was at play. Termed transfusion-related immunomodulation (or TRIM), the clinical sequelae of this include include febrile nonhemolytic transfusion reaction, RBC alloimmunization, and CMV transmission. Prestorage leukoreduction (i.e., in the blood bank versus at the bedside with a filter) substantially decreases the number of white blood cells, and may decrease some of these risks, although the data is not entirely supportive of these claims. Multiple studies have also investigated rates of tumor recurrence with leukoreduction, with both positive and negative results.

The strongest evidence to date supporting leukoreduction is with postoperative infection. Multiple studies have shown a several-fold decrease in bacterial wound infections and central venous line infections when using RBCs that had been leukoreduced.

Ref: Butterworth JF IV, Mackey DC, Wasnick JD. *Morgan and Mikhail's Clinical Anesthesiology.* 5th ed. New York, NY: McGraw Hill; 2013.

CHAPTER 7

Endocrine Physiology

1. Which of the following hormones is produced in the hypothalamus?

    (A) adrenocorticotropic hormone

    (B) growth hormone

    (C) oxytocin

    (D) prolactin

    (E) thyroid-stimulating hormone

2. Hormone secretion is regulated via a complex array of mechanisms including feedback regulation. The feedback substrate may be another hormone, nutrient, or ion. Which of the following hormones is paired correctly with its feedback substrate?

    (A) ACTH: IGF-1

    (B) GH: triiodothyronine

    (C) aldosterone: plasma K^+ levels

    (D) insulin: plasma Ca^{2+} levels

    (E) TSH: cortisol

3. Which of the following treatments for thyroid storm (severe thyrotoxicosis) relies on a mechanism known as the Wolff-Chaikoff effect?

    (A) propranolol

    (B) hydrocortisone

    (C) propylthiouracil

    (D) Lugol's iodine

    (E) methimazole

4. Which of the following hormones acts to decrease plasma Ca^{2+} levels and decrease bone resorption?

    (A) PTH

    (B) vitamin D

    (C) calcitonin

    (D) cortisol

    (E) triiodothyronine

5. In the adrenal gland, which of the following enzymes catalyzes the conversion of norepinephrine to epinephrine?

    (A) tyrosine hydroxylase

    (B) dopa decarboxylase

    (C) dopamine β-hydroxylase

    (D) phenylethanolamine N-methyltransferase

    (E) catechol-O-methyltransferase

6. The zona glomerulosa of the adrenal cortex is the sole source of production for which of the following hormones?

    (A) aldosterone

    (B) cortisol

    (C) dehydroepiandrosterone

    (D) androstenedione

    (E) corticosterone

7. Produced in the endocrine pancreas, which of the following hormones acts to decrease appetite and inhibit gluconeogenesis?

    (A) insulin

    (B) glucagon

    (C) somatostatin

    (D) pancreatic polypeptide

    (E) ghrelin

8. Under anaerobic conditions, lactate formed in the muscles may be converted back into glucose via which of the following pathways?

    (A) citric acid cycle

    (B) pentose phosphate pathway

    (C) Cori cycle

    (D) alanine cycle

    (E) glycolysis

9. Pyruvate is a versatile substrate that can participate in various enzymatic reactions to directly produce all of the following molecules EXCEPT:

    (A) lactate
    (B) alanine
    (C) oxaloacetate
    (D) acetyl-CoA
    (E) glucose-6-phosphate

10. Insulin has which of the following metabolic effects?

    (A) stimulates gluconeogenesis
    (B) stimulates protein catabolism
    (C) stimulates glycogenolysis
    (D) stimulates lipolysis
    (E) stimulates glycolysis

11. Epinephrine stimulates which of the following metabolic processes?

    (A) lipolysis in adipose tissue
    (B) glycolysis in the liver
    (C) glycogen synthesis in the liver
    (D) fatty acid synthesis in the liver
    (E) triglyceride release from skeletal muscle

12. Chronic stress has which of the following physiologic effects?

    (A) increased levels of TSH
    (B) decreased levels of cortisol
    (C) decreased levels of catecholamines
    (D) increased gluconeogenesis
    (E) increased levels of growth hormone

13. Which of the following is a catabolic product of protein?

    (A) glucose
    (B) creatine
    (C) thyroxine
    (D) dopamine
    (E) DNA

14. Of the following neurotransmitters, hormones, or drugs, which of the following uses cGMP as an intracellular second messenger?

    (A) thyroxine
    (B) ANP
    (C) cocaine
    (D) acetylcholine
    (E) epinephrine

15. Which of the following enzymes is critical in the regulation of cholesterol synthesis?

    (A) HMG-CoA reductase
    (B) acetyl-CoA carboxylase
    (C) triacylglycerol synthase
    (D) lipoprotein lipase
    (E) β-hydroxybutyrate dehydrogenase

16. Which of the following tissues exclusively utilizes glucose as its metabolic substrate?

    (A) liver
    (B) brain
    (C) heart
    (D) erythrocytes
    (E) adipose tissue

Answers and Explanations: Endocrine Physiology

1. Which of the following hormones is produced in the hypothalamus?

   (A) adrenocorticotropic hormone
   (B) growth hormone
   (C) **oxytocin**
   (D) prolactin
   (E) thyroid-stimulating hormone

Oxytocin and arginine vasopressin are both produced by magnocellular neurons in the hypothalamus. These neurons originate in the paraventricular and supraoptic nuclei of the hypothalamus and terminate in the posterior pituitary.

Parvicellular neurons of the hypothalamus release hypophysiotropic hormones that regulate the anterior pituitary. Hormones released include: corticotropin-releasing hormone (CRH), gonadotropin-releasing hormone (GnRH), thyrotropin-releasing hormone (TRH), growth hormone-releasing hormone (GHRH), and dopamine. The parvicellular neurons terminate in the median eminence of the hypothalamus, and the hypophysiotropic hormones travel via a plexus of capillaries and hypophysial portal veins to reach the anterior pituitary.

Ref: Molina PE. *Endocrine Physiology*. 4th ed. New York, NY: McGraw Hill; 2013.

2. Hormone secretion is regulated via a complex array of mechanisms including feedback regulation. The feedback substrate may be another hormone, nutrient, or ion. Which of the following hormones is paired correctly with its feedback substrate?

   (A) ACTH: IGF-1
   (B) GH: triiodothyronine
   (C) **aldosterone: plasma K$^+$ levels**
   (D) insulin: plasma Ca^{2+} levels
   (E) TSH: cortisol

Plasma K$^+$ concentration plays a role in the feedback regulation of aldosterone secretion. Aldosterone release is stimulated by an increase in plasma K$^+$ concentration and also by angiotensin II (as part of the renin-angiotensin-aldosterone system). Aldosterone then acts to increase K$^+$ excretion via the kidney (and increase Na$^+$ and water reabsorption).

The anterior pituitary produces three different families of hormones:

- Glycoproteins: thyroid-stimulating hormone (TSH), follicle-stimulating hormone (FSH), and luteinizing hormone (LH)
- Pro-opiomelanocortin (POMC): adrenocorticotropic hormone (ACTH), β-endorphin, and melanocyte-stimulating hormones (MSH)
- Growth hormone and prolactin

Typically, hormones released by the anterior pituitary are under negative feedback control via the hormones released by their target organs. For example, TSH binds to receptors in the thyroid gland and stimulates release of thyroxine (T$_4$) and triiodothyronine (T$_3$). TSH secretion is then decreased via negative feedback inhibition by T$_3$. Another example of negative feedback inhibition, glucocorticoids (cortisol) will inhibit the secretion of corticotropin-releasing hormone CRH and adrenocorticotropic hormone ACTH (part of the hypothalamic-pituitary-adrenal [HPA] axis). Similarly, GH release is inhibited by insulin-like growth factor-1 (IGF-1) and somatostatin.

Insulin is under control of a variety of feedback mechanisms including neural control (sympathetic stimulation inhibits release and parasympathetic stimulation stimulates release), hormonal control (somatostatin inhibits release), and nutrient control (increased plasma glucose and amino acid levels stimulate release).

Ref: Molina PE. *Endocrine Physiology*. 4th ed. New York, NY: McGraw Hill; 2013.

3. Which of the following treatments for thyroid storm (severe thyrotoxicosis) relies on a mechanism known as the Wolff-Chaikoff effect?

(A) propranolol

(B) hydrocortisone

(C) propylthiouracil

(D) **Lugol's iodine**

(E) methimazole

Oral iodides, such as Lugol's iodine (a mixture of iodine and potassium iodide), act via the Wolff-Chaikoff effect to decrease thyroid hormone levels. Iodine is a fundamental requirement for thyroid hormone synthesis. Ingested iodine is converted to iodide, absorbed in the small intestine, and then taken up by the thyroid gland. The Wolff-Chaikoff effect describes how large doses of iodine inhibit many of the steps involved in uptake, production, and release of thyroid hormones. Control of thyrotoxicosis is best achieved if propylthiouracil or methimazole (see below) are given first, before administration of oral iodides. Oral iodide therapy usually works for short-term control of hyperthyroidism or thyroid storm (10–15 days).

Propylthiouracil (PTU) and methimazole both inhibit the synthesis of thyroid hormones. Either may used to treat thyroid storm, but PTU may be advantageous, as it also partially inhibits conversion of thyroxine (T_4) to triiodothyronine (T_3). Note that PTU administration is sometimes associated with severe hepatic failure requiring liver transplantation.

Propranolol, a nonselective β-blocker, is often used to treat the sympathomimetic symptoms of thyroid storm such as hypertension, tachycardia, and tremors. Propranolol also may also inhibit conversion of thyroxine (T_4) to triiodothyronine (T_3). Hydrocortisone inhibits the conversion of thyroxine (T_4) to triiodothyronine (T_3). Glucocorticoid administration also treats any relative adrenal insufficiency associated with thyroid storm. Other treatments for severe thyrotoxicosis include supportive measures such as active cooling, antipyretics, and intravenous fluids.

Ref: Brunton LL, Chabner BA, Knollman BC. *Goodman and Gilman's The Pharmacological Basis of Therapeutics.* 12th ed. New York, NY: McGraw Hill; 2011.

4. Which of the following hormones acts to decrease plasma Ca^{2+} levels and decrease bone resorption?

(A) PTH

(B) vitamin D

(C) **calcitonin**

(D) cortisol

(E) triiodothyronine

Bone metabolism and plasma Ca^{2+} levels are regulated by a number of hormones, including parathyroid hormone (PTH) and vitamin D. An increase in plasma Ca^{2+} levels acts via negative feedback inhibition to decrease release of PTH, decrease release of 1-25-hydroxyvitamin D (calcitriol), and increase release of calcitonin.

The release of PTH is triggered by a decrease in plasma Ca^{2+} levels. In bones, PTH acts to increase osteoclast activity, increase bone resorption, and increase release of Ca^{2+} and phosphate. At the kidney, PTH acts to increase Ca^{2+} reabsorption, increase phosphate excretion, and increase the rate of hydroxylation of 25-hydroxyvitamin D to active 1,25-hydroxyvitamin D (calcitriol).

Dietary vitamin D requires hydroxylation in the liver and kidney to become 1,25-hydroxyvitamin D (calcitriol). Calcitriol increases reabsorption of Ca^{2+} from both the intestine and the kidneys. In bones, calcitriol stimulates osteoclasts and increases bone resorption and increases circulating plasma Ca^{2+} levels.

Calcitonin has the opposite effects of PTH. It inhibits osteoclasts, decreases plasma Ca^{2+} levels, and decreases bone resorption.

Cortisol plays a catabolic role. It increases bone resorption and decreases bone synthesis (increases risk of fractures).

Triiodothyronine is required for bone remodeling. Excess thyroid hormone will increase bone resorption.

Growth hormone (GH) and insulin-like growth factor (IGF-1) stimulate bone synthesis and growth.

Androgens and estrogens increase 1α-hydroxylation of vitamin D and decrease bone resorption.

Ref: Molina PE. *Endocrine Physiology.* 4th ed. New York, NY: McGraw Hill; 2013.

5. In the adrenal gland, which of the following enzymes catalyzes the conversion of norepinephrine to epinephrine?

(A) tyrosine hydroxylase

(B) dopa decarboxylase

(C) dopamine β-hydroxylase

(D) **phenylethanolamine N-methyltransferase**

(E) catechol-O-methyltransferase

In the adrenal medulla, four enzymatic reactions occur to convert the amino acid tyrosine into epinephrine:

• hydroxylation of tyrosine to L-dopa by tyrosine hydroxylase.

- decarboxylation of L-dopa to dopamine by dopa decarboxylase.
- hydroxylation of dopamine to norepinephrine by dopamine β-hydroxylase.
- methylation of norepinephrine to epinephrine by phenylethanolamine N-methyltransferase (note the prefix nor- of norepinephrine comes from a German abbreviation indicating "without methyl").

Epinephrine and norepinephrine are metabolized by either catechol-*O*-methyltransferase (COMT) into metanephrine and normetanephrine, or by monoamine oxidase eventually forming vanillylmandelic acid (VMA). Metabolic products are excreted via the urine.

Ref: Molina PE. *Endocrine Physiology.* 4th ed. New York, NY: McGraw Hill; 2013.

6. The zona glomerulosa of the adrenal cortex is the sole source of production for which of the following hormones?

   (A) **aldosterone**
   (B) cortisol
   (C) dehydroepiandrosterone
   (D) androstenedione
   (E) corticosterone

The zona glomerulosa, zona fasciculata, and zona reticularis form the three layers of the adrenal cortex. **The zona glomerulosa produces aldosterone** (it lacks 17α-hydroxylase and cannot produce androgens or cortisol). The zona fasciculata and zona reticularis both produce cortisol and androgens (dehydroepiandrosterone [DHEA] and androstenedione). Corticosterone is produced during the biosynthesis of both aldosterone and glucocorticoids. However, only the zona glomerulosa has the enzyme P450aldo to catalyze the formation of aldosterone.

Ref: Gardner DG, Shoback D. *Greenspan's Basic and Clinical Endocrinology.* 9th ed. New York, NY: McGraw Hill; 2011.

7. Produced in the endocrine pancreas, which of the following hormones acts to decrease appetite and inhibit gluconeogenesis?

   (A) **insulin**
   (B) glucagon
   (C) somatostatin
   (D) pancreatic polypeptide
   (E) ghrelin

The endocrine pancreas is formed from Islets of Langerhans cells spread throughout the exocrine pancreas (which is involved in digestion). The Islets of Langerhans contain a variety of cell types:

- α cells—produce glucagon
- β cells—produce insulin
- δ cells—produce somatostatin
- ε cells—produce ghrelin

PP cells—produce pancreatic polypeptide

Insulin release, triggered by an increase in glucose, promotes glycogen, protein, and triglyceride synthesis. Insulin also inhibits glycogenolysis, inhibits gluconeogenesis, and in the brain acts to decrease appetite. Glucagon release is inhibited by glucose, insulin, and somatostatin. Glucagon promotes gluconeogenesis, ketogenesis, and increases release of energy stores from the liver (glycogenolysis).

Somatostatin release is stimulated by glucose. In the pancreas, somatostatin is thought to have mainly a paracrine role. (In the hypothalamus somatostatin inhibits release of growth hormone, while in the gastrointestinal tract it decreases gastric emptying, decreases gastric acid production, and decreases splanchnic blood flow.)

The role of pancreatic ghrelin is not clear. (In the stomach, ghrelin secretion promotes gastric emptying, acid secretion, and stimulates appetite.) The role of pancreatic polypeptide is also unclear. It appears to be under the influence of both neural (vagal) and nutrient signals.

Ref: Gardner DG, Shoback D. *Greenspan's Basic and Clinical Endocrinology.* 9th ed. New York, NY: McGraw Hill; 2011.

8. Under anaerobic conditions, lactate formed in the muscles may be converted back into glucose via which of the following pathways?

   (A) citric acid cycle
   (B) pentose phosphate pathway
   (C) **Cori cycle**
   (D) alanine cycle
   (E) glycolysis

Under low oxygen conditions, anaerobic glycolysis provides exercising muscles a source of ATP. The endproduct of glycolysis, pyruvate, is converted into lactate by lactate dehydrogenase. Lactate may be transported to the liver and serve as a substrate for gluconeogenesis, with the glucose produced returning to the muscles. This movement of lactate from the muscles with the return of glucose is known as the Cori cycle. (Note: Metformin inhibits hepatic gluconeogenesis and as a result may lead to lactic acidosis, particularly in those patients with renal failure.)

The alanine cycle is similar to the Cori cycle in that it "recycles" the products of anaerobic glycolysis in the muscles and returns glucose. The end-product of glycolysis, pyruvate, is transaminated in the muscles to alanine. The alanine can circulate to the liver where it is deaminated back to pyruvate which serves as a substrate for gluconeogenesis.

Glycolysis is the metabolic process that converts glucose to pyruvate and forms both ATP and NADH. It is part of both anaerobic and aerobic cellular respiration. The citric acid cycle (Krebs cycle) is part of aerobic cellular respiration and converts acetyl-CoA (derived from pyruvate) into CO_2 and energy (ATP, $FADH_2$, and NADH). The pentose phosphate pathway produces substrates for nucleotide synthesis.

Ref: Janson LW, Tischler M. *Medical Biochemistry: The Big Picture.* New York, NY: McGraw Hill; 2012.

9. Pyruvate is a versatile substrate that can participate in various enzymatic reactions to directly produce all of the following molecules EXCEPT:

(A) lactate

(B) alanine

(C) oxaloacetate

(D) acetyl-CoA

(E) **glucose-6-phosphate**

Pyruvate can be directly converted into four different molecules:

- Lactate
- Alanine
- Oxaloacetate
- Acetyl-CoA

Glucose-6-phosphate (G6P), pyruvate, and acetyl-CoA are all important metabolic control points (Figure 7-1). Dietary glucose is converted to G6P by the enzyme glucokinase. G6P can participate in a variety of metabolic pathways including glycolysis, glycogenesis, and the pentose phosphate pathway. Pyruvate may be utilized for gluconeogenesis, the Cori cycle, the alanine cycle, or conversion to acetyl-CoA. Acetyl-CoA plays a role in the citric acid cycle (Krebs cycle), ketone body synthesis, and fatty acid metabolism.

Ref: Janson LW, Tischler M. *Medical Biochemistry: The Big Picture.* New York, NY: McGraw Hill; 2012.

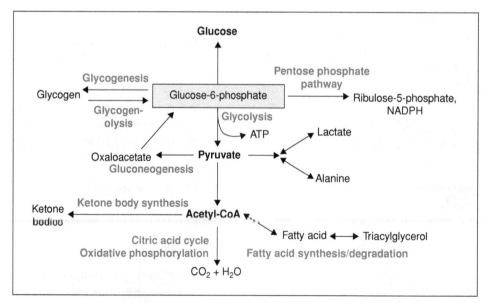

FIG. 7-1. Summary of Important Control Points of Metabolism. The three important intermediaries, glucose-6-phosphate, pyruvate, and acetyl-CoA are indicated. Metabolic pathways of importance are indicated in red. ATP, adenosine triphosphate; CoA, coenzyme A; NADPH, nicotinamide adenine dinucleotide phosphate. (Adapted with permission from Naik P: *Biochemistry,* 3rd edition, Jaypee Brothers Medical Publishers (P) Ltd. 2009.)

10. Insulin has which of the following metabolic effects?

    (A) stimulates gluconeogenesis

    (B) stimulates protein catabolism

    (C) stimulates glycogenolysis

    (D) stimulates lipolysis

    (E) **stimulates glycolysis**

Insulin has a variety of metabolic effects. In the liver, it stimulates glycolysis, glycogenesis, fatty acid synthesis, and pentose phosphate pathway. In the adipose tissue, it stimulates glucose uptake, stimulates fatty acid uptake, and triglyceride synthesis. In the skeletal muscle, it stimulates glucose uptake, glycogenesis, and protein synthesis In general, insulin inhibits gluconeogenesis, glycogenolysis, protein catabolism, and lipolysis.

Ref: Janson LW, Tischler M. *Medical Biochemistry: The Big Picture*. New York, NY: McGraw Hill; 2012.

11. Epinephrine stimulates which of the following metabolic processes?

    (A) **lipolysis in adipose tissue**

    (B) glycolysis in the liver

    (C) glycogen synthesis in the liver

    (D) fatty acid synthesis in the liver

    (E) triglyceride release from skeletal muscle

In many ways, epinephrine, glucagon, cortisol, and growth hormone play a counter-regulatory role to insulin in energy metabolism. Insulin is an anabolic hormone involved in storage of energy in the form of lipogenesis and glycogen synthesis.
Epinephrine has the following metabolic effects:

- Liver: Inhibits glycolysis, glycogen synthesis, and fatty acid synthesis. Stimulates gluconeogenesis and glycogenolysis.
- Adipose tissue: Stimulates lipolysis and inhibits triglyceride uptake.
- Skeletal muscle: Inhibits glycogen synthesis and stimulates glycolysis, glycogenolysis, and triglyceride uptake.

Epinephrine also inhibits insulin release from pancreas.
  Glucagon has the following metabolic effects:

- Liver: Inhibits glycolysis, glycogen synthesis, and fatty acid synthesis. Stimulates gluconeogenesis and glycogenolysis.

In this way, glucagon and epinephrine have the same effects on the liver and act to increase hepatic glucose production.

Cortisol and growth hormone complement the actions of glucagon and catecholamines: they both stimulate lipolysis, glycogenolysis, and gluconeogenesis. (Note: For protein synthesis growth hormone has the opposite action of epinephrine, glucagon, and cortisol. Growth hormone promotes protein synthesis, while epinephrine, glucagon, and cortisol promote proteolysis.)

Ref: Janson LW, Tischler M. *Medical Biochemistry: The Big Picture*. New York, NY: McGraw Hill; 2012.

12. Chronic stress has which of the following physiologic effects?

    (A) increased levels of TSH

    (B) decreased levels of cortisol

    (C) decreased levels of catecholamines

    (D) **increased gluconeogenesis**

    (E) increased levels of GH

The stress or "fight-or-flight" response activates the hypothalamic-pituitary-adrenal (HPA) axis and the sympathetic nervous system. This increases the circulating levels of cortisol and catecholamines. Acute activation of the stress response increases the amount of energy substrates available. Chronic activation of these mechanisms can lead to pathologic conditions. Alterations include:

- Inhibition of reproductive function: Glucocorticoids, corticotropin-releasing hormone (CRH), and β-endorphin suppress the release of gonadotropin-releasing hormone (GnRH), luteinizing hormone (LH), and follicle-stimulating hormone (FSH).
- Inhibition of growth hormone (GH): Activation of HPA axis directly suppresses GH release and also inhibits end-organ effects of IGF-1.
- Inhibition of thyroid function: CRH and cortisol inhibit thyroid-stimulating hormone (TSH) production.
- Altered energy metabolism: Catecholamines and cortisol **stimulate gluconeogenesis**, lipolysis, hepatic glycogenolysis, peripheral insulin resistance, muscle proteolysis, and bone resorption.
- Altered immune response: Glucocorticoids inhibit the immune response and have anti-inflammatory effects.

Ref: Molina PE. *Endocrine Physiology*. 4th ed. New York, NY: McGraw Hill; 2013.

13. Which of the following is a catabolic product of protein?

(A) **glucose**
(B) creatine
(C) thyroxine
(D) dopamine
(E) DNA

Amino acids derived from dietary proteins are basic building blocks for a variety of many important molecules including: enzymes, hormones, neurotransmitters, channel proteins, structural proteins, and motor proteins. Amino acids are found in:

- DNA/RNA: Derived from glycine, glutamine, and aspartate.
- Dopamine, epinephrine, and norepinephrine: Derived from tyrosine.
- Serotonin: Derived from tryptophan.
- Heme: Derived from glycine.
- Thyroxine: Derived from tyrosine.
- Creatine: Derived from glycine and arginine.

The catabolic products of amino acids include glucose, glycogen, ketone bodies, and fatty acids (all derived from the carbon skeletons); CO_2, H_2O, and urea (principal form of nitrogenous waste).

Ref: Janson LW, Tischler M. *Medical Biochemistry: The Big Picture.* New York, NY: McGraw Hill; 2012.

14. Of the following neurotransmitters, hormones, or drugs, which of the following uses cGMP as an intracellular second messenger?

(A) thyroxine
(B) **ANP**
(C) cocaine
(D) acetylcholine
(E) epinephrine

Activation of receptors by neurotransmitters, hormones, or drugs may lead to a cascade of events (signal transduction pathways) that involve second messenger systems. Second messenger pathways include:

1. cAMP: G protein-coupled receptors, acting via a G_s subunit, activate adenylyl cyclase and increase cAMP formation (e.g., β_1 and β_2 adrenergic receptor activation). G_i subunit activation **inhibits** adenylyl cyclase and cAMP formation (e.g., α_2 adrenergic receptor activation and M_2 cholinergic receptor activation).

2. cGMP: Atrial natriuretic peptide (ANP) binds to transmembrane receptors, activates guanylate cyclase, and increases the formation of cGMP. Nitric oxide (NO) also mediates its actions via cGMP: NO stimulates a soluble form of guanylate cyclase, increases the formation of cGMP, and ultimately induces a cascade of intracellular events leading to smooth muscle relaxation.

3. Inositol triphosphate: G protein-coupled receptors, acting via a G_q subunit, activate phospholipase C (PLC). PLC activation leads to conversion of phosphatidylinositol-4,5-bisphosphate to inositol-1,4,5-trisphosphate (IP_3) and diacylglycerol (DAG) (e.g., α_1 adrenergic receptor activation and M_1 and M_3 cholinergic receptors).

4. Ions: Voltage-gated ion channels (e.g., for Na^+, Ca^{2+}, K^+) and ligand-gated ion channels (e.g., nicotinic cholinergic receptor) regulate passive ion fluxes, which are established by cellular electrochemical gradients.

Thyroxine and a number of other hormones (e.g., androgens, estrogens, and glucocorticoids) act via nuclear receptors. Receptors are located either in the cytoplasm or nucleus. Activation leads to alterations in gene transcription.

Cocaine has local anesthetic properties (via blockade of sodium channels in nerve fibers) and also acts via blockade of catecholamine reuptake in the nervous system.

Refs: Rodwell VW, Bender DA, Botham KM, Kennelly PJ, Weil PA. *Harpers Illustrated Biochemistry.* 30th ed. New York, NY: McGraw Hill; 2015.

Kasper D, Fauci A, Hauser S, Longo D, Jameson J, Loscalzo J. *Harrison's Principles of Internal Medicine.* 19th ed. New York, NY: McGraw Hill; 2015.

Brunton LL, Chabner BA, Knollman BC. *Goodman and Gilman's The Pharmacological Basis of Therapeutics.* 12th ed. New York, NY: McGraw Hill; 2011.

15. Which of the following enzymes is critical in the regulation of cholesterol synthesis?

(A) **HMG-CoA reductase**
(B) acetyl-CoA carboxylase
(C) triacylglycerol synthase
(D) lipoprotein lipase
(E) β-hydroxybutyrate dehydrogenase

HMG-CoA reductase (3-hydroxy-3-methyl-glutaryl-CoA reductase) is the critical enzyme in the synthesis of cholesterol. Cholesterol may be obtained from the diet or synthesized from acetyl-CoA:

1 acetyl-CoA + 1 acetoacetyl-CoA + H_2O
= 3-hydroxy-3-methyl-glutaryl-CoA (3-HMG-CoA).

In the liver, mitochondrial 3-HMG-CoA may be utilized to produce ketone bodies (see below), while cytoplasmic 3-HMG-CoA may be utilized to produce cholesterol. The first step in cholesterol synthesis requires the enzyme HMG-CoA reductase to catalyze the conversion of 3-HMG-CoA to mevalonic acid. HMG-CoA reductase is inhibited by cholesterol, glucagon, epinephrine, and low ATP levels; while insulin increases its activity. The cholesterol medications known as statins are competitive inhibitors of HMG-CoA reductase.

Acetyl-CoA carboxylase catalyzes the first step of fatty acid synthesis: acetyl-CoA + HCO_3^- = malonyl-CoA. Acetyl-CoA is a versatile substrate and plays a role in the citric acid cycle (Krebs cycle), ketone body synthesis, cholesterol synthesis, and fatty acid metabolism. Acetyl-CoA carboxylase is activated by high levels of citrate. Citrate is the first intermediate of the Krebs cycle (citric acid cycle) and high levels reflect a situation of plentiful carbohydrate/sugar supplies. Insulin also activates acetyl-CoA carboxylase (promotes storage of energy in the form of fatty acids) while epinephrine and glucagon inhibit its activity (promote energy production).

Triacylglycerol synthase catalyzes the formation of triacylglycerols (triglycerides or fat). In the liver, triacylglycerols, cholesterol, and apolipoproteins form very-low-density lipoprotein (VLDL). VLDL enters the circulation and delivers fatty acids to muscle and adipose tissue. Lipoprotein lipase, found in capillary walls of muscle and adipose tissue, catalyzes the lipolysis of triacylglycerols in VLDL to liberate the fatty acids. Insulin increases the activity of lipoprotein lipase (promotes storage of energy).

Ketone bodies (acetoacetate, acetone, and β-hydroxybutyrate) can be used as an alternative to carbohydrates as an energy source. (Note: From a structural point of view, only acetoacetate and acetone are ketones!) Ketone bodies are formed in the liver from acetyl-CoA (acetyl-CoA may be derived from glucose, fatty acids, or ketogenic amino acids). Ketone bodies can be transported from the liver to other tissues such as the brain, heart, and muscle and can be converted back into acetyl-CoA and enter the citric acid cycle to produce ATP. The enzyme, β-hydroxybutyrate dehydrogenase catalyzes the conversion of acetoacetate to β-hydroxybutyrate.

Ref: Janson LW, Tischler M. *Medical Biochemistry: The Big Picture*. New York, NY: McGraw Hill; 2012.

16. Which of the following tissues exclusively utilizes glucose as its metabolic substrate?

(A) liver
(B) brain
(C) heart
(D) erythrocytes
(E) adipose tissue

Erythrocytes (red blood cells) do not have mitochondria and can only generate ATP via anaerobic glycolysis. They utilize glucose exclusively for their metabolic requirements, as they cannot utilize fatty acids or ketone bodies.

The liver may utilize a variety of different substrates for its energy requirements including: glucose, fatty acids, lactate, glycerol, and amino acids.

The brain utilizes glucose for the majority of its energy demands (approximately 80%) with ketone bodies for accounting for the remainder (approximately 20%).

The heart utilizes mainly fatty acids and glucose for its energy demands. It may also utilize ketone bodies and lactate.

Adipose tissue mainly utilizes glucose and triacylglycerol for its energy demands.

Ref: Rodwell VW, Bender DA, Botham KM, Kennelly PJ, Weil PA. *Harpers Illustrated Biochemistry*. 30th ed. New York, NY: McGraw Hill; 2015.

PART 2

Pharmacology

CHAPTER 8

General Pharmacology

1. An adult farm worker requires treatment for exposure to an insecticide containing parathion (cholinesterase inhibitor). To reverse the potentially dangerous side effects of parathion, a tertiary amine muscarinic antagonist such as atropine is recommended over a quaternary amine muscarinic antagonist such as glycopyrrolate. This choice of atropine is based on which pharmacokinetic or pharmacodynamic parameter?

   (A) Atropine has a larger volume of distribution than glycopyrrolate.
   (B) Atropine is a competitive muscarinic antagonist while glycopyrrolate is a noncompetitive muscarinic antagonist.
   (C) Atropine has a shorter terminal half-life than glycopyrrolate.
   (D) Atropine has a slower rate of clearance than glycopyrrolate.
   (E) Atropine has decreased oral bioavailability compared to glycopyrrolate.

2. An oral dose of morphine is subject to metabolism in the liver. After hepatic extraction, approximately 33% of the morphine enters the systemic circulation unchanged. Which of the following terms best describes this fraction of drug that reaches the systemic circulation?

   (A) volume of distribution
   (B) first-pass elimination
   (C) extraction ratio
   (D) clearance
   (E) bioavailability

3. A patient is taking atenolol, a beta-adrenoceptor antagonist, to control his hypertension. During surgery, the patient's heart rate is increased with the administration of atropine. In this situation, the use of atropine to reverse the heart rate effects of atenolol is an example of a:

   (A) chemical antagonist
   (B) physiologic antagonist
   (C) partial agonist
   (D) noncompetitive antagonist
   (E) competitive antagonist

4. Regarding inhaled anesthetics, the speed of induction is dependent on an increase of F_A/F_I (alveolar concentration/inspired concentration). Which factor will increase F_A/F_I?

   (A) decreased minute ventilation
   (B) low blood:gas partition coefficient
   (C) increased cardiac output
   (D) low minimum alveolar concentration (MAC)
   (E) low rate of metabolism

5. In a one compartment pharmacokinetic model, half-life ($T_{1/2}$) is directly proportional to:

   (A) clearance
   (B) rate of elimination
   (C) volume of distribution
   (D) bioavailability
   (E) hepatic blood flow

6. The degree of ionization of a drug can markedly alter its lipid solubility. Which of these weak bases will be the most lipid soluble at pH 7.9?

   (A) codeine (pK$_a$ = 8.2)
   (B) methadone (pK$_a$ = 8.4)
   (C) chlordiazepoxide (pK$_a$ = 4.6)
   (D) lidocaine (pK$_a$ = 7.9)
   (E) propranolol (pK$_a$ = 9.4)

7. The addition of epinephrine (1:200,000) to a lumbar epidural injection of morphine will cause:

   (A) increased rate of epidural morphine clearance.
   (B) increased peak plasma concentration of morphine.
   (C) decreased time to peak plasma concentration of morphine.
   (D) increased bioavailability of intrathecal morphine.
   (E) increased elimination half-time of intrathecal morphine.

8. Which mechanism of transport is most important for drugs to redistribute from the epidural space to the spinal cord?

   (A) endocytosis
   (B) active transport
   (C) facilitated diffusion
   (D) passive diffusion
   (E) exocytosis

9. Ephedrine produces indirect effects by displacing norepinephrine from nerve terminals into the extracellular fluid. Repeated doses of ephedrine can lead to rapidly decreased effectiveness. What is this effect known as?

   (A) hyporeactivity
   (B) hyperreactivity
   (C) hypersensitivity
   (D) tolerance
   (E) tachyphylaxis

10. Most medications are biotransformed by either a phase I or phase II reaction. Which of the following is an example of a **phase II** reaction?

    (A) acetylation
    (B) oxidation
    (C) deamination
    (D) desulfuration
    (E) reduction

11. After a prolonged intravenous infusion of an anesthetic, which pharmacokinetic parameter is the most useful to predict time to recovery?

    (A) elimination half-life
    (B) context-sensitive half-time
    (C) volume of distribution
    (D) clearance
    (E) loading dose

12. For most drugs at clinical concentrations, drug elimination is directly proportional to drug clearance and drug concentration. What is this referred to as?

    (A) intrinsic clearance
    (B) flow-dependent elimination
    (C) capacity-limited elimination
    (D) first-order elimination
    (E) first-pass elimination

13. In a clinical dose range, renal failure will significantly alter the termination of action of which drug?

    (A) vecuronium
    (B) succinylcholine
    (C) sevoflurane
    (D) fentanyl
    (E) propofol

14. Hepatic cirrhosis can have complex effects on drug pharmacokinetics. For a patient with significant hepatic cirrhosis, what is a possible reason for delayed termination of drug action?

    (A) increased levels of plasma binding proteins
    (B) increased hepatocyte metabolism
    (C) decreased total body water content
    (D) presence of portosystemic shunts
    (E) increased hepatic blood flow

15. A patient is prescribed, and compliant with, a standard dose of codeine for postoperative analgesia. The patient becomes unusually drowsy and requires resuscitation for a near respiratory arrest. Subsequent evaluation determines that plasma levels of morphine were abnormally elevated. Which of the following is the most likely explanation for this toxicity?

    (A) The patient has increased N-acetylation activity.
    (B) The patient is a "poor metabolizer" of codeine.
    (C) The patient is an "extensive metabolizer" of codeine.
    (D) The patient is an "ultrarapid metabolizer" of codeine.
    (E) The patient has impaired glutathione transferase activity.

16. Cytochrome P450 3A4 (CYP3A4) is inhibited by grapefruit juice and medications such as ketoconazole and fluoxetine. This can result in increased plasma concentrations of drugs metabolized by CYP3A4. If a patient is taking food or medications that inhibit CYP3A4, which analgesic would be an appropriate choice to minimize the risk of analgesic toxicity?

    (A) fentanyl
    (B) alfentanil
    (C) sufentanil
    (D) methadone
    (E) hydromorphone

17. Total hepatic blood flow decreases as volatile anesthetic concentration is increased from 1 MAC to 2 MAC. Which drug's hepatic clearance will be relatively unaffected by this decrease in hepatic blood flow?

    (A) fentanyl
    (B) morphine
    (C) propofol
    (D) midazolam
    (E) diazepam

18. Possible drug-drug interactions include synergistic interactions and additive interactions. Which of the following drug-drug interactions causes an **additive** clinical effect?

    (A) desflurane and nitrous oxide
    (B) ketorolac and fentanyl
    (C) sevoflurane and rocuronium
    (D) cis-atracurium and vecuronium
    (E) fentanyl and midazolam

19. A patient is hypertensive with myocardial ischemia thought to be due to acute cocaine intoxication. Which of the following initial medical treatments should be **avoided?**

    (A) phentolamine
    (B) aspirin
    (C) nitroglycerin
    (D) propranolol
    (E) lorazepam

20. Which of the following herbal medicines may increase the sedative effects of anesthetics?

    (A) garlic
    (B) ginkgo
    (C) ginseng
    (D) kava
    (E) ephedra (ma huang)

21. Which herbal medicine can inhibit reuptake of serotonin, norepinephrine, and dopamine and potentially interact with serotonin reuptake inhibitors to cause serotonin syndrome?

    (A) valerian
    (B) saw palmetto
    (C) St. John's wort
    (D) echinacea
    (E) ginseng

22. A patient is given haloperidol to manage postoperative agitation. Afterward, the patient develops extrapyramidal symptoms. Which medication should be used to treat this dystonic reaction?

    (A) diphenhydramine
    (B) dantrolene
    (C) calcium gluconate
    (D) atropine
    (E) acetylcysteine

23. Which class of medications is the most common cause of anesthetic drug-induced anaphylaxis?

    (A) muscle relaxants
    (B) propofol
    (C) opioids
    (D) ester local anesthetics
    (E) antibiotics

24. During general anesthesia, initial treatment of an anesthetic drug-induced anaphylactic or anaphylactoid reaction includes which of the following?

    (A) intravascular volume expansion
    (B) antihistamines
    (C) inhaled bronchodilators
    (D) corticosteroids
    (E) vasopressin

25. A patient under general anesthesia develops an anaphylactic or anaphylactoid reaction. In an anesthetized patient, what is the most common clinical sign of anaphylaxis?

    (A) wheezing
    (B) diaphoresis
    (C) urticaria
    (D) perioral edema
    (E) hypotension

Answers and Explanations: General Pharmacology

1. An adult farm worker requires treatment for exposure to an insecticide containing parathion (cholinesterase inhibitor). To reverse the potentially dangerous side effects of parathion, a tertiary amine muscarinic antagonist such as atropine is recommended over a quaternary amine muscarinic antagonist such as glycopyrrolate. This choice of atropine is based on which pharmacokinetic or pharmacodynamic parameter?

    (A) **Atropine has a larger volume of distribution than glycopyrrolate.**

    (B) Atropine is a competitive muscarinic antagonist while glycopyrrolate is a noncompetitive muscarinic antagonist.

    (C) Atropine has a shorter terminal half-life than glycopyrrolate.

    (D) Atropine has a slower rate of clearance than glycopyrrolate.

    (E) Atropine has decreased oral bioavailability compared to glycopyrrolate.

    Atropine is a tertiary amine alkaloid while glycopyrrolate is a quaternary amine. Both are competitive antagonists of acetylcholine at muscarinic receptors. However, the structure of glycopyrrolate means that is it positively charged and unable to cross the blood-brain barrier as easily as atropine. This means atropine is more widely distributed than glycopyrrolate and can reverse both the peripheral and CNS effects of parathion.

    Atropine has a longer half-life, an increased rate of clearance, and greater oral bioavailability than glycopyrrolate.

    Ref: Katzung BG, Masters SB, Trevor AJ. *Basic and Clinical Pharmacology.* 12th ed. (LANGE Basic series). New York, NY: McGraw Hill; 2012.

2. An oral dose of morphine is subject to metabolism in the liver. After hepatic extraction, approximately 33% of the morphine enters the systemic circulation unchanged.

Which of the following terms best describes this fraction of drug that reaches the systemic circulation?

    (A) volume of distribution

    (B) first-pass elimination

    (C) extraction ratio

    (D) clearance

    (E) **bioavailability**

    Bioavailability is the portion of drug that reaches the systemic circulation unchanged.

    Volume of distribution (Vd) is the ratio of drug in the body to concentration in plasma or blood.

    First-pass elimination is the metabolism of drug before it reaches the systemic circulation. Extraction ratio is the clearance of drug from the liver divided by the hepatic blood flow. Clearance is the rate of drug elimination divided by the drug concentration.

    Ref: Katzung BG, Masters SB, Trevor AJ. *Basic and Clinical Pharmacology.* 12th ed. (LANGE Basic series). New York, NY: McGraw Hill; 2012.

3. A patient is taking atenolol, a beta-adrenoceptor antagonist, to control his hypertension. During surgery, the patient's heart rate is increased with the administration of atropine. In this situation, the use of atropine to reverse the heart rate effects of atenolol is an example of a:

    (A) chemical antagonist

    (B) **physiologic antagonist**

    (C) partial agonist

    (D) noncompetitive antagonist

    (E) competitive antagonist

    Atropine is a competitive antagonist of acetylcholine at muscarinic receptors. However, in this example, atropine's effect on the heart rate is used to reverse the effects of atenolol. This is an example of physiologic antagonism, where a common pathway (the heart rate) can be manipulated by different receptor types.

A chemical antagonist binds the other drug and makes it unavailable for receptor binding. A partial agonist, in contrast to a full agonist, can only produce a submaximal pharmacologic response even when all receptors are occupied. A noncompetitive antagonist binds to a receptor at a separate site than the agonist. This leads to altered receptor activity even though agonist binding is not directly affected (also termed allosteric modulation).

A competitive antagonist reversibly competes with an agonist for receptor occupancy.

Ref: Katzung BG, Masters SB, Trevor AJ. *Basic and Clinical Pharmacology.* 12th ed. (LANGE Basic series). New York, NY: McGraw Hill; 2012.

4. Regarding inhaled anesthetics, the speed of induction is dependent on an increase of F_A/F_I (alveolar concentration/inspired concentration). Which factor will increase F_A/F_I?

    (A)   decreased minute ventilation
    (B)   **low blood:gas partition coefficient**
    (C)   increased cardiac output
    (D)   low minimum alveolar concentration (MAC)
    (E)   low rate of metabolism

The rate of rise of F_A/F_I is dependent on a number of factors:

A low blood: gas partition coefficient means the anesthetic has low solubility and F_A/F_I will increase faster than for an anesthetic with increased solubility.

Increased cardiac output will slow the rate of rise of F_A/F_I, as will decreased minute ventilation. Minimum alveolar concentration (MAC) and metabolism of volatile anesthetics do not play a significant role in speed of induction.

Ref: Katzung BG, Masters SB, Trevor AJ. *Basic and Clinical Pharmacology.* 12th ed. (LANGE Basic series). New York, NY: McGraw Hill; 2012.

5. In a one compartment pharmacokinetic model, half-life ($T_{1/2}$) is directly proportional to:

    (A)   clearance
    (B)   rate of elimination
    (C)   **volume of distribution**
    (D)   bioavailability
    (E)   hepatic blood flow

Half-life ($T_{1/2}$) is directly proportional to volume of distribution ($T_{1/2} = (\ln 2 \times Vd)/C_L$; Vd = volume of distribution; C_L = clearance).

$T_{1/2}$ is inversely proportional to clearance.

Rate of elimination = $C_L \times$ (drug concentration).

Bioavailability is the portion of drug that reaches the systemic circulation unchanged; it is proportional to the area under the curve for a blood concentration versus time graph. Hepatic blood flow is a determinant of first-pass elimination.

Ref: Katzung BG, Masters SB, Trevor AJ. *Basic and Clinical Pharmacology.* 12th ed. (LANGE Basic series). New York, NY: McGraw Hill; 2012.

6. The degree of ionization of a drug can markedly alter its lipid solubility. Which of these weak bases will be the most lipid soluble at pH 7.9?

    (A)   codeine (pK_a = 8.2)
    (B)   methadone (pK_a = 8.4)
    (C)   chlordiazepoxide (pK_a = 4.6)
    (D)   lidocaine (pK_a = 7.9)
    (E)   **propranolol (pK_a = 9.4)**

pK_a is the pH at which 50% of the drug is in its ionized form and 50% is in its unionized form. Weak bases are neutral (lipid soluble) in their unprotonated (unionized) form. In an alkaline environment more of a weak base will be in its unprotonated form. At a pH of 7.9, propranolol (pK_a = 9.4) will be the most unionized medication.

Ref: Katzung BG, Masters SB, Trevor AJ. *Basic and Clinical Pharmacology.* 12th ed. (LANGE Basic series). New York, NY: McGraw Hill; 2012.

7. The addition of epinephrine (1:200,000) to a lumbar epidural injection of morphine will cause:

    (A)   increased rate of epidural morphine clearance.
    (B)   increased peak plasma concentration of morphine.
    (C)   decreased time to peak plasma concentration of morphine.
    (D)   **increased bioavailability of intrathecal morphine.**
    (E)   increased elimination half-time of intrathecal morphine.

Epinephrine (1:200,000) added to a lumbar epidural injection of morphine will alter morphine pharmacokinetics in the following manner:

Epinephrine decreases morphine's rate of clearance from the epidural space. Epidural epinephrine also decreases the peak plasma concentration of morphine and delays the time to peak plasma concentration significantly. At the intrathecal site, epidural epinephrine will increase the bioavailability of morphine injected epidurally and decrease elimination half-time.

Ref: Bernards CM, et al. Epidural, CSF, and plasma pharmacokinetics of epidural opioids (Part 2). *Anesthesiology.* 2003; 99:466–75.

8. Which mechanism of transport is most important for drugs to redistribute from the epidural space to the spinal cord?

    (A) endocytosis
    (B) active transport
    (C) facilitated diffusion
    (D) **passive diffusion**
    (E) exocytosis

Drugs in the epidural space passively diffuse across the spinal meninges to the spinal cord. In general, other mechanisms for drugs to permeate tissues include active transport, facilitated diffusion, endocytosis, and exocytosis.

Ref: Katzung BG, Masters SB, Trevor AJ. *Basic and Clinical Pharmacology.* 12th ed. (LANGE Basic series). New York, NY: McGraw Hill; 2012.

9. Ephedrine produces indirect effects by displacing norepinephrine from nerve terminals into the extracellular fluid. Repeated doses of ephedrine can lead to rapidly decreased effectiveness. What is this effect known as?

    (A) hyporeactivity
    (B) hyperreactivity
    (C) hypersensitivity
    (D) tolerance
    (E) **tachyphylaxis**

Repeated doses of a drug that rapidly causes diminished effectiveness is known as tachyphylaxis. Hyporeactivity is a diminished drug response as compared to the general population. Hyperreactivity is an increased drug response as compared to the general population. Hypersensitivity refers to allergic responses to a drug. Tolerance is a diminished response to a drug; in contrast to tachyphylaxis, tolerance develops over a longer time period.

Refs: Katzung BG, Masters SB, Trevor AJ. *Basic and Clinical Pharmacology.* 12th ed. (LANGE Basic series). New York, NY: McGraw Hill; 2012.
Brunton LL, Chabner BA, Knollman BC. *Goodman and Gilman's The Pharmacological Basis of Therapeutics.* 12th ed. New York, NY: McGraw Hill; 2011.

10. Most medications are biotransformed by either a phase I or phase II reaction. Which of the following is an example of a **phase II** reaction?

    (A) **acetylation**
    (B) oxidation
    (C) deamination
    (D) desulfuration
    (E) reduction

Phase I reactions usually produce a polar metabolite. Typical phase I reactions include oxidation (including deamination and desulfuration), reduction, and hydrolysis. A phase II reaction is typically a conjugation reaction to form a highly polar metabolite. Typical phase II reactions are glucuronidation, acetylation, sulfation, methylation, and glutathione conjugation.

Ref: Katzung BG, Masters SB, Trevor AJ. *Basic and Clinical Pharmacology.* 12th ed. (LANGE Basic series). New York, NY: McGraw Hill; 2012.

11. After a prolonged intravenous infusion of an anesthetic, which pharmacokinetic parameter is the most useful to predict time to recovery?

    (A) elimination half-life
    (B) **context-sensitive half-time**
    (C) volume of distribution
    (D) clearance
    (E) loading dose

Recovery depends on both drug elimination and drug redistribution. The relative importance of each of these factors also depends on the overall duration of the intravenous infusion. Context-sensitive half-time incorporates all of these aspects and is a measure of how long it takes for a 50% decrease in the plasma drug concentration.

Elimination half-life does not consider the effects of drug redistribution. Elimination half-life measures the rate of drug removal from the systemic circulation.

Volume of distribution (Vd) is the ratio of drug in the body to concentration in plasma or blood.

Clearance is the rate of drug elimination divided by the drug concentration.

A loading dose quickly raises the concentration of drug in the plasma to a targeted level.

Ref: Brunton LL, Chabner BA, Knollman BC. *Goodman and Gilman's The Pharmacological Basis of Therapeutics.* 12th ed. New York, NY: McGraw Hill; 2011.

12. For most drugs at clinical concentrations, drug elimination is directly proportional to drug clearance and drug concentration. What is this referred to as?

 (A) intrinsic clearance
 (B) flow-dependent elimination
 (C) capacity-limited elimination
 (D) **first-order elimination**
 (E) first-pass elimination

Saturation of drug metabolism results in nonlinear pharmacokinetics where a constant amount of drug is eliminated per unit of time (zero-order kinetics). However, the metabolism of most drugs, at clinical concentrations, is not saturated and follows first-order kinetics, where a constant fraction of drug is eliminated per unit of time. This is termed first-order elimination (rate of elimination = clearance × drug concentration).

Intrinsic clearance reflects the absolute metabolic capacity of an organ to clear a drug, irrespective of actual blood flow.

Flow-dependent elimination usually refers to drugs that are efficiently metabolized by the liver. For these "high-extraction" drugs, blood flow to the liver is the rate limiting step for elimination.

Capacity-limited elimination is another term for saturable (nonlinear) elimination.

First-pass elimination refers to drug metabolism in the liver before the drug reaches the systemic circulation.

Refs: Katzung BG, Masters SB, Trevor AJ. *Basic and Clinical Pharmacology.* 12th ed. (LANGE Basic series). New York, NY: McGraw Hill; 2012.
Brunton LL, Chabner BA, Knollman BC. *Goodman and Gilman's The Pharmacological Basis of Therapeutics.* 12th ed. New York, NY: McGraw Hill; 2011.

13. In a clinical dose range, renal failure will significantly alter the termination of action of which drug?

 (A) **vecuronium**
 (B) succinylcholine
 (C) sevoflurane
 (D) fentanyl
 (E) propofol

Renal elimination accounts for approximately 30% of a dose of vecuronium. Renal failure results in delayed elimination and a longer duration of neuromuscular blockade.

Succinylcholine is metabolized by pseudocholinesterase, and renal failure does not prolong neuromuscular blockade.

The termination of action of sevoflurane (and all volatile anesthetics) is due to pulmonary excretion rather than renal elimination.

Fentanyl pharmacokinetics and clinical effects are not significantly altered by renal failure. Propofol undergoes liver metabolism to less active metabolites, which are renally excreted.

Ref: Brunton LL, Chabner BA, Knollman BC. *Goodman and Gilman's The Pharmacological Basis of Therapeutics.* 12th ed. New York, NY: McGraw Hill; 2011.

14. Hepatic cirrhosis can have complex effects on drug pharmacokinetics. For a patient with significant hepatic cirrhosis, what is a possible reason for delayed termination of drug action?

 (A) increased levels of plasma binding proteins
 (B) increased hepatocyte metabolism
 (C) decreased total body water content
 (D) **presence of portosystemic shunts**
 (E) increased hepatic blood flow

The effects of liver disease on drug termination of action are not always intuitive. In general, liver cirrhosis can alter drug pharmacokinetics due to the following changes:

• presence of portosystemic shunts,
• decreased levels of plasma binding proteins and albumin,
• decreased hepatocyte metabolism,
• increased total body water content and altered volume of distribution, and
• decreased hepatic blood flow.

Ref: Miller RD. Miller's *Anesthesia.* 8th ed. Philadelphia, PA: Elsevier; 2015.

15. A patient is prescribed, and compliant with, a standard dose of codeine for postoperative analgesia. The patient becomes unusually drowsy and requires resuscitation for a near respiratory arrest. Subsequent evaluation determines that plasma levels of morphine were abnormally elevated. Which of the following is the most likely explanation for this toxicity?

    (A) The patient has increased N-acetylation activity.
    (B) The patient is a "poor metabolizer" of codeine.
    (C) The patient is an "extensive metabolizer" of codeine.
    (D) The patient is an "ultrarapid metabolizer" of codeine.
    (E) The patient has impaired glutathione transferase activity.

    Codeine is converted to morphine in the liver by a cytochrome 2D6 (CYP2D6) *O*-demethylation reaction. Genetic polymorphisms of CYP2D6 exist: poor metabolizers have reduced production of morphine and reduced analgesia, extensive metabolizers are considered normal, and ultrarapid metabolizers have increased production of morphine and are at higher risk of respiratory depression. Other cytochrome P450 polymorphisms exist including altered glutathione transferase activity and altered *N*-acetylation, but they do not affect codeine metabolism.

    Ref: Katzung BG, Masters SB, Trevor AJ. *Basic and Clinical Pharmacology.* 12th ed. (LANGE Basic series). New York, NY: McGraw Hill; 2012.

16. Cytochrome P450 3A4 (CYP3A4) is inhibited by grapefruit juice and medications such as ketoconazole and fluoxetine. This can result in increased plasma concentrations of drugs metabolized by CYP3A4. If a patient is taking food or medications that inhibit CYP3A4, which analgesic would be an appropriate choice to minimize the risk of analgesic toxicity?

    (A) fentanyl
    (B) alfentanil
    (C) sufentanil
    (D) methadone
    (E) hydromorphone

    Hydromorphone is metabolized by CYP2D6 and inhibitors of CYP3A4 will not affect it significantly. Other

opioids metabolized by CYP2D6 include prodrugs such as codeine, oxycodone, and hydrocodone. CYP3A4 metabolizes many anesthetic drugs, including opioids (fentanyl, alfentanil, sufentanil, methadone), benzodiazepines, lidocaine, ropivacaine, and haloperidol.

Ref: Miller RD. Miller's *Anesthesia.* 8th ed. Philadelphia, PA: Elsevier; 2015.

17. Total hepatic blood flow decreases as volatile anesthetic concentration is increased from 1 MAC to 2 MAC. Which drug's hepatic clearance will be relatively unaffected by this decrease in hepatic blood flow?

    (A) fentanyl
    (B) morphine
    (C) propofol
    (D) midazolam
    (E) diazepam

    Since diazepam is a drug with a low intrinsic hepatic clearance, changes in hepatic blood flow will cause minimal changes in hepatic clearance.

    Clearance (mL/min/kg):

    $$Fentanyl = 13$$
    $$Morphine = 24$$
    $$Propofol = 27$$
    $$Midazolam = 6.6$$
    $$Diazepam = 0.38$$

    For drugs that are efficiently cleared by the liver (>6 mL/min/kg), the rate limiting metabolic step is hepatic blood flow, rather than intrinsic hepatic metabolic capacity. This is termed flow-limited hepatic clearance (hepatic clearance = hepatic blood flow × hepatic extraction ratio). Drugs with a high hepatic clearance include fentanyl, meperidine, morphine, propofol, ketamine, and lidocaine. Drugs with a low hepatic clearance include diazepam, lorazepam, methadone, and rocuronium.

    Refs: Brunton LL, Chabner BA, Knollman BC. *Goodman and Gilman's The Pharmacological Basis of Therapeutics.* 12th ed. New York, NY: McGraw Hill; 2011.

    Miller RD. Miller's *Anesthesia.* 8th ed. Philadelphia, PA: Elsevier; 2015.

    Katzung BG, Masters SB, Trevor AJ. *Basic and Clinical Pharmacology.* 12th ed. (LANGE Basic series). New York, NY: McGraw Hill; 2012.

18. Possible drug-drug interactions include synergistic interactions and additive interactions. Which of the following drug-drug interactions causes an **additive** clinical effect?

(A) desflurane and nitrous oxide

(B) ketorolac and fentanyl

(C) sevoflurane and rocuronium

(D) cis-atracurium and vecuronium

(E) fentanyl and midazolam

Volatile anesthetics and nitrous oxide have an additive interaction to cause unconsciousness. NSAIDs and opioids have a synergistic interaction to cause analgesia. Volatile anesthetics and nondepolarizing muscle relaxants have a synergistic interaction to cause paralysis. Aminosteroid and benzylisoquinoline muscle relaxants have a synergistic interaction to cause paralysis. Opioids have a synergistic interaction with benzodiazepines to cause hypnosis.

Ref: Rosow CE. Anesthetic drug interaction: An overview. *J Clin Anesth.* 1997; 9(6 Suppl):27S–32S.

19. A patient is hypertensive with myocardial ischemia thought to be due to acute cocaine intoxication. Which of the following initial medical treatments should be **avoided**?

(A) phentolamine

(B) aspirin

(C) nitroglycerin

(D) propranolol

(E) lorazepam

Initial treatments for cocaine associated myocardial ischemia include benzodiazepines, aspirin, nitroglycerin, and phentolamine. Propranolol is not recommended, as beta-blockade can lead to unopposed alpha-adrenergic activity and coronary vasoconstriction.

Ref: Schwartz BG, Rezkalla S, Kloner RA. Cardiovascular effects of cocaine. *Circulation.* 2010; 122:2558–69.

20. Which of the following herbal medicines may increase the sedative effects of anesthetics?

(A) garlic

(B) ginkgo

(C) ginseng

(D) kava

(E) ephedra (ma huang)

Kava may increase the sedative effects of anesthetics. Garlic, ginkgo, ginseng, and kava all may increase the risk of bleeding. Ephedra (ma huang) may cause intraoperative hemodynamic instability via direct and indirect sympathomimetic effects.

Ref: Katzung BG, Masters SB, Trevor AJ. *Basic and Clinical Pharmacology. 12th ed. (LANGE Basic series).* New York, NY: McGraw Hill; 2012.

21. Which herbal medicine can inhibit reuptake of serotonin, norepinephrine, and dopamine and potentially interact with serotonin reuptake inhibitors to cause serotonin syndrome?

(A) valerian

(B) saw palmetto

(C) St. John's wort

(D) echinacea

(E) ginseng

St. John's wort inhibits reuptake of serotonin, norepinephrine, and dopamine. It can interact with serotonin reuptake inhibitors to cause serotonin syndrome. It should be discontinued 5 days before surgery. Valerian is a sedative that modulates GABA neurotransmission. It is often used to treat insomnia. It should not be acutely withheld, as benzodiazepine-like withdrawal can occur. Saw palmetto is often used by men to relieve symptoms of benign prostatic hypertrophy. The mechanism of action is not known. Echinacea is often used for prevention and treatment of infections. The mechanism of action is not fully understood, but short-term use is associated with immunostimulatory effects.

Ref: Katzung BG, Masters SB, Trevor AJ. *Basic and Clinical Pharmacology. 12th ed. (LANGE Basic series).* New York, NY: McGraw Hill; 2012.

22. A patient is given haloperidol to manage postoperative agitation. Afterward, the patient develops extrapyramidal symptoms. Which medication should be used to treat this dystonic reaction?

(A) diphenhydramine

(B) dantrolene

(C) calcium gluconate

(D) atropine

(E) acetylcysteine

Haloperidol is a conventional antipsychotic often used to treat agitation. Extrapyramidal side effects such as torticollis, opisthotonis, and oculogyric crisis can be treated with an anticholinergic agent such as benztropine or diphenhydramine.

Haloperidol can also cause neuroleptic malignant syndrome (NMS): hyperthermia, rigidity, altered mental status, autonomic lability. The treatment of NMS can include dantrolene. Dantrolene is also used to treat malignant hyperthermia.

Calcium gluconate is used to treat an overdose of calcium channel blocking drugs.

Atropine, a muscarinic antagonist, can be used in conjunction with the administration of acetylcholinesterase inhibitors. Atropine is also used to treat organophosphorus pesticide poisoning. Acetylcysteine is used to treat acetaminophen overdose.

Ref: Brunton LL, Chabner BA, Knollman BC. *Goodman and Gilman's The Pharmacological Basis of Therapeutics.* 12th ed. New York, NY: McGraw Hill; 2011.

23. Which class of medications is the most common cause of anesthetic drug-induced anaphylaxis?

    (A) muscle relaxants
    (B) propofol
    (C) opioids
    (D) ester local anesthetics
    (E) antibiotics

Muscle relaxants are the most common cause of anesthetic drug-induced anaphylaxis (60% to 80% of all reactions). Less frequently, induction agents (propofol, etomidate), opioids, ester local anesthetics, and antibiotics can all potentially cause anaphylaxis.

Ref: Longnecker DE, Brown DL, Newman MF, Zapol WM. *Anesthesiology.* 2nd ed. New York, NY: McGraw Hill; 2012.

24. During general anesthesia, initial treatment of an anesthetic drug-induced anaphylactic or anaphylactoid reaction includes which of the following?

    (A) intravascular volume expansion
    (B) antihistamines
    (C) inhaled bronchodilators
    (D) corticosteroids
    (E) vasopressin

Initial therapy of anaphylaxis during general anesthesia includes:

- Stop administration of antigen.
- Maintain airway and administer 100% oxygen.
- Discontinue anesthetic agents.
- Intravascular volume expansion.
- Epinephrine.

Secondary treatment includes:

- Antihistamines.
- Bronchodilators.
- Corticosteroids.
- Sodium bicarbonate.
- Vasopressin.

Ref: Longnecker DE, Brown DL, Newman MF, Zapol WM. *Anesthesiology.* 2nd ed. New York, NY: McGraw Hill; 2012.

25. A patient under general anesthesia develops an anaphylactic or anaphylactoid reaction. In an anesthetized patient, what is the most common clinical sign of anaphylaxis?

    (A) wheezing
    (B) diaphoresis
    (C) urticaria
    (D) perioral edema
    (E) hypotension

Anaphylaxis refers to life-threatening allergic reactions. The most common clinical sign of anaphylaxis in an anesthetized patient is hypotension. Under anesthesia, other signs of anaphylaxis may include:

- Respiratory—coughing, wheezing, decreased pulmonary compliance, acute respiratory failure.
- Cardiovascular—diaphoresis, tachycardia, dysrhythmias, cardiac arrest.
- Cutaneous—urticaria, flushing, perioral edema.

Ref: Longnecker DE, Brown DL, Newman MF, Zapol WM. *Anesthesiology.* 2nd ed. New York, NY: McGraw Hill; 2012.

CHAPTER 9

Gases and Vapors

1. Which of the following statements regarding the physical properties of nitrous oxide is FALSE?

   (A) Nitrous oxide is colorless.

   (B) Nitrous oxide is odorless.

   (C) Nitrous oxide cannot support combustion.

   (D) Nitrous oxide has a boiling point below room temperature.

   (E) Nitrous oxide is nonflammable.

2. Which of the following potent volatile agents is most likely to evaporate when left in an open container in the operating room?

   (A) desflurane

   (B) enflurane

   (C) halothane

   (D) isoflurane

   (E) sevoflurane

3. Which of the following physical properties best correlates with volatile anesthetic potency?

   (A) boiling point

   (B) density

   (C) lipid solubility

   (D) molecular mass

   (E) viscosity

4. Nitrous oxide and xenon are both thought to inhibit which of the following receptors in the central nervous system?

   (A) acetylcholine

   (B) GABA

   (C) glycine

   (D) N-methyl-D-aspartate

   (E) neurokinin 1

5. Halothane, desflurane, isoflurane, and sevoflurane all produce which of the following effects on cerebrovascular physiology and metabolism?

   (A) an increase in cerebral blood flow, decrease in metabolic rate

   (B) an increase in cerebral blood flow, no change in metabolic rate

   (C) a decrease in cerebral blood flow, decrease in metabolic rate

   (D) a decrease in cerebral blood flow, no change in metabolic rate

   (E) a decrease in cerebral blood flow, increase in metabolic rate

6. Nitrous oxide exerts which of the following effects on the central nervous system?

   (A) decreased cerebral blood flow

   (B) decreased cerebral blood volume

   (C) ablation of the cerebrovascular response to CO_2

   (D) decrease in intracranial pressure

   (E) increase in cerebral metabolic rate

7. Which of the following inhaled anesthetics is most likely to produce seizure-like activity on the electroencephalogram (EEG)?

   (A) desflurane

   (B) enflurane

   (C) halothane

   (D) isoflurane

   (E) sevoflurane

8. Which of the following statements is TRUE regarding the effect of inhaled anesthetics on the cardiovascular system?

   (A) Desflurane has the greatest negative inotropic effect compared to other volatile agents.

   (B) halothane at 1 MAC results in tachycardia.

   (C) nitrous oxide has no effect on myocardial contractility.

   (D) isoflurane causes a reflex increase in heart rate.

   (E) sevoflurane exerts a greater decrease in systemic vascular resistance than isoflurane.

9. Which of the following inhaled gases is most likely to sensitize the myocardium to the arrhythmogenic effects of epinephrine?

   (A) desflurane

   (B) enflurane

   (C) halothane

   (D) isoflurane

   (E) sevoflurane

10. A 20-year-old healthy patient is undergoing a bunionectomy using sevoflurane anesthesia and a laryngeal mask. Which of the following pulmonary effects is most likely to occur?

    (A) an increase in tidal volume

    (B) an increase in respiratory rate

    (C) an increase in alveolar ventilation

    (D) an increase in bronchial smooth motor tone

    (E) an increase in functional residual capacity

11. A patient is emerging from anesthesia with an end-tidal concentration of isoflurane of 0.12% (0.1 MAC). Which of the following pulmonary effects would you most likely expect in this situation?

    (A) decreased ventilatory response to hypoxemia

    (B) decreased respiratory rate

    (C) inhibition of hypoxic pulmonary vasodilation

    (D) increased airway resistance

    (E) increased risk of laryngospasm

12. Which of the following inhaled anesthetics has the greatest effect on potentiation of neuromuscular blockade?

    (A) desflurane

    (B) halothane

    (C) isoflurane

    (D) nitrous oxide

    (E) sevoflurane

13. A woman is undergoing cesarean delivery under general anesthesia with 1 MAC of isoflurane in oxygen/air. Which of the following best describes the effect of this gas mixture on the uterus?

    (A) increased permeability of the placenta to polarized molecules

    (B) a 20% decrease in uterine smooth muscle tone

    (C) a 40% increase in uterine blood flow

    (D) decreased responsiveness to tocolytic agents

    (E) augmentation of the effect of oxytocin

14. Which of the following statements regarding compound A is true?

    (A) Its generation is increased when using soda lime instead of Baralyme.

    (B) Toxicity is dose-dependent.

    (C) Injury to renal cells is largely irreversible.

    (D) The likelihood of renal injury is independent of inspired gas flow.

    (E) It is formed by the breakdown product of desflurane.

15. Which of the following statements regarding the inhaled anesthetics and the liver is TRUE?

    (A) Sevoflurane has no effect on portal blood flow.

    (B) Nitrous oxide decreases hepatic arterial blood flow.

    (C) Halothane hepatitis is fatal in >50% of cases.

    (D) Enflurane is the volatile agent that undergoes the highest degree of hepatic metabolism.

    (E) Isoflurane causes direct vasoconstriction of the hepatic artery.

16. Oxidation of the cobalt atom of vitamin B12 by nitrous oxide may lead to which of the following?

    (A) microcytic anemia
    (B) thrombocytopenia
    (C) erythrocytosis and increased risk for DVT
    (D) megaloblastic anemia
    (E) leukocytosis

17. Which of the following immunologic effects has been demonstrated with volatile anesthetics?

    (A) They are bacteriostatic at clinical concentrations.
    (B) They decrease the ability of leukocytes to phagocytize bacteria.
    (C) Increased risk of viral infection.
    (D) Increased chemotaxis of leukocytes to the lung leading to inflammatory acute lung injury.
    (E) Suppression of natural killer cells.

18. Which one of the following statements regarding the formation of carbon monoxide during inhalational anesthesia is TRUE?

    (A) Carbon monoxide may be produced by isoflurane, enflurane, and sevoflurane.
    (B) Dry carbon dioxide absorbent is a risk factor for carbon monoxide formation.
    (C) Soda lime is more likely to produce carbon monoxide than Baralyme.
    (D) High fresh gas flows reduce the risk of carbon monoxide formation.
    (E) Carbon monoxide toxicity is highest during the last case of the day.

19. Which of the following inhaled anesthetics has the lowest extent of metabolism?

    (A) desflurane
    (B) halothane
    (C) isoflurane
    (D) nitrous oxide
    (E) sevoflurane

20. A patient undergoing a vascular procedure is switched from isoflurane to sevoflurane. Fifteen minutes later, the monitor display shows that his end-tidal isoflurane is 0.55%, and his end-tidal sevoflurane concentration is 0.5%. What is his minimum alveolar concentration (MAC)?

    (A) 0.25 MAC
    (B) 0.33 MAC
    (C) 0.5 MAC
    (D) 0.75 MAC
    (E) 1 MAC

21. Which of the following factors increases MAC for an individual undergoing general anesthesia?

    (A) acute alcohol intoxication
    (B) acute cocaine intoxication
    (C) age >70
    (D) hyperthyroidism
    (E) pregnancy

22. Which of the following health outcomes in operating room personnel has been associated with exposure to waste anesthetic gases?

    (A) increased incidence of hypertension
    (B) increased incidence of reactive airways disease
    (C) increased incidence of noninfectious hepatitis
    (D) increased incidence of neuropsychiatric disease
    (E) increased incidence of spontaneous abortions

23. Which of the following regarding the inhaled anesthetic xenon is TRUE?

    (A) Only 0.5% of xenon is metabolized.
    (B) It is a naturally occurring gas.
    (C) It has a MAC of 1.17.
    (D) It is very soluble compared to other inhaled anesthetic agents.
    (E) It causes a dose-dependent reduction in arterial blood pressure.

Answers and Explanations: Gases and Vapors

1. Which of the following statements regarding the physical properties of nitrous oxide is FALSE?

   (A) Nitrous oxide is colorless.
   (B) Nitrous oxide is odorless.
   (C) Nitrous oxide cannot support combustion.
   (D) Nitrous oxide has a boiling point below room temperature.
   (E) Nitrous oxide is nonflammable.

Nitrous oxide is a colorless and odorless gas. While it is nonflammable, it is an oxidizing agent and does support combustion. For this reason, its concentration should be kept to a minimum in cases where the risk of surgical or airway fire are elevated. Its boiling point is well below room temperature ($-88°C$), meaning that at standard temperature and pressure, nitrous oxide exists in a gaseous form, in contrast to the potent volatile anesthetic agents. However, because its critical temperature is above room temperature ($36°C$), nitrous oxide can be liquified when sufficient pressure exists inside a cylinder.

Ref: Butterworth JF IV, Mackey DC, Wasnick JD. *Morgan and Mikhail's Clinical Anesthesiology.* 5th ed. New York, NY: McGraw Hill; 2013.

2. Which of the following potent volatile agents is most likely to evaporate when left in an open container in the operating room?

   (A) desflurane
   (B) enflurane
   (C) halothane
   (D) isoflurane
   (E) sevoflurane

The degree to which a liquid will evaporate depends on the vapor pressure, or the pressure exerted by a vapor when it is in equilibrium with the liquid phase. The boiling point of a liquid is the temperature at which vapor pressure equals atmospheric pressure. A high vapor pressure and/or a low boiling point will favor evaporation of the liquid phase into a vapor phase. As can be seen from Table 9-1, desflurane has the highest vapor pressure and lowest boiling point. In fact, at high altitudes, where boiling points are not as high, desflurane may boil at normal room temperature of $20°C$.

TABLE 9-1. Vapor pressures and boiling points for the potent volatile anesthetic agents.

Volatile agent	Vapor pressure at 20°C (mm Hg)	Boiling point (°C)
Desflurane	669	22.8
Enflurane	172	56.5
Halothane	243	50.2
Isoflurane	238	48.5
Sevoflurane	157	58.5

Ref: Butterworth JF IV, Mackey DC, Wasnick JD. *Morgan and Mikhail's Clinical Anesthesiology.* 5th ed. New York, NY: McGraw Hill; 2013.

3. Which of the following physical properties best correlates with volatile anesthetic potency?

   (A) boiling point
   (B) density
   (C) lipid solubility
   (D) molecular mass
   (E) viscosity

Of all the physicochemical properties of volatile anesthetics, lipid solubility correlates the best with anesthetic potency. This discovery, made at the turn of the 20th century, was termed the Meyer-Overton theory of anesthesia. Meyer was able to show that there was a strong correlation between the solubility of known anesthetics in olive oil and their potency in tadpoles. When plotted in a log:log format, the relationship between minimum alveolar concentration and oil:gas

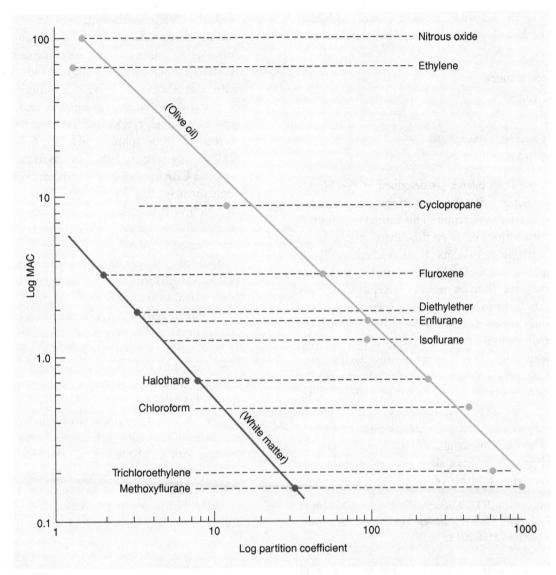

FIG. 9-1. There is a good but not perfect correlation between anesthetic potency and lipid solubility. MAC, minimum alveolar concentration. (Modified and reproduced, with permission, from Lowe HJ, Hagler K: *Gas Chromatography in Biology and Medicine.* Churchill, 1969.)

partition coefficient is inverse and linear (Figure 9-1). For example, halothane has an oil:gas partition coefficient of 224, and a MAC of 0.75; on the other end of the spectrum, nitrous oxide has a very small oil:gas partition coefficient of 1.4, but a MAC of 104. Sevoflurane, isoflurane, and desflurane all fall in the middle of these values.

The implication of this relationship is that inhaled anesthetics appear to be hydrophobic and may exert their action in part by binding to a hydrophobic site in the central nervous system. It has long been postulated that the lipid bilayer of neurons was the site of action;

the so-called "critical volume hypothesis" suggests that when a certain mass of hydrophobic anesthetic molecules are absorbed into the membrane, it becomes deformed to the extent that protein channels no longer function properly and conduction of action potentials ceases. While this may be part of the explanation for the mechanism of anesthetic action, it is likely an oversimplification, as inhaled anesthetics have been shown to influence other targets, such as proteins themselves.

Ref: Butterworth JF IV, Mackey DC, Wasnick JD. *Morgan and Mikhail's Clinical Anesthesiology.* 5th ed. New York, NY: McGraw Hill; 2013.

4. Nitrous oxide and xenon are both thought to inhibit which of the following receptors in the central nervous system?

   (A) acetylcholine

   (B) GABA

   (C) glycine

   (D) N-methyl-D-aspartate

   (E) neurokinin 1

Besides the lipid bilayer (as described in the Meyer-Overton hypothesis), there are several other putative targets for anesthetic action in the central nervous system. Both nitrous oxide and the inert anesthetic gas xenon are believed to inhibit NMDA receptors. This is one putative mechanism by which nitrous oxide provides analgesia. These are excitatory receptors, and their inhibition leads to decreased neuronal activity. Many anesthetics appear to enhance the GABA-ergic inhibition of the central nervous system by hyperpolarizing cell membranes. This is supported by the fact that GABA agonists enhance anesthesia, whereas GABA antagonists partially reverse anesthetic effect. Other receptors that are sites of anesthetic action probably include those that bind to glycine, calcium, and glutamate. The exact mechanism of anesthetic action of inhaled gases is far from clear and probably involves many overlapping pathways.

   Ref: Butterworth JF IV, Mackey DC, Wasnick JD. *Morgan and Mikhail's Clinical Anesthesiology.* 5th ed. New York, NY: McGraw Hill; 2013.

5. Halothane, desflurane, isoflurane, and sevoflurane all produce which of the following effects on cerebrovascular physiology and metabolism?

   (A) an increase in cerebral blood flow, decrease in metabolic rate

   (B) an increase in cerebral blood flow, no change in metabolic rate

   (C) a decrease in cerebral blood flow, decrease in metabolic rate

   (D) a decrease in cerebral blood flow, no change in metabolic rate

   (E) a decrease in cerebral blood flow, increase in metabolic rate

All of the volatile anesthetics increase cerebral blood flow (CBF) in a dose-dependent manner by acting as direct vasodilators of the cerebral vasculature. However,

while the CBF increases with the volatile agents, cerebral metabolism decreases, a phenomenon known as "uncoupling," since the decrease in metabolic demand ($CMRO_2$) is not proportionally met with a decrease in CBF. This effect is most potent for halothane but still occurs with isoflurane, sevoflurane, and desflurane, especially at levels >1.5 MAC. For example, halothane increases CBF by approximately 200% but decreases $CMRO_2$ by about 10%. In contrast, isoflurane increases CBF by about 20% and reduces $CMRO_2$ by approximately 50% (Figure 9-2). The increase in CBF seen with volatile agents (and halothane in particular) is typically associated with an increase in cerebral blood volume. In patients with normal intracranial compliance, this does not appear to be an issue; however, in patients with reduced intracranial compliance (e.g., related to traumatic brain injury or tumor), the use of volatile agent can significantly increase the intracranial pressure. Hyperventilation and the induction of hypocapnia may not attenuate this effect. For this reason, patients with reduced intracranial compliance are typically anesthetized with a total intravenous anesthetic (TIVA) technique.

The cerebrovascular responsiveness to carbon dioxide is preserved (in patients with normal intracerebral compliance) with all of the volatile anesthetics. However, autoregulation in response to increased systemic arterial pressures is impaired due to the direct vasodilation. Instead of compensatory vasoconstriction to maintain a constant CBF between a MAP of 50 and 150 mm Hg,

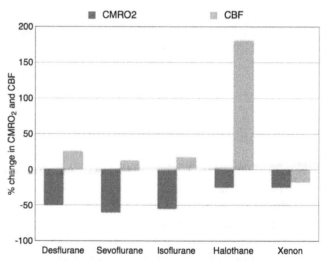

FIG. 9-2. Anticipated changes in cerebral metabolic rate of oxygen consumption ($CMRO_2$) and cerebral blood flow (CBF) with approximately 1 minimum alveolar concentration (MAC) of selected anesthetic gases. (Reproduced with permission from Miller RD. *Miller's Anesthesia*, 8th edition. Philadelphia, PA: Elsevier, 2015).

the CBF is directly tied to systemic pressures. The lower part of the autoregulation curve is not affected, since the cerebral vessels are already maximally dilated.

Ref: Miller RD. Miller's *Anesthesia*. 8th ed. Philadelphia, PA: Elsevier; 2015.

6. Nitrous oxide exerts which of the following effects on the central nervous system?

    (A) decreased cerebral blood flow
    (B) decreased cerebral blood volume
    (C) ablation of the cerebrovascular response to CO_2
    (D) decrease in intracranial pressure
    (E) **increase in cerebral metabolic rate**

Unlike the other inhaled anesthetics, nitrous oxide increases the cerebral metabolic rate ($CMRO_2$). In addition, it also increases cerebral blood flow, cerebral blood volume, and intracranial pressure when administered alone. This is likely due to the sympathomimetic effect of the gas. In combination with the volatile agents, this effect on ICP is preserved. However, the co-administration of intravenous anesthetics such as barbiturates, propofol, opioids, or benzodiazepines greatly reduces or completely ablates this effect, and ICP is not increased. Despite this, its use in neurosurgery is no longer routine, and especially in cases where intracranial compliance is decreased, its negative effects outweigh any potential benefits.

Ref: Miller RD. Miller's *Anesthesia*. 8th ed. Philadelphia, PA: Elsevier; 2015.

7. Which of the following inhaled anesthetics is most likely to produce seizure-like activity on the electroencephalogram (EEG)?

    (A) desflurane
    (B) **enflurane**
    (C) halothane
    (D) isoflurane
    (E) sevoflurane

Most volatile anesthetics have a marked effect on the EEG, decreasing the high-frequency activity and increasing the slow-frequency activity. Burst suppression and isoelectric EEG patterns are possible with 1.5 MAC to 2 MAC of isoflurane, desflurane, or sevoflurane. $CMRO_2$ is typically about 50% of baseline at this level (remember that cerebral oxygen requirements are still present with isoelectric activity in order to

maintain cellular integrity and homeostasis). Halothane requires very high concentrations to produce burst suppression in animals (4 MAC); this concentration is clearly not clinically applicable.

Enflurane is an exception to this pattern. High concentrations of enflurane cause a high-voltage, high-frequency EEG pattern that can progress to spike and dome complexes and frank seizure activity. This property can be leveraged when administering anesthesia for mapping of seizure foci. In contrast, enflurane is typically avoided in patients with seizure disorders.

Nitrous oxide has no inhibitory effect on the EEG, and may increase the frequency slightly.

Refs: Longnecker DE, Brown DL, Newman MF, Zapol WM. *Anesthesiology*. 2nd ed. New York, NY: McGraw Hill; 2012.
Brunton LL, Chabner BA, Knollman BC. *Goodman & Gilman's the Pharmacological Basis of Therapeutics*. 12th ed. New York, NY: McGraw Hill; 2011.

8. Which of the following statements is TRUE regarding the effect of inhaled anesthetics on the cardiovascular system?

    (A) Desflurane has the greatest negative inotropic effect compared to other volatile agents.
    (B) Halothane at 1 MAC results in tachycardia.
    (C) Nitrous oxide has no effect on myocardial contractility.
    (D) **Isoflurane causes a reflex increase in heart rate.**
    (E) Sevoflurane exerts a greater decrease in systemic vascular resistance than isoflurane.

Nitrous oxide has a direct negative inotropic effect on the myocardium. Despite this, it has the least overall effect on the cardiovascular system of all the inhaled gases (Table 9-2). This is because nitrous oxide is a sympathetic stimulator, and the increased level of catecholamines present during nitrous anesthesia produces a slight compensatory increase in arterial blood pressure and heart rate so that cardiac output is essentially unchanged from baseline. Desflurane is also a weak stimulator of the sympathetic system, and tachycardia is frequently seen during the "ramp-up" phase of desflurane anesthesia, when rapid increases in the partial pressure are occurring. Isoflurane also produces an increase in heart rate, but this is because of a baroreceptor-mediated reflex in response to vasodilation. Halothane causes either no effect on heart rate or a slight decrease due to a blunting of the baroreceptor reflexes.

TABLE 9-2. **Cardiovascular effects of anesthetic gases.**

	Nitrous oxide	Halothane	Isoflurane	Desflurane	Sevoflurane
Blood pressure	↔	↓↓	↓↓	↓↓	↓
Heart rate	↔	↔ or ↓	↑	↔ or ↑	↔
Systemic vascular resistance	↔	↔	↓↓	↓↓	↓
Cardiac output	↔	↓	↔	↔ or ↓	↓

Sevoflurane, desflurane, and isoflurane are all vasodilators and decrease the SVR, with isoflurane and desflurane producing a greater effect than sevoflurane. These reductions in SVR are associated with a decrease in blood pressure. Halothane also causes a decrease in blood pressure, but this is due to direct myocardial depression, not vasodilation.

All volatile anesthetics are mild coronary vasodilators. Some concern has been expressed regarding the potential for a steal phenomenon, whereby vasodilation in nonstenosed areas diverts flow from stenotic areas that are unable to vasodilate. This concern is probably largely overstated, and providing that tachycardia and hypotension are avoided in patients with coronary disease, volatiles do not appear to cause abnormal myocardial perfusion resulting in ischemia.

Ref: Miller RD. Miller's *Anesthesia*. 8th ed. Philadelphia, PA: Elsevier; 2015.

9. Which of the following inhaled gases is most likely to sensitize the myocardium to the arrhythmogenic effects of epinephrine?

(A) desflurane

(B) enflurane

(C) halothane

(D) isoflurane

(E) sevoflurane

Halothane has long been known to sensitize the myocardium to catecholamines and predispose to arrhythmias. Other volatile agents can produce the same effect but to a much lesser extent. Halothane reduces the threshold for both atrial and ventricular arrhythmias. The effect appears to be related to the dose of epinephrine, starting with premature ventricular contractions at low doses and escalating through to sustained ventricular tachyarrhythmias. Epinephrine doses above 1.5 mcg/kg during halothane anesthesia should be avoided. This phenomenon is attenuated by the pretreatment with sodium thiopental.

Ref: Miller RD. Miller's *Anesthesia*. 8th ed. Philadelphia, PA: Elsevier; 2015.

10. A 20-year-old healthy patient is undergoing a bunionectomy using sevoflurane anesthesia and a laryngeal mask. Which of the following pulmonary effects is most likely to occur?

(A) an increase in tidal volume

(B) an increase in respiratory rate

(C) an increase in alveolar ventilation

(D) an increase in bronchial smooth motor tone

(E) an increase in functional residual capacity

All volatile anesthetics depress respiration via central effects on the medullary respiratory center, as well as relaxant effects on skeletal muscles of respiration. Volatile agents cause rapid, shallow breathing with increased respiratory rate and decreased tidal volumes. Despite the increase in rate, the overall alveolar ventilation is decreased, producing an increase in PaCO$_2$. The anesthetic gases all result in a decreased FRC and atelectasis in the spontaneously breathing patient.

Isoflurane, sevoflurane, and halothane are all potent bronchodilating agents, relaxing smooth muscle in the airway, and decreasing airway resistance (sevo > halo > iso). Desflurane has little bronchodilating effect and in patients with reactive airways disease can in fact provoke bronchospasm. Inhalational induction with desflurane is associated with an increased risk of salivation, laryngospasm, bronchospasm, and coughing due to its pungency. This effect is greatest at high concentrations (> 1 MAC). Its use in asthmatics and for inhalational induction is discouraged.

Nitrous oxide also causes an increase in respiratory rate and decrease in tidal volume, but the overall alveolar ventilation appears to be preserved, with a normal PaCO$_2$.

Ref: Longnecker DE, Brown DL, Newman MF, Zapol WM. *Anesthesiology*. 2nd ed. New York, NY: McGraw Hill; 2012.

11. A patient is emerging from anesthesia with an end-tidal concentration of isoflurane of 0.12% (0.1 MAC). Which of the following pulmonary effects would you most likely expect in this situation?

(A) **decreased ventilatory response to hypoxemia**

(B) decreased respiratory rate

(C) inhibition of hypoxic pulmonary vasodilation

(D) increased airway resistance

(E) increased risk of laryngospasm

The volatile gases and nitrous oxide are potent inhibitors of the ventilatory response to hypoxemia and hypercarbia. This is a dose- and agent-dependent effect (halo > iso > sevo > des) but overall still exists at sub-anesthetic concentrations such as 0.1 MAC. The effect is mediated via the peripheral chemoreceptors in the carotid bodies.

This is a critical consideration during emergence when patients typically have small amounts of residual volatile agent on-board, but little in the way of stimulation. These patients may become hypercarbic and hypoxic during transport or in the recovery room. Hypoxic pulmonary vasodilation is inhibited by volatile agents but not at clinical concentrations and certainly not at 0.1 MAC.

Ref: Longnecker DE, Brown DL, Newman MF, Zapol WM. *Anesthesiology.* 2nd ed. New York, NY: McGraw Hill; 2012.

12. Which of the following inhaled anesthetics has the greatest effect on potentiation of neuromuscular blockade?

(A) **desflurane**

(B) halothane

(C) isoflurane

(D) nitrous oxide

(E) sevoflurane

The volatile agents all produce a dose-dependent potentiation of neuromuscular blockade (Figure 9-3). The mechanism is not entirely clear but may be related to inhibition of postsynaptic acetylcholine receptors, an effect on the motor neurons themselves, or enhancement of the neuromuscular antagonist at the receptor site. Inhaled anesthetics decrease the dose of non-depolarizing neuromuscular blockers required, increase the duration, and depress the train-of-four and tetanus responses. The ability of the volatile agent to potentiate this effect is inversely related to potency; therefore, the

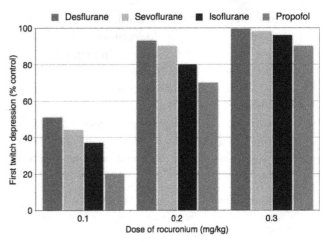

FIG. 9-3. Effect of 1.5 minimum alveolar concentration (MAC) anesthesia with desflurane, sevoflurane, isoflurane, as well as propofol total intravenous anesthesia on first twitch depression during rocuronium-induced neuromuscular blockade. (Reproduced with permission from Miller RD, *Miller's Anesthesia,* 8th edition. Philadelphia, PA: Elsevier, 2015).

order of potentiation from strongest to weakest is desflurane > sevoflurane > isoflurane > halothane. Nitrous oxide potentiates the least of the inhaled gases.

Ref: Miller RD. Miller's *Anesthesia.* 8th ed. Philadelphia, PA: Elsevier; 2015.

13. A woman is undergoing cesarean delivery under general anesthesia with 1 MAC of isoflurane in oxygen/air. Which of the following best describes the effect of this gas mixture on the uterus?

(A) increased permeability of the placenta to polarized molecules

(B) **a 20% decrease in uterine smooth muscle tone**

(C) a 40% increase in uterine blood flow

(D) decreased responsiveness to tocolytic agents

(E) augmentation of the effect of oxytocin

The volatile agents all produce a dose-dependent decrease in uterine smooth muscle contractility. This effect may be somewhat less pronounced with desflurane. Traditionally, following delivery of the fetus during a cesarean delivery under general anesthesia, the volatile agent was decreased to 0.5 MAC and nitrous oxide was added or increased up to 0.5 MAC to reduce this effect and facilitate contraction of the uterus, thereby reducing the risk of uterine atony and postpartum hemorrhage. The volatile agents impair the ability of oxytocin to contract the uterus. In contrast, volatile agents have been used in the past to facilitate uterine relaxation for manual removal of placenta or in difficult deliveries (such as twins). Since general anesthetics are rare these days for cesarean deliveries, other uterine relaxant agents such as nitroglycerin have almost completely supplanted the use of volatile agents. Nitrous oxide has no effect on uterine smooth muscle tone.

Note that there is also a dose-dependent decrease in uterine blood flow as well with the inhaled volatile gases. This is related to vasodilation and arterial hypotension.

Ref: Butterworth JF IV, Mackey DC, Wasnick JD. *Morgan and Mikhail's Clinical Anesthesiology.* 5th ed. New York, NY: McGraw Hill; 2013.

14. Which of the following statements regarding compound A is true?

(A) Its generation is increased when using soda lime instead of Baralyme.

(B) Toxicity is dose-dependent.

(C) Injury to renal cells is largely irreversible.

(D) The likelihood of renal injury is independent of inspired gas flow.

(E) It is formed by the breakdown product of desflurane.

Compound A is a degradation product of sevoflurane that occurs when the gas is exposed to carbon dioxide absorbent. Compound A has been shown to cause acute tubular necrosis in rats, but the clinical implication of this in humans is unknown. In experimental conditions where volunteers were exposed to long durations of sevoflurane anesthesia, levels of compound A did increase, as did enzymatic markers of renal injury and BUN and creatinine levels. However, these typically return to normal within several days, and there are no cases of irreversible renal injury reported in humans.

The risk of incurring nephrotoxicity appears to be dose dependent, with 150 ppm-hours as an accepted threshold (i.e., 50 ppm × 3 hours, or 25 ppm × 6 hours). Compound A is generated more when Baralyme is used in place of soda lime, and especially when low fresh gas flows are utilized. For this reason, the FDA advises that flow rates <2 L/min be avoided when using sevoflurane. Although it is a primarily a theoretical concern, patient with preexisting renal injury should probably avoid sevoflurane, as other volatile options exist.

15. Which of the following statements regarding the inhaled anesthetics and the liver is TRUE?

(A) Sevoflurane has no effect on portal blood flow.

(B) Nitrous oxide decrease hepatic arterial blood flow.

(C) Halothane hepatitis is fatal in >50% of cases.

(D) Enflurane is the volatile agent that undergoes the highest degree of hepatic metabolism.

(E) Isoflurane causes direct vasoconstriction of the hepatic artery.

All volatile anesthetics decrease mean arterial pressure and portal blood flow, and hence total hepatic blood flow. Hepatic artery blood flow is decreased by halothane and enflurane through direct vasoconstriction, whereas isoflurane and sevoflurane cause increased flow velocity in the hepatic sinusoids. When administered to volunteers not undergoing surgery, these newer volatile agents appear to produce no elevations in markers of liver injury, suggesting that surgical factors (i.e., further decreases in hepatic blood flow related to positioning or retraction) may be responsible for any transient elevations in enzymes observed. Nitrous oxide has no significant effect on hepatic hemodynamics.

Halothane undergoes metabolism by the liver (15%–20%), more than any other volatile anesthetic (sevoflurane 5%, enflurane = 3%, isoflurane = 0.2%, desflurane = 0.02%). The breakdown products, trifluoroacetic acid and trifluoroacetic chloride, are able to bind to proteins in the liver, where they are recognized by the immune system as antigens. The resulting immune response is known as halothane hepatitis, and typically results in fulminant hepatic necrosis, fatal in 50% to 75% of cases. Multiple exposures increase the likelihood of this response, in line with an immune mechanism. Halothane hepatitis is 10 to 20 times more prevalent in adults than in the pediatric population.

Ref: Longnecker DE, Brown DL, Newman MF, Zapol WM. *Anesthesiology.* 2nd ed. New York, NY: McGraw Hill; 2012.

16. Oxidation of the cobalt atom of vitamin B12 by nitrous oxide may lead which of the following?

(A) microcytic anemia

(B) thrombocytopenia

(C) erythrocytosis and increased risk for DVT

(D) megaloblastic anemia

(E) leukocytosis

Nitrous oxide irreversibly oxides the cobalt atom of vitamin B_{12}, thereby inhibiting the vitamin B_{12} dependent enzyme methionine synthetase. Methionine synthetase is necessary for the formation of myelin (through the conversion of homocysteine to methionine) and DNA synthesis. The clinical effects of the impairment of DNA synthesis are primarily observed as megaloblastic bone marrow changes and agranulocytosis. Besides the hematologic effects, the inhibition of methionine synthetase may result in neurologic effects related to the decreased production of myelin, including posterior lateral spinal cord degeneration, polyneuropathy, and ataxia.

The duration of exposure of 50% nitrous oxide to cause these changes is probably >6 hours but has been reliably observed at about 12 hours. Exposure to nitrous oxide for longer than 4 days leads to agranulocytosis. Most patients are not affected given the brief, single exposure, but repeated exposures can be harmful, especially given the rapid inactivation of the enzymes and the long time required for new production. Dental personnel have a higher incidence of abnormal bone marrow and neurologic disease than operating room personnel, which may relate to the type of scavenging equipment used and the inhaled concentration the clinicians are exposed to.

Ref: Longnecker DE, Brown DL, Newman MF, Zapol WM. *Anesthesiology.* 2nd ed. New York, NY: McGraw Hill; 2012.

17. Which of the following immunologic effects has been demonstrated with volatile anesthetics?

(A) They are bacteriostatic at clinical concentrations.

(B) They decrease the ability of leukocytes to phagocytize bacteria.

(C) Increased risk of viral infection.

(D) Increased chemotaxis of leukocytes to the lung leading to inflammatory acute lung injury.

(E) **Suppression of natural killer cells.**

Volatile anesthetics have been shown to suppress the function of natural killer (NK) cells in experimental models. One of the roles of NK cells is to "mop up" the neoplastic cells that are not excised and/or are hematogenously spread during the course of surgical excision of a tumor. It has been argued that the suppressive effect on NK cell populations is one of the mechanisms by which general anesthesia using volatile anesthetic agents fails to reduce the incidence of cytologic recurrence in several cancer models compared to total intra-venous anesthesia (with or without regional anesthesia). However, the strength of the evidence supporting avoidance of volatile agents in patients with cancer is weak. The effect that the general stress response to surgery has on NK cells is probably much greater.

Inhaled anesthetics (including nitrous oxide) decrease the chemotactic migration of leukocytes necessary for inflammatory reactions. There is evidence that anesthesia with volatile agents decreases the incidence and severity of acute lung injury in at-risk patients.

Ref: Hemmings HC, Egan TD. *Pharmacology and Physiology for Anesthesia: Foundations and Clinical Application.* 1st ed. Philadelphia, PA: Elsevier; 2013.

18. Which one of the following statements regarding the formation of carbon monoxide during inhalational anesthesia is TRUE?

(A) Carbon monoxide may be produced by isoflurane, enflurane, and sevoflurane.

(B) **Dry carbon dioxide absorbent is a risk factor for carbon monoxide formation.**

(C) Soda lime is more likely to produce carbon monoxide than Baralyme.

(D) High fresh gas flows reduce the risk of carbon monoxide formation.

(E) Carbon monoxide toxicity is highest during the last case of the day.

Volatile anesthetics can be degraded by the strong bases present in carbon dioxide absorbent materials into carbon monoxide (CO). CO is a colorless, odorless gas that has a high affinity for hemoglobin, preventing oxygen carriage and delivery. In addition, it is difficult to detect because the pulse oximeter cannot differentiate between oxyhemoglobin and carboxyhemoglobin. Prolonged or high levels of CO can lead to delayed neurologic effects such as cognitive effects, personality changes, and ataxia.

Desflurane produces the highest concentration of CO on exposure to carbon dioxide absorbent, followed in order by enflurane and isoflurane. Sevoflurane and halothane produce a negligible amount of CO. The most important modifiable risk factor for production of CO during an anesthetic is the dryness of the absorbent. Several cases have been reported of first case starts on Monday incurring CO toxicity. In looking for a cause, it was noted that the fresh gas was left on with high flow rates over the weekend, drying out the absorbent and priming it for such a reaction.

Soda lime and Baralyme are 15% and 13% water by weight, respectively. Soda lime must be dried out to a hydration level of 1.4% before noticeable CO production will occur; in contrast, the hydration threshold for CO production with Baralyme is about 5%. Therefore, an increased margin of safety exists with soda lime with respect to desiccation.

Ref: Longnecker DE, Brown DL, Newman MF, Zapol WM. *Anesthesiology.* 2nd ed. New York, NY: McGraw Hill; 2012.

19. Which of the following inhaled anesthetics has the lowest extent of metabolism?

(A) desflurane

(B) halothane

(C) isoflurane

(D) **nitrous oxide**

(E) sevoflurane

Inhaled anesthetics undergo metabolism in the body to varying degrees. Xenon is the exception, in that truly no metabolic conversion exists. Halothane is the agent with the highest degree of metabolism: approximately 15% to 20% of the gas is either reduced or oxidized by the liver (see question 15 regarding halothane hepatitis). Other gases that undergo oxidative metabolism via the cytochrome P450 pathway include sevoflurane (5%), enflurane (3%), isoflurane (0.2%), and desflurane (0.02%).

Nitrous oxide is also an interesting exception. Although it is miniscule, there is a measurable amount of the gas that undergoes reductive metabolism (0.004%). This is not carried out by a metabolic pathway in the liver but is converted to nitrogen in the gastrointestinal tract by anaerobic bacteria such as Pseudomonas. Oxygen concentrations >10% in the GI tract tend to inhibit this reaction.

Ref: Miller RD. Miller's *Anesthesia.* 8th ed. Philadelphia, PA: Elsevier; 2015.

20. A patient undergoing a vascular procedure is switched from isoflurane to sevoflurane. Fifteen minutes later, the monitor display shows that his end-tidal isoflurane is 0.55%, and his end-tidal sevoflurane concentration is 0.5%. What is his minimum alveolar concentration (MAC)?

(A) 0.25 MAC

(B) 0.33 MAC

(C) 0.5 MAC

(D) **0.75 MAC**

(E) 1 MAC

Minimum alveolar concentration (MAC) is the concentration of inhaled anesthetic in the alveoli that inhibits movement in 50% of patients upon surgical stimulus. There are different MAC derivatives for different goals. The concentration required to prevent movement with surgical stimulus in 99% of patients is approximately 1.3 MAC (or 1.3 × the MAC value for that anesthetic gas). For example, to prevent movement in 99% of patients upon incision when using sevoflurane (MAC 2.0%), an alveolar concentration of 2.6% would be required. Other derivatives of MAC include:

- MAC_{BAR} (MAC required to abolish sympathetic response to incision in 50%). Approximately 1.5 MAC.
- MAC_{AWAKE} (MAC required to abolish eye opening on command in 50%). Approximately 0.5 MAC.
- MAC_{AWARE} (MAC required to abolish memory and consciousness in 50%). This is a less well-defined concept, but is generally accepted to be less than MAC awake (~0.2–0.3 MAC).

There are two keys to answering this problem. The first is the recognition that MAC is roughly additive. The other is knowing the MAC of common anesthetic gases. The MAC values for halothane, isoflurane, sevoflurane, and desflurane are 0.75%, 1.1%, 2%, and 6%, respectively. In the above example, 0.55% isoflurane is equivalent to 0.5 MAC; 0.5% sevoflurane is 25% of its MAC value of 2%. Adding these up, we get 0.5 MAC plus 0.25 MAC equals 0.75 MAC.

Ref: Butterworth JF IV, Mackey DC, Wasnick JD. *Morgan and Mikhail's Clinical Anesthesiology.* 5th ed. New York, NY: McGraw Hill; 2013.

21. Which of the following factors increases MAC for an individual undergoing general anesthesia?

(A) acute alcohol intoxication

(B) **acute cocaine intoxication**

(C) age > 70

(D) hyperthyroidism

(E) pregnancy

Multiple physiologic and pharmacologic factors affect MAC (Table 9-3). In general, CNS depressants (acute alcohol intoxication, opioids, barbiturates, benzodiazepines, clonidine, ketamine, etc.) decrease MAC; there-

TABLE 9-3. **Factors affecting MAC.**[a]

Variable	Effect on MAC	Comments	Variable	Effect on MAC	Comments
Temperature			Electrolytes		
Hypothermia	↓		Hypercalcemia	↓	
Hyperthermia	↓	↑ if > 42°C	Hypernatremia	↑	Caused by altered CSF[b]
			Hyponatremia	↓	Caused by altered CSF
Age			Pregnancy	↓	MAC decreased by
Young	↑				one-third at 8 weeks'
Elderly	↓				gestation; normal by
					72 h postpartum
Alcohol			Drugs		
Acute intoxication	↓		Local anesthetics	↓	Except cocaine
Chronic abuse	↑		Opioids	↓	
			Ketamine	↓	
			Barbiturates	↓	
Anemia			Benzodiazepines	↓	
Hematocrit <10%	↓		Verapamil	↓	
PaO_2	↓		Lithium	↓	
<40 mm Hg			Sympatholytics		
$PaCO_2$			Methyldopa	↓	
>95 mm Hg	↓	Caused by < pH in CSF	Clonidine	↓	
Thyroid			Dexmedetomidine	↓	
Hyperthyroid	No change		Sympathomimetics		
Hypothyroid	No change		Amphetamine		
Blood pressure			Chronic	↓	
Mean arterial pressure	↓		Acute	↑	
<40 mm Hg			Cocaine	↑	
			Ephedrine	↑	

[a]These conclusions are based on human and animal studies.
[b]CSF, cerebrospinal fluid.
From: Butterworth JF IV, Mackey DC, Wasnick JD. *Morgan and Mikhail's Clinical Anesthesiology*. 5th ed. New York, NY: McGraw Hill; 2013.

fore, the amount of inhaled anesthetic required to achieve the same depth of anesthesia. In contrast, CNS stimulants (amphetamines, cocaine, and ephedrine) all increase MAC. MAC also decreases with advancing age (at a rate of 6% per decade of life), pregnancy, hypothermia, and profound hypoxemia, hypercarbia, or hypotension. Chronic alcohol ingestion increases MAC.

Several factors have no effect of MAC, including sex, thyroid gland dysfunction, hyper/hypokalemia, and hypertension.

Ref: Butterworth JF IV, Mackey DC, Wasnick JD. *Morgan and Mikhail's Clinical Anesthesiology*. 5th ed. New York, NY: McGraw Hill; 2013.

22. Which of the following health outcomes in operating room personnel has been associated with exposure to waste anesthetic gases?

(A) increased incidence of hypertension
(B) increased incidence of reactive airways disease
(C) increased incidence of noninfectious hepatitis
(D) increased incidence of neuropsychiatric disease
(E) **increased incidence of spontaneous abortions**

Several epidemiologic studies have demonstrated an increased association of exposure to waste anesthetic gases with reduced fecundity (ability to conceive) and an increased incidence of spontaneous abortions and congenital defects. In general, these studies show a relative risk for reproductive problems between 20% and 90% compared to groups of other hospital workers that were not exposed. However, these studies have multiple limitations that mandate caution in their interpretation. Many of them are older studies, conducted in an era where scavenging was not as sophisticated as it is today. The methodology of several of these studies was poor, prone to multiple confounders and recall bias on the part of the respondents. Several other surveys have suggested that it is in fact the workplace conditions inherent to operating room jobs that are associated (e.g., standing for long hours, fatigue, long work hours). However, given that these increased odds ratios have been repeatedly demonstrated in several large studies, the evidence as a whole suggests a slight increase in this adverse health outcome exists.

Ref: Barash PG. Clinical anesthesia. 7th ed. Philadelphia, PA: Lippincott Williams and Wilkins; 2013.

23. Which of the following regarding the inhaled anesthetic xenon is TRUE?

    (A)   Only 0.5% of xenon is metabolized.
    (B)   **It is a naturally occurring gas.**
    (C)   It has a MAC of 1.17.
    (D)   It is very soluble compared to other inhaled anesthetic agents.
    (E)   It causes a dose-dependent reduction in arterial blood pressure.

Xenon is a naturally occurring odorless, inert gas that has been used as an anesthetic. Because it is inert, it does not combine with other molecules, and is completely eliminated without any metabolism. Xenon is relatively insoluble (blood:gas partition coefficient 0.115), meaning that it reaches equilibrium with the tissues quickly and provides a rapid onset and emergence. The MAC of xenon is 0.71. Its mechanism of action is thought to be antagonism of the NMDA receptors in the central nervous system. Xenon is expensive (it cannot be manufactured and in fact has to be extracted from air) and in limited supply, two factors that have limited its use.

Xenon has minimal cardiorespiratory effects, and blood pressure, contractility, heart rate, and systemic vascular resistance are all essentially unchanged. It does cause a slight increase in airway pressure, an effect that is due to its increased viscosity compared to oxygen and not due to an increase in bronchial tone. Xenon has shown promise as a neuroprotective agent.

Refs: Butterworth JF IV, Mackey DC, Wasnick JD. *Morgan and Mikhail's Clinical Anesthesiology.* 5th ed. New York, NY: McGraw Hill; 2013.

Brunton LL, Chabner BA, Knollman BC. *Goodman & Gilman's the Pharmacological Basis of Therapeutics.* 12th ed. New York, NY: McGraw Hill; 2011.

CHAPTER 10

Opioids

1. Mu (μ) opioid receptor activation leads to supraspinal analgesia via which of the following mechanisms?

   (A) decreased release of substance P from primary afferent inputs

   (B) increased release of dopamine in the nucleus accumbens

   (C) decreased activity in the ventrolateral medulla

   (D) decreased release of GABA from periaqueductal gray matter

   (E) decreased release of dopamine in the arcuate nucleus

2. Activation of opioid receptors leads to activation of which intracellular transduction mechanism?

   (A) G proteins

   (B) adenylate cyclase

   (C) voltage gated calcium channels

   (D) voltage gated sodium channels

   (E) outward rectifying potassium channels

3. Which of the following opioids is the most hydrophilic?

   (A) morphine

   (B) fentanyl

   (C) codeine

   (D) methadone

   (E) heroin

4. In patients with reduced renal function, morphine administration has altered duration and potency. Which metabolite of morphine is responsible for this?

   (A) morphine-3-glucuronide

   (B) morphine-6-glucuronide

   (C) morphine-3,6-diglucuronide

   (D) normorphine

   (E) morphine

5. An adult is administered a single dose of fentanyl (100 micrograms intravenously). The clinical effects of fentanyl are terminated mainly by:

   (A) redistribution

   (B) hydroxylation

   (C) N-dealkylation

   (D) conjugation

   (E) demethylation

6. After a 3-hour intravenous infusion, which opioid has the longest context sensitive half-time?

   (A) fentanyl

   (B) sufentanil

   (C) alfentanil

   (D) remifentanil

   (E) propofol

7. Which opioid has the longest duration of action after epidural injection?

   (A) alfentanil

   (B) fentanyl

   (C) hydromorphone

   (D) methadone

   (E) morphine

8. The addition of 20 micrograms of fentanyl to a low-dose bupivacaine spinal will decrease the likelihood of:

   (A) respiratory depression

   (B) pruritus

   (C) a failed block

   (D) urinary retention

   (E) nausea and vomiting

9. A patient has significant hepatic and renal impairment. To avoid dosage adjustment due to this impairment, which opioid would be the best choice for intraoperative analgesia?

   (A) methadone
   (B) fentanyl
   (C) sufentanil
   (D) hydromorphone
   (E) remifentanil

10. Which opioid must be converted from a prodrug to an active form?

    (A) morphine
    (B) codeine
    (C) fentanyl
    (D) hydromorphone
    (E) remifentanil

11. In large doses, which opioid will likely produce the most hypotension?

    (A) fentanyl
    (B) sufentanil
    (C) alfentanil
    (D) morphine
    (E) remifentanil

12. Which opioid is most likely to cause tachycardia?

    (A) morphine
    (B) meperidine
    (C) codeine
    (D) fentanyl
    (E) alfentanil

13. Which factor is LEAST likely to increase the risk of opioid related respiratory depression?

    (A) natural sleep
    (B) chronic renal failure
    (C) benzodiazepines
    (D) clonidine
    (E) alcohol

14. Low doses of opioids tend to have the greatest effect on which respiratory activity?

    (A) decreased tidal volume
    (B) decreased respiratory rate
    (C) decreased chest wall rigidity
    (D) increased CO_2 responsiveness
    (E) increased O_2 responsiveness

15. Which of the following is a side effect of morphine?

    (A) diarrhea
    (B) peripheral vasoconstriction
    (C) biliary spasm
    (D) hyperthermia
    (E) mydriasis

16. Which opioid metabolite is most likely to cause seizures?

    (A) meperidinic acid
    (B) norfentanyl
    (C) normeperidine
    (D) morphine-3,6-glucuronide
    (E) morphine-6-glucuronide

17. Sustained administration of an opiate agonist (days to weeks) leads to loss of drug effect. This is best described as:

    (A) desensitization
    (B) tolerance
    (C) dependence
    (D) withdrawal
    (E) addiction

18. The combination of monoamine oxidase inhibitors (MAOIs) and opiate receptor agonists can lead to potentially fatal serotonin syndrome. Which opiate is the best choice to provide analgesia for a patient who is taking a MAOI?

    (A) meperidine
    (B) dextromethorphan
    (C) tramadol
    (D) tapentadol
    (E) morphine

19. Which opioid is most useful for a surgical procedure that requires rapid recovery?

    (A) fentanyl
    (B) sufentanil
    (C) morphine
    (D) remifentanil
    (E) methadone

20. Which opioid is relatively contraindicated in a patient with prolonged QT syndrome?

    (A) fentanyl
    (B) sufentanil
    (C) morphine
    (D) remifentanil
    (E) methadone

Answers and Explanations: Opioids

1. Mu (μ) opioid receptor activation leads to supraspinal analgesia via which of the following mechanisms?

   (A) decreased release of substance P from primary afferent inputs

   (B) increased release of dopamine in the nucleus accumbens

   (C) decreased activity in the ventrolateral medulla

   (D) **decreased release of GABA from periaqueductal gray matter**

   (E) decreased release of dopamine in the arcuate nucleus

   Mu (μ) opioid receptor activation at the spinal level decreases release of substance P from primary afferent inputs. Euphoria and mood-altering properties of opiates are mediated by increased release of dopamine in the nucleus accumbens. Respiratory rate and tidal volume are decreased by mu (μ) opioid receptor activation in the ventrolateral medulla. Prolactin release is increased by mu (μ) opioid receptor activation; this is due to presynaptically decreased release of dopamine in the arcuate nucleus.

   Refs: Brunton LL, Chabner BA, Knollman BC. *Goodman & Gilman's the Pharmacological Basis of Therapeutics.* 12th ed. New York, NY: McGraw Hill; 2011.
   Miller RD. Miller's *Anesthesia.* 8th ed. Philadelphia, PA: Elsevier; 2015.

2. Activation of opioid receptors leads to activation of which intracellular transduction mechanism?

   (A) **G proteins**
   (B) adenylate cyclase
   (C) voltage gated calcium channels
   (D) voltage gated sodium channels
   (E) outward rectifying potassium channels

   G proteins (G_i and/or G_o) are activated, as are inward rectifying potassium channels. Adenylate cyclase and voltage-gated calcium channels are inhibited by activation of the opioid receptor. Voltage-gated sodium channels are not involved in opioid receptor-activated intracellular transduction mechanisms.

   Refs: Brunton LL, Chabner BA, Knollman BC. *Goodman & Gilman's the Pharmacological Basis of Therapeutics.* 12th ed. New York, NY: McGraw Hill; 2011.
   Miller RD. Miller's *Anesthesia.* 8th ed. Philadelphia, PA: Elsevier; 2015.

3. Which of the following opioids is the most hydrophilic?

   (A) **morphine**
   (B) fentanyl
   (C) codeine
   (D) methadone
   (E) heroin

   Morphine has a relatively low lipid solubility. Fentanyl, codeine, methadone, and heroin are all more lipophilic than morphine.

   Refs: Brunton LL, Chabner BA, Knollman BC. *Goodman & Gilman's the Pharmacological Basis of Therapeutics.* 12th ed. New York, NY: McGraw Hill; 2011.
   Miller RD. Miller's *Anesthesia.* 8th ed. Philadelphia, PA: Elsevier; 2015.

4. In patients with reduced renal function, morphine administration has altered duration and potency. Which metabolite of morphine is responsible for this?

   (A) morphine-3-glucuronide
   (B) **morphine-6-glucuronide**
   (C) morphine-3,6-diglucuronide
   (D) normorphine
   (E) morphine

Morphine-6-glucuronide is approximately twice as potent as morphine and can accumulate in renal failure. Morphine-3-glucuronide may mediate the excitatory effects of morphine. Morphine-3,6-diglucuronide is formed in small amounts, as is normorphine. Very small amounts of morphine are excreted unchanged.

Refs: Brunton LL, Chabner BA, Knollman BC. *Goodman & Gilman's the Pharmacological Basis of Therapeutics.* 12th ed. New York, NY: McGraw Hill; 2011.

Miller RD. Miller's *Anesthesia.* 8th ed. Philadelphia, PA: Elsevier; 2015.

5. An adult is administered a single dose of fentanyl (100 micrograms intravenously). The clinical effects of fentanyl are terminated mainly by:

(A) **redistribution**

(B) hydroxylation

(C) N-dealkylation

(D) conjugation

(E) demethylation

After a small bolus of fentanyl the plasma and CSF levels of fentanyl rapidly diminish due to redistribution to muscle and fat. Fentanyl undergoes N-dealkylation and hydroxylation in the liver.

Refs: Brunton LL, Chabner BA, Knollman BC. *Goodman & Gilman's the Pharmacological Basis of Therapeutics.* 12th ed. New York, NY: McGraw Hill; 2011.

Miller RD. Miller's *Anesthesia.* 8th ed. Philadelphia, PA: Elsevier; 2015.

6. After a 3-hour intravenous infusion, which opioid has the longest context sensitive half-time?

(A) **fentanyl**

(B) sufentanil

(C) alfentanil

(D) remifentanil

(E) propofol

Recovery from an opioid infusion depends on both drug redistribution and drug elimination. The duration of the infusion plays an important role. Context-sensitive half-time is the time for the plasma concentration of drug to decrease by 50% (after a maintenance

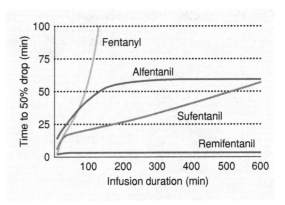

FIG. 10-1. In contrast to other opioids, the time necessary to achieve a 50% decrease in the plasma concentration of remifentanil (its **context-sensitive half-time**) is very short and is not influenced by the duration of the infusion. (Reproduced with permission from Egan TD. The pharmacokinetics of the new short-acting opiod remifentanil [GI87084B] in healthy adult male volunteers. *Anesthesiology.* 1993;79:881.)

infusion). After a 3-hour intravenous infusion, fentanyl will have the longest context sensitive half-time, followed by alfentanil, sufentanil, and remifentanil (Figure 10-1).

Ref: Brunton LL, Chabner BA, Knollman BC. *Goodman & Gilman's the Pharmacological Basis of Therapeutics.* 12th ed. New York, NY: McGraw Hill; 2011.

7. Which opioid has the longest duration of action after epidural injection?

(A) alfentanil

(B) fentanyl

(C) hydromorphone

(D) methadone

(E) **morphine**

Morphine is relatively hydrophilic compared to the other listed opioids (Table 10-1). This means morphine will remain in the CSF for a longer period of time—up to 24 hours after a single bolus.

Refs: Brunton LL, Chabner BA, Knollman BC. *Goodman & Gilman's the Pharmacological Basis of Therapeutics.* 12th ed. New York, NY: McGraw Hill; 2011.

Miller RD. Miller's *Anesthesia.* 8th ed. Philadelphia, PA: Elsevier; 2015.

TABLE 10-1. Epidural or intrathecal opioids for the treatment of acute (bolus) or chronic (infusion) pain.

Drug	Single dose (mg)[a]	Infusion rate (mg/h)[b]	Onset (min)	Duration of effect of a single dose (h)[c]
Epidural				
Morphine	1–6	0.1–1.0	30	6–24
Meperidine	20–150	5–20	5	4–8
Methadone	1–10	0.3–0.5	10	6–10
Hydromorphone	1–2	0.1–0.2	15	10–16
Fentanyl	0.025–0.1	0.025–0.10	5	2–4
Sufentanil	0.01–0.06	0.01–0.05	5	2–4
Alfentanil	0.5–1	0.2	15	1–3
Subarachnoid (Intrathecal)				
Morphine	0.1–0.3		15	8–24+
Fentanyl	0.005–0.025		5	3–6

[a]Low doses may be effective when administered to the elderly or when injected in the thoracic region.
[b]If combining with a local anesthetic, consider using 0.0625% bupivacaine.
[c]Duration of analgesia varies widely; higher doses produce longer duration. With the exception of epidural/intrathecal morphine or epidural sufentanil, all other spinal opioid use is considered to be off label.
(Reprinted from Brunton LL, Chabner BA, Knollman BC. *Goodman & Gilman's the Pharmacological Basis of Therapeutics.* 12th ed. New York, NY: McGraw Hill; 2011, after the International Association for the Study of Pain, 1992.)

8. The addition of 20 micrograms of fentanyl to a low-dose bupivacaine spinal will decrease the likelihood of:

    (A) respiratory depression

    (B) pruritus

    (C) a failed block

    (D) urinary retention

    (E) nausea and vomiting

    Spinal opioids have side effects such as pruritus, nausea, vomiting, urinary retention, and respiratory depression. The benefit of spinal opioids includes increasing the likelihood of a successful spinal anesthetic when used in conjunction with low-dose bupivacaine or lidocaine.

    Ref: Brunton LL, Chabner BA, Knollman BC. *Goodman & Gilman's the Pharmacological Basis of Therapeutics.* 12th ed. New York, NY: McGraw Hill; 2011.

9. A patient has significant hepatic and renal impairment. To avoid dosage adjustment due to this impairment, which opioid would be the best choice for intraoperative analgesia?

    (A) methadone

    (B) fentanyl

    (C) sufentanil

    (D) hydromorphone

    (E) remifentanil

    Remifentanil is metabolized by plasma esterases. No adjustment is required for hepatic or renal impairment.

    Ref: Brunton LL, Chabner BA, Knollman BC. *Goodman & Gilman's the Pharmacological Basis of Therapeutics.* 12th ed. New York, NY: McGraw Hill; 2011.

10. Which opioid must be converted from a prodrug to an active form?

    (A) morphine

    (B) codeine

    (C) fentanyl

    (D) hydromorphone

    (E) remifentanil

    Approximately 10% of administered codeine is metabolized in the liver to morphine. It is this morphine fraction that provides the analgesic effect of codeine.

    Ref: Brunton LL, Chabner BA, Knollman BC. *Goodman & Gilman's the Pharmacological Basis of Therapeutics.* 12th ed. New York, NY: McGraw Hill; 2011.

11. In large doses, which opioid will likely produce the most hypotension?

    (A) fentanyl

    (B) sufentanil

    (C) alfentanil

    (D) morphine

    (E) remifentanil

    Morphine (and meperidine) can cause histamine release. High doses of morphine can cause a greater degree of hypotension than fentanyl, sufentanil, alfentanil, or remifentanil.

    Refs: Brunton LL, Chabner BA, Knollman BC. *Goodman & Gilman's the Pharmacological Basis of Therapeutics.* 12th ed. New York, NY: McGraw Hill; 2011.
    Miller RD. Miller's *Anesthesia.* 8th ed. Philadelphia, PA: Elsevier; 2015.

12. Which opioid is most likely to cause tachycardia?

    (A) morphine

    (B) **meperidine**

    (C) codeine

    (D) fentanyl

    (E) alfentanil

Opioids usually cause bradycardia. However, meperidine rarely causes bradycardia, and it can cause tachycardia. This may be due to normeperidine's similarity to atropine.

Refs: Brunton LL, Chabner BA, Knollman BC. *Goodman & Gilman's the Pharmacological Basis of Therapeutics.* 12th ed. New York, NY: McGraw Hill; 2011.

Miller RD, Miller's *Anesthesia.* 8th ed. Philadelphia, PA: Elsevier; 2015.

13. Which factor is LEAST likely to increase the risk of opioid related respiratory depression?

    (A) natural sleep

    (B) chronic renal failure

    (C) benzodiazepines

    (D) **clonidine**

    (E) alcohol

Numerous factors increase the risk of opioid related respiratory depression: medications, general anesthetics, alcohol, benzodiazepines, barbiturates; natural sleep, obstructive sleep apnea, the very young and the elderly, chronic renal or cardiopulmonary disease, and pain relief. Clonidine does not affect opioid-related respiratory depression.

TABLE 10-2. Factors known to increase the duration or magnitude of opioid-related respiratory depression.

Elderly
Increased dose
Sleeping state
Other central nervous system depressants (volatile anesthetics, benzodiazepines, barbiturates, alcohol)
Renal insufficiency
Hypocarbia
Respiratory acidosis
Reduced hepatic clearance (e.g., reduced hepatic blood flow)
Pain

Refs: Brunton LL, Chabner BA, Knollman BC. *Goodman & Gilman's the Pharmacological Basis of Therapeutics.* 12th ed. New York, NY: McGraw Hill; 2011.

Miller RD. Miller's *Anesthesia.* 8th ed. Philadelphia, PA: Elsevier; 2015.

14. Low doses of opioids tend to have the greatest effect on which respiratory activity?

    (A) decreased tidal volume

    (B) **decreased respiratory rate**

    (C) decreased chest wall rigidity

    (D) increased CO_2 responsiveness

    (E) increased O_2 responsiveness

Opioids depress respiratory rate, tidal volume, CO_2 responsiveness, and hypoxic stimulation (Figure 10-2). Chest wall rigidity is often increased by opioids. Generally, opioids cause a more significant reduction in respiratory rate than tidal volume.

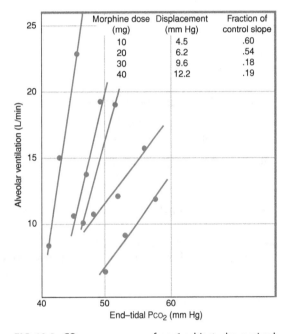

FIG. 10-2. CO_2 response curves from 1 subject who received 4 doses of morphine 10 mg intravenously at 40-minute intervals. (Reprinted with permission from Keats AS. The effect of drugs on respiration in man. *Ann Rev Pharmacol Toxicol.* 1985;25:41.)

Refs: Brunton LL, Chabner BA, Knollman BC. *Goodman & Gilman's the Pharmacological Basis of Therapeutics.* 12th ed. New York, NY: McGraw Hill; 2011.

Miller RD. Miller's *Anesthesia.* 8th ed. Philadelphia, PA: Elsevier; 2015.

15. Which of the following is a side effect of morphine?

    (A) diarrhea

    (B) peripheral vasoconstriction

    (C) **biliary spasm**

    (D) hyperthermia

    (E) mydriasis

Morphine can cause biliary spasm by increasing contraction at the sphincter of Oddi. Morphine also slows GI activity and causes constipation. It also causes skin flushing via cutaneous vasodilation. Opioids alter heat regulation, and body temperature can decrease. Opioids cause miosis (pupillary constriction).

Refs: Brunton LL, Chabner BA, Knollman BC. *Goodman & Gilman's the Pharmacological Basis of Therapeutics.* 12th ed. New York, NY: McGraw Hill; 2011.

Miller RD. Miller's *Anesthesia.* 8th ed. Philadelphia, PA: Elsevier; 2015.

16. Which opioid metabolite is most likely to cause seizures?

(A) meperidinic acid

(B) norfentanyl

(C) **normeperidine**

(D) morphine-3,6-glucuronide

(E) morphine-6-glucuronide

Normeperidine can cause excitatory symptoms including seizures. Morphine-3-glucuronide may contribute to the excitatory effects of morphine.

Refs: Brunton LL, Chabner BA, Knollman BC. *Goodman & Gilman's the Pharmacological Basis of Therapeutics.* 12th ed. New York, NY: McGraw Hill; 2011.

Miller RD. Miller's *Anesthesia.* 8th ed. Philadelphia, PA: Elsevier; 2015.

17. Sustained administration of an opiate agonist (days to weeks) leads to loss of drug effect. This is best described as:

(A) desensitization

(B) **tolerance**

(C) dependence

(D) withdrawal

(E) addiction

Loss of effect with exposure to opiates as a result of transient activation (minutes to hours) is termed desensitization. Dependence occurs during the state of tolerance. It refers to the withdrawal syndrome that occurs with drug abstinence or use of opiate antagonist.

Addiction is a behavior of drug-seeking that occurs despite negative social and/or physical outcomes.

Ref: Brunton LL, Chabner BA, Knollman BC. *Goodman & Gilman's the Pharmacological Basis of Therapeutics.* 12th ed. New York, NY: McGraw Hill; 2011.

18. The combination of monoamine oxidase inhibitors (MAOIs) and opiate receptor agonists can lead to potentially fatal serotonin syndrome. Which opiate is the best choice to provide analgesia for a patient who is taking a MAOI?

(A) meperidine

(B) dextromethorphan

(C) tramadol

(D) tapentadol

(E) **morphine**

Meperidine, dextromethorphan, tramadol, and tapentadol all inhibit uptake of norepinephrine and serotonin and should be avoided in patients taking MAOIs. Morphine is not a serotonin reuptake inhibitor.

Refs: Brunton LL, Chabner BA, Knollman BC. *Goodman & Gilman's the Pharmacological Basis of Therapeutics.* 12th ed. New York, NY: McGraw Hill; 2011.

Miller RD. Miller's *Anesthesia.* 8th ed. Philadelphia, PA: Elsevier; 2015.

19. Which opioid is most useful for a surgical procedure that requires rapid recovery?

(A) fentanyl

(B) sufentanil

(C) morphine

(D) **remifentanil**

(E) methadone

Remifentanil has a rapid onset and offset, making it ideal for procedures requiring rapid recovery.

Refs: Brunton LL, Chabner BA, Knollman BC. *Goodman & Gilman's the Pharmacological Basis of Therapeutics.* 12th ed. New York, NY: McGraw Hill; 2011.

Miller RD. Miller's *Anesthesia.* 8th ed. Philadelphia, PA: Elsevier; 2015.

20. Which opioid is relatively contraindicated in a patient with prolonged QT syndrome?

(A) fentanyl

(B) sufentanil

(C) morphine

(D) remifentanil

(E) **methadone**

Methadone is associated with prolonged QT syndrome; other opioids are not.

Ref: Brunton LL, Chabner BA, Knollman BC. *Goodman & Gilman's the Pharmacological Basis of Therapeutics.* 12th ed. New York, NY: McGraw Hill; 2011.

CHAPTER 11

Barbiturates

1. The principal mechanism of action of the barbiturate class of drugs is best described as:

   (A) blockade of CNS sodium channels
   (B) inhibition of NMDA receptors
   (C) potentiation of GABA-mediated chloride currents
   (D) stimulation of mu- and kappa-opioid receptors
   (E) stimulation of alpha-$_2$ adrenergic receptors

2. In which of the following circumstances should the induction dose of barbiturates be reduced?

   (A) neonates
   (B) plasma pH of 7.25
   (C) plasma pH of 7.55
   (D) nonpregnant female patients
   (E) patients taking barbiturates regularly

3. The primary mechanism by which a patient awakens following an induction dose of thiopental is:

   (A) binding of drug to proteins in the CSF
   (B) metabolism by microsomal enzymes in the liver
   (C) metabolism by plasma esterases
   (D) clearance by the kidneys
   (E) redistribution of drug to lean tissues

4. Which of the following best describes the pharmacokinetics when using large doses of thiopental?

   (A) hepatic extraction ratio increases
   (B) rate of hepatic clearance increases
   (C) rate of oxidative transformation increases
   (D) kinetics change from zero order to first order
   (E) kinetics change from first order to zero order

5. Compared to thiopental, the reason a patient awakens more rapidly from an intravenous infusion of methohexital is that:

   (A) methohexital has a higher rate of hepatic clearance
   (B) methohexital has a higher volume of distribution
   (C) methohexital is less potent
   (D) methohexital is less highly protein bound
   (E) methohexital has a lower pH

6. A 48-year-old woman is brought to the emergency room with a witnessed overdose of phenobarbital, a short-acting barbiturate. She is confused and somnolent, and her vital signs are BP 85/40 mm Hg, HR 104 bpm, RR 6/min. Which of the following is the most appropriate agent to accelerate the elimination of the drug?

   (A) flumazenil
   (B) naloxone
   (C) physostigmine
   (D) sodium bicarbonate
   (E) sodium thiosulfate

7. Which of the following best characterizes the cardiovascular effect following an induction dose of thiopental in a healthy adult?

   (A) arterial vasodilation
   (B) peripheral venodilation
   (C) bradycardia
   (D) decreased myocardial oxygen supply
   (E) increase in cardiac index

8. Which of the following best describes the effect of barbiturates on the pulmonary system?

   (A) profound apnea lasting 8–10 minutes
   (B) brief period of apnea lasting 30–45 seconds
   (C) increase in the rate of salivation
   (D) bronchospasm
   (E) inhibition of hypoxic pulmonary vasoconstriction

9. Which of the following best describes the effect of uremia on the free fraction of thiopental?

   (A) an increase in the free fraction by 10%
   (B) an increase in the free fraction by 25%
   (C) an increase in the free fraction by 50%
   (D) an increase in the free fraction by 75%
   (E) an increase in the free fraction by 100%

10. During therapeutic brain protection, thiopental cannot reduce the cerebral metabolic rate of oxygen consumption (CMRO$_2$) below 50% because:

   (A) the cardiac output would be too low to support arterial blood pressure
   (B) thiopental would create a steal phenomenon, worsening flow to ischemic tissue
   (C) thiopental only affects the neuron's functional cellular processes
   (D) thiopental's maximum effect on CMRO$_2$ is approximately 25%
   (E) an isoelectric EEG cannot be achieved with thiopental

11. A pregnant woman at 39 weeks gestation is given 4.5 mg/kg of thiopental for induction of general anesthesia for cesarean delivery. Which of the following is NOT a likely explanation as to why the fetus is delivered in an awake state 3 minutes later?

   (A) a rapid decrease in maternal plasma levels
   (B) nonhomogeneity of blood in the intervillous space
   (C) thiopental diffuses poorly across the placenta
   (D) fetal extraction of the drug from umbilical venous blood
   (E) shunting in the fetal circulation

12. Which of the following best describes the reason for the decreased requirement of thiopental in elderly patients?

   (A) the decreased size of the central compartment
   (B) the presence of polypharmacy
   (C) increased sensitivity of the aged brain
   (D) increased rate of redistribution
   (E) impaired autonomic reflexes

DIRECTIONS: Use the following scenario to answer questions 13 and 14:
A 45-year-old woman with a history of depression receives two courses of electroconvulsive therapy 48 hours apart as an inpatient. Methohexital 1 mg/kg is used for induction of general anesthesia on both occasions for its epileptogenic effect. One day following the second treatment, the floor nurse states that the patient is complaining of nausea, vomiting, severe abdominal pain, anxiety, and weakness in her arms and legs. Her heart rate is 110 bpm, her blood pressure is 160/95 mm Hg, and her respiratory rate is 24/min. She is afebrile and is acting confused. Abdominal examination reveals pain to palpation but no peritoneal signs or rebound tenderness. The nurse states that the patient passed some reddish-colored urine early this morning.

13. Given the presentation above, which of the following is the most likely diagnosis?

   (A) malingering
   (B) impacted kidney stones
   (C) acute appendicitis
   (D) acute porphyria
   (E) salmonella poisoning

14. Which of the following is the most appropriate next step in the management of this patient?

   (A) administration of midazolam
   (B) administration of labetalol
   (C) administration of fentanyl
   (D) administration of ondansetron
   (E) administration of hemin

15. Following the bolus of 5 mL of thiopental through an intravenous line placed at the wrist, a patient complains of intense burning pain in his hand. This is immediately followed by blanching of the hand and a blueish discoloration of the fingertips. Which of the following is NOT an appropriate next step in the management of this patient?

    (A) systemic heparinization
    (B) intravenous bicarbonate
    (C) axillary brachial plexus block
    (D) intra-arterial lidocaine
    (E) intra-arterial urokinase

16. Thiopental is compatible with which of the following substances?

    (A) rocuronium
    (B) meperidine
    (C) oxytocin
    (D) ephedrine
    (E) Ringer's lactate

Answers and Explanations: Barbiturates

1. The principal mechanism of action of the barbiturate class of drugs is best described as:

   (A) blockade of CNS sodium channels

   (B) inhibition of NMDA receptors

   (C) **potentiation of GABA-mediated chloride currents**

   (D) stimulation of mu- and kappa-opioid receptors

   (E) stimulation of alpha-$_2$ adrenergic receptors

The mechanisms by which barbiturates produce unconsciousness have been extensively researched. Barbiturates exert their effect at the GABA$_A$ receptor, but appear to have a concentration-dependent effect. At low concentrations, barbiturates bind to the receptor, preventing the dissociation of GABA from the receptor and thereby prolonging its effect; at higher concentrations, there appears to be a direct activation of the chloride channels, mimicking GABA without requiring its binding to the receptor. Either mechanism increases the flow of chloride through the central pore of the receptor. This hyperpolarizes the postsynaptic cell membrane and results in inhibition of postsynaptic neuron.

Barbiturates are known to have an inhibitory effect on excitatory neurotransmitters (including glutamate and acetylcholine), although the extent to which these contribute to sedation and hypnosis is unclear.

Ref: Longnecker DE, Brown DL, Newman MF, Zapol WM. *Anesthesiology.* 2nd ed. New York, NY: McGraw Hill; 2012.

2. In which of the following circumstances should the induction dose of barbiturates be reduced?

   (A) neonates

   (B) **plasma pH of 7.25**

   (C) plasma pH of 7.55

   (D) nonpregnant female patients

   (E) patients taking barbiturates regularly

The usual induction dose for thiopental (the most commonly used barbiturate) in adults is 3–4 mg/kg. Neonates and small children often require more due to increased clearance (5–8 mg/kg), whereas pregnant patients and the elderly require less (1–3 mg/kg). When dosed for lean body mass rather than total body mass, no adjustments need to be made for sex, age, or obesity.

The concentration of barbiturate in the CNS is influenced by the degree of unbound drug. Therefore, disease states that reduce overall plasma protein levels (e.g., cirrhosis, renal failure) increase the concentration of free barbiturate, necessitating a reduction in dose by approximately 40–50%.

Chronic use of barbiturates is known to induce the same oxidative microsomal enzymes that are responsible for metabolism. For this reason, patients that take barbiturates often require a higher induction dose.

Barbiturates are weak acids, and both thiopental (7.6) and methohexital (7.9) have a pK$_A$ slightly above normal physiologic pH. Thiopental and methohexital are approximately 40% and 25% ionized at physiologic pH, respectively. Acidosis will **increase** the **nonionized** fraction and favor transfer of these agents into the brain. In patients who are acidemic, a dose reduction of approximately 50% is often recommended in order to achieve an appropriate effect. In contrast, patients who are alkalemic frequently require an increased dose.

Ref: Miller RD. *Miller's Anesthesia.* 8th ed. Philadelphia, PA: Elsevier; 2015.

3. The primary mechanism by which a patient awakens following an induction dose of thiopental is:

   (A) binding of drug to proteins in the CSF

   (B) metabolism by microsomal enzymes in the liver

   (C) metabolism by plasma esterases

   (D) clearance by the kidneys

   (E) **redistribution of drug to lean tissues**

After a single intravenous bolus, the plasma level of thiopental rapidly declines as drug moves from blood to various tissue compartments. Thiopental will initially be taken up by those compartments that have high blood flow (i.e., brain, heart, liver, and kidney). Drug is also taken up by muscle and, at a much slower rate, fat. As the plasma levels decline from the tissue uptake, the concentration gradient reverses in the brain and drug moves back into the plasma, to be redistributed to the other two compartments. Equilibration occurs in the muscle group in approximately 15–30 minutes, while equilibrium in the fat compartment takes 200–300 minutes; therefore, it is redistribution to the muscle group that leads to awakening. Since thiopental is quite lipid soluble, large doses and/or prolonged infusions tend to result in accumulation in the fat compartment, which prolong the terminal clearance. This is why, compared to propofol, patients who are anesthetized with thiopental experience a prolonged "hangover."

Ultimately, all of the drug is metabolized in the liver, but this has little effect on the awakening. Thiopental is not metabolized by plasma esterases. Protein binding is not an important mechanism of effect termination, as there is little protein in the CSF, although there is protein in the brain tissue.

Ref: Longnecker DE, Brown DL, Newman MF, Zapol WM. *Anesthesiology.* 2nd ed. New York, NY: McGraw Hill; 2012.

4. Which of the following best describes the pharmacokinetics when using large doses of thiopental?

(A) hepatic extraction ratio increases

(B) rate of hepatic clearance increases

(C) rate of oxidative transformation increases

(D) kinetics change from zero order to first order

(E) kinetics change from first order to zero order

The hepatic extraction ratio for thiopental is low (0.1–0.2). This means that hepatic blood flow has little effect on the clearance of drug by the liver, and clearance is instead dependent more on intrinsic metabolic processes in the hepatic parenchyma. However, large doses of thiopental have been shown to saturate receptors and change the kinetics from first order to zero order. As such, only a constant *amount* of drug is extracted per unit of time, in contrast to a constant *fraction*, as in first-order kinetics. The result is a further decrease in the extraction ratio, a decline in overall clearance, and accumulation of drug. Answers B and C are nonsensical in this context.

Ref: Longnecker DE, Brown DL, Newman MF, Zapol WM. *Anesthesiology,* 2nd ed. New York, NY: McGraw Hill; 2012.

5. Compared to thiopental, the reason a patient awakens more rapidly from an intravenous infusion of methohexital is that:

(A) methohexital has a higher rate of hepatic clearance

(B) methohexital has a higher volume of distribution

(C) methohexital is less potent

(D) methohexital is less highly protein bound

(E) methohexital has a lower pH

Methohexital and thiopental have similar pharmacokinetics, including volume of distribution, distribution half-lives, and rates of protein binding. Methohexital is a more potent drug, requiring only 1–1.5 mg/kg to achieve unconsciousness versus 3–5 mg/kg for thiopental. Both drugs are alkaline solutions of pH 10–11. The reason that patients awaken more quickly from a methohexital infusion relates to its roughly threefold higher rate of hepatic clearance (Table 11-1).

Both thiopental and methohexital are biotransformed hepatically into inactive, water-soluble metabolites that are either conjugated to glucuronic acid and excreted in the bile, or excreted directly into the urine.

Ref: Miller RD. *Miller's Anesthesia.* 8th ed. Philadelphia, PA: Elsevier; 2015.

TABLE 11-1. Pharmacologic properties of methohexital and thiopental.

Drug	Formulation	Typical induction dose (mg/kg)	Vss (L/kg)	Protein binding (%)	$t_{1/2}\alpha$ (distribution half-life)	$t_{1/2}\beta$ (terminal half-life)
Methohexital	2.5% solution, pH 10–11	1–1.5	2.2	70–80	6	3.9
Thiopental	1% solution, pH 10–11	3–5	2.5	75–85	8	11.6

6. A 48-year-old woman is brought to the emergency room with a witnessed overdose of phenobarbital, a short-acting barbiturate. She is confused and somnolent, and her vital signs are BP 85/40 mm Hg, HR 104 bpm, RR 6/min. Which of the following is the most appropriate agent to accelerate the elimination of the drug?

    (A) flumazenil
    (B) naloxone
    (C) physostigmine
    (D) sodium bicarbonate
    (E) sodium thiosulfate

    There is no specific antidote to barbiturate toxicity, and treatment is supportive. In addition to activated charcoal and hemodynamic support, this patient should receive sodium bicarbonate to alkalinize the urine. Since barbiturates are weak acids, a more alkaline environment in the renal tubule promotes dissociation of the molecule and a greater proportion of ionized drug on the tubule side of the membrane (ion trapping). Goals should include maintaining a urine pH >7.5 and a urine output of ≥2 mL/kg/hr. Hypokalemia should also be treated as it will hamper efforts to alkalinize the urine due to H^+-K^+ exchange in the kidney.

    Flumazenil is the antidote for benzodiazepines, while naloxone is a specific opioid-antagonist. Physostigmine is used to treat anticholinergic symptoms. Sodium thiosulfate is used in the treatment of cyanide poisoning.

    Ref: Longnecker DE, Brown DL, Newman MF, Zapol WM. *Anesthesiology*. 2nd ed. New York, NY: McGraw Hill; 2012.

7. Which of the following best characterizes the cardiovascular effect following an induction dose of thiopental in a healthy adult?

    (A) arterial vasodilation
    (B) peripheral venodilation
    (C) bradycardia
    (D) decreased myocardial oxygen supply
    (E) increase in cardiac index

    Barbiturates consistently produce a reduction in *venous* tone due primarily to a central sympatholytic effect, and to a lesser extent a direct effect on venous smooth muscle. This results in an increase in venous capacitance and a decrease in ventricular filling. There is also an associated direct negative inotropic effect on the heart due to a decrease in calcium influx into the myocytes. The arterial circulation is often only minimally affected; however, in cases where sympathetic tone is high (e.g., hypovolemia, shock), even small doses of thiopental may result in profound decreases in arterial pressure and cardiac output. The heart rate usually increases upon induction with thiopental (10–36%), due to baroreceptor-mediated reflex stimulation following a decrease in cardiac output and arterial pressure. This relative tachycardia partially offsets the decrease in cardiac output, but also increases myocardial work, and therefore care must be taken in patients who have ischemic heart disease. However, the arterio-coronary venous oxygen difference is typically unchanged, providing the patient has normal coronary arteries that can increase flow to meet demand, and providing arterial diastolic pressure is not significantly reduced.

    Ref: Longnecker DE, Brown DL, Newman MF, Zapol WM. *Anesthesiology*. 2nd ed. New York, NY: McGraw Hill; 2012.

8. Which of the following best describes the effect of barbiturates on the pulmonary system?

    (A) profound apnea lasting 8–10 minutes
    (B) brief period of apnea lasting 30–45 seconds
    (C) increase in the rate of salivation
    (D) bronchospasm
    (E) inhibition of hypoxic pulmonary vasoconstriction

    Barbiturates produce a transient depression of respiratory drive, with apnea occurring in at least 20% of patients induced with thiopental alone; the concomitant use of opioids increases the incidence and duration of apnea significantly. By themselves, barbiturates should be expected to produce apnea occurring at 60–90 seconds after the bolus, lasting approximately 30–45 seconds, with full respiratory recovery after approximately 15 minutes.

    Unlike ketamine, barbiturates do not promote excess salivation. While barbiturates are not bronchodilators, they are not associated with bronchospasm and are safe to use in asthmatics. As is the case with intravenous anesthetics as a whole, hypoxic pulmonary vasoconstriction is not impaired with the use of barbiturates.

    Ref: Longnecker DE, Brown DL, Newman MF, Zapol WM. *Anesthesiology*. 2nd ed. New York, NY: McGraw Hill; 2012.

9. Which of the following best describes the effect of uremia on the free fraction of thiopental?

(A) an increase in the free fraction by 10%

(B) an increase in the free fraction by 25%

(C) an increase in the free fraction by 50%

(D) an increase in the free fraction by 75%

(E) **an increase in the free fraction by 100%**

Uremia causes a decrease in the protein binding of thiopental. In one study of the effect of chronic renal and hepatic disease on the unbound fraction of thiopental, it was found that compared to a baseline free fraction of 28%, these diseases led to an increase in the unbound fraction to 53% and 56%, respectively. This doubling (i.e., a 100% increase) in the free fraction necessitates a 50% reduction in the dose of thiopental on induction in both these populations.

A further reason to reduce the dose of thiopental in renal disease is the preexisting cardiac depression.

Ref: Longnecker DE, Brown DL, Newman MF, Zapol WM. *Anesthesiology*. 2nd ed. New York, NY: McGraw Hill; 2012.

10. During therapeutic brain protection, thiopental cannot reduce the cerebral metabolic rate of oxygen consumption ($CMRO_2$) below 50% because:

(A) the cardiac output would be too low to support arterial blood pressure

(B) thiopental would create a steal phenomenon, worsening flow to ischemic tissue

(C) **thiopental only affects the neuron's functional cellular processes**

(D) thiopental's maximum effect on $CMRO_2$ is approximately 25%

(E) an isoelectric EEG cannot be achieved with thiopental

Barbiturates are one of several pharmacologic agents capable of brain protection, and have conclusively been shown to beneficially affect outcomes during focal cerebral ischemia. They exert their effect by reducing the metabolic demand of the *functioning* brain and, if administered in sufficient doses, slow the EEG down to burst suppression and finally electrical silence. At this stage, the $CMRO_2$ is approximately 50%. Further increases in thiopental concentration will not affect $CMRO_2$ because the remaining oxygen demand is for constitutive cellular metabolic processes.

These can only be reduced through the application of hypothermia, such as in the use of deep hypothermic circulatory arrest, where temperatures of $<18°C$ result in a $CMRO_2$ of $<10\%$.

Thiopental is an anticonvulsant, and may also confer protection by free radical scavenging, membrane stabilization, NMDA antagonism, Ca channel blockade, and maintenance of protein synthesis.

Thiopental has been shown to result in a reverse steal phenomenon, where the vasoconstriction and reduction in cerebral blood flow that accompanies the decreased $CMRO_2$ leads to shunting of blood away from healthy brain toward those ischemic areas that cannot vasoconstrict.

Ref: Miller RD. Miller's *Anesthesia*. 8th ed. Philadelphia, PA: Elsevier; 2015.

11. A pregnant woman at 39 weeks gestation is given 4.5 mg/kg of thiopental for induction of general anesthesia for cesarean delivery. Which of the following is NOT a likely explanation as to why the fetus is delivered in an awake state 3 minutes later?

(A) a rapid decrease in maternal plasma levels

(B) nonhomogeneity of blood in the intervillous space

(C) **thiopental diffuses poorly across the placenta**

(D) fetal extraction of the drug from umbilical venous blood

(E) shunting in the fetal circulation

As a lipid-soluble drug, thiopental is readily transported across the placenta, with reported fetal-to-maternal ratios between 0.4 and 1.1. However, events occur in both the mother and fetus to reduce the concentration of thiopental that reaches the brain.

Just as in nonpregnant adults, the plasma thiopental concentration in the central compartment rapidly declines after a bolus from redistribution to the brain and other highly perfused viscera, and subsequently the muscle tissue. This decline aids in the reduction of drug transfer across the placenta.

Maternal blood enters the intervillous space from the endometrial spiral arterioles in high-pressure spurts that are nonuniform and dependent on several factors (e.g., intrauterine pressure, contour of the contraction wave) for patency. This results in a nonuniform character of the villous blood—in other words, fetal blood in villous capillaries from certain underperfused areas of the placenta may return to the umbilical vein with little thiopental. This explains the time lag in peak umbilical vein thiopental concentration compared to the maternal arterial concentration that exists (up to 3 minutes).

The umbilical vein travels first through the liver, where a large portion of thiopental is extracted before it can reach the central circulation. The drug concentration is further reduced by admixture with venous blood from the gastrointestinal tract, extremities, and head before reaching the left heart. Finally, much of the cardiac output is diverted through the ductus arteriosus, thereby returning to the placenta having not contributed to perfusion of the fetal brain.

Ref: Chestnut DH. *Chestnut's Obstetric Anesthesiology: Principles and Practice.* 5th ed. Philadelphia, PA: Elsevier; 2014.

12. Which of the following best describes the reason for the decreased requirement of thiopental in elderly patients?

    (A) **the decreased size of the central compartment**
    (B) the presence of polypharmacy
    (C) increased sensitivity of the aged brain
    (D) increased rate of redistribution
    (E) impaired autonomic reflexes

Elderly patients experience increased peak plasma levels of thiopental compared to younger adults for a given dose. This is not a pharmacodynamic effect (e.g., sensitivity of the CNS). Rather, it is primarily due to a reduced volume of the central compartment into which the drug initially distributes due to reduced total body water. In addition, decreased albumin levels lead to a 20% increase in free fraction of thiopental. Finally, the elderly have a decreased rate of redistribution (not increased) due to age-related decline in cardiac output. Together these factors contribute to an increased level of free drug presented to the geriatric brain. It is recommended that for patients older than 65 years of age, an appropriate induction dose would be 2–2.5 mg/kg. Impaired autonomic reflexes and potential drug interactions from polypharmacy do not necessarily affect the required dose.

Ref: Longnecker DE, Brown DL, Newman MF, Zapol WM. *Anesthesiology.* 2nd ed. New York, NY: McGraw Hill; 2012.

DIRECTIONS: Use the following scenario to answer questions 13 and 14:
A 45-year-old woman with a history of depression receives two courses of electroconvulsive therapy 48 hours apart as an inpatient. Methohexital 1 mg/kg is used for induction of general anesthesia on both occasions for its epileptogenic effect. One day following the second treatment, the floor nurse states that the patient is complaining of nausea, vomiting, severe abdominal pain, anxiety, and weakness in her arms and legs. Her heart rate is 110 bpm, her blood pressure is 160/95 mm Hg, and her respiratory rate is 24/min. She is afebrile and is acting confused. Abdominal examination reveals pain to palpation but no peritoneal signs or rebound tenderness. The nurse states that the patient passed some reddish-colored urine early this morning.

13. Given the presentation above, which of the following is the most likely diagnosis?

    (A) malingering
    (B) impacted kidney stones
    (C) acute appendicitis
    (D) **acute porphyria**
    (E) salmonella poisoning

The clinical picture of severe abdominal pain, neurologic symptoms, autonomic instability, and dark urine following barbiturate use strongly suggests an acute porphyric crisis. Barbiturates are the classic anesthetic trigger agent for porphyrias, and should be avoided in cases of known porphyria.

Porphyrias are a group of diseases that have in common an enzymatic defect that leads to the accumulation of various intermediary products of heme synthesis. Heme is a ubiquitous molecule that is a component of various compounds including hemoglobin, myoglobin, and the cytochromes. The initial step in the heme synthesis pathway is catalyzed by the enzyme ALA synthetase, which normally has a low activity level due to negative feedback by intracellular free heme. However, in cases where additional heme is required (such as when the cytochrome p450 enzyme system is induced with barbiturates), ALA synthetase is readily inducible, and precursors are generated. Patients with porphyrias cannot process the precursors, leading to a buildup and the development of the clinical syndrome. The most important type of porphyria in anesthetic practice is acute intermittent porphyria (AIP) as it is most likely to be fulminant, and in some cases fatal. AIP is so named because patients experience lengthy periods of quiescence between attacks.

Acute crises are characterized by severe abdominal pain, nausea, vomiting and diarrhea, autonomic and peripheral neuropathy, cardiovascular instability (tachycardia and hypertension), electrolyte disturbances (hyponatremia, hypokalemia, hypomagnesemia), neuromuscular weakness, and psychiatric symptoms.

Ref: Miller RD. Miller's *Anesthesia*. 8th ed. Philadelphia, PA: Elsevier; 2015.

14. Which of the following is the most appropriate next step in the management of this patient?

    (A) administration of midazolam

    (B) administration of labetalol

    (C) administration of fentanyl

    (D) administration of ondansetron

    (E) **administration of hemin**

Treatment of a porphyric crisis is largely supportive, and correction of fluid and electrolyte deficits should be a priority. The prompt administration of glucose or other simple carbohydrates can reduce the duration and intensity of an attack, and should be another first measure. Pain can often be severe, and opioids are frequently required for management. Beta-blockers may be administered to control tachycardia and hypertension. Antiemetics such as ondansetron may also be required.

Despite the above, hemin is the only specific form of therapy. It is a lyophylized form of heme that supplements the intracellular heme pool. This inhibits ALA synthetase, thereby slowing the production of heme precursors. It is best given early in an attack, in a dose of 3–4 mg/kg IV daily × 4 days.

Ref: Miller RD. Miller's *Anesthesia*. 8th ed. Philadelphia, PA: Elsevier; 2015.

15. Following the bolus of 5 mL of thiopental through an intravenous line placed at the wrist, a patient complains of intense burning pain in his hand. This is immediately followed by blanching of the hand and a blueish discoloration of the fingertips. Which of the following is NOT an appropriate next step in the management of this patient?

    (A) systemic heparinization

    (B) **intravenous bicarbonate**

    (C) axillary brachial plexus block

    (D) intra-arterial lidocaine

    (E) intra-arterial urokinase

Inadvertent arterial injection of thiopental is a serious matter. This is usually heralded by the patient's complaint of intense, burning pain, followed by the development of blanching and/or blisters. Thiopental causes profound vasoconstriction of the artery, crystal formation, endarteritis, ADP release, and thrombosis and norepinephrine release, all of which promote eventual ischemia and necrosis of the distal structures if perfusion is sufficiently impaired. Gangrene in the forearm, hand, or fingers may necessitate amputation. Treatment includes administration of intra-arterial lidocaine or procaine to dilate the vessel, systemic heparinization to prevent/attenuate thrombosis, intra-arterial injection of thrombolytics to reverse thrombosis, local injection of alpha-adrenergic blockers in the affected area, and performance of a brachial plexus or stellate ganglion block to reverse the vasospasm. There is no role for intravenous bicarbonate.

Ref: Longnecker DE, Brown DL, Newman MF, Zapol WM. *Anesthesiology*. 2nd ed. New York, NY: McGraw Hill; 2012.

16. Thiopental is compatible with which of the following substances?

    (A) rocuronium

    (B) meperidine

    (C) **oxytocin**

    (D) ephedrine

    (E) Ringer's lactate

Due to its strong alkalinity (pH 10.6), thiopental is known to precipitate as a free acid when mixed with many drugs and solutions of lower pH. Examples include nearly all of the neuromuscular blocking agents, Ringer's lactate solution, atropine, glycopyrrolate, diphenhydramine, meperidine, hydromorphone, codeine, morphine, and ephedrine. Drugs used in anesthesia that are reportedly compatible include hydrocortisone, neostigmine, oxytocin, and aminophylline.

Precipitation can result in a "concrete-like" blocked intravenous line, rendering it useless. This can be disastrous in an emergency situation, and should thiopental be used, the recommendation is to flush the intravenous line liberally until the thiopental is cleared with confidence before administering a subsequent drug. Use of a separate IV port is also a prudent step.

Ref: Miller RD. Miller's *Anesthesia*. 8th ed. Philadelphia, PA: Elsevier; 2015.

CHAPTER 12

Propofol

1. Which of the following is NOT a direct central nervous system effect of propofol?

   (A) $GABA_A$ receptor activation in the hippocampus
   (B) widespread NMDA glutamate receptor inhibition
   (C) decreased serotonin levels in the area postrema
   (D) activation of glycine-gated chloride channels in the spinal cord
   (E) activation of α_2 adrenergic receptors in the locus ceruleus

2. Fospropofol is a prodrug that is converted to propofol by:

   (A) hydrolysis by alkaline phosphatases
   (B) hydrolysis by blood and tissue esterases
   (C) hydrolysis by butyrylcholinesterases
   (D) a Hofmann elimination reaction
   (E) intramolecular rearrangement at physiologic pH

3. The pharmacokinetics and pharmacodynamics of propofol are altered by age. Based on a mg/kg dose, which of the following patients requires the largest induction dose of propofol?

   (A) preterm neonate
   (B) 1-year-old
   (C) 6-year-old
   (D) 15-year-old
   (E) 40-year-old

4. The rapid termination of action after a single intravenous dose of propofol is due to propofol's:

   (A) high hepatic extraction ratio
   (B) high degree of protein binding
   (C) renal clearance of glucuronic acid metabolites
   (D) redistribution to the periphery
   (E) small volume of distribution

5. Propofol is metabolized mainly by the liver. However, since clearance of propofol exceeds hepatic blood flow, extra-hepatic metabolism also occurs. The organ most responsible for the extra-hepatic metabolism of propofol is the:

   (A) kidneys
   (B) large intestine
   (C) spleen
   (D) brain
   (E) pancreas

6. Which age-related change in the drug disposition of propofol explains the slower recovery from a propofol infusion in the elderly?

   (A) increased lean body mass
   (B) increased total body water
   (C) decreased V_d
   (D) increased hepatic clearance
   (E) increased $T_{1/2}\beta$

7. Which hemodynamic variable decreases the most after induction of anesthesia with propofol?

   (A) heart rate
   (B) systolic blood pressure
   (C) systemic vascular resistance
   (D) cardiac output
   (E) stroke volume

8. Which intravenous anesthetic, after an induction dose, typically causes the greatest decrease in mean blood pressure?

   (A) midazolam
   (B) propofol
   (C) ketamine
   (D) etomidate
   (E) thiopental

9. After an induction dose of propofol, what is the most frequent effect on the respiratory system?

   (A) apnea
   (B) increased tidal volume
   (C) bronchoconstriction
   (D) unchanged minute ventilation
   (E) increase in the slope of the CO_2-response curve

10. A surgical procedure requires monitoring of sensory evoked responses. Maintenance of anesthesia is provided by propofol infusion. Which sensory evoked response is most resistant to propofol-induced change that could be mistaken for surgically induced change?

    (A) visual evoked potentials (VEPs)
    (B) transcranial motor evoked potentials (MEPs)
    (C) brainstem auditory evoked potentials (BAEPs)
    (D) somatosensory evoked potentials (SSEPs)
    (E) electroencephalogram (EEG)

11. Many intravenous anesthetics have been reported to cause seizure-like activity, yet many of these same anesthetics also have anticonvulsant properties. Which of the following intravenous anesthetics is most likely to cause epileptogenic activity?

    (A) methohexital
    (B) propofol
    (C) etomidate
    (D) ketamine
    (E) midazolam

12. Propofol infusion syndrome (PRIS) has been described after prolonged, high-dose, infusions of propofol. PRIS is characterized by:

    (A) hypokalemia
    (B) metabolic alkalosis
    (C) splenomegaly
    (D) rhabdomyolysis
    (E) hyperglycemia

13. During induction of anesthesia, the most common side effect of propofol is:

    (A) pain on injection
    (B) myoclonus
    (C) apnea
    (D) hypotension
    (E) tingling/discomfort in the genital areas

14. Propofol administered at a dose of 25–75 mcg/kg/min is appropriate for:

    (A) induction of general anesthesia
    (B) maintenance of general anesthesia
    (C) sedation
    (D) antiemesis
    (E) enhancement of neuromuscular blockade

15. Which anesthetic is the best choice for maintenance of anesthesia to ensure rapid recovery?

    (A) propofol
    (B) thiopental
    (C) isoflurane
    (D) sevoflurane
    (E) desflurane

Answers and Explanations: Propofol

1. Which of the following is NOT a direct central nervous system effect of propofol?

   (A) GABA$_A$ receptor activation in the hippocampus
   (B) widespread NMDA glutamate receptor inhibition
   (C) decreased serotonin levels in the area postrema
   (D) activation of glycine-gated chloride channels in the spinal cord
   (E) activation of α_2 adrenergic receptors in the locus ceruleus

   Dexmedetomidine is an agonist of α_2 adrenergic receptors. Activation of these receptors in the locus ceruleus results in sedation. Alpha$_2$ adrenergic receptors may have an indirect role in propofol's sedative effects.

   Propofol has many CNS effects including:

   • GABA$_A$ receptor activation in the hippocampus, which is a probable site of propofol's amnestic effects
   • Widespread NMDA glutamate receptor inhibition
   • Decreased serotonin levels in the area postrema, an action mediated by GABA receptor activation, which may mediate the antiemetic effects of propofol
   • Activation of glycine-gated chloride channels in the spinal cord.

   Ref: Miller RD. *Miller's Anesthesia*. 8th ed. Philadelphia, PA: Elsevier; 2015.

2. Fospropofol is a prodrug that is converted to propofol by:

   (A) hydrolysis by alkaline phosphatases
   (B) hydrolysis by blood and tissue esterases
   (C) hydrolysis by butyrylcholinesterases
   (D) a Hofmann elimination reaction
   (E) intramolecular rearrangement at physiologic pH

   Fospropofol is converted to propofol by hydrolysis by endothelial cell surface alkaline phosphatases.

   Remifentanil is hydrolyzed by blood and tissue esterases.

   Succinylcholine is hydrolyzed by butyrylcholinesterases.

   Atracurium and cis-atracurium are metabolized via a Hofmann elimination reaction.

   Midazolam undergoes intramolecular rearrangement at physiologic pH.

   Ref: Brunton LL, Chabner BA, Knollman BC. *Goodman & Gilman's the Pharmacological Basis of Therapeutics*. 12th ed. New York, NY: McGraw Hill; 2011.

3. The pharmacokinetics and pharmacodynamics of propofol are altered by age. Based on a mg/kg dose, which of the following patients requires the largest induction dose of propofol?

   (A) preterm neonate
   (B) 1-year-old
   (C) 6-year-old
   (D) 15-year-old
   (E) 40-year-old

   The induction dose of propofol for children younger than 2 years of age is 2.9 mg/kg. Preterm neonates require less propofol, given their reduced fat content, reduced protein binding, and immature renal and hepatic systems. For children 6–12 years of age, the induction dose of propofol is 2.2 mg/kg. The typical adult induction dose of propofol is 2–2.5 mg/kg, while after the age of 60, 1–1.75 mg/kg is recommended.

   Ref: Miller RD. *Miller's Anesthesia*. 8th ed. Philadelphia, PA: Elsevier; 2015.

4. The rapid termination of action after a single intravenous dose of propofol is due to propofol's:

   (A) high hepatic extraction ratio
   (B) high degree of protein binding
   (C) renal clearance of glucuronic acid metabolites
   (D) redistribution to the periphery
   (E) small volume of distribution

The termination of action of a propofol bolus is due to rapid redistribution from the central compartment (brain) to the periphery (fat). Propofol has a high hepatic extraction ratio, is highly protein bound (98%), and is renally cleared via glucuronic acid metabolites, but these are not as influential in determining termination of action after a single bolus. Propofol has a relatively large volume of distribution ($V_d = 2–10$ L/kg).

Ref: Miller RD. *Miller's Anesthesia*. 8th ed. Philadelphia, PA: Elsevier; 2015.

5. Propofol is metabolized mainly by the liver. However, since clearance of propofol exceeds hepatic blood flow, extra-hepatic metabolism also occurs. The organ most responsible for the extra-hepatic metabolism of propofol is the:

(A) **kidneys**
(B) large intestine
(C) spleen
(D) brain
(E) pancreas

The kidneys play a role in the extra-hepatic metabolism of propofol, with some studies indicating they are responsible for 30% of total body clearance. Other studies suggest that the small intestine and lungs may also be involved in the extra-hepatic metabolism of propofol.

Ref: Miller RD. *Miller's Anesthesia*. 8th ed. Philadelphia, PA: Elsevier; 2015.

6. Which age-related change in the drug disposition of propofol explains the slower recovery from a propofol infusion in the elderly?

(A) increased lean body mass
(B) increased total body water
(C) decreased V_d
(D) increased hepatic clearance
(E) **increased $T_{1/2}\beta$**

Age-related increase in elimination half-time, $T_{1/2}\beta$, results in slower recovery from a propofol infusion in the elderly. Other age-related changes include decreased lean body mass, decreased total body water content, increased V_d, and decreased hepatic clearance.

Ref: Miller RD. *Miller's Anesthesia*. 8th ed. Philadelphia, PA: Elsevier; 2015.

7. Which hemodynamic variable decreases the most after induction of anesthesia with propofol?

(A) heart rate
(B) **systolic blood pressure**
(C) systemic vascular resistance
(D) cardiac output
(E) stroke volume

After induction with propofol (2–2.5 mg/kg), systolic blood pressure will decrease 25–40%. Cardiac output, systemic vascular resistance, and stroke volume all decrease to a lesser degree, while heart rate does not change.

Ref: Miller RD. *Miller's Anesthesia*. 8th ed. Philadelphia, PA: Elsevier; 2015.

8. Which intravenous anesthetic, after an induction dose, typically causes the greatest decrease in mean blood pressure?

(A) midazolam
(B) **propofol**
(C) ketamine
(D) etomidate
(E) thiopental

Propofol will decrease mean blood pressure (MBP) up to 40% after an induction dose. Midazolam, ketamine, etomidate, and thiopental can all decrease MBP after induction but to a lesser extent.

Ref: Miller RD. *Miller's Anesthesia*. 8th ed. Philadelphia, PA: Elsevier; 2015.

9. After an induction dose of propofol, what is the most frequent effect on the respiratory system?

(A) **apnea**
(B) increased tidal volume
(C) bronchoconstriction
(D) unchanged minute ventilation
(E) increase in the slope of the CO_2-response curve

The incidence of apnea after an induction dose of propofol is 25–30%. Other effects of an induction dose of propofol can include reduced tidal volume and tachypnea. An infusion of propofol results in decreased tidal volume, increased respiratory rate, and a variable effect on minute ventilation. Propofol decreases ventilatory response to CO_2 and the slope of the CO_2-response curve is decreased. Propofol is a bronchodilator.

Ref: Miller RD. *Miller's Anesthesia.* 8th ed. Philadelphia, PA: Elsevier; 2015.

10. A surgical procedure requires monitoring of sensory evoked responses. Maintenance of anesthesia is provided by propofol infusion. Which sensory evoked response is most resistant to propofol-induced change that could be mistaken for surgically induced change?

    (A) visual evoked potentials (VEPs)

    (B) transcranial motor evoked potentials (MEPs)

    (C) **brainstem auditory evoked potentials (BAEPs)**

    (D) somatosensory evoked potentials (SSEPs)

    (E) electroencephalogram (EEG)

    BAEPs are relatively resistant to change induced by propofol. Propofol can alter SSEPs, VEPs, and transcranial MEPs such that the change could be mistaken for surgically induced change. Propofol also causes EEG changes in a dose-dependent manner; initially amplitude increases then markedly decreases, while alpha activity initially increases then shifts to delta waves.

    Ref: Miller RD. *Miller's Anesthesia.* 8th ed. Philadelphia, PA: Elsevier; 2015.

11. Many intravenous anesthetics have been reported to cause seizure-like activity, yet many of these same anesthetics also have anticonvulsant properties. Which of the following intravenous anesthetics is most likely to cause epileptogenic activity?

    (A) **methohexital**

    (B) propofol

    (C) etomidate

    (D) ketamine

    (E) midazolam

    Methohexital can cause epileptogenic activity, whereas propofol, etomidate, and ketamine are more likely to cause myoclonic activity. Benzodiazepines such as midazolam are anticonvulsants.

    Ref: Barash PG. *Clinical Anesthesia.* 7th ed. Philadelphia, PA: Lippincott Williams & Wilkins; 2013.

12. Propofol infusion syndrome (PRIS) has been described after prolonged, high-dose, infusions of propofol. PRIS is characterized by:

    (A) hypokalemia

    (B) metabolic alkalosis

    (C) splenomegaly

    (D) **rhabdomyolysis**

    (E) hyperglycemia

    Propofol infusion syndrome (PRIS) may present as acute refractory bradycardia or asystole in the setting of metabolic acidosis, hepatomegaly, hyperlipidemia, and rhabdomyolysis. Other features include hyperkalemia, acute cardiac failure, lipemia, and skeletal myopathy.

    Ref: Brunton LL, Chabner BA, Knollman BC. *Goodman & Gilman's the Pharmacological Basis of Therapeutics.* 12th ed. New York, NY: McGraw Hill; 2011.

13. During induction of anesthesia, the most common side effect of propofol is:

    (A) pain on injection

    (B) myoclonus

    (C) apnea

    (D) **hypotension**

    (E) tingling/discomfort in the genital areas

    Side effects of propofol induction include pain on injection, myoclonus, apnea, thrombophlebitis of the vein, and tingling/discomfort in the genital area. The most common side effect of propofol on induction is hypotension.

    Ref: Miller RD. *Miller's Anesthesia.* 8th ed. Philadelphia, PA: Elsevier; 2015.

14. Propofol administered at a dose of 25–75 mcg/kg/min is appropriate for:

    (A) induction of general anesthesia

    (B) maintenance of general anesthesia

    (C) **sedation**

    (D) antiemesis

    (E) enhancement of neuromuscular blockade

    Propofol administered at 25–75 mcg/kg/hr is typical for sedation. Propofol administered at 1–2.5 mg/kg is typical for induction of general anesthesia; 50–150 mcg/kg/min for maintenance of general anesthesia; 10–20 mg IV or infusion of 10 mcg/kg/min for antiemesis. Propofol does not enhance neuromuscular blockade produced by neuromuscular blocking drugs.

    Ref: Miller RD. *Miller's Anesthesia.* 8th ed. Philadelphia, PA: Elsevier; 2015.

15. Which anesthetic is the best choice for maintenance of anesthesia to ensure rapid recovery?

   (A) propofol
   (B) thiopental
   (C) isoflurane
   (D) sevoflurane
   (E) desflurane

With respect to rapid recovery from anesthesia, propofol is superior to thiopental and equal to isoflurane and sevoflurane. Use of desflurane for maintenance of anesthesia results in a faster recovery compared to propofol.

Ref: Miller RD. *Miller's Anesthesia.* 8th ed. Philadelphia, PA: Elsevier; 2015.

CHAPTER 13

Etomidate

1. The principal mechanism of action of etomidate is best described as:

   (A) potentiation of GABA-mediated chloride currents
   (B) stimulation of μ- and κ-opioid receptors
   (C) stimulation of α_2-adrenergic receptors
   (D) inhibition of NMDA receptors
   (E) blockade of CNS sodium channels

2. In order to increase its water solubility, etomidate is formulated with which of the following compounds?

   (A) glycerol
   (B) benzyl alcohol
   (C) sodium bisulfite
   (D) propylene glycol
   (E) methylparaben

DIRECTIONS: Use the following scenario to answer questions 3 and 4:
A 60-year-old, 80-kg man presents for exploratory laparotomy after he was stabbed in the left upper quadrant of his abdomen. He has no other injuries. Chest X-ray reveals free air under the diaphragm. His past medical history includes hypercholesterolemia treated with atorvastatin and an appendectomy at age 15 years. Physical exam reveals blood pressure is 95/45 mm Hg and his heart rate is 112 bpm. He is pale and appears to be in mild respiratory distress as well as moderate pain. He has received 1,200 ml of lactated Ringer's solution intravenously since admission from the emergency department 45 minutes ago.

3. The most appropriate induction dose of etomidate for this patient is:

   (A) 5 mg
   (B) 12 mg
   (C) 32 mg
   (D) 64 mg
   (E) 100 mg

4. The expected duration of anesthesia following the above single induction dose would be expected to be:

   (A) 1 minute
   (B) 2 minutes
   (C) 4 minutes
   (D) 7 minutes
   (E) 10 minutes

5. Which of the following best describes the method of inactivation of etomidate?

   (A) metabolism in the liver by ester hydrolysis
   (B) metabolism in the bloodstream by ester hydrolysis
   (C) elimination by Hofmann degradation
   (D) deactivation by the lungs, followed by renal excretion
   (E) elimination via the fecal route

6. A 50-year-old man with a history of coronary disease and mild aortic stenosis is scheduled for knee replacement. He is induced with 0.3 mg/kg of etomidate. Which of the following hemodynamic effects best describe the expected response?

(A) increased heart rate, increased cardiac index, no change in PCWP

(B) increased heart rate, decreased cardiac index, decreased PCWP

(C) no change in heart rate, increased cardiac index, decreased PCWP

(D) decreased heart rate, no change in cardiac index, increased PCWP

(E) no change in heart rate, no change in cardiac index, no change in PCWP

7. Which of the following statements best describes the cardiac effects following induction and intubation with etomidate as the sole agent?

(A) etomidate is likely to prolong the QT interval

(B) hypertension and tachycardia commonly follow intubation

(C) myocardial oxygen demand is likely to exceed supply

(D) arrhythmias such as PVCs are common

(E) reflex bradycardia often occurs

8. A patient is sedated with etomidate for DC cardioversion. Which of the following best describes the ventilatory effect of etomidate during the case?

(A) more episodes of apnea than equipotent propofol sedation

(B) greater respiratory drive than equipotent methohexital sedation

(C) higher $PaCO_2$ than equipotent propofol sedation

(D) reduced respiratory drive than equipotent methohexital sedation

(E) a decrease in PaO_2 compared to thiopental sedation

9. Which of the following best describes the effect of etomidate on bronchial tone?

(A) etomidate promotes bronchial histamine release, but only in doses >0.4 mg/kg

(C) etomidate can promote bronchial histamine release with any dose

(D) etomidate has minimal effect on histamine release

(E) etomidate effectively prevents histamine release during bronchospasm

(F) etomidate is more effective than propofol at preventing acetylcholine-induced tracheal constriction

10. Which of the following best describes the effect of an induction dose of etomidate on the central nervous system?

(A) a decrease in $CMRO_2$, a decrease in CBF, and a decrease in CPP

(B) a decrease in $CMRO_2$, an increase in CBF, and a decrease in CPP

(C) a decrease in $CMRO_2$, a decrease in CBF, and an increase in CPP

(D) an increase in $CMRO_2$, a decrease in CBF, and a decrease in CPP

(E) an increase in $CMRO_2$, an increase in CBF, and a decrease in CPP

11. Which of the following is NOT associated with the use of etomidate?

(A) grand mal seizures

(B) decreased latency of somatosensory evoked potentials

(C) the absence of beta waves on EEG

(D) disruption of intraoperative mapping of seizure foci

(E) increased amplitude of somatosensory evoked potentials

12. Which of the following best describes the effect of an induction dose of etomidate on the endocrine system?

    (A) a dose-dependent, reversible inhibition of the enzyme 11β-hydroxylase

    (B) a dose-dependent, reversible inhibition of the enzyme tyrosine hydroxylase

    (C) a dose-dependent, reversible inhibition of the enzyme catechol-*O*-methyltransferase

    (D) a dose-dependent, reversible inhibition of the enzyme 5α-reductase

    (E) a dose-dependent, reversible inhibition of the enzyme aldosterone synthase

13. The lethality of an anesthetic induction drug can be quantified by relating the lethal dose to the effective hypnotic dose (LD50/ED50). Which of the following best describes the LD50/ED50 of etomidate?

    (A) 3
    (B) 4
    (C) 6
    (D) 9
    (E) 12

14. Which of the following is NOT a reported side effect of etomidate?

    (A) nausea and vomiting
    (B) increased intraocular pressure
    (C) superficial thrombophlebitis
    (D) myoclonic movements
    (E) pain on injection

15. Which of the following is the best explanation for why etomidate is a poor choice for long-term sedation in the critical care setting?

    (A) it precipitates in intravenous lines when added to acidic drugs

    (B) it is associated with an increase in ICP

    (C) it causes adrenocortical suppression

    (D) recovery is prolonged after infusion compared to other drugs

    (E) it causes an increase in serum lipids

16. A 20-year-old otherwise healthy male is brought to the operating room for decompressive craniotomy following a motor vehicle accident. He also has a left femur fracture, but no intra-abdominal or intrathoracic injuries. Paramedics report a good deal of blood loss from the thigh in the field. His blood pressure is 85/50 mm Hg, his heart rate is 110 bpm, and his respiratory rate is 28/min. Glasgow Coma Scale score is 8. Which of the following is the most appropriate intravenous induction agent for this patient?

    (A) etomidate
    (B) ketamine
    (C) methohexital
    (D) propofol
    (E) thiopental

Answers and Explanations: Etomidate

1. The principal mechanism of action of etomidate is best described as:

   (A) **potentiation of GABA-mediated chloride currents**

   (B) stimulation of μ- and κ-opioid receptors

   (C) stimulation of α_2-adrenergic receptors

   (D) inhibition of NMDA receptors

   (E) blockade of CNS sodium channels

Etomidate is an imidazole-containing anesthetic that is structurally unlike other intravenous anesthetics (Figure 13-1).

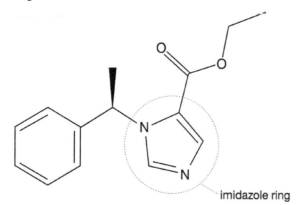

imidazole ring

FIG. 13-1. Structural formula of etomidate showing imidazole ring with two nitrogen atoms.

The mechanisms by which etomidate produce unconsciousness are somewhat unclear, but appear to primarily involve activation of $GABA_A$ receptor, increasing transmembrane chloride conductance. This hyperpolarizes the postsynaptic cell membrane and results in inhibition of postsynaptic neuron. While the $GABA_A$ receptor is made up of a combination of five subunits, the β_2- and β_3-subunits appear to be most important for its effect, and etomidate will selectively potentiate receptors containing these subunits. Etomidate has no analgesic activity.

Ref: Miller RD. *Miller's Anesthesia.* 8th ed. Philadelphia, PA: Elsevier; 2015.

2. In order to increase its water solubility, etomidate is formulated with which of the following compounds?

   (A) glycerol

   (B) benzyl alcohol

   (C) sodium bisulfite

   (D) **propylene glycol**

   (E) methylparaben

Glycerol is one component of the aqueous emulsion used to carry propofol (the other being soy oil and egg phosphatide). Benzyl alcohol and methylparaben are both preservative agents used in intravenous medications. Sodium bisulfite is a reducing agent used to prevent oxidation of drugs.

   In the United States, etomidate is supplied as a 2 mg/mL solution in 35% propylene glycol. It has a pH of 6.9 and, unlike sodium thiopental, does not precipitate when mixed with other drugs. Propylene glycol is associated with pain on injection, and the incidence of pain with this formulation of etomidate is up to 50%. A lipid formulation available in Europe may decrease this side effect.

   Ref: Miller RD. *Miller's Anesthesia.* 8th ed. Philadelphia, PA: Elsevier; 2015.

DIRECTIONS: Use the following scenario to answer questions 3 and 4:

A 60-year-old, 80-kg man presents for exploratory laparotomy after he was stabbed in the left upper quadrant of his abdomen. He has no other injuries. Chest X-ray reveals free air under the diaphragm. His past medical history includes hypercholesterolemia treated with atorvastatin and an appendectomy at age 15 years. Physical exam reveals blood pressure is 95/45 mm Hg and his heart rate is 112 bpm. He is pale and appears to be in mild respiratory distress as well as moderate pain. He has received 1,200 mL of lactated Ringer's solution intravenously since admission from the emergency department 45 minutes ago.

3. The most appropriate induction dose of etomidate for this patient is:

(A) 5 mg

(B) 12 mg

(C) **32 mg**

(D) 64 mg

(E) 100 mg

The typical range for induction of anesthesia when using etomidate is 0.2–0.6 mg/kg IV. In this case, 12 mg represents a dose of 0.15 mg/kg, which is likely inadequate; 64 mg represents a dose of 0.8 mg/kg, which is excessive; and 32 mg represents a dose of 0.4 mg/kg, which falls within the appropriate range. In marked contrast to most other intravenous anesthetic agents (e.g., propofol, thiopental, fentanyl, and remifentanil), hypovolemia does not alter the pharmacodynamics of etomidate. Hypovolemic patients such as this one require no dosage adjustment when inducing with etomidate, whereas the dose of propofol should be reduced by 30–50% to account for increased central compartment concentration and effect.

Ref: Longnecker DE, Brown DL, Newman MF, Zapol WM. *Anesthesiology.* 2nd ed. New York, NY: McGraw Hill; 2012.

4. The expected duration of anesthesia following the above single induction dose would be expected to be:

(A) 1 minute

(B) 2 minutes

(C) 4 minutes

(D) **7 minutes**

(E) 10 minutes

The onset of anesthesia after a typical induction dose (0.2–0.6 mg/kg) is rapid and similar to that seen with propofol or thiopental (one arm-brain circulation time). The duration after a single bolus is linearly related to the dose and is approximately 100 seconds per 0.1 mg/kg. In this case, 0.4 mg/kg should result in 400 seconds, or approximately 7 minutes, of unconsciousness.

Ref: Longnecker DE, Brown DL, Newman MF, Zapol WM. *Anesthesiology.* 2nd ed. New York, NY: McGraw Hill; 2012.

5. Which of the following best describes the method of inactivation of etomidate?

(A) **metabolism in the liver by ester hydrolysis**

(B) metabolism in the bloodstream by ester hydrolysis

(C) elimination by Hofmann degradation

(D) deactivation by the lungs, followed by renal excretion

(E) elimination via the fecal route

Etomidate is metabolized in the liver by two mechanisms. The principal reaction is ester hydrolysis, which leads to the production of the carboxylic acid of etomidate, an inactive metabolite. The less important hepatic metabolic process is N-dealkylation. While 2% of the drug is excreted unchanged, most is cleared as metabolites via the kidneys (85%) or via the biliary route (13%).

Ref: Miller RD. *Miller's Anesthesia.* 8th ed. Philadelphia, PA: Elsevier; 2015.

6. A 50-year-old man with a history of coronary disease and mild aortic stenosis is scheduled for knee replacement. He is induced with 0.3 mg/kg of etomidate. Which of the following hemodynamic effects best describe the expected response?

(A) increased heart rate, increased cardiac index, no change in PCWP

(B) increased heart rate, decreased cardiac index, decreased PCWP

(C) no change in heart rate, increased cardiac index, decreased PCWP

(D) decreased heart rate, no change in cardiac index, increased PCWP

(E) **no change in heart rate, no change in cardiac index, no change in PCWP**

Etomidate is unique in its ability to minimally affect hemodynamics over a wide induction dose range (0.2–0.6 mg/kg), even in patients with cardiovascular disease. A typical induction dose of 0.3 mg/kg appears to have little effect on heart rate, mean arterial pressure, CVP, PCWP, PAP, stroke volume, cardiac index, and both SVR and PVR. Some small studies have reported that patients with aortic or mitral valve disease may demonstrate some decrease (<20%) in MAP, but other studies show minimal change.

Ref: Longnecker DE, Brown DL, Newman MF, Zapol WM. *Anesthesiology.* 2nd ed. New York, NY: McGraw Hill; 2012.

7. Which of the following statements best describes the cardiac effects following induction and intubation with etomidate as the sole agent?

(A)   etomidate is likely to prolong the QT interval

(B)   **hypertension and tachycardia commonly follow intubation**

(C)   myocardial oxygen demand is likely to exceed supply

(D)   arrhythmias such as PVCs are common

(E)   reflex bradycardia often occurs

Etomidate has minimal effect on the QT interval, and arrhythmias (such as PVCs) are not associated with its use. Etomidate produces a parallel decrease in both myocardial consumption and blood flow, so that the supply-demand ratio is preserved. Reflex bradycardia does not occur with the use of etomidate since baroreceptors are not activated. However, since etomidate does not provide any analgesia, patients who are not pretreated with analgesics do tend to exhibit tachycardia and hypertension in response to laryngoscopy. This can be largely prevented with the administration of fentanyl 1–5 mcg/kg prior to induction.

Ref: Longnecker DE, Brown DL, Newman MF, Zapol WM. *Anesthesiology*. 2nd ed. New York, NY: McGraw Hill; 2012.

8.   A patient is sedated with etomidate for DC cardioversion. Which of the following best describes the ventilatory effect of etomidate during the case?

(A)   more episodes of apnea than equipotent propofol sedation

(B)   **greater respiratory drive than equipotent methohexital sedation**

(C)   higher $PaCO_2$ than equipotent propofol sedation

(D)   reduced respiratory drive than equipotent methohexital sedation

(E)   a decrease in PaO_2 compared to thiopental sedation

Etomidate has little effect on the respiratory system. There is no histamine release, and as such it is a safe agent to administer in patients with reactive airways disease. The ventilatory response to carbon dioxide is depressed compared to baseline, but is greater for a given $PaCO_2$ than an equipotent dose of methohexital. Many patients continue to breathe spontaneously following an induction dose of etomidate, making it an attractive agent for cases required brief sedation. In contrast, propofol and the barbiturate class of drugs very quickly lead to apnea in clinical doses. PaO_2 is

typically preserved. Hiccups are common following etomidate induction.

Ref: Miller RD. *Miller's Anesthesia*. 8th ed. Philadelphia, PA: Elsevier; 2015.

9.   Which of the following best describes the effect of etomidate on bronchial tone?

(A)   etomidate promotes bronchial histamine release, but only in doses >0.4 mg/kg

(C)   etomidate can promote bronchial histamine release with any dose

(D)   **etomidate has minimal effect on histamine release**

(E)   etomidate effectively prevents histamine release during bronchospasm

(F)   etomidate is more effective than propofol at preventing acetylcholine-induced tracheal constriction

Etomidate does not promote histamine release at any dose, and therefore it is a good choice for use in those with reactive airways disease. However, it does not prevent histamine release during active bronchospasm. Etomidate has been shown to prevent muscarinic-induced constriction of the tracheobronchial tree, but not as effectively as propofol.

Ref: Miller RD. *Miller's Anesthesia*. 8th ed. Philadelphia, PA: Elsevier; 2015.

10.   Which of the following best describes the effect of an induction dose of etomidate on the central nervous system?

(A)   a decrease in $CMRO_2$, a decrease in CBF, and a decrease in CPP

(B)   a decrease in $CMRO_2$, an increase in CBF, and a decrease in CPP

(C)   **a decrease in $CMRO_2$, a decrease in CBF, and an increase in CPP**

(D)   an increase in $CMRO_2$, a decrease in CBF, and a decrease in CPP

(E)   an increase in $CMRO_2$, an increase in CBF, and a decrease in CPP

An induction dose of etomidate (0.2–0.4 mg/kg) reduces both cerebral blood flow and $CMRO_2$ by 30–45%. Etomidate also reduces elevated ICP, but unlike induction doses of propofol or thiopental, MAP is preserved without the need for additional vasopressor therapy. As a result, cerebral perfusion pressure is increased (CPP = MAP − ICP), and there is a beneficial net increase in the cerebral oxygen supply-demand ratio. Etomidate is an appropriate agent to use for induction and maintenance of anesthesia during most neurosurgical procedures.

Ref: Miller RD. *Miller's Anesthesia*. 8th ed. Philadelphia, PA: Elsevier; 2015.

11. Which of the following is NOT associated with the use of etomidate?

   (A) grand mal seizures

   (B) decreased latency of somatosensory evoked potentials

   (C) the absence of beta waves on EEG

   (D) **disruption of intraoperative mapping of seizure foci**

   (E) increased amplitude of somatosensory evoked potentials

Etomidate produces changes in the EEG similar to thiopental, except that there is an absence of increased beta wave activity at induction that is typically seen with thiopental. Increased EEG activity in epileptogenic foci is common with its use, and grand mal seizures have been reported. For this reason it is probably best avoided in patients with seizure disorders. However, this property makes it useful as an aid to intraoperative mapping of seizure foci before surgical ablation. Despite this, like thiopental and propofol, etomidate is an anticonvulsant, and has been used to treat status epilepticus.

Unlike barbiturates, propofol, and the volatile gases, etomidate does not have a negative effect on amplitude or latency of somatosensory evoked potentials. Rather, etomidate has the unique ability to cause increases in the amplitude of cortical SSEPs. Etomidate infusions have been used to enhance monitoring capability in patients with poor baseline recordings due to pathology.

Ref: Miller RD. *Miller's Anesthesia*. 8th ed. Philadelphia, PA: Elsevier; 2015.

12. Which of the following best describes the effect of an induction dose of etomidate on the endocrine system?

   (A) **a dose-dependent, reversible inhibition of the enzyme 11β-hydroxylase**

   (B) a dose-dependent, reversible inhibition of the enzyme tyrosine hydroxylase

   (C) a dose-dependent, reversible inhibition of the enzyme catechol-*O*-methyltransferase

   (D) a dose-dependent, reversible inhibition of the enzyme 5α-reductase

   (E) a dose-dependent, reversible inhibition of the enzyme aldosterone synthase

Tyrosine hydroxylase catalyzes the conversion of L-tyrosine to L-DOPA, an important step in the synthesis of catecholamines. In contrast, catechol-*O*-methyltransferase inactivates dopamine, norepinephrine, and epinephrine. 5α-reductase is involved in the synthesis of androgens and estrogens. Aldosterone synthase converts corticosterone to aldosterone. None of these are affected by the use of etomidate.

Etomidate is known to cause a reversible inhibition of 11β-hydroxylase (and, to a lesser extent, 17α-hydroxylase), which is responsible for converting 11-deoxycortisol to cortisol in the zona fasciculata of the adrenal cortex. This results in a temporary reduction in circulating cortisol levels, and a corresponding increase in ACTH levels (6–8 hours after a single bolus, up to 24 hours after infusion). The effect is dose dependent. Controversy exists regarding the clinical significance of this effect. Typically the lowest cortisol level postoperatively can still be expected to be in the normal range. Even in high-stress surgical procedures, where a normal cortisol level is critical for maintenance of hemodynamic function, the native stress response is usually robust enough to overcome any temporary inhibition of the enzyme. One exception may be in critically ill patients with septic shock; some studies have shown increased mortality in this population despite the use of supplemental steroids, while others have found no difference in outcome. This has to be balanced against the fact that intraoperative hypotension is a strong predictor of mortality in critically ill patients; since etomidate is the induction agent with the most stable hemodynamic effects, some argue that it should still be used in this population to prevent a large drop in the mean arterial pressure.

Ref: Miller RD. *Miller's Anesthesia*. 8th ed. Philadelphia, PA: Elsevier; 2015.

13. The lethality of an anesthetic induction drug can be quantified by relating the lethal dose to the effective hypnotic dose (LD50/ED50). Which of the following best describes the LD50/ED50 of etomidate?

   (A) 3

   (B) 4

   (C) 6

   (D) 9

   (E) **12**

Etomidate appears to be the least lethal of the commonly used anesthetic induction drugs, based on therapeutic index studies in rodents (Table 13-1).

TABLE 13-1. LD50/ED50 for commonly used induction agents.

Intravenous Anesthetic Agent	LD50/ED50
Etomidate (racemic)	12
Ketamine (racemic)	6.3
Methohexital	4.8–9.5
Thiopental	3.6–4.6
Propofol	3.4

Source: Miller RD. *Miller's Anesthesia*. 8th ed. Philadelphia, PA: Elsevier; 2015.

Ref: Miller RD. *Miller's Anesthesia*. 8th ed. Philadelphia, PA: Elsevier; 2015.

14. Which of the following is NOT a reported side effect of etomidate?

    (A) nausea and vomiting

    (B) increased intraocular pressure

    (C) superficial thrombophlebitis

    (D) myoclonic movements

    (E) pain on injection

Nausea and vomiting occur commonly (30–40%) with etomidate. Pain on injection carries a similar incidence as propofol but can be attenuated with the injection of lidocaine in advance. Superficial thrombophlebitis is also relatively common (up to 20%) and can occur as much as 24–72 hours after injection, usually through a small gauge cannula. Etomidate is commonly associated with involuntary myoclonic movements during induction. Myoclonus is not thought to be related to cortical seizure activity, but rather to subcortical disinhibition. The movements can be largely prevented or attenuated by pretreatment with opioids or benzodiazepines prior to induction.

Intraocular pressure is rapidly reduced by 30%–60% after induction with etomidate, and lasts about 5 minutes, but can be maintained using an infusion.

Ref: Miller RD. *Miller's Anesthesia*. 8th ed. Philadelphia, PA: Elsevier; 2015.

15. Which of the following is the best explanation for why etomidate is a poor choice for long-term sedation in the critical care setting?

    (A) it precipitates in intravenous lines when added to acidic drugs

    (B) it is associated with an increase in ICP

    (C) it causes adrenocortical suppression

    (D) recovery is prolonged after infusion compared to other drugs

    (E) it causes an increase in serum lipids

Etomidate does not precipitate in intravenous lines (unlike thiopental, which does in the presence of solutions with low pH). Etomidate is known to effectively reduce ICP and is used frequently in patients with reduced intracranial compliance. Compared to other common intravenous sedatives and hypnotic agents, etomidate has a very short context-sensitive half-time (Figure 13-2), making it a good choice for long-term infusions that can be turned off and titrated relatively quickly. While propofol has been shown to elevate serum lipid levels after long-term infusion, no such problem has been reported with etomidate.

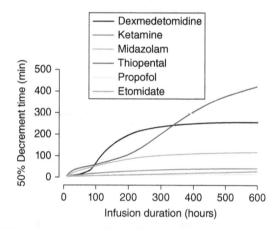

FIG. 13-2. Context-sensitive half-time as a function of infusion duration for common intravenous anesthetics. (Reproduced with permission from Johnson KB. *Clinical Pharmacology for Anesthesiology*. 1st ed. New York, NY: McGraw Hill; 2015.)

As discussed above, etomidate does cause reversible suppression of cortisol production, and while it is likely of little clinical significance for elective perioperative use, it is no longer commonly used as a long-term sedative agent in the ICU for fear of worsened outcomes.

Ref: Johnson KB. *Clinical Pharmacology for Anesthesiology*. 1st ed. New York, NY: McGraw Hill; 2015.

16. A 20-year-old otherwise healthy male is brought to the operating room for decompressive craniotomy following a motor vehicle accident. He also has a left femur fracture, but no intra-abdominal or intrathoracic injuries. Paramedics report a good deal of blood loss from the thigh in the field. His blood pressure is 85/50 mm Hg, his heart rate is 110 bpm, and his respiratory rate is 28/min. Glasgow Coma Scale score is 8.

Which of the following is the most appropriate intravenous induction agent for this patient?

(A) **etomidate**

(B) ketamine

(C) methohexital

(D) propofol

(E) thiopental

The primary hemodynamic goal for this induction is to maintain cerebral perfusion pressure (CPP). CPP = mean arterial pressure − intracranial pressure. Methohexital, thiopental, and propofol all decrease MAP as well as ICP; while CPP could be expected to be preserved if both MAP and ICP decrease proportionally, this may not always be the case, especially in a hypovolemic patient such as this one where arterial blood pressure is tenuous. Ketamine preserves MAP, but it is known to increase ICP, making it a poor choice. Etomidate is attractive for two reasons in this case: it reduces ICP by decreasing $CMRO_2$ and CBF, and at the same time preserves MAP, leading to a preservation or augmentation of cerebral perfusion pressure.

Ref: Longnecker DE, Brown DL, Newman MF, Zapol WM. *Anesthesiology*. 2nd ed. New York, NY: McGraw Hill; 2012.

CHAPTER 14

Benzodiazepines

1. Which of the following is NOT a pharmacologic property of benzodiazepines?

   (A) sedation
   (B) muscle relaxation
   (C) amnesia
   (D) analgesia
   (E) anticonvulsant

2. What is the mechanism of action of midazolam at the $GABA_A$ receptor?

   (A) direct activation of the $GABA_A$ receptor and increased chloride conductance
   (B) direct activation of the $GABA_A$ receptor and increased potassium conductance
   (C) competitive inhibition at the acetylcholine binding site
   (D) allosteric modulation of GABA binding to $GABA_A$ receptor
   (E) increased transmembrane sodium conductance

3. Which of the following benzodiazepines is considered long-lasting?

   (A) midazolam
   (B) lorazepam
   (C) diazepam
   (D) triazolam
   (E) temazepam

4. Why is midazolam prepared in a solution with the pH adjusted to <4?

   (A) this increases the volume of distribution (V_d)
   (B) this increases pK_a
   (C) this increases hepatic clearance
   (D) this increases water solubility
   (E) this increases lipid solubility

5. Which of the following patient characteristics will significantly **increase** the metabolism of midazolam?

   (A) increased age
   (B) cigarette smoking
   (C) chronic alcohol consumption
   (D) decreased renal function
   (E) use of cimetidine

6. Which benzodiazepine is considered to have **inactive** metabolites?

   (A) diazepam
   (B) midazolam
   (C) lorazepam
   (D) alprazolam
   (E) chlordiazepoxide

7. After an induction dose of midazolam, which of the following hemodynamic changes is **most** likely?

   (A) decreased cardiac index
   (B) increased systemic vascular resistance
   (C) increased mean blood pressure
   (D) decreased heart rate
   (E) decreased pulmonary vascular resistance

8. The incidence of ventilatory depression after the administration of midazolam is associated with all of the following factors EXCEPT:

   (A) speed of injection
   (B) geriatric patient
   (C) co-administration of opioids
   (D) ASA 4 patient
   (E) obstructive sleep apnea

9. In which of the following ways do benzodiazepines usually affect sleep?

   (A) increased length of REM sleep
   (B) decreased number of REM cycles
   (C) increased Stage 0 sleep
   (D) increased Stage 3 and 4 sleep
   (E) increased Stage 2 sleep

10. A patient is taking chronic benzodiazepines to treat symptoms of anxiety. Perioperatively the benzodiazepine is acutely stopped. Which of the following signs is associated with benzodiazepine withdrawal syndrome?

   (A) bradycardia
   (B) myoclonic jerks
   (C) increased sensitivity to pain
   (D) increased appetite
   (E) hypertension

11. Midazolam is a versatile intravenous anesthetic and may be used in a variety of clinical situations. A reason for selecting midazolam may include:

   (A) reduced PONV
   (B) superior analgesia
   (C) relatively shorter period of amnesia
   (D) reduced seizure threshold
   (E) relatively faster emergence from anesthesia

12. A patient is taking chronic benzodiazepines to treat symptoms of anxiety. The patient takes an intentional overdose of the benzodiazepine and a tricyclic antidepressant. In this situation flumazenil should be avoided due to the risk of:

   (A) tachycardia
   (B) seizures
   (C) hearing loss
   (D) malignant hypertension
   (E) severe nausea

13. How does flumazenil act to reverse the effects of benzodiazepines?

   (A) competitive antagonist
   (B) uncompetitive antagonist
   (C) physiologic antagonist
   (D) chemical antagonist
   (E) noncompetitive antagonist

Answers and Explanations: Benzodiazepines

1. Which of the following is NOT a pharmacologic property of benzodiazepines?

   (A) sedation
   (B) muscle relaxation
   (C) amnesia
   (D) analgesia
   (E) anticonvulsant

   Although there is some experimental evidence regarding benzodiazepines' ability to modify pain transmission in the spinal cord, benzodiazepines are clinically not considered to have analgesic properties. Benzodiazepines have all of the following properties:
   - Sedation
   - Hypnosis
   - Anxiolysis
   - Amnesia
   - Anticonvulsant
   - Muscle relaxant

   Ref: Miller RD. *Miller's Anesthesia*. 8th ed. Philadelphia, PA: Elsevier; 2015.

2. What is the mechanism of action of midazolam at the $GABA_A$ receptor?

   (A) direct activation of the $GABA_A$ receptor and increased chloride conductance
   (B) direct activation of the $GABA_A$ receptor and increased potassium conductance
   (C) competitive inhibition at the acetylcholine binding site
   (D) allosteric modulation of GABA binding to $GABA_A$ receptor
   (E) increased transmembrane sodium conductance

   Midazolam (and other benzodiazepines) act at the benzodiazepine receptor on the $GABA_A$ receptor complex. The binding of midazolam results in increased binding affinity of GABA for the $GABA_A$ receptor (allosteric modulation). $GABA_A$ activation causes influx of chloride ions and hyperpolarization of the cell membrane. Direct activation of the $GABA_A$ receptor can occur with barbiturates and etomidate. NMDA receptor activation alters sodium and potassium conductance. Barbiturates such as thiopental are also thought to act as a competitive inhibitors at CNS acetylcholine (and glutamate) receptors.

   Ref: Miller RD. *Miller's Anesthesia*. 8th ed. Philadelphia, PA: Elsevier; 2015.

3. Which of the following benzodiazepines is considered long-lasting?

   (A) midazolam
   (B) lorazepam
   (C) diazepam
   (D) triazolam
   (E) temazepam

   Diazepam is considered long-lasting as its elimination half-life is 20–50 hours. Midazolam and triazolam are short-acting (midazolam elimination half-life = 1.7–2.6 hours). Lorazepam and temazepam are intermediate-acting (lorazepam elimination half-life = 11–22 hours).

   Ref: Miller RD. *Miller's Anesthesia*. 8th ed. Philadelphia, PA: Elsevier; 2015.

4. Why is midazolam prepared in a solution with the pH adjusted to <4?

   (A) this increases the volume of distribution (V_d)
   (B) this increases pK_a
   (C) this increases hepatic clearance
   (D) this increases water solubility
   (E) this increases lipid solubility

   Midazolam is formulated in an acidic medium (pH 3.5) to increase its water solubility. Its imidazole ring structure means that midazolam can be both lipid and water soluble depending on the pH of the solution. At pH <4, the imidazole ring is in a ring-open form and the midazolam formulation is water soluble. At physiologic pH of 7.4, the imidazole ring is in a ring-closed form and midazolam is lipid soluble.

Refs: Miller RD. *Miller's Anesthesia.* 8th ed. Philadelphia, PA: Elsevier; 2015.
Gerecke M. Chemical structure and properties of midazolam compared with other benzodiazepines. *Br J Clin Pharmac.* 1983;16:11S–16S.

5. Which of the following patient characteristics will significantly **increase** the metabolism of midazolam?

   (A) increased age
   (B) cigarette smoking
   (C) chronic alcohol consumption
   (D) decreased renal function
   (E) use of cimetidine

Chronic alcohol consumption increases the metabolism of midazolam. Cigarette smoking and increased age have no significant effect on midazolam metabolism (cigarette smoking increases the clearance of diazepam, while increased age decreases the clearance of diazepam). Decreased renal function may lead to the accumulation of midazolam metabolites. Cimetidine will inhibit the hydroxylation of midazolam.

Ref: Miller RD. *Miller's Anesthesia.* 8th ed. Philadelphia, PA: Elsevier; 2015.

6. Which benzodiazepine is considered to have **inactive** metabolites?

   (A) diazepam
   (B) midazolam
   (C) lorazepam
   (D) alprazolam
   (E) chlordiazepoxide

Benzodiazepines are metabolized in the liver by cytochrome P450 enzymes. Many benzodiazepines have active metabolites and these metabolites can be an important determinant of the drug's clinical duration of action. Lorazepam does not have active metabolites; it is metabolized via glucuronidation to inactive forms. Chlordiazepoxide and diazepam are *N*-dealkylated to form products including nordazepam, which is biologically active. Alprazolam and midazolam form

hydroxylated compounds that are active. In certain circumstances, such as repeated dosing in patients with renal failure, metabolites of midazolam may accumulate and have a significant clinical effect.

Refs: Miller RD. *Miller's Anesthesia.* 8th ed. Philadelphia, PA: Elsevier; 2015.
Barash PG. *Clinical Anesthesia.* 7th ed. Philadelphia, PA: Lippincott Williams & Wilkins; 2013.

7. After an induction dose of midazolam, which of the following hemodynamic changes is **most** likely?

   (A) decreased cardiac index
   (B) increased systemic vascular resistance
   (C) increased mean blood pressure
   (D) decreased heart rate
   (E) decreased pulmonary vascular resistance

The hemodynamic effects of midazolam are modest, but after an induction dose of midazolam cardiac index may decrease by up to 25%. Other hemodynamic changes associated with an induction dose of midazolam include:

* variable effect on heart rate (slight increase or decrease)
* decreased systemic vascular resistance
* decreased mean blood pressure
* unchanged pulmonary vascular resistance

Ref: Miller RD. *Miller's Anesthesia.* 8th ed. Philadelphia, PA: Elsevier; 2015.

8. The incidence of ventilatory depression after the administration of midazolam is associated with all of the following factors EXCEPT:

   (A) speed of injection
   (B) geriatric patient
   (C) co-administration of opioids
   (D) ASA 4 patient
   (E) obstructive sleep apnea

The speed of midazolam injection affects the onset time of peak respiratory depression rather than the overall incidence of respiratory depression. Other factors associated with ventilatory depression after administration of midazolam are:

* geriatric patients
* debilitating disease
* use of other respiratory depressants (opioids)
* obstructive sleep apnea

Ref: Miller RD. *Miller's Anesthesia.* 8th ed. Philadelphia, PA: Elsevier; 2015.

9. In which of the following ways do benzodiazepines usually affect sleep?

   (A) increased length of REM sleep
   (B) decreased number of REM cycles
   (C) increased Stage 0 sleep
   (D) increased Stage 3 and 4 sleep
   (E) **increased Stage 2 sleep**

Benzodiazepines increase the amount of time spent in Stage 2 sleep. Benzodiazepines usually decrease the amount of time spent in Stage 0, 1, 3, 4, and REM sleep. They also decrease sleep latency and usually increase the number of REM cycles. Overall, benzodiazepines usually increase total sleep time. When benzodiazepines are discontinued, a "rebound" in the amount of REM sleep may occur.

Ref: Brunton LL, Chabner BA, Knollman BC. *Goodman & Gilman's the Pharmacological Basis of Therapeutics.* 12th ed. New York, NY: McGraw Hill; 2011.

10. A patient is taking chronic benzodiazepines to treat symptoms of anxiety. Perioperatively the benzodiazepine is acutely stopped. Which of the following signs is associated with benzodiazepine withdrawal syndrome?

   (A) bradycardia
   (B) **myoclonic jerks**
   (C) increased sensitivity to pain
   (D) increased appetite
   (E) hypertension

Benzodiazepine withdrawal symptoms and signs include:
   • myoclonic jerks
   • muscle cramps
   • sleep disturbance
   • anxiety, agitation
   • seizures
   • delirium

Bradycardia is associated with cocaine withdrawal; increased sensitivity to pain and hypertension are associated with opioid withdrawal; and increased appetite is associated with nicotine withdrawal.

Ref: Brunton LL, Chabner BA, Knollman BC. *Goodman & Gilman's the Pharmacological Basis of Therapeutics.* 12th ed. New York, NY: McGraw Hill; 2011.

11. Midazolam is a versatile intravenous anesthetic and may be used in a variety of clinical situations. A reason for selecting midazolam may include:

   (A) **reduced PONV**
   (B) superior analgesia
   (C) relatively shorter period of amnesia
   (D) reduced seizure threshold
   (E) relatively faster emergence from anesthesia

Although the exact mechanism of action is not completely understood, there is evidence that midazolam can reduce the incidence of PONV. Other effects of midazolam include:
   • relatively longer period of amnesia
   • increased seizure threshold
   • relatively slower emergence from anesthesia

Midazolam is not considered to have clinically significant analgesic action.

Ref: Miller RD. *Miller's Anesthesia.* 8th ed. Philadelphia, PA: Elsevier; 2015.

12. A patient is taking chronic benzodiazepines to treat symptoms of anxiety. The patient takes an intentional overdose of the benzodiazepine and a tricyclic antidepressant. In this situation flumazenil should be avoided due to the risk of:

   (A) tachycardia
   (B) **seizures**
   (C) hearing loss
   (D) malignant hypertension
   (E) severe nausea

Flumazenil should be avoided in the setting of chronic benzodiazepine use or in cases of tricyclic antidepressant overdose, as seizures have been reported. In general, other side effects of flumazenil administration include tachycardia, hypertension, hearing changes, and nausea.

Ref: Brunton LL, Chabner BA, Knollman BC. *Goodman & Gilman's the Pharmacological Basis of Therapeutics.* 12th ed. New York, NY: McGraw Hill; 2011.

13. How does flumazenil act to reverse the effects of benzodiazepines?

   (A) **competitive antagonist**
   (B) uncompetitive antagonist

(C) physiologic antagonist

(D) chemical antagonist

(E) noncompetitive antagonist

Flumazenil is a competitive antagonist at the benzodiazepine receptor. It can reverse undesirable effects of benzodiazepines, including excessive sedation and respiratory depression. Patient monitoring is important, particularly if long-lasting benzodiazepines are reversed, as re-sedation can occur if flumazenil is cleared before the benzodiazepine.

Ref: Miller RD. *Miller's Anesthesia.* 8th ed. Philadelphia, PA: Elsevier; 2015.

CHAPTER 15

Ketamine

1. The principal mechanism of action of ketamine is best described as:

   (A) potentiation of GABA-mediated chloride currents
   (B) stimulation of μ- and κ-opioid receptors
   (C) stimulation of α_2-adrenergic receptors
   (D) inhibition of NMDA receptors
   (E) blockade of CNS sodium channels

2. The typical anesthetic state observed following an induction dose of ketamine is best characterized by which of the following?

   (A) catalepsy
   (B) miosis
   (C) hypoventilation
   (D) flaccid paralysis
   (E) ablation of protective reflexes

3. Which of the following statements regarding the pharmacokinetics of ketamine is true?

   (A) ketamine is poorly lipid soluble
   (B) the duration of action of a single induction bolus is 2–3 minutes
   (C) ketamine has a relatively low degree of protein binding
   (D) the elimination clearance of the R- enantiomer is larger than the S+ enantiomer
   (E) clearance is independent of hepatic blood flow

4. The time to peak effect of a 5 mg/kg dose of ketamine administered via the intramuscular route is expected to be:

   (A) 1 minute
   (B) 3 minutes
   (C) 5 minutes
   (D) 10 minutes
   (E) 20 minutes

5. The metabolite resulting from N-demethylation of ketamine in the liver by microsomal enzymes that still carries some degree of activity is:

   (A) hydroxyketamine
   (B) oxyketamine
   (C) norketamine
   (D) hydroxynorketamine
   (E) oxynorketamine

6. Which of the following cardiovascular responses would be expected following an induction dose of ketamine?

   (A) a decrease in heart rate
   (B) an increase in the pulmonary capillary wedge pressure
   (C) a decrease in cardiac index
   (D) an increase in right atrial pressure
   (E) a decrease in left ventricular stroke work

7. A 68-year-old woman with mild pulmonary hypertension receives intravenous ketamine 2 mg/kg. Which of the following best describes the expected cardiovascular response?

   (A) a decrease in myocardial oxygen consumption
   (B) an increase in pulmonary vascular resistance
   (C) a decrease in the heart rate
   (D) a decrease in pulmonary vascular resistance
   (E) a decrease in contractility

8. The cardiovascular stimulatory effects of ketamine can best be blunted by the pre-administration of:

    (A) vasopressin
    (B) midazolam
    (C) neostigmine
    (D) ondansetron
    (E) fenoldopam

9. A 20-year-old male patient receives 1.5 mg/kg of intravenous ketamine. Which of the following best describes the expected respiratory effect?

    (A) a decrease in respiratory rate only
    (B) a decrease in tidal volume only
    (C) a decrease in respiratory rate with an increase in tidal volume
    (D) an increase in respiratory rate with a decrease in tidal volume
    (E) no change in respiratory rate or tidal volume

10. Ketamine would most likely be helpful in the treatment of which of the following respiratory conditions?

    (A) status asthmaticus
    (B) laryngospasm
    (C) pulmonary hypertension
    (D) bronchiectasis
    (E) atelectasis

11. Which of the following effects on the central nervous system would be most likely to result from an induction dose of ketamine?

    (A) a decrease in $CMRO_2$
    (B) an increase in theta wave activity
    (C) a decrease in cerebral blood flow
    (D) an attenuation of the cerebrovascular response to carbon dioxide
    (E) a decrease in intracranial pressure

12. Which of the following factors increases the risk for emergence reactions related to ketamine anesthesia?

    (A) playing music during anesthesia
    (B) age under 18 years
    (C) low dose of ketamine
    (D) female sex
    (E) pretreatment with benzodiazepines

13. An 8-year-old child receives 2 mg/kg of ketamine intravenously. The factor that most likely places her at risk for laryngospasm is:

    (A) an absence of protective reflexes
    (B) excessive salivation
    (C) an insufficient induction dose
    (D) apnea due to an excessive dose
    (E) increased bulbar muscle spasticity

14. In which of the following patients would ketamine be most indicated?

    (A) a 21-year-old with an open eye injury
    (B) a 35-year-old with a closed head injury
    (C) a 59-year-old with a gunshot wound to the abdomen
    (D) a 60-year-old with a history of coronary artery disease
    (E) a 72-year-old with an abdominal aortic aneurysm

15. During acute pericardial tamponade, which of the following best describes the physiologic rationale for the use of ketamine as an induction agent?

    (A) a reduction in left ventricular stroke volume
    (B) a decrease in pulmonary vascular resistance
    (C) a reduction in systemic vascular resistance
    (D) an increase in right atrial pressure
    (E) an increase in contractility

16. At which of following locations is ketamine postulated to exert its antihyperalgesic or antiallodynic effects?

    (A) the peripheral nervous system
    (B) the dorsal horn of the spinal cord
    (C) the frontal cortex
    (D) the medullary reticular formation
    (E) the thalamoneocortical projection system

Answers and Explanations:
Ketamine

1. The principal mechanism of action of ketamine is best described as:

    (A) potentiation of GABA-mediated chloride currents
    (B) stimulation of μ- and κ-opioid receptors
    (C) stimulation of α_2-adrenergic receptors
    (D) **inhibition of NMDA receptors**
    (E) blockade of CNS sodium channels

While many intravenous anesthetics exert their effect by potentiating the effect of GABA, the principal analgesic and anesthetic mechanism of ketamine is blockade of the NMDA receptor. Ketamine is known to have effects on a wide variety of receptors, including AMPA, adenosine, μ-opioid, and cholinergic receptors, but the relative contribution of these players is substantially less significant than the NMDA inhibition.

It is generally accepted that the main role of ketamine (when used in subhypnotic doses) is as an anti-hyperalgesic, antiallodynic drug, reducing the temporal summation of nociceptive afferent input that leads to central sensitization and windup.

Ketamine is quite versatile in terms of its route of administration. It can be given via the intravenous, intramuscular, rectal, subcutaneous, transdermal, topical, oral, intranasal, sublingual, transmucosal, epidural, or intrathecal route. Ketamine has been gargled as a local throat analgesic, locally infiltrated, and used in intravenous regional anesthesia. The oral bioavailability of ketamine is low, and since so many other routes are available, this method is not particularly common. Intramuscular ketamine 4–5 mg/kg is very effective in the preoperative sedation in patients who are uncooperative.

Ref: Miller RD. *Miller's Anesthesia.* 8th ed. Philadelphia, PA: Elsevier; 2015.

2. The typical anesthetic state observed following an induction dose of ketamine is best characterized by which of the following?

    (A) **catalepsy**
    (B) miosis
    (C) hypoventilation
    (D) flaccid paralysis
    (E) ablation of protective reflexes

Ketamine produces unconsciousness and analgesia in a dose-related manner. The anesthetic state produced by ketamine has been termed "dissociative anesthesia." Rather than normal sleep, patients appear dissociated from their environment in an apparent cataleptic state. Patients may move, vocalize, and exhibit ocular tracking movements, but have profound analgesia and do not react to surgical stimuli or recall any of the events that occurred during the anesthetic. Amnesia, while part of the ketamine experience, is not as predictable as it is with benzodiazepines. Corneal, cough, and swallow reflexes may be present, but these should not be assumed to be protective. Skeletal muscle tone is also maintained and in some cases increased, with seemingly purposeless movements of the arms, legs, trunk, and head.

Miosis is not a consistent feature with ketamine administration; the tendency of ketamine to antagonize the cholinergic system produces a relative increase in sympathetic tone, bronchodilation, and mydriasis. Ketamine has no effect on minute ventilation.

Ref: Longnecker DE, Brown DL, Newman MF, Zapol WM. *Anesthesiology.* 2nd ed. New York, NY: McGraw Hill; 2012.

3. Which of the following statements regarding the pharmacokinetics of ketamine is true?

    (A) ketamine is poorly lipid soluble
    (B) the duration of action of a single induction bolus is 2–3 minutes
    (C) **ketamine has a relatively low degree of protein binding**
    (D) the elimination clearance of the R- enantiomer is larger than the S+ enantiomer
    (E) clearance is independent of hepatic blood flow

Ketamine is highly lipid soluble and has a pKa of 7.5 (near physiologic pH), resulting in rapid delivery to the brain. It has a large volume of distribution (approximately 3 L/kg). Bolus doses are rapidly distributed, with a distribution half-life of about 15 minutes. Clearance of ketamine is also relatively high (12–17 mL/kg/min), which helps explain its fairly brisk elimination half-life of 2.5 hours. Total body clearance is approximately equal to hepatic blood flow; this means that changes in liver blood flow affect clearance of ketamine. In contrast to nearly every other intravenous anesthetic agent, ketamine is poorly protein bound, at about 12%. In contrast, barbiturates, propofol, and benzodiazepines are all 85–98% protein bound, and etomidate is 75% protein bound. Ketamine just has to be different.

The ketamine that is available in the United States is a racemic mixture, but in some countries the S+ enantiomer is available for clinical use. S+ enantiomer has approximately four times the potency of the R-enantiomer, with fewer psychomimetic side effects than the racemic drug. It also has a larger clearance compared to the R- enantiomer.

Refs: Miller RD. *Miller's Anesthesia.* 8th ed. Philadelphia, PA: Elsevier; 2015.

Longnecker DE, Brown DL, Newman MF, Zapol WM. *Anesthesiology.* 2nd ed. New York, NY: McGraw Hill; 2012.

4. The time to peak effect of a 5 mg/kg dose of ketamine administered via the intramuscular route is expected to be:

(A) 1 minute
(B) 3 minutes
(C) 5 minutes
(D) 10 minutes
(E) 20 minutes

Ketamine can be administered by a variety of routes. In children or adults with mental disabilities who will not tolerate a mask or an intravenous catheter placement, intramuscular ketamine can facilitate a (relatively speaking) smooth induction. An IM dose of 4–6 mg/kg will induce unconsciousness in about 20 minutes. It is important to have appropriate monitors, suction, and airway equipment at bedside while the patient gradually loses consciousness and his/her airway reflexes. Once the patient is sedated enough, the airway can begin to be managed and an IV secured.

Ref: Miller RD. *Miller's Anesthesia.* 8th ed. Philadelphia, PA: Elsevier; 2015.

5. The metabolite resulting from N-demethylation of ketamine in the liver by microsomal enzymes that still carries some degree of activity is:

(A) hydroxyketamine
(B) oxyketamine
(C) norketamine
(D) hydroxynorketamine
(E) oxynorketamine

Ketamine is metabolized in the liver by N-demethylation to form norketamine. This is then hydroxylated to hydroxynorketamine. Both of these intermediate metabolites are conjugated to glucuronide and excreted in the urine. Norketamine apparently has about 70%–80% of the activity of the original drug. Although it does not last very long providing the glucuronidation pathway is not impaired, research does suggest that it contributes somewhat to a prolongation of the effect.

Ref: Miller RD. *Miller's Anesthesia.* 8th ed. Philadelphia, PA: Elsevier; 2015.

6. Which of the following cardiovascular responses would be expected following an induction dose of ketamine?

(A) a decrease in heart rate
(B) an increase in the pulmonary capillary wedge pressure
(C) a decrease in cardiac index
(D) an increase in right atrial pressure
(E) a decrease in left ventricular stroke work

Ketamine is unique among intravenous anesthetics in that it stimulates the cardiovascular system rather than depresses it. Hemodynamic changes following an intravenous induction dose of 0.5–2 mg/kg are seen in Table 15-1. Interestingly, using an equianesthetic dose of the S+ enantiomer produces the same effect as the racemic mixture, despite an overall dose reduction of 50%. Moreover, the hemodynamic changes appear NOT to be dose-related; a dose of 1 mg/kg appears to produce the same increase in blood pressure, heart rate, etc. as a dose of 2 mg/kg or 0.5 mg/kg. Ketamine appears to act centrally by stimulating the sympathetic system, rather than by a peripheral mechanism such as inhibition of the baroreceptor reflex.

TABLE 15-1. Cardiovascular effects of ketamine.

Hemodynamic variable	Effect of ketamine
Mean blood pressure	Up to 35% increase
Heart rate	Up to 60% increase
Cardiac output	Up to 50% increase
Systemic vascular resistance	Up to 35% increase
Pulmonary artery pressure	Up to 50% increase
Right atrial pressure	Up to 35% increase
Pulmonary artery occlusion ("wedge") pressure	No change
Left ventricular stroke work index	Up to 30% increase

However, a repeated dose of ketamine often produces a less pronounced or even opposite effect. This may be because of its direct myocardial depressant action, as evidenced by some in vitro studies. This phenomenon is not typically seen clinically unless the patient is completely depleted of catecholamines, as the sympathetic stimulation overrides any direct negative inotropic effect.

These cardiovascular stimulatory effects result in increased myocardial work, which may not be well tolerated in patients with severe coronary atherosclerotic disease.

Ref: Miller RD. *Miller's Anesthesia*. 8th ed. Philadelphia, PA: Elsevier; 2015.

7. A 68-year-old woman with mild pulmonary hypertension receives intravenous ketamine 2 mg/kg. Which of the following best describes the expected cardiovascular response?

  (A) a decrease in myocardial oxygen consumption
  (B) **an increase in pulmonary vascular resistance**
  (C) a decrease in the heart rate
  (D) a decrease in pulmonary vascular resistance
  (E) a decrease in contractility

This patient would be expected to exhibit all of the usual hemodynamic responses to ketamine listed in Table 15-1. In addition, patients with preexisting pulmonary arterial hypertension are thought to exhibit an exaggerated increase in pulmonary artery pressure, which, if severe enough, may precipitate acute right ventricular failure. Most textbooks recommend against using ketamine in this population for this reason. However, these recommendations have largely been made on the basis of older case reports and series. In particular, children may fare better than adults. A recent retrospective analysis of 68 children with pulmonary hypertension undergoing a variety of procedures using ketamine as the anesthetic agent showed that the drug could be used safely with no complications.

Refs: Miller RD. *Miller's Anesthesia*. 8th ed. Philadelphia, PA: Elsevier; 2015.
Williams GD, et al. Perioperative complications in children with pulmonary hypertension undergoing general anesthesia with ketamine. *Paediatric Anaesth*. 2010;20:28–37.

8. The cardiovascular stimulatory effects of ketamine can best be blunted by the pre-administration of:

  (A) vasopressin
  (B) **midazolam**
  (C) neostigmine
  (D) ondansetron
  (E) fenoldopam

Increases in blood pressure, heart rate, and other hemodynamic parameters can be mitigated with the use of vasoactive medications such as alpha- and beta-blockers, nitrates, and/or clonidine. These are often difficult to precisely titrate in relation to the cardiovascular effect of ketamine, especially for those drugs with a longer duration of action. Other anesthetic agents, either intravenous or inhaled, tend to blunt the hemodynamic effect of ketamine as well. Another strategy to avoid the increased myocardial workload is to deliver ketamine as an infusion instead of a bolus (if appropriate).

Interestingly, benzodiazepines may be the most effective and practical means to balance these cardiovascular effects. Judicious doses of either midazolam and diazepam have the effect of blunting the hypertension and tachycardia associated with ketamine induction.

Ref: Miller RD. *Miller's Anesthesia*. 8th ed. Philadelphia, PA: Elsevier; 2015.

9. A 20-year-old male patient receives 1.5 mg/kg of intravenous ketamine. Which of the following best describes the expected respiratory effect?

  (A) a decrease in respiratory rate only
  (B) a decrease in tidal volume only
  (C) a decrease in respiratory rate with an increase in tidal volume
  (D) an increase in respiratory rate with a decrease in tidal volume
  (E) **no change in respiratory rate or tidal volume**

One of the reasons for ketamine's continued popularity as an anesthetic and sedative agent is the fact that is has virtually no effect on ventilatory drive. This is true in adult patients with normal pulmonary physiology as well as in those with COPD. High-induction bolus doses (>2 mg/kg IV) may produce a transient (1–3 minutes) decrease in minute ventilation, but in general it is a useful analgesic and sedative agent in cases where hypercarbia from respiratory depression would be dangerous or undesirable.

Ketamine's effect on the ventilatory drive in children is similar to that in adults, and it is used extensively for procedural sedation in children in the emergency room setting, particularly because of its predictable effect with a wide safety margin following intramuscular injection.

Refs: Longnecker DE, Brown DL, Newman MF, Zapol WM. *Anesthesiology.* 2nd ed. New York, NY: McGraw Hill; 2012.

10. Ketamine would most likely be helpful in the treatment of which of the following respiratory conditions?

(A) status asthmaticus

(B) laryngospasm

(C) pulmonary hypertension

(D) bronchiectasis

(E) atelectasis

Ketamine is a potent bronchial smooth muscle relaxant. Isolated smooth muscle preparations demonstrate relaxation in the presence of ketamine, indicating that the decrease in bronchial tone is at least partially due to a direct effect rather than solely to an indirect sympathetic effect. Ketamine is useful in the induction of patients who are actively bronchospastic and those who have severe "brittle" reactive airways disease. It is occasionally used to treat status asthmaticus unresponsive to conventional therapy due to its bronchodilating action.

One of the undesired side effects of ketamine is salivation. If left untreated, this may provoke laryngospasm. Pretreatment with an antisialagogue such as glycopyrrolate typically ameliorates this effect.

Refs: Miller RD. *Miller's Anesthesia.* 8th ed. Philadelphia, PA: Elsevier; 2015.
Longnecker DE, Brown DL, Newman MF, Zapol WM. *Anesthesiology.* 2nd ed. New York, NY: McGraw Hill; 2012.

11. Which of the following effects on the central nervous system would be most likely to result from an induction dose of ketamine?

(A) a decrease in $CMRO_2$

(B) an increase in theta wave activity

(C) a decrease in cerebral blood flow

(D) an attenuation of the cerebrovascular response to carbon dioxide

(E) a decrease in intracranial pressure

Ketamine is a different anesthetic agent in several respects. While most intravenous anesthetics exert their effect by the inhibition of GABA channels, ketamine blocks the NMDA receptor. This results in a "dissociative" state where patients may move, vocalize, and track movement with their eyes, demonstrate corneal and cough reflexes, and yet do not respond to pain or have explicit recall.

Most intravenous agents decrease $CMRO_2$, cerebral blood flow, and intracranial pressure; in contrast, ketamine causes *increases* in all three of these variables. Ketamine is therefore a poor choice for patients with a noncompliant intracranial compartment, such as those with space-occupying lesions or recent head trauma. However, ketamine has little effect on the cerebrovascular response to carbon dioxide. Therefore, the increases in cerebral volume and pressure caused by ketamine can be mitigated to a certain extent by reducing $PaCO_2$ through hyperventilation.

Ketamine produces EEG changes that are again different from other intravenous anesthetics. Monitors of the depth of anesthesia that rely on EEG recordings are therefore unreliable during ketamine anesthesia. Light anesthesia with ketamine produces beta waves, whereas deep anesthesia (i.e., that depth associated with analgesia) is marked predominantly by theta wave activity. Even profound ketamine anesthesia does not produce an isoelectric EEG.

Ref: Longnecker DE, Brown DL, Newman MF, Zapol WM. *Anesthesiology.* 2nd ed. New York, NY: McGraw Hill; 2012.

12. Which of the following factors increases the risk for emergence reactions related to ketamine anesthesia?

(A) playing music during anesthesia

(B) age under 18 years

(C) low dose of ketamine

(D) female sex

(E) pretreatment with benzodiazepines

An emergence reaction is an undesirable psychological experience occurring during awakening from anesthesia. Patients that have emergence reactions report a variety of manifestations including vivid dreaming, "out-of-body" feelings, and hallucinations. Fear, excitement, and confusion are commonly associated with the hallucinations. These typically occur within the first hour after awakening, and rarely persist longer than 2–3 hours. The cause of emergence reactions is unclear, but may be related to ketamine-induced depression of auditory and visual pathways in the brain, resulting in "misinterpretation" of stimuli. When ketamine is used as a sole technique, or is a major part of the anesthetic, the incidence may be as high as 30%.

Several factors have been shown to increase the incidence of emergence reactions. These include female sex, adult (vs. pediatric) patients, and large and/or rapidly administered doses of ketamine. Patients who dream frequently at home may also be at higher risk for vivid dreaming after ketamine anesthesia. Playing music during anesthesia has been postulated by some to increase the incidence due to a possible pro-hallucinatory effect, but this has been disproven.

Benzodiazepines (including midazolam, lorazepam, and diazepam) are very effective at reducing the incidence of emergence reactions following ketamine.

Ref: Miller RD. *Miller's Anesthesia*. 8th ed. Philadelphia, PA: Elsevier; 2015.

13. An 8-year-old child receives 2 mg/kg of ketamine intravenously. The factor that most likely places her at risk for laryngospasm is:

(A) an absence of protective reflexes

(B) excessive salivation

(C) an insufficient induction dose

(D) apnea due to an excessive dose

(E) increased bulbar muscle spasticity

One of the attractive properties of ketamine is the relative preservation of the protective reflexes, such as the swallow, cough, sneeze, and gag reflexes. In addition, ketamine used in routine doses does not typically depress the ventilatory drive. However, ketamine is known to promote salivation, especially in children, and these excessive secretions can lead to outright upper airway obstruction in addition to laryngospasm. This may be particularly true for the child who is recovering from an upper respiratory tract infection. This is not just a pediatric problem; many adults who are receiving even modest doses of ketamine for pain as part of their multimodal analgesic plan are "juicy" during anesthesia or sedation, which can lead to coughing, laryngospasm, or other airway issues. For this reason, many anesthesiologists co-administer an antisialagogue such as atropine or glycopyrrolate when using ketamine.

Ref: Miller RD. *Miller's Anesthesia*. 8th ed. Philadelphia, PA: Elsevier; 2015.

14. In which of the following patients would ketamine be most indicated?

(A) a 21-year-old with an open eye injury

(B) a 35-year-old with a closed head injury

(C) a 59-year-old with a gunshot wound to the abdomen

(D) a 60-year-old with a history of coronary artery disease

(E) a 72-year-old with an abdominal aortic aneurysm

Ketamine is usually not a first-line induction agent for routine, elective cases. However, the classical teaching has been that there are several specific circumstances in which a ketamine induction may be desirable. The severely hypovolemic, hypotensive patient (e.g., one who is exsanguinating) is one example, since the sympathomimetic effect of ketamine will help maintain blood pressure and cardiac output pending resuscitation. The other classic example is the patient with severe acute bronchospasm (see question 10), since the adrenergic release will aid in bronchodilation.

On the other hand, there are reasons to consider avoiding ketamine. Since the drug is known to increase intraocular pressure, patients with open eye injuries or acute angle glaucoma are generally poor candidates for ketamine. Similarly, patients with reduced intracranial compliance may not tolerate the increase in intracranial pressure, and ketamine should be used with caution, if at all, in these patients. Patients who will not tolerate a sudden increase in blood pressure or left ventricular work (e.g., those with aortic aneurysmal disease or coronary atherosclerotic disease) may be better served by induction with another agent.

Ref: Longnecker DE, Brown DL, Newman MF, Zapol WM. *Anesthesiology*. 2nd ed. New York, NY: McGraw Hill; 2012.

15. During acute pericardial tamponade, which of the following best describes the physiologic rationale for the use of ketamine as an induction agent?

(A) a reduction in left ventricular stroke volume

(B) a decrease in pulmonary vascular resistance

(C) a reduction in systemic vascular resistance

(D) an increase in right atrial pressure

(E) an increase in contractility

During acute pericardial tamponade, the key problem is restriction of cardiac chamber size during diastole due to the expansion of the pericardial sac. This is especially true of the more compliant, thin-walled right heart. This restriction limits the right-sided stroke volume, which effectively lowers overall cardiac output. The goals of anesthetic management during tamponade are to maintain the preload as much as possible, and to promote the ejection of whatever stroke volume is in the ventricles. This gives rise to the phrase "fast, full, and forward"—a rapid heart rate and full preload will give the cardiac output a fighting chance until the pressure can be relieved. Bradycardia and a low CVP are not well tolerated in these circumstances.

Since ketamine accelerates heart rate and maintains or increases right atrial pressure (see Table 15-1), this makes it an ideal agent for providing analgesia and/or anesthesia during emergent decompression of the pericardium either via a pericardial window or with a needle. A further advantage is that ketamine typically preserves spontaneous respiration, which may obviate the need for positive pressure ventilation and its associated deleterious effect on right ventricular preload.

Bear in mind that with *in vitro* animal heart models, ketamine does not have the same stimulatory effect as in the intact patient. This has led some to question its efficacy in the setting of a patient whose catecholamine stores are depleted due to stress, shock, or sepsis, since ketamine relies on the indirect release of these adrenergic compounds. On the other hand, ketamine is still the least cardiodepressant of all the induction agents in these heart models. The point to take home here is that ketamine alone is not a replacement for appropriate resuscitation with fluids and judicious use of vasoactive medications in the critically ill patient.

Ref: Miller RD. *Miller's Anesthesia.* 8th ed. Philadelphia, PA: Elsevier; 2015.

16. At which of following locations is ketamine postulated to exert its antihyperalgesic or antiallodynic effects?

(A) the peripheral nervous system

(B) the dorsal horn of the spinal cord

(C) the frontal cortex

(D) the medullary reticular formation

(E) the thalamoneocortical projection system

Ketamine is a potent analgesic agent, and has enjoyed a renaissance for its proven effect of reducing both postoperative pain scores and the amount of postoperative opioids that patients consume, while extending the time until first request of analgesia. It turns out that not a lot of ketamine is required to exert a beneficial effect: many authors recommend a bolus dose of 0.25–0.5 mg/kg at the beginning of the procedure. Some protocols call for an infusion of ketamine throughout the case, especially in patients with preexisting chronic pain or during certain procedures (e.g., spine surgery).

Persistent afferent nociceptive input to the spinal cord results in activation and upregulation of NMDA receptors in the dorsal horn. This promotes the enhanced and amplified transmission of pain signals to the brain, an effect known as central sensitization or "windup." As an NMDA receptor blocker, ketamine stops the excessive barrage of nociceptive input and helps prevent windup from occurring. There is a positive feedback loop that exists in the dorsal horn in the setting of neuropathic pain states whereby more afferent input leads to more recruitment of wide dynamic range neurons, which amplifies the pain signal, resulting in even more recruitment. The attenuation of this cycle and the consequent reduction in the development of hyperalgesia helps explain why the analgesic effect of ketamine far outlasts its pharmacologic duration of action in the body.

Ref: Longnecker DE, Brown DL, Newman MF, Zapol WM. *Anesthesiology.* 2nd ed. New York, NY: McGraw Hill; 2012.

CHAPTER 16

Local Anesthetics

1. For which one of the following sodium channel conformational states do local anesthetics have the MOST affinity?

    (A) rest
    (B) closed intermediate
    (C) open
    (D) inactivated

2. Which of the following local anesthetic factors has the MOST effect on speed of onset of neural blockade?

    (A) pKa
    (B) baricity
    (C) protein binding
    (D) presence of an ester-linkage
    (E) volume of distribution

3. Which of the following represents the correct order of blockade of nerve fibers in response to a peripheral nerve block?

    (A) A∝ → Aβ → Aδ → Aγ → B → C
    (B) C → Aβ → A∝ → Aγ → Aδ → B
    (C) C → Aβ → Aδ → Aγ → B → A∝
    (D) B → Aδ → Aγ → Aβ → A∝ → C
    (E) B → C → A∝ → Aβ → Aδ → Aγ

4. For a given dose of local anesthetic, which of the following routes of administration would result in the highest plasma level of the drug?

    (A) intercostal
    (B) epidural
    (C) brachial plexus
    (D) subcutaneous
    (E) sciatic

5. Which of the following best describes the route of elimination for spinal lidocaine?

    (A) excreted unchanged in the urine
    (B) spontaneous breakdown of the drug in the CSF
    (C) biotransformation by spinal cord glial cells
    (D) metabolism by plasma cholinesterase
    (E) hepatic oxidative metabolism

6. Which of the following is the principal blood protein that binds local anesthetics?

    (A) albumin
    (B) lipoprotein
    (C) gamma globulin
    (D) $\alpha 1$-acid glycoprotein
    (E) C-reactive protein

7. Which of the following accounts for the relatively rapid plasma clearance of chloroprocaine?

    (A) The presence of an amide group
    (B) The presence of a butyl group
    (C) The presence of a carbonyl group
    (D) The presence of an ester group
    (E) The presence of a hydroxyl group

8. Which of the following drugs is synthesized specifically as a single enantiomer?

    (A) benzocaine
    (B) lidocaine
    (C) procaine
    (D) ropivacaine
    (E) tetracaine

9. For which of the following local anesthetics will the addition of epinephrine add the LEAST benefit in terms of prolonging the duration of action?

   (A) lidocaine
   (B) mepivacaine
   (C) ropivacaine
   (D) bupivacaine
   (E) chloroprocaine

10. Which of the following additives to the local anesthetic solution is not associated with prolongation of the sensory block?

    (A) epinephrine
    (B) corticosteroids
    (C) clonidine
    (D) phenylephrine
    (E) bicarbonate

11. Which of the following factors is NOT associated with increased risk for seizures following injection of local anesthetic into the axillary brachial plexus?

    (A) Increased potency of the local anesthetic
    (B) Increased rate of injection
    (C) Elevated $PaCO_2$
    (D) The use of an ester-linked local anesthetic (compared with amide-linked)
    (E) Decreased arterial pH

12. Which of the following presenting signs/symptoms is most common during central nervous system toxicity from local anesthetics?

    (A) dizziness
    (B) agitation
    (C) perioral numbness
    (D) tinnitus
    (E) seizures

13. Which of the following is a characteristic clinical finding with transient neurologic symptoms (TNS) following spinal anesthesia?

    (A) paresthesias
    (B) motor weakness
    (C) posterior thigh pain
    (D) numbness
    (E) prompt onset upon resolution of the spinal block

14. Which of the following factors is MOST associated with an increased risk of developing transient neurologic symptoms following a spinal anesthetic?

    (A) BMI <20 kg/m²
    (B) high concentration of local anesthetic
    (C) use of hyperbaric solutions
    (D) surgery in the lithotomy position
    (E) use of chloroprocaine

15. Cauda equina syndrome following neuraxial anesthesia is associated with which of the following risk factors?

    (A) small-gauge spinal catheters
    (B) lidocaine spinal anesthesia
    (C) lithotomy position
    (D) pencil-point needles
    (E) obesity

16. What is the approximate ratio of the dose of lidocaine required to cause irreversible cardiac collapse compared to seizures?

    (A) 1:1
    (B) 2:1
    (C) 3:1
    (D) 5:1
    (E) 7:1

17. Systemic hypotension after an inadvertent large dose of bupivacaine is MOST likely to result from which of the following mechanisms?

    (A) myocardial depression
    (B) cardiac conduction system blockade
    (C) autonomic nervous system blockade
    (D) arterial vasodilation
    (E) venodilation and preload reduction

18. Which one of the following local anesthetics is MOST likely to cause a true allergic reaction?

   (A) bupivacaine
   (B) chloroprocaine
   (C) lidocaine
   (D) mepivacaine
   (E) ropivacaine

19. You are selecting a solution to use for a femoral block in a patient undergoing an ACL repair. Which of the following is NOT an appropriate additive for use in local anesthetic solutions?

   (A) sodium bisulfite
   (B) methylparaben
   (C) glucose
   (D) phenol
   (E) phenylephrine

20. Which of the following local anesthetic drugs is NOT associated with methemoglobinemia?

   (A) benzocaine
   (B) bupivacaine
   (C) lidocaine
   (D) prilocaine
   (E) tetracaine

21. Treatment of symptomatic methemoglobinemia is best achieved with which one of the following?

   (A) indocyanine green
   (B) indigo carmine
   (C) vitamin C
   (D) methylene blue
   (E) 100% oxygen

22. You have just completed a brachial plexus block in the preoperative area for a patient undergoing fixation of a wrist fracture. Suddenly, the monitor begins to alarm, and you note that there are multiple short runs of ventricular tachycardia, and what appears to be QRS widening. The blood pressure is 82/46 mm Hg. The patient reports feeling dizzy and unwell. Which of the following is the BEST initial treatment option?

   (A) Amiodarone 150 mg IV slow push
   (B) Lidocaine 1 mg/kg IV
   (C) Lipid emulsion 20% 1.5 mL/kg bolus
   (D) Immediate synchronized DC cardioversion
   (E) Vasopressin 40 units IV

Answers and Explanations: Local Anesthetics

1. For which one of the following sodium channel conformational states do local anesthetics have the MOST affinity?

   (A) rest
   (B) closed intermediate
   (C) open
   (D) inactivated

   According to the modulated receptor hypothesis, sodium channels respond to membrane depolarization by undergoing a series of conformational changes in their physical state (Figure 16-1). Each receptor is composed of an α-subunit and two β-subunits. The cycle begins at rest, with none of the four domains on the alpha-subunit activated. Once each of these change shape in sequence (closed intermediate stage), the sodium channel is activated (open stage), allowing sodium ions to enter the cell. Several milliseconds later, the channel becomes inactivated by yet another conformational change (inactivated stage), after which no further sodium ions can pass through.

   Local anesthetics bind to amino acid residue within the sodium channel receptors in the open state with high affinity. In contrast, the affinity for the sodium channel in the inactivated state is relatively low; there is weak binding at the closed state. Many studies have shown that the rate of blockade of nerve impulse propagation is dependent on the rate of depolarization. In other words, the more rapidly the nerve is firing, the more frequently the sodium channels will exist in an open state momentarily, and the faster the onset of the block. This has been termed "use-dependent blockade."

   Ref: Hadzic A. *NYSORA Textbook of Regional Anesthesia and Acute Pain Medicine.* 1st ed. New York, NY: McGraw Hill; 2007.

2. Which of the following local anesthetic factors has the MOST effect on speed of onset of neural blockade?

   (A) pKa
   (B) baricity
   (C) protein binding
   (D) presence of an ester-linkage
   (E) volume of distribution

   Local anesthetics are weak bases. As such, the higher the pKa, the greater the proportion of the drug that exists in its free base (unionized) state compared to the charged cationic (ionized) state. Uncharged local anesthetic salts diffuse more easily across lipid bilayers, increasing the mass of the drug inside the axon.

   Most local anesthetics have a pKa between 7 and 9 (Table 16-1). The closer the pKa to physiologic pH, the more drug will exist in an uncharged state, and (in general) the faster the onset.

   TABLE 16-1. Commonly used local anesthetics and their physicochemical properties.

Local anesthetic	pKa	Lipid solubility	Protein binding
Mepivacaine	7.7	0.8	75%
Lidocaine	7.8	2.9	70%
Ropivacaine	8.1	2.8	94%
Bupivacaine	8.1	28	96%
Tetracaine	8.4	12	76%
Chloroprocaine	9.1	2.3	N/A

   Lipid solubility also plays a role in the speed of onset, as highly lipophilic local anesthetics cross the membrane more easily than hydrophilic ones do, and are therefore more potent (i.e., less drug is required to cause blockade). In addition, mass of the drug (i.e., the number of molecules) is important; this is why, despite a higher pKa, 20 mL of 3% chloroprocaine has a similar onset (or even a slight speed advantage) when

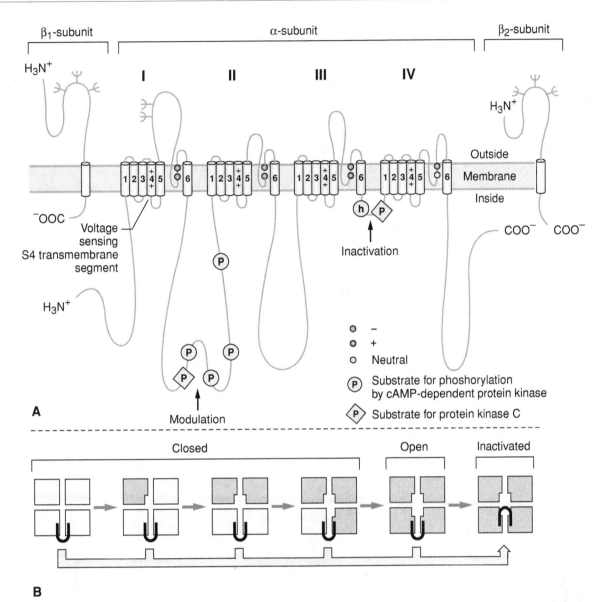

FIG. 16-1. Structure and function of voltage-gated Na+ channels. **A.** A 2-dimensional representation of the α (center), β₁ (left), and β₂ (right) subunits of the voltage-gated Na+ channel from mammalian brain. The polypeptide chains are represented by continuous lines with length approximately proportional to the actual length of each segment of the channel protein. Cylinders represent regions of transmembrane α helices. Ψ indicates sites of demonstrated *N*-linked glycosylation. Note the repeated structure of the 4 homologous domains (I through IV) of the α-subunit. Voltage sensing: The S4 transmembrane segments in each homologous domain of the α-subunit serve as voltage sensors. (+) Represents the positively charged amino acid residues at every third position within these segments. An electrical field (negative inside) exerts a force on these charged amino acid residues, pulling them toward the intracellular side of the membrane. Pore: The S5 and S6 transmembrane segments and the short membrane-associated loops between them (segments SS1 and SS2) form the walls of the pore in the center of an approximately symmetrical square array of the 4 homologous domains (see *B*). The amino acid residues indicated by circles in segment SS2 are critical for determining the conductance and ion selectivity of the Na+ channel and its ability to bind the extracellular pore blocking toxins tetrodotoxin and saxitoxin. Inactivation: The short intracellular loop connecting homologous domains III and IV serves as the inactivation gate of the Na+ channel. It is thought to fold into the intracellular mouth of the pore and occlude it within a few milliseconds after the channel opens. Three hydrophobic residues (isoleucine–phenylalanine–methionine [IFM]) at the position marked *H* appear to serve as an inactivation particle, entering the intracellular mouth of the pore and binding to an inactivation gate receptor there. Modulation: The gating of the Na+ channel can be modulated by protein phosphorylation. Phosphorylation of the inactivation gate between homologous domains III and IV by protein kinase C slows inactivation. Phosphorylation of sites in the intracellular loop between homologous domains I and II by either protein kinase C ◇P or cyclic adenosine monophosphate (AMP)–dependent protein kinase ⓟ reduces Na+ channel activation. **B.** The 4 homologous domains of the Na+ channel α-subunit are illustrated as a square array as viewed looking down on the membrane. The sequence of conformational changes that the Na+ channel undergoes during activation and inactivation is diagrammed. Upon depolarization, each of the 4 homologous domains undergoes a conformational change in sequence to an activated state. After all 4 domains have activated, the Na+ channel can open. Within a few milliseconds after opening, the inactivation gate between domains III and IV closes over the intracellular mouth of the channel and occludes it, preventing further ion conductance. (Reproduced with permission from Catterall W, Mackie K. Local anesthetics. In: Hardman JG, Limbird LE, Gilman AF, eds. Goodman and Gilman's *The Pharmacological Basis of Therapeutics* 10th edition. New York: McGraw-Hill, 2001:370.)

injected in the epidural space compared to 20 mL of 2% lidocaine. This dose of chloroprocaine simply contains more moles of the drug: 2.2 mM compared to 1.7 for lidocaine. Finally, protein binding does not affect onset of the block. A common misconception is that protein binding influences the duration of the block. This is incorrect, although there is an association: lipid-soluble drugs are more highly protein bound by nature. It is the lipid solubility that prevents lipophilic drugs from diffusing away from lipid rich environments such as the lipid bilayer of a nerve.

Ref: Hadzic A. *NYSORA Textbook of Regional Anesthesia and Acute Pain Medicine.* 1st ed. New York, NY: McGraw Hill; 2007.

3. Which of the following represents the correct order of blockade of nerve fibers in response to a peripheral nerve block?

(A) Aα → Aβ → Aδ → Aγ → B → C
(B) C → Aβ → Aα → Aγ → Aδ → B
(C) C → Aβ → Aδ → Aγ → B → Aα
(D) B → Aδ → Aγ → Aβ → Aα → C
(E) B → C → Aα → Aβ → Aδ → Aγ

Nerve fibers are classified into three major categories: myelinated somatic fibers (A-fibers), myelinated preganglionic autonomic fibers (B-fibers), and nonmyelinated fibers (C-fibers). In general, B- and C-fibers are relatively small (<1–2 µm in diameter), whereas

A-fibers vary between 4 and 20 µm. A-fibers are further subdivided based on diameter and conduction velocity. Each type of fiber plays a specific role in propagating impulses. Aα are motor afferents, Aβ transmit sensation of touch and pressure, Aδ are responsible for conducting fast pain impulses as well as temperature and touch, and Aγ are muscle spindle efferents. C-fibers subserve pain and temperature and have a much slower conduction velocity (and are therefore responsible for so-called "slow pain" transmission).

Two general rules apply regarding susceptibility of nerve fibers to local anesthetics (Figure 16-2). First, smaller nerves are more easily blocked than larger nerves because a shorter length of the axon is required to be blocked to halt the conduction completely. Second, myelinated fibers are more easily blocked than nonmyelinated fibers. This is because in the presence of the fatty, insulating myelin sheath, local anesthetic tends to be concentrated near the axonal membrane at the nodes, rather than being spread thinly along the length of the fiber. This explains why C-fibers, which are quite small, are more resistant to local anesthetic blockade than larger, but myelinated, fibers. This can be observed clinically when a patient reports no sharp pain in response to a pinprick (A-delta fibers), yet groans in pain when the surgeon manipulates the broken wrist during skin prep due to delayed blockade of slow-pain C-fibers.

Ref: Hadzic A. *NYSORA Textbook of Regional Anesthesia and Acute Pain Medicine.* 1st ed. New York, NY: McGraw Hill; 2007.

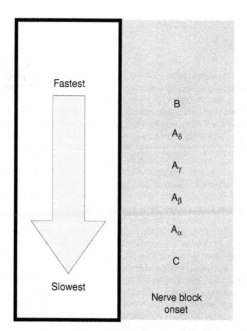
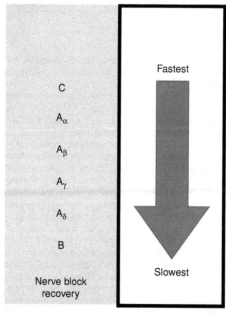

FIG. 16-2. Differential rate of nerve blockade. (Reproduced with permission from Hadzic A. *Hadzic's Peripheral Nerve Blocks and Anatomy for Ultrasound Guided Regional Anesthesia.* 2nd ed. New York, NY: McGraw Hill; 2012.)

4. For a given dose of local anesthetic, which of the following routes of administration would result in the highest plasma level of the drug?

(A) **intercostal**
(B) epidural
(C) brachial plexus
(D) subcutaneous
(E) sciatic

The plasma concentration of local anesthetic following injection depends on several factors, including tissue vascularity, the presence of fat that can bind local anesthetic, and the use of vasoconstrictors. Several studies have confirmed that, independent of the local anesthetic used, intercostal deposition results in the largest Cmax, followed, in order, by caudal, epidural, brachial plexus, and sciatic and femoral block. This is likely the result of the presence of rich intercostal vascularity as well as a large surface area over which the local anesthetic spreads. These factors combined lead to a rapid rise in plasma concentrations.

Ref: Hadzic A. *NYSORA Textbook of Regional Anesthesia and Acute Pain Medicine.* 1st ed. New York, NY: McGraw Hill; 2007.

5. Which of the following best describes the route of elimination for spinal lidocaine?

(A) excreted unchanged in the urine
(B) spontaneous breakdown of the drug in the CSF
(C) biotransformation by spinal cord glial cells
(D) metabolism by plasma cholinesterase
(E) **hepatic oxidative metabolism**

As a member of the amide group, lidocaine is primarily metabolized by the liver. The metabolic pathways and intermediates for each amide vary. Lidocaine is dealkylated in the liver to monoethylglycine-xylide (MEGX), which is an active metabolite that is equipotent for seizures. MEGX is then further dealkylated to the inactive metabolite glycine-xylide (GX).

Renal excretion of unchanged local anesthetics is a very minor contributor to clearance, representing less than 5% of the total dose. There is no role for biotransformation of amide local anesthetics in the CSF, spinal cord, or plasma. As such, spinally administered amide local anesthetics must first be absorbed systemically and extracted by the liver prior to metabolism.

Ref: Hadzic A. *NYSORA Textbook of Regional Anesthesia and Acute Pain Medicine.* 1st ed. New York, NY: McGraw Hill; 2007.

6. Which of the following is the principal blood protein that binds local anesthetics?

(A) albumin
(B) lipoprotein
(C) gamma globulin
(D) **α1-acid glycoprotein**
(E) C-reactive protein

As weak bases, local anesthetics are highly protein bound to α_1-acid glycoprotein (AAG). This plasma protein is an acute phase reactant, and is upregulated during periods of stress and inflammation, as well as during uremia. Conversely, levels of AAG decrease in pregnancy, newborns, and in those with liver disease, resulting in the potential for an increased free fraction of local anesthetic. This is likely to be of little clinical significance for the single-injection peripheral nerve block; however, continuous epidural or perineural techniques may place these patients at risk for systemic toxicity due to accumulation of drug and decreased hepatic metabolism.

Ref: Hadzic A. *NYSORA Textbook of Regional Anesthesia and Acute Pain Medicine.* 1st ed. New York, NY: McGraw Hill; 2007.

7. Which of the following accounts for the relatively rapid plasma clearance of chloroprocaine?

(A) The presence of an amide group
(B) The presence of a butyl group
(C) The presence of a carbonyl group
(D) **The presence of an ester group**
(E) The presence of a hydroxyl group

All local anesthetics contain hydrophilic and hydrophobic domains separated by an intermediate chain of either the ester type or the amide type. This linkage gives name to the two principal types of local anesthetics, the esters and the amides. Procaine is considered the original synthetic ester-linked local anesthetic, while lidocaine is the prototypical amide (Figure 16-3). The ester linkage is rapidly hydrolyzed by plasma cholinesterase (also known as pseudocholinesterase or butyrylcholinesterase) and liver esterases. This accounts for its rapid clearance almost immediately after the drug is absorbed into the bloodstream. For example,

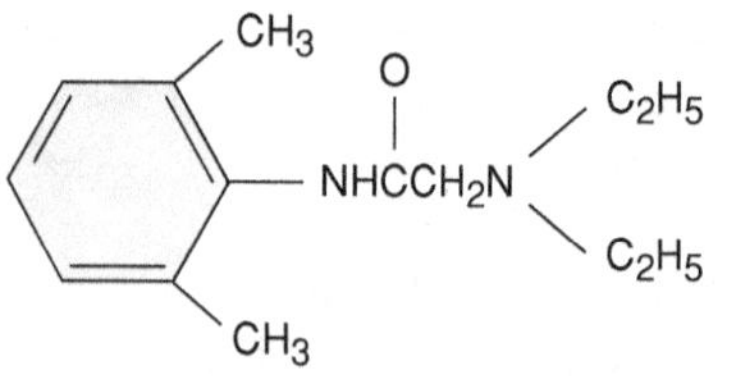

Lidocaine

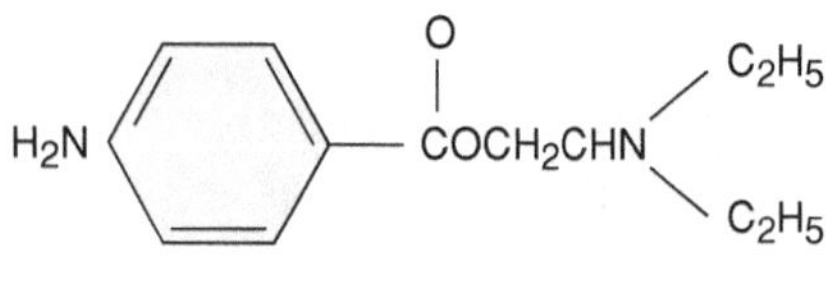

Procaine

FIG. 16-3. Structure of lidocaine and procaine. (Reproduced with permission from Longnecker DE, Brown DL, Newman MF, Zapol WM. *Anesthesiology*. 2nd ed. New York, NY: McGraw Hill; 2012.)

the *in vitro* half-life of procaine is approximately 40 seconds in healthy individuals. Chloroprocaine is metabolized even faster (*in vitro* half-life of approximately 20 seconds). The clearance of ester-linked local anesthetics is prolonged in those with severe hepatic disease, homozygotes for atypical plasma cholinesterase, and neonates (plasma cholinesterase activity is ~50% in the neonate and does not reach adult values until approximately 1 year of age).

Ref: Hadzic A. *NYSORA Textbook of Regional Anesthesia and Acute Pain Medicine*. 1st ed. New York, NY: McGraw Hill; 2007.

8. Which of the following drugs is synthesized specifically as a single enantiomer?

(A) benzocaine
(B) lidocaine
(C) procaine
(D) ropivacaine
(E) tetracaine

The pipecoloxylidides are a group of local anesthetics that include mepivacaine, bupivacaine, and ropivacaine. All of these are chiral drugs because they contain an asymmetric carbon atom and have a left-handed and right-handed configuration. Both mepivacaine and bupivacaine are prepared as racemic mixtures containing equal proportions of both S- and R-forms, whereas ropivacaine is manufactured as a pure S-enantiomer (Figure 16-4). Receptors (such as those found on the sodium channel) are stereospecific, meaning that half of the racemic dose administered is not contributing to the

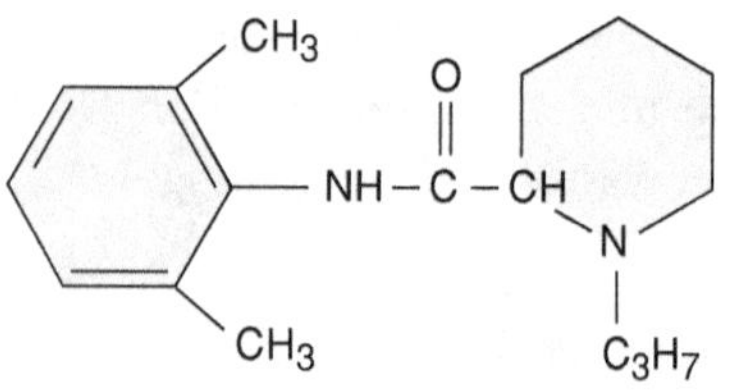

S-Ropivacaine

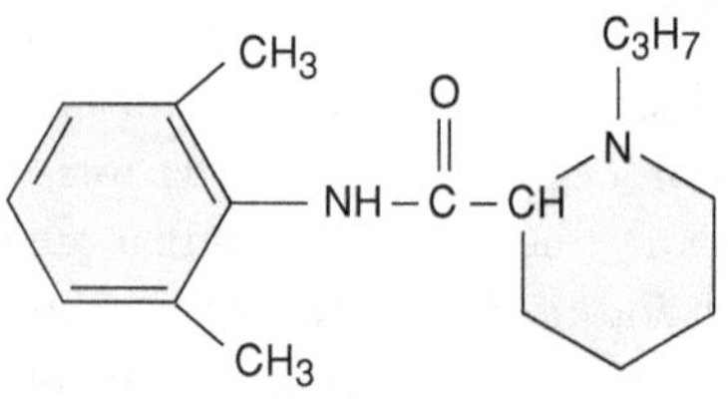

R-Ropivacaine

FIG. 16-4. Clinical forms of ropivacaine. The only difference between the S- and R-isomers is their spatial orientation. (Reproduced with permission from Longnecker DE, Brown DL, Newman MF, Zapol WM. *Anesthesiology*. 2nd ed. New York, NY: McGraw Hill; 2012.)

clinical effect. In fact, these "other" enantiomers may have negative or toxic effects on other membrane channel receptors. As such, the advantage of a pure stereoisomeric preparation of ropivacaine is a higher threshold for cardiotoxicity and central nervous system toxicity than the racemic mixture. Similarly, the intravascular dose of levo-bupivacaine required to cause lethality in animals is higher than racemic bupivacaine.

Ref: Longnecker DE, Brown DL, Newman MF, Zapol WM. *Anesthesiology*. 2nd ed. New York, NY: McGraw Hill; 2012.

9. For which of the following local anesthetics will the addition of epinephrine add the LEAST benefit in terms of prolonging the duration of action?

(A) lidocaine
(B) mepivacaine
(C) ropivacaine
(D) bupivacaine
(E) chloroprocaine

The duration of neural block depends on the physical characteristics of the local anesthetic and the presence or absence of vasoconstrictors. The most important physical characteristic is lipid solubility; the more lipophilic the agent, the longer it will remain in a lipid-rich environment such as the neurolemma, and the less rapidly it will be uptaken by the vasculature. In general, local anesthetics can be divided into three categories: short-acting (e.g., 2-chloroprocaine, 45–90 minutes), intermediate duration (e.g., lidocaine, mepivacaine, 90–180 minutes), and long-acting (e.g., bupivacaine, levobupivacaine, ropivacaine, 4–18 hours).

Vasoconstrictors are thought to decrease local blood flow to the block area and reduce the uptake and redistribution of the local anesthetic, thereby prolonging the block duration. The degree of block prolongation with the addition of a vasoconstrictor appears to be related to the intrinsic vasodilatory properties of the local anesthetic; the more intrinsic vasodilatory action the local anesthetic has, the more prolongation is achieved with addition of a vasoconstrictor. For example, lidocaine is a potent vasodilator, and the addition of an adrenergic agonist such as epinephrine has a significant effect on the block prolongation. Chloroprocaine and mepivacaine behave in a manner similar to lidocaine. Bupivacaine is a mild vasodilator, and epinephrine will add some benefit, although not as much as the short/intermediate-acting drugs. In contrast, ropivacaine and levo-bupivacaine are themselves mild vasoconstrictors, and adding epinephrine will not extend the block duration by the same proportion. Remember that cocaine is the only local anesthetic that has substantial vasoconstrictive properties independent of the dose.

Ref: Hadzic A. *NYSORA Textbook of Regional Anesthesia and Acute Pain Medicine.* 1st ed. New York, NY: McGraw Hill; 2007.

10. Which of the following additives to the local anesthetic solution is not associated with prolongation of the sensory block?

(A) epinephrine

(B) corticosteroids

(C) clonidine

(D) phenylephrine

(E) bicarbonate

Epinephrine and phenylephrine are both α-adrenergic agonists, and promote vasoconstriction at the site of deposition, reducing uptake and prolonging the duration of the block. Clonidine is an α_2-agonist and therefore is not a vasoconstrictor. However, it is known that α-adrenergic receptors are present in the dorsal horn of the spinal cord, and these are thought to be responsible for the prolongation of sensory blockade seen when clonidine is added to the local anesthetic for spinal anesthesia.

Corticosteroids have been shown in multiple models to prolong sensory blockade for peripheral nerve block; the exact mechanism is unclear, but may relate to the suppression of inflammation, blockade of C-fiber transmission, and the suppression of ectopic neural discharges.

Bicarbonate is used to raise the pH of epinephrine-containing solutions of local anesthetics in order to increase the proportion of drug that exists in the unionized form. This has been proposed to increase the speed of block onset, but it does not prolong the duration of the blockade.

Ref: Hadzic A. *NYSORA Textbook of Regional Anesthesia and Acute Pain Medicine.* 1st ed. New York, NY: McGraw Hill; 2007.

11. Which of the following factors is NOT associated with increased risk for seizures following injection of local anesthetic into the axillary brachial plexus?

(A) Increased potency of the local anesthetic

(B) Increased rate of injection

(C) Elevated $PaCO_2$

(D) The use of an ester-linked local anesthetic (compared with amide-linked)

(E) Decreased arterial pH

Ester-linked local anesthetics are inherently safer than amides are with respect to systemic toxicity because they are metabolized by plasma cholinesterase and have a very short plasma half-life compared to the amide group. For example, the plasma half-life of chloroprocaine is several minutes, compared to 3.5 hours for bupivacaine.

The toxic potency of local anesthetics directly mirrors their anesthetic potency. Therefore, bupivacaine is roughly 4 times as potent as lidocaine (think about using 0.5% bupivacaine and 2% lidocaine to achieve surgical anesthesia; since you can use 4 times less bupivacaine to achieve the same motor and sensory block, it is 4 times more potent). Rate of injection has been shown to lower the toxic threshold, highlighting the thought that the rate of rise in the concentration curve of plasma local anesthetics is a more important factor than overall dose is.

Both hypercarbia and acidosis (either respiratory or metabolic) are risk factors for CNS toxicity. Hypercarbia is particularly dangerous because it increases cerebral blood flow and uptake of local anesthetic by the brain. A vicious cycle can occur during CNS toxicity, starting with the onset of a seizure and the production of excess CO_2 due to neuronal and muscular excitatory activity. This vasodilates the cerebral arterial tree, leading to increased delivery of drug to the brain, which prolongs the seizure. Clearly a priority during CNS toxicity is to maintain adequate oxygenation and ventilation. Acidosis decreases the plasma binding of local anesthetics, which leads to more unbound drug available for uptake by the brain (and heart).

Ref: Hadzic A. *NYSORA Textbook of Regional Anesthesia and Acute Pain Medicine.* 1st ed. New York, NY: McGraw Hill; 2007.

12. Which of the following presenting signs/symptoms is most common during central nervous system toxicity from local anesthetics?

    (A) dizziness

    (B) agitation

    (C) perioral numbness

    (D) tinnitus

    (E) **seizures**

The classical teaching regarding clinical presentation of local anesthetic systemic toxicity (LAST) is that with increasing plasma concentrations of drug, there is a corresponding worsening of the clinical profile (Figure 16-5). These start from premonitory signs such as numbness of the tongue and perioral area, metallic taste in the mouth, dizziness, and tinnitus through to muscular twitching, unconsciousness, seizures and finally coma. With further

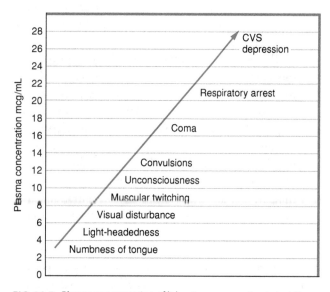

FIG. 16-5. Plasma concentration of lidocaine versus systemic toxicity. CVS, cardiovascular system. (Reproduced with permission from Longnecker DE, Brown DL, Newman MF, Zapol WM. *Anesthesiology.* 2nd ed. New York, NY: McGraw Hill; 2012.)

increases in local anesthetic concentration, respiratory and cardiovascular depression occurs.

However, the clinical presentation is not so straightforward, and the initial presenting sign can in fact be seizures or cardiovascular collapse. In a 2010 review of the previous 30 years worth of reported cases of LAST, 68% of cases with CNS toxicity described seizures as part of the clinical picture. In contrast, only 18% reported dizziness, drowsiness, tinnitus, perioral numbness, confusion, dysphoria, or dysarthria; 11% reported agitation; and 7% reported loss of consciousness.

Ref: Longnecker DE, Brown DL, Newman MF, Zapol WM. *Anesthesiology.* 2nd ed. New York, NY: McGraw Hill; 2012.

13. Which of the following is a characteristic clinical finding with transient neurologic symptoms (TNS) following spinal anesthesia?

    (A) paresthesias

    (B) motor weakness

    (C) **posterior thigh pain**

    (D) numbness

    (E) prompt onset upon resolution of the spinal block

TNS is a syndrome of symptoms that have their onset from within a few hours until approximately 24 hour after a complete recovery from spinal blockade. The cardinal symptom is pain, usually originating in the lower back or gluteal region and often radiating down the posterior thighs. The pain is described as burning, aching, or crampy. The intensity is variable and ranges from barely noticeable to severe (average is 6.2 on a scale of 1 to 10). TNS is not characterized by any neurologic symptoms—in other words, if a patient complains of numbness, paresthesia, weakness, or bowel/bladder dysfunction, the diagnosis of TNS should be excluded and another cause identified. Similarly, investigations such as magnetic resonance imaging and electropathological testing are always normal in patients with TNS. Unlike most neurologic problems arising from neuraxial blockade where pain and/or neurologic symptoms exist upon resolution of the block, TNS is characterized by full recovery from spinal, followed by onset of the symptoms within the next 24 hours.

In general, the syndrome is self-limiting, and most cases disappear after 4 days. NSAIDs are the mainstay of symptomatic treatment, although some patients may require a weak opioid analgesic. In cases where muscle spasm accompanies the pain, a muscle relaxant such as cyclobenzaprine may accelerate recovery. Other therapies include leg elevation, heating pads, TENS, and trigger point injections.

Ref: Cousins MJ, Carr DB, Horlocker TT, Bridenbaugh PO. *Cousins & Bridenbaugh's Neural Blockade in Clinical Anesthesia and Pain Medicine.* 4th ed. Philadelphia, PA: Lippincott Williams & Wilkins; 2009.

14. Which of the following factors is MOST associated with an increased risk of developing transient neurologic symptoms following a spinal anesthetic?

    (A) BMI <20 kg/m^2

    (B) high concentration of local anesthetic

    (C) use of hyperbaric solutions

    (D) **surgery in the lithotomy position**

    (E) use of chloroprocaine

The primary risk factors for the development of TNS include the use of lidocaine and the lithotomy position. Lidocaine is approximately 7 times more likely to cause TNS than is bupivacaine, procaine, or prilocaine. Mepivacaine is less well studied but may carry a higher risk as well, compared to bupivacaine.

Postulated factors that have conflicting evidence but may contribute include ambulatory surgical status, arthroscopic knee surgery, and obesity. Pregnant patients undergoing cesarean delivery under spinal anesthesia have a similar incidence of TNS as non-pregnant patients undergoing surgical procedures in the supine position.

Neither the baricity nor the concentration of the solution appears to play a role in predicting which patients will develop TNS.

Ref: Cousins MJ, Carr DB, Horlocker TT, Bridenbaugh PO. *Cousins & Bridenbaugh's Neural Blockade in Clinical Anesthesia and Pain Medicine.* 4th ed. Philadelphia, PA: Lippincott Williams & Wilkins; 2009.

15. Cauda equina syndrome following neuraxial anesthesia is associated with which of the following risk factors?

    (A) **small-gauge spinal catheters**

    (B) lidocaine spinal anesthesia

    (C) lithotomy position

    (D) pencil-point needles

    (E) obesity

Cauda equina syndrome is an inflammatory lesion of the lumbosacral nerve roots, and has multiple possible etiologies, including trauma, tumors, rheumatologic disease, and spinal stenosis, among others. Features include severe back, thigh, or leg pain (or combinations of the three); numbness/paresthesia of the perineum, bowel, bladder, and/or sexual dysfunction; and weakness and/or numbness of the lower limbs.

Cauda equina syndrome has occurred following neuraxial (especially spinal) anesthesia. Various causes have been proposed, including unintentional intrathecal injection of substances during epidural anesthesia and repeated intrathecal injection after failed spinal block with lidocaine. However, two principal factors have been implicated in recent decades. First, in the late 1980s, clinicians began to use 27- to 32-gauge microcatheters for continuous spinal anesthesia. After a short period, 11 cases of cauda equina syndrome prompted the FDA to remove these devices from the market. The explanation for their culpability was that injection (and perhaps especially infusion or reinjection) of local anesthetics resulted in pooling around a specific area of the intrathecal space, leading to direct toxicity of the nerves. Most of these patients received hyperbaric 5% lidocaine.

The second factor was a series of 8 cases of inadvertent intrathecal injection of large doses of chloroprocaine meant for the epidural space. The neurotoxicity in these cases was attributed to the preservative, sodium bisulfite. Chloroprocaine spinal anesthesia was unpopular for several years until a series of studies using preservative-free chloroprocaine demonstrated that it provided quality anesthesia with no neurologic sequelae.

Ref: Cousins MJ, Carr DB, Horlocker TT, Bridenbaugh PO. *Cousins & Bridenbaugh's Neural Blockade in Clinical Anesthesia and Pain Medicine.* 4th ed. Philadelphia, PA: Lippincott Williams & Wilkins; 2009.

16. What is the approximate ratio of the dose of lidocaine required to cause irreversible cardiac collapse compared to seizures?

    (A) 1:1

    (B) 2:1

    (C) 3:1

    (D) 5:1

    (E) **7:1**

The CC:CNS ratio is a marker of the margin between convulsions and fatal cardiovascular collapse. Its value varies between local anesthetics. For example, lidocaine has a CC:CNS ratio of 7:1, meaning that it requires roughly 7 times the amount of lidocaine to cause cardiac arrest than it does to cause a seizure. This represents a relatively high margin between these two toxic events. The CC:CNS ratio for bupivacaine is approximately

3.5:1, indicating a much lower dose required to cause a fatal cardiovascular event compared to a seizure.

Ref: Cousins MJ, Carr DB, Horlocker TT, Bridenbaugh PO. *Cousins & Bridenbaugh's Neural Blockade in Clinical Anesthesia and Pain Medicine.* 4th ed. Philadelphia, PA: Lippincott Williams & Wilkins; 2009.

17. Systemic hypotension after an inadvertent large dose of bupivacaine is MOST likely to result from which of the following mechanisms?

   (A) myocardial depression

   (B) cardiac conduction system blockade

   (C) autonomic nervous system blockade

   (D) arterial vasodilation

   (E) venodilation and preload reduction

In general, concentrations of local anesthetics that produce CNS toxicity will increase systemic blood pressure, heart rate, and cardiac output in direct relation to the duration of the seizure. However, at higher doses, cardiovascular depression occurs, although the mechanisms will vary depending on the specific agent. For example, bupivacaine is much more likely to produce ventricular arrhythmias (and eventually ventricular fibrillation) by inhibition of fast sodium channels in the cardiac membrane. In contrast, ventricular arrhythmias are virtually impossible to produce with lidocaine or mepivacaine. High concentrations of these agents are more often associated with depression of myocardial contractility and increases in LVEDP.

Ref: Cousins MJ, Carr DB, Horlocker TT, Bridenbaugh PO. *Cousins & Bridenbaugh's Neural Blockade in Clinical Anesthesia and Pain Medicine.* 4th ed. Philadelphia, PA: Lippincott Williams & Wilkins; 2009.

18. Which one of the following local anesthetics is MOST likely to cause a true allergic reaction?

   (A) bupivacaine

   (B) chloroprocaine

   (C) lidocaine

   (D) mepivacaine

   (E) ropivacaine

While allergic reactions to amide-linked local anesthetics have been reported, these events are extremely rare, and are often confused with other more frequent events such as systemic toxicity and epinephrine-induced tachycardia. Many patients who have experienced wheal and flare responses, and even anaphylactoid reactions, have gone on to have negative intradermal testing to the purported local anesthetic allergen. Allergy to the ester group of local anesthetics (e.g., chloroprocaine) has long been thought to be much more common, since these are derivatives of p-aminobenzoic acid, a known allergen. Other patients are allergic to metabisulfite, a preservative in epinephrine-containing solutions. Cross-reactivity can occur because metabisulfite is present in several other drugs and foods.

Ref: Cousins MJ, Carr DB, Horlocker TT, Bridenbaugh PO. *Cousins & Bridenbaugh's Neural Blockade in Clinical Anesthesia and Pain Medicine.* 4th ed. Philadelphia, PA: Lippincott Williams & Wilkins; 2009.

19. You are selecting a solution to use for a femoral block in a patient undergoing an ACL repair. Which of the following is NOT an appropriate additive for use in local anesthetic solutions?

   (A) sodium bisulfite

   (B) methylparaben

   (C) glucose

   (D) phenol

   (E) phenylephrine

Local anesthetics are frequently manufactured with additives and/or preservatives. For example, lidocaine or bupivacaine are frequently available in solutions containing epinephrine for its vasoconstrictive properties. However, epinephrine becomes oxidized in the presence of light and degrades quickly. Sodium bisulfite is a common antioxidant that is added to epinephrine-containing solutions in order to prevent this process. While it is safe to use for nerve blocks, it has been implicated in causing cauda equina syndrome, and caution should be used when considering local anesthetics containing bisulfites during epidural blockade in case of inadvertent subarachnoid administration.

Methylparaben is an antimicrobial and antifungal agent that is added to many multidose vials. It has no intrinsic neural toxicity, and nerve blocks can be done safely using these solutions. Methylparaben is metabolized to p-amino benzoic acid (PABA), which is an allergen, and as such has been implicated in being the true cause of suspected allergic reactions to local anesthetics.

Glucose is frequently added to solutions of local anesthetics in order to render them hyperbaric. Phenylephrine, like epinephrine, is a vasoconstrictor that can be added to prolong the duration of neural blockade.

Phenol is a chemical mixture consisting of several compounds and is used for permanent, neurolytic blocks, primarily for cancer-related pain. This is not an appropriate additive for clinical nerve blockade for surgical analgesia.

Ref: Cousins MJ, Carr DB, Horlocker TT, Bridenbaugh PO. *Cousins & Bridenbaugh's Neural Blockade in Clinical Anesthesia and Pain Medicine.* 4th ed. Philadelphia, PA: Lippincott Williams & Wilkins; 2009.

20. Which of the following local anesthetic drugs is NOT associated with methemoglobinemia?

   (A) benzocaine

   (B) bupivacaine

   (C) lidocaine

   (D) prilocaine

   (E) tetracaine

Methemoglobinemia is a condition that results when iron in the hemoglobin molecule exists in the oxidized (Fe^{3+}) state. In this state, the hemoglobin complex is incapable of binding oxygen. Methemoglobin also shifts the oxyhemoglobin dissociation curve to the left and converts the normal sigmoid shape of the curve to a hyperbolic one; both of these actions impair unloading of oxygen to the tissues. In addition, oxidized heme is cytotoxic and is much more readily released from the globin molecule, causing direct tissue damage.

Normally, methemoglobin levels account for only 1–2% of total hemoglobin, due to the action of cytochrome b5 methemoglobin reductase found in red blood cells. In the presence of certain toxins, reduced hemoglobin may be oxidized at a greater rate than the enzyme can handle, and clinical methemoglobinemia results. The signs and symptoms are to a degree nonspecific, and relate principally to the deficit in oxygen-carrying capacity: cyanosis, tachypnea, tachycardia, hypertension, coronary ischemia, altered consciousness/agitation, hypotension, syncope/coma, and apnea. A discrepancy between the pulse oximeter saturation and the measured PaO_2 is suggestive of methemoglobinemia. A

SpO_2 of <90% and a PaO_2 >70 mm Hg is especially typical. However, a wide range of discrepancies had been reported, and the SpO_2 can substantially underestimate the degree of hypoxia. In order to diagnose methemoglobinemia correctly, a co-oximeter must be used, which will discriminate various hemoglobin species.

While other agents exist that can provoke sufficient oxidative stress (e.g., nitrates), certain local anesthetics have been implicated. Benzocaine and prilocaine together account for more than 90% of cases of local anesthetic-induced methemoglobinemia. The remaining few reported cases involve only lidocaine or tetracaine. Benzocaine 20% is still commonly used for topical preparation of the airway for awake intubation, although many experts have called for a ban on its use since it is impossible to predict which patients will develop methemoglobinemia during benzocaine administration, and only one spray may be sufficient to cause the condition. Prilocaine is commonly encountered as a component of EMLA cream. Unexplained cyanosis or altered cardiopulmonary status in a young child where EMLA has been used should prompt consideration of methemoglobinemia as part of the differential.

Ref: Cousins MJ, Carr DB, Horlocker TT, Bridenbaugh PO. *Cousins & Bridenbaugh's Neural Blockade in Clinical Anesthesia and Pain Medicine.* 4th ed. Philadelphia, PA: Lippincott Williams & Wilkins; 2009.

21. Treatment of symptomatic methemoglobinemia is best achieved with which one of the following?

   (A) indocyanine green

   (B) indigo carmine

   (C) vitamin C

   (D) methylene blue

   (E) 100% oxygen

In cases of symptomatic methemoglobinemia, the definitive therapy is methylene blue, which accelerates the reduction of methemoglobin to deoxyhemoglobin promptly. The dose is 0.5 mg/kg for newborns (up to 2 months) and 1–2 mg/kg in older patients, repeated every 60 minutes up to a total dose of 7 mg/kg. Patients that have G6PD-deficiency will not respond to the methylene blue therapy, however, and may in fact develop hemolysis in response to it; for these patients, ascorbic acid (vitamin C), an antioxidant that effectively reverses methemoglobinemia, is the treatment of choice. Its action is slower than that of methylene blue.

While a deficiency in oxygen-carrying capacity is the principal problem, supplemental oxygen therapy is not effective in symptomatic methemoglobinemia, as it will not reverse the hypoxemia and tissue hypoxia. Hyperbaric oxygen therapy also has not been shown to be effective.

Indigo carmine and indocyanine green are both dyes that can artifactually lower the pulse oximetry reading in the same manner as methylene blue can, but they play no role in therapy for methemoglobinemia.

Ref: Cousins MJ, Carr DB, Horlocker TT, Bridenbaugh PO. *Cousins & Bridenbaugh's Neural Blockade in Clinical Anesthesia and Pain Medicine.* 4th ed. Philadelphia, PA: Lippincott Williams & Wilkins; 2009.

22. You have just completed a brachial plexus block in the preoperative area for a patient undergoing fixation of a wrist fracture. Suddenly, the monitor begins to alarm, and you note that there are multiple short runs of ventricular tachycardia, and what appears to be QRS widening. The blood pressure is 82/46 mm Hg. The patient reports feeling dizzy and unwell. Which of the following is the BEST initial treatment option?

(A) Amiodarone 150 mg IV slow push

(B) Lidocaine 1 mg/kg IV

(C) **Lipid emulsion 20% 1.5 mL/kg bolus**

(D) Immediate synchronized DC cardioversion

(E) Vasopressin 40 units IV

Local anesthetic systemic toxicity (LAST) is a serious and potentially fatal complication following the administration of local anesthetics. Some fun facts about LAST:

- The incidence of LAST is completely unknown. The reported incidence is somewhere around 1–2 per 1,000 peripheral nerve blocks, but there are undoubtedly many, many more cases that go unreported. Perform enough blocks and it will happen to you.

- LAST may present with neurologic signs (confusion, hallucination, seizure, coma) or cardiovascular signs (tachy- or bradyarrhythmias, QRS widening, hypotension, cardiac arrest), or both at the same time. LAST does not always follow the commonly

described progression of neurologic followed by cardiovascular signs.

- Do NOT count on the "classic" premonitory symptoms—tinnitus, perioral numbness, metallic taste—being reported in advance of more serious signs, particularly when patients are sedated for block procedures. If they ARE present, that can be helpful, but their absence is not reassuring.

- Have a high index of suspicion for LAST. If the patient has received a bolus of local anesthetic recently, or is receiving a continuous infusion, keep LAST at the top of your differential while you work through other causes of any neurologic or cardiovascular changes.

- Lipid emulsion is a life-saving therapy. If you have ANY suspicion of LAST, give it, and give it early. There are virtually no downsides to administering lipid emulsion in this setting. Prolonged infusions of lipid have been associated with pancreatitis and lung injury, but these theoretical concerns are irrelevant with this dose and in this resuscitation situation.

Here is how to make sure your patients never have a complication from LAST:

- Ensure lipid emulsion is stocked by the pharmacy wherever local anesthetic is used: operating room, preop block area, PACU, labor floor, ICU, and any patient floor where epidural/perineural catheters or IV lidocaine infusions are administered.

- Lipid emulsion has a shelf life. Make sure it is replaced accordingly.

- Know how to use it, and make it easy for others. Ensure that each bag of lipid emulsion has a label with easy-to-follow instructions. I recommend having a 500-mL bag rather than 250 mL: it gets used up pretty quickly.

- Memorize the dose: the recommended dose is 1.5 mL/kg (note: mL, not mg), followed by an infusion of 0.25 mL/kg/min. That will get you started. Have a problem doing math and programming a pump while doing chest compressions? Yup, same here. That is why some have advocated for *SIMPLE* instructions based on an assumed lean body weight of 70 kg. One easy-to-remember, mathematics-free approximation of the formula is:

Immediate IV bolus of 100 mL of intralipid, followed by 1000 mL/hr (Figure 16-6)

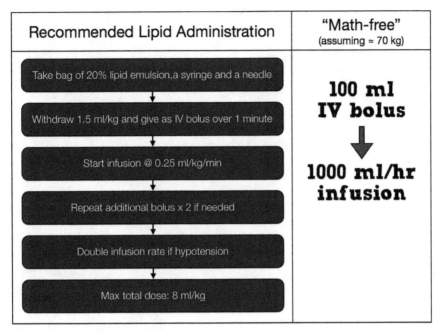

FIG. 16-6. Recommended instructions for administration of lipid emulsion during suspected local anesthetic systemic toxic event, along with a simplified "math-free" version based on a lean body mass of 70 kg.

Once things have cooled off and you have stabilized things, you can check the math and make sure the lipid is being administered appropriately.

Ref: Longnecker DE, Brown DL, Newman MF, Zapol WM. *Anesthesiology.* 2nd ed. New York, NY: McGraw Hill; 2012.

CHAPTER 17

Muscle Relaxants

1. How does succinylcholine cause neuromuscular block-ade at the neuromuscular junction?

   (A) competitive inhibition of acetylcholine

   (B) sensitization of the nicotinic acetylcholine receptor (nAChR)

   (C) inactivation of voltage gated sodium channels

   (D) decreased potassium permeability

   (E) decreased depolarization of the end-plate

2. A nondepolarizing muscle relaxant (NDMR) binds to which subunit of the nicotinic acetylcholine receptor (nAChR)?

   (A) alpha

   (B) beta

   (C) delta

   (D) epsilon

   (E) gamma

3. Concurrent disease states can alter the response to non-depolarizing muscle relaxants (NDMRs). Which disease state results in a hypersensitive response to NDMRs?

   (A) burn injury

   (B) cerebral palsy

   (C) peripheral nerve injury

   (D) hemiplegia

   (E) myasthenia gravis

4. Liver failure will have the most significant effect on the duration of action of which nondepolarizing muscle relaxant (NDMR)?

   (A) vecuronium

   (B) cisatracurium

   (C) rocuronium

   (D) atracurium

   (E) succinylcholine

5. Which of the following drugs does NOT decrease butyrylcholinesterase (pseudocholinesterase) activity?

   (A) ranitidine

   (B) echothiophate

   (C) neostigmine

   (D) esmolol

   (E) oral contraceptives

6. Which of the following medications will cause resistance to a nondepolarizing muscle relaxant (NDMR)?

   (A) amlodipine

   (B) gentamicin

   (C) desflurane

   (D) magnesium

   (E) carbamazepine

7. A patient has received a nondepolarizing muscle relaxant (NDMR) for many hours in the ICU and becomes hypotensive. The hypotension is thought to be due to elevated levels of laudanosine. Which NDMR did the patient receive?

   (A) vecuronium

   (B) rocuronium

   (C) atracurium

   (D) cis-atracurium

   (E) pancuronium

8. Which nondepolarizing muscle relaxant (NDMR) has the most potent active metabolites?

   (A) cisatracurium
   (B) pancuronium
   (C) rocuronium
   (D) vecuronium
   (E) gantacurium

9. During surgery an adult patient is given a second dose of succinylcholine approximately 5 minutes after the first dose. This scenario increases the risk of which of the following side effects of succinylcholine?

   (A) malignant hyperthermia
   (B) prolonged paralysis
   (C) postoperative myalgias
   (D) bradycardia
   (E) histamine release

10. A patient has a history of severe asthma. Which nondepolarizing muscle relaxant (NDMR) should be avoided?

    (A) vecuronium
    (B) rocuronium
    (C) atracurium
    (D) cisatracurium
    (E) pancuronium

11. Administration of succinylcholine can increase potassium levels, and in susceptible patients this can lead to significant hyperkalemia. In which of the following conditions is succinylcholine safe to use?

    (A) burn injury
    (B) Guillain-Barré syndrome
    (C) massive trauma
    (D) chronic renal failure
    (E) closed head injury

12. For which patient is succinylcholine contraindicated?

    (A) patient with an "open" eye injury
    (B) patient at risk of pulmonary aspiration
    (C) patient with increased intracranial pressure
    (D) routine pediatric patient
    (E) patient who requires a rapid sequence induction

13. A patient is tested for butyrylcholinesterase (pseudo-cholinesterase) activity and has a dibucaine number of 80. She is given succinylcholine during surgery. Which of the following scenarios is most likely?

    (A) normal response to succinylcholine
    (B) slightly prolonged 20–30 minute response to succinylcholine
    (C) prolonged 4–8 hour response to succinylcholine
    (D) abnormally rapid recovery from succinylcholine
    (E) impossible to determine clinical effect without knowing the quantity of enzyme

14. Neostigmine is given to reverse the effects of a nondepolarizing muscle relaxant (NDMR). The anesthesiologist does not administer adequate glycopyrrolate to the patient. Which of the following side effects of neostigmine is most likely?

    (A) tachycardia
    (B) pupillary dilation
    (C) bronchodilation
    (D) dry mouth
    (E) intestinal spasm

15. Inhaled anesthetics and TIVA can potentiate the effects of nondepolarizing muscle relaxants (NDMRs). Which of the following agents is the most potent?

    (A) desflurane
    (B) sevoflurane
    (C) isoflurane
    (D) nitrous oxide
    (E) propofol

16. Many antibiotics can potentiate the effects of nondepolarizing muscle relaxants (NDMRs). Which antibiotic has NO effect on neuromuscular blockade?

    (A) gentamicin
    (B) lincomycin
    (C) clindamycin
    (D) cefazolin
    (E) tetracycline

17. A patient with pre-eclampsia is treated with magnesium sulfate. The patient requires a general anesthetic and vecuronium is used to provide neuromuscular blockade. How does magnesium sulfate alter the pharmacokinetics/pharmacodynamics of vecuronium?

    (A) decreased ED_{95}

    (B) increased onset of action

    (C) decreased recovery time

    (D) enhanced recovery with neostigmine administration

    (E) no effect

18. Which drug will augment the effects of nondepolarizing muscle relaxants (NDMRs)?

    (A) lithium

    (B) carbamazepine

    (C) azathioprine

    (D) hydrocortisone

    (E) mannitol

Answers and Explanations: Muscle Relaxants

1. How does succinylcholine cause neuromuscular blockade at the neuromuscular junction?

   (A) competitive inhibition of acetylcholine
   (B) sensitization of the nicotinic acetylcholine receptor (nAChR)
   (C) inactivation of voltage gated sodium channels
   (D) decreased potassium permeability
   (E) decreased depolarization of the end-plate

   Succinylcholine's mechanism of action remains incompletely understood. Succinylcholine binds to the nAChR and causes prolonged depolarization of the end-plate. This leads to:

   • inactivation of voltage gated sodium channels
   • desensitization of the nAChR
   • increased potassium permeability

   Nondepolarizing muscle relaxants are competitive inhibitors of acetylcholine.

   Ref: Miller RD. *Miller's Anesthesia.* 8th ed. Philadelphia, PA: Elsevier; 2015.

2. A nondepolarizing muscle relaxant (NDMR) binds to which subunit of the nicotinic acetylcholine receptor (nAChR)?

   (A) alpha
   (B) beta
   (C) delta
   (D) epsilon
   (E) gamma

   The nAChR is made up of 2 alpha-subunits, 1 beta-subunit, 1 delta-subunit, and either 1 gamma-subunit or 1 epsilon-subunit. A NDMR binds to the alpha-subunit of the nAChR. The adult nAChR contains the gamma-subunit and the fetal nAChR contains the epsilon-subunit.

   Ref: Miller RD. *Miller's Anesthesia.* 8th ed. Philadelphia, PA: Elsevier; 2015.

3. Concurrent disease states can alter the response to nondepolarizing muscle relaxants (NDMRs). Which disease state results in a hypersensitive response to NDMRs?

   (A) burn injury
   (B) cerebral palsy
   (C) peripheral nerve injury
   (D) hemiplegia
   (E) myasthenia gravis

   Myasthenia gravis results in a hypersensitive response to nondepolarizing muscle relaxants (NDMRs). Burn injury, cerebral palsy, peripheral nerve injury, and hemiplegia cause resistance to NDMRs.

   Ref: Butterworth JF IV, Mackey DC, Wasnick JD. *Morgan & Mikhail's Clinical Anesthesiology.* 5th ed. New York, NY: McGraw Hill; 2013.

4. Liver failure will have the most significant effect on the duration of action of which nondepolarizing muscle relaxant (NDMR)?

   (A) vecuronium
   (B) cisatracurium
   (C) rocuronium
   (D) atracurium
   (E) succinylcholine

   Liver failure will prolong the duration of action of rocuronium, pancuronium, and, to a lesser extent, vecuronium. Liver failure has no effect on atracurium and cisatracurium. Liver disease can result in decreased butyrylcholinesterase (pseudocholinesterase) activity and modestly prolong the duration of action of succinylcholine (depolarizing muscle relaxant).

Ref: Butterworth JF IV, Mackey DC, Wasnick JD. *Morgan & Mikhail's Clinical Anesthesiology.* 5th ed. New York, NY: McGraw Hill; 2013.

5. Which of the following drugs does NOT decrease butyrylcholinesterase (pseudocholinesterase) activity?

    (A) **ranitidine**

    (B) echothiophate

    (C) neostigmine

    (D) esmolol

    (E) oral contraceptives

A number of medical conditions and drugs can decrease butyrylcholinesterase (pseudocholinesterase) activity: pregnancy, liver disease, renal failure, advanced age, echothiophate, neostigmine, metoclopramide, esmolol, pancuronium, and oral contraceptives. Clinically, these factors only modestly increase the duration of action of succinylcholine. Ranitidine and cimetidine (H_2 antagonists) do not have any effect on butyrylcholinesterase (pseudocholinesterase) activity.

Ref: Butterworth JF IV, Mackey DC, Wasnick JD. *Morgan & Mikhail's Clinical Anesthesiology.* 5th ed. New York, NY: McGraw Hill; 2013.

6. Which of the following medications will cause resistance to a nondepolarizing muscle relaxant (NDMR)?

    (A) amlodipine

    (B) gentamicin

    (C) desflurane

    (D) magnesium

    (E) **carbamazepine**

Anticonvulsants such as carbamazepine, phenytoin, and sodium valproate cause resistance to the effects of nondepolarizing muscle relaxants (NDMRs). A variety of medications can increase (potentiate) the effects of NDMRs: antibiotics including aminoglycosides and clindamycin; calcium channel blockers; inhalational anesthetics; magnesium sulfate; high doses of local anesthetics; and dantrolene.

Ref: Butterworth JF IV, Mackey DC, Wasnick JD. *Morgan & Mikhail's Clinical Anesthesiology.* 5th ed. New York, NY: McGraw Hill; 2013.

7. A patient has received a nondepolarizing muscle relaxant (NDMR) for many hours in the ICU and becomes hypotensive. The hypotension is thought to be due to elevated levels of laudanosine. Which NDMR did the patient receive?

    (A) vecuronium

    (B) rocuronium

    (C) **atracurium**

    (D) cis-atracurium

    (E) pancuronium

There are reports of CNS excitation and cardiovascular effects such as hypotension associated with the use of atracurium. Atracurium and cis-atracurium are both metabolized by Hofmann elimination and ester hydrolysis. Hofmann elimination results in laudanosine formation. Laudanosine can have CNS-stimulating properties and cardiovascular effects. Since cis-atracurium is approximately 5 times more potent than atracurium, laudanosine accumulation is not thought to be clinically relevant.

Ref: Miller RD. *Miller's Anesthesia.* 8th ed. Philadelphia, PA: Elsevier; 2015.

8. Which nondepolarizing muscle relaxant (NDMR) has the most potent active metabolites?

    (A) cisatracurium

    (B) pancuronium

    (C) rocuronium

    (D) **vecuronium**

    (E) gantacurium

The 3-OH metabolite of vecuronium is approximately 80% as potent as vecuronium. The 3-OH metabolite of pancuronium is approximately 66% as potent as pancuronium. Cisatracurium, rocuronium, and gantacurium do not have active metabolites.

Ref: Miller RD. *Miller's Anesthesia.* 8th ed. Philadelphia, PA: Elsevier; 2015.

9. During surgery an adult patient is given a second dose of succinylcholine approximately 5 minutes after the first dose. This scenario increases the risk of which of the following side effects of succinylcholine?

    (A) malignant hyperthermia

    (B) prolonged paralysis

    (C) postoperative myalgias

    (D) **bradycardia**

    (E) histamine release

Bradycardia can occur with administration of succinylcholine. Pediatric patients are more prone to bradycardia, as are adults given a second dose of succinylcholine approximately 5 minutes after the first dose. Prophylactic administration of atropine can prevent the bradycardia.

Refs: Miller RD. *Miller's Anesthesia*. 8th ed. Philadelphia, PA: Elsevier; 2015; Butterworth JF IV, Mackey DC, Wasnick JD. *Morgan & Mikhail's Clinical Anesthesiology*. 5th ed. New York, NY: McGraw Hill; 2013.

10. A patient has a history of severe asthma. Which nondepolarizing muscle relaxant (NDMR) should be avoided?

    (A) vecuronium
    (B) rocuronium
    (C) atracurium
    (D) cisatracurium
    (E) pancuronium

Histamine release is more common with benzylisoquinolinium neuromuscular relaxants. Although relatively rare, bronchospasm can occur. Of the listed NDMRs, atracurium causes the most histamine release and should be avoided in asthmatics. Cisatracurium, vecuronium, rocuronium, and pancuronium do not cause histamine release.

Refs: Miller RD. *Miller's Anesthesia*. 8th ed. Philadelphia, PA: Elsevier; 2015; Butterworth JF IV, Mackey DC, Wasnick JD. *Morgan & Mikhail's Clinical Anesthesiology*. 5th ed. New York, NY: McGraw Hill; 2013.

11. Administration of succinylcholine can increase potassium levels, and in susceptible patients this can lead to significant hyperkalemia. In which of the following conditions is succinylcholine safe to use?

    (A) burn injury
    (B) Guillain-Barré syndrome
    (C) massive trauma
    (D) chronic renal failure
    (E) closed head injury

Succinylcholine will increase potassium levels by 0.5 mEq/dL. Patients with chronic renal failure do not have a higher risk of a hyperkalemic response to succinylcholine than do patients with normal renal function. Conditions that increase risk of hyperkalemic response to succinylcholine include:

- burn injury
- Guillain-Barré syndrome

- massive trauma
- closed head injury
- myopathies
- spinal cord injury
- shock and metabolic acidosis

Refs: Miller RD. *Miller's Anesthesia*. 8th ed. Philadelphia, PA: Elsevier; 2015; Butterworth JF IV, Mackey DC, Wasnick JD. *Morgan & Mikhail's Clinical Anesthesiology*. 5th ed. New York, NY: McGraw Hill; 2013.

12. For which patient is succinylcholine contraindicated?

    (A) patient with an "open" eye injury
    (B) patient at risk of pulmonary aspiration
    (C) patient with increased intracranial pressure
    (D) routine pediatric patient
    (E) patient who requires a rapid sequence induction

In patients with undiagnosed myopathies, succinylcholine can cause hyperkalemic cardiac arrest. Because of this, succinylcholine is not used routinely for pediatric patients. Succinylcholine will increase intraocular pressure, intragastric pressure, and intracranial pressure. However, there is little evidence that succinylcholine increases risk or worsens outcomes for patients with "open" eye injuries, patients at risk of pulmonary aspiration, or patients with increased intracranial pressure. Despite its number of side effects, succinylcholine's short onset and duration of action mean that it is still indicated for patients who require a rapid-sequence induction.

Refs: Miller RD. *Miller's Anesthesia*. 8th ed. Philadelphia, PA: Elsevier; 2015; Butterworth JF IV, Mackey DC, Wasnick JD. *Morgan & Mikhail's Clinical Anesthesiology*. 5th ed. New York, NY: McGraw Hill; 2013.

13. A patient is tested for butyrylcholinesterase (pseudocholinesterase) activity and has a dibucaine number of 80. She is given succinylcholine during surgery. Which of the following scenarios is most likely?

    (A) normal response to succinylcholine
    (B) slightly prolonged 20–30 minute response to succinylcholine
    (C) prolonged 4–8 hour response to succinylcholine
    (D) abnormally rapid recovery from succinylcholine
    (E) impossible to determine clinical effect without knowing the quantity of enzyme

A patient with a dibucaine number of 80 will have a normal response to succinylcholine. Butyrylcholinesterase (pseudocholinesterase) metabolizes succinylcholine. Dibucaine inhibits normal butyrylcholinesterase activity by 80%. A patient with normal butyrylcholinesterase activity has a dibucaine number of 80, while a homozygote with abnormal alleles will have a dibucaine number of 20. The dibucaine number is a qualitative measure of butyrylcholinesterase function rather than a quantitative measure of the amount of enzyme. A patient with a dibucaine number of 20 will have a prolonged 4–8-hour response to succinylcholine. A heterozygote patient with one abnormal gene and one normal gene will have a slightly prolonged 20–30-minute response to succinylcholine.

Ref: Butterworth JF IV, Mackey DC, Wasnick JD. *Morgan & Mikhail's Clinical Anesthesiology.* 5th ed. New York, NY: McGraw Hill; 2013.

14. Neostigmine is given to reverse the effects of a nondepolarizing muscle relaxant (NDMR). The anesthesiologist does not administer adequate glycopyrrolate to the patient. Which of the following side effects of neostigmine is most likely?

(A) tachycardia
(B) pupillary dilation
(C) bronchodilation
(D) dry mouth
(E) **intestinal spasm**

Muscarinic side effects of cholinesterase inhibitors include: intestinal spasm, bradycardia, bronchospasm, increased bladder tone, and pupillary constriction.

Ref: Butterworth JF IV, Mackey DC, Wasnick JD. *Morgan & Mikhail's Clinical Anesthesiology.* 5th ed. New York, NY: McGraw Hill; 2013.

15. Inhaled anesthetics and TIVA can potentiate the effects of nondepolarizing muscle relaxants (NDMRs). Which of the following agents is the most potent?

(A) **desflurane**
(B) sevoflurane
(C) isoflurane
(D) nitrous oxide
(E) propofol

Inhaled anesthetics and TIVA can potentiate the effects of NDMRs in the following order of potency: desflurane > sevoflurane > isoflurane > nitrous oxide or propofol.

Ref: Miller RD. *Miller's Anesthesia.* 8th ed. Philadelphia, PA: Elsevier; 2015.

16. Many antibiotics can potentiate the effects of nondepolarizing muscle relaxants (NDMRs). Which antibiotic has NO effect on neuromuscular blockade?

(A) gentamicin
(B) lincomycin
(C) clindamycin
(D) **cefazolin**
(E) tetracycline

Aminoglycosides, polymyxins, lincomycin, clindamycin, and tetracyclines all potentiate the effects of NDMRs. Cephalosporins (cefazolin) and penicillins do not potentiate the effects of NDMRs.

Ref: Miller RD. *Miller's Anesthesia.* 8th ed. Philadelphia, PA: Elsevier; 2015.

17. A patient with pre-eclampsia is treated with magnesium sulfate. The patient requires a general anesthetic and vecuronium is used to provide neuromuscular blockade. How does magnesium sulfate alter the pharmacokinetics/pharmacodynamics of vecuronium?

(A) **decreased ED_{95}**
(B) increased onset of action
(C) decreased recovery time
(D) enhanced recovery with neostigmine administration
(E) no effect

Magnesium sulfate will enhance the effects of vecuronium and other nondepolarizing muscle relaxants (NDMRs), and the ED_{95} will be decreased. Other effects of magnesium sulfate on NDMR pharmacokinetics include decreased onset of action, increased recovery time, and diminished recovery with neostigmine administration.

Refs: Miller RD. *Miller's Anesthesia.* 8th ed. Philadelphia, PA: Elsevier; 2015; Butterworth JF IV, Mackey DC, Wasnick JD. *Morgan & Mikhail's Clinical Anesthesiology.* 5th ed. New York, NY: McGraw Hill; 2013.

18. Which drug will augment the effects of nondepolarizing muscle relaxants (NDMRs)?

    (A) lithium
    (B) carbamazepine
    (C) azathioprine
    (D) hydrocortisone
    (E) mannitol

Lithium, via both presynaptic and postsynaptic effects, augment the neuromuscular blockade of NDMRs. Steroids, anticonvulsants, and, to a lesser degree, azathioprine cause resistance to nondepolarizing muscle relaxants (NDMRs). Mannitol has no effect on NDMRs.

Ref: Miller RD. *Miller's Anesthesia.* 8th ed. Philadelphia, PA: Elsevier; 2015.

CHAPTER 18

Cardiovascular and Respiratory Pharmacology

1. A patient with atrial fibrillation and left ventricular dysfunction is prescribed digoxin. Unfortunately, the patient misreads the prescription and takes significantly more than the recommended dose. The result is acute digoxin intoxication. Which of the following therapeutic options will reverse the effects of digoxin?

   (A) potassium chloride
   (B) lidocaine
   (C) cardioversion
   (D) immunotherapy
   (E) dialysis

2. Which of the following medications is a positive inotrope **without** activating the β_1-receptor?

   (A) isoproterenol
   (B) glucagon
   (C) dobutamine
   (D) dopamine
   (E) norepinephrine

3. A postoperative patient is noted to have severe heart failure. In an attempt to improve cardiac output, an infusion of milrinone is initiated. In this patient, which of the following side effects is most likely to limit the use of milrinone?

   (A) pulmonary artery hypertension
   (B) thrombocytopenia
   (C) hypotension
   (D) peripheral vasoconstriction
   (E) bronchospasm

4. A patient with rapid atrial fibrillation requires medical intervention. Which of the following antiarrhythmics can be administered to maintain normal sinus rhythm?

   (A) amiodarone
   (B) digoxin
   (C) verapamil
   (D) adenosine
   (E) metoprolol

5. A patient with chronic stable angina and sinus bradycardia requires medical therapy for his anginal symptoms. Initially, which of the following therapies is recommended?

   (A) metoprolol
   (B) diltiazem
   (C) verapamil
   (D) labetalol
   (E) amlodipine

6. At clinical doses, which of the following vasodilators acts mainly on venous capacitance vessels?

   (A) nitroprusside
   (B) nesiritide
   (C) nitroglycerin
   (D) verapamil
   (E) hydralazine

7. A patient with hypertension is treated with an ACE inhibitor. Unfortunately, the patient develops angioedema, and the medication is discontinued. Which of the following effects of ACE inhibitors is considered a likely cause of the angioedema?

   (A) decreased renin
   (B) inhibition of AT_1 receptors
   (C) activation of AT_2 receptors
   (D) increased angiotensin II
   (E) increased bradykinin

8. A hardworking anesthesiology resident rarely, if ever, is relieved from the operating room and unfortunately, over the course of many months, develops an electrolyte imbalance. The resident's electrocardiogram shows prolonged PR interval, prolonged QRS interval, and peaked T waves. Which of the following electrolytes is abnormal?

   (A) Ca^{2+}
   (B) K^+
   (C) Mg^{2+}
   (D) PO_4^{2-}
   (E) Na^+

9. A patient with sepsis is placed on an infusion of norepinephrine to maintain mean arterial pressure (MAP) of at least 65 mm Hg. As per the surviving sepsis guidelines, the addition of which of the following vasopressors may help to raise MAP and allow the norepinephrine infusion to be decreased?

   (A) epinephrine
   (B) dopamine
   (C) dobutamine
   (D) vasopressin
   (E) phenylephrine

10. Which of the following statements regarding beta-$_2$ (β_2) agonists is TRUE?

   (A) Inhalation of albuterol via a metered-dose inhaler typically results in 50%–60% of the drug deposited in the lungs.
   (B) Compared to short-acting β_2-agonists (SABAs), long-acting β_2-agonists (LABAs) are more lipid soluble.
   (C) Binding of β_2-agonists to the pulmonary epithelial membrane receptor leads to a decrease in cyclic AMP.
   (D) β_2-agonists are ineffective when administered orally.
   (E) Side effects include hyperkalemia.

11. Which of the following statements regarding nebulized ipratropium is TRUE?

   (A) Ipratropium is slightly more effective in asthma than in COPD.
   (B) Ipratropium is only available in a nebulized form.
   (C) Ipratropium has no impact on mucociliary clearance.
   (D) Due to its pharmacology, ipratropium cannot be co-administered together with a β_2-agonist.
   (E) Activity is maximal at 2–3 hours after inhalation.

DIRECTIONS: For each of the numbered phrases or statements below, select the ONE lettered heading that is most closely associated with it. Each lettered heading may be selected once, more than once, or not at all.

   (A) albuterol
   (B) antihistamines
   (C) anti-IgE receptor therapy
   (D) corticosteroids
   (E) cromolyn
   (F) dextromethorphan
   (G) magnesium sulfate
   (H) methylxanthines
   (I) leukotriene antagonists
   (J) phosphodiesterase inhibitors

12. Side effects include osteoporosis and cataracts.

13. A second-line anti-inflammatory agent that blocks the arachidonic acid pathway.

14. An injectable medication indicated for severe asthma that reduces corticosteroid requirements.

Answers and Explanations: Cardiovascular and Respiratory Pharmacology

1. A patient with atrial fibrillation and left ventricular dysfunction is prescribed digoxin. Unfortunately, the patient misreads the prescription and takes significantly more than the recommended dose. The result is acute digoxin intoxication. Which of the following therapeutic options will reverse the effects of digoxin?

   (A) potassium chloride
   (B) lidocaine
   (C) cardioversion
   (D) **immunotherapy**
   (E) dialysis

   Digoxin is a cardiac glycoside that inhibits myocyte Na^+, K^+-ATPase, which results in increased intracellular calcium and positive inotropy.

   Acute overdose may present with: vomiting, hyperkalemia, and cardiac arrhythmias (sinus bradycardia, second- or third-degree AV block, asystole, ventricular tachycardia, or ventricular fibrillation).

   Treatment of acute digoxin intoxication includes:

   - **Immunotherapy with digoxin-specific antibodies, which will reverse the effects of digoxin.** These antibodies bind digoxin to form inactive complexes that are excreted in the urine.
   - Hyperkalemia should be treated with calcium gluconate, $+/-$ sodium bicarbonate, $+/-$ sodium polystyrene sulfonate.
   - Bradyarrhythmias may be treated with atropine or pacemaker (note: pacing or cardioversion for arrhythmia management in these patients may induce even more severe arrhythmias).
   - Ventricular tachyarrhythmias may be treated with lidocaine.
   - Digoxin is NOT effectively removed by dialysis.

   Chronic intoxication with digoxin may present with: altered mental status, brady- or tachyarrhythmias, and electrolyte abnormalities due to concomitant diuretic use (hypokalemia and hypomagnesemia).

Refs: Brunton LL, Chabner BA, Knollman BC. *Goodman & Gilman's the Pharmacological Basis of Therapeutics.* 12th ed. New York, NY: McGraw Hill; 2011.

Benowitz NL. Chapter 61. Digoxin and Other Cardiac Glycosides. In: Olson KR. eds. *Poisoning & Drug Overdose, 6e.* New York, NY: McGraw-Hill; 2012.

2. Which of the following medications is a positive inotrope **without** activating the β_1-receptor?

   (A) isoproterenol
   (B) **glucagon**
   (C) dobutamine
   (D) dopamine
   (E) norepinephrine

   Glucagon acts via a G-protein-coupled receptor (GPCR), independent of the β_1-receptor, to cause both positive chronotropic and inotropic effects on the heart. It has been used to treat patients with a β-blocker overdose.

   The positive inotropic effects of isoproterenol, dobutamine, dopamine, and norepinephrine are all due to activation of the β_1-receptor. β_1-receptors are GPCRs that cause activation of adenylyl cyclase, increased intracellular levels of cAMP and protein kinase A, and activation of L-type Ca^{2+} channels.

Ref: Brunton LL, Chabner BA, Knollman BC. *Goodman & Gilman's the Pharmacological Basis of Therapeutics.* 12th ed. New York, NY: McGraw Hill; 2011.

3. A postoperative patient is noted to have severe heart failure. In an attempt to improve cardiac output, an infusion of milrinone is initiated. In this patient, which of the following side effects is most likely to limit the use of milrinone?

   (A) pulmonary artery hypertension
   (B) thrombocytopenia
   (C) **hypotension**

(D) peripheral vasoconstriction

(E) bronchospasm

Milrinone is an example of a phosphodiesterase III inhibitor that acts as an inodilator (positive inotropy with decreased pre- and afterload). Phosphodiesterase III inhibition maintains intracellular levels of cAMP in smooth and cardiac muscle and increases contractility, improves lusitropy (myocardial relaxation), and causes arterial and venous dilatation. Milrinone may be indicated for patients with heart failure, as it can improve cardiac output. **However, its use in heart failure patients may be limited due its arterial and venous vasodilatory effects and resultant hypotension.** Phosphodiesterase (PDE) inhibitors decrease pulmonary and systemic vascular resistance. (Sildenafil is PDE-5 inhibitor with increased specificity for the pulmonary artery and is used in the treatment of pulmonary hypertension.) Other relatively rare complications of milrinone therapy may include thrombocytopenia and bronchospasm (or anaphylaxis).

Ref: Brunton LL, Chabner BA, Knollman BC. *Goodman & Gilman's the Pharmacological Basis of Therapeutics.* 12th ed. New York, NY: McGraw Hill; 2011.

4. A patient with rapid atrial fibrillation requires medical intervention. Which of the following antiarrhythmics can be administered to maintain normal sinus rhythm?

(A) amiodarone

(B) digoxin

(C) verapamil

(D) adenosine

(E) metoprolol

Options for management of atrial fibrillation include either ventricular rate control with AV nodal blocking agents or maintenance of sinus rhythm with Class I or III antiarrhythmics. **Amiodarone is predominantly a Class III antiarrhythmic drug.** AV nodal blocking agents include adenosine, calcium channel blockers, β blockers, and digoxin (by increasing vagal tone).

Antiarrhythmic drugs may be classified in a variety of ways, including type of electrophysiologic action, mechanism of arrhythmia, or genetics. The traditional Vaughan Williams classification is based on electrophysiologic properties of the drug:

• Class I—Na$^+$ channel block

• Class II—β blockade

• Class III—action potential prolongation (usually K$^+$ channel block)

• Class IV—Ca^{2+} channel block

Ref: Brunton LL, Chabner BA, Knollman BC. *Goodman & Gilman's the Pharmacological Basis of Therapeutics.* 12th ed. New York, NY: McGraw Hill; 2011.

5. A patient with chronic stable angina and sinus bradycardia requires medical therapy for his anginal symptoms. Initially, which of the following therapies is recommended?

(A) metoprolol

(B) diltiazem

(C) verapamil

(D) labetalol

(E) amlodipine

For a patient with angina and sinus bradycardia, a dihydropyridine Ca^{2+} channel blocker (DHP CCB) such as amlodipine is indicated. Other examples of DHP CCBs include nifedipine, felodipine, and nicardipine. As a class, DHP CCBs are relatively more selective for coronary vasculature with fewer cardiac effects such as suppression of SA node automaticity or AV conduction.

CCBs inhibit voltage-sensitive Ca^{2+} channels (L-type), thus preventing entry of extracellular Ca^{2+} into smooth and cardiac muscle. A variety of different CCBs are available:

• Phenylalkylamine: verapamil

• Benzothiazepine: diltiazem

• Dihydropyridines: nifedipine, amlodipine, felodipine, nicardipine, nimodipine

In general, DHPs cause coronary vasodilation with minimal or no effect on cardiac contractility, SA node automaticity, or AV node conduction. DHPs are more potent vasodilators than verapamil or diltiazem is. DHPs cause direct arterial dilation and reflex increases in sympathetic tone (which mitigates any direct effects on contractility, SA node automaticity, or AV node conduction).

Verapamil and diltiazem suppress SA node automaticity and AV node conduction; they also significantly suppress cardiac contractility and cause coronary vasodilation.

Ref: Brunton LL, Chabner BA, Knollman BC. *Goodman & Gilman's the Pharmacological Basis of Therapeutics.* 12th ed. New York, NY: McGraw Hill; 2011.

6. At clinical doses, which of the following vasodilators acts mainly on venous capacitance vessels?

(A) nitroprusside

(B) nesiritide

(C) **nitroglycerin**

(D) verapamil

(E) hydralazine

Nitrates, via formation of nitric oxide (NO), cause smooth muscle relaxation and vasodilation. **Although the exact mechanism is unclear, nitroglycerin mainly acts as a venodilator on venous capacitance vessels.** Higher doses of nitroglycerin may also directly decrease arteriolar resistance and afterload, but reflex sympathetic activation tends to mitigate this effect.

Other vasodilators include:

- Nitroprusside—a direct NO donor; causes both arterial and venodilation. Metabolism is notable for cyanide production, which is then metabolized to thiocyanate and excreted renally. NO-mediated oxidation of hemoglobin can also cause methemoglobinemia.

- Hydralazine—direct-acting vasodilator that causes significant afterload reduction via an unknown mechanism. Both intravenous and oral formulations are used; intravenous hydralazine is relatively slow to reach maximal effect.

- Nesiritide—a form of recombinant brain natriuretic peptide (BNP). An agonist at natriuretic peptide receptors that causes increased sodium and water excretion and vasodilation. Used in the treatment of heart failure, nesiritide decreases both systemic and pulmonary vascular resistance, mean blood pressure, and pulmonary capillary wedge pressure.

- Verapamil—a phenylalkylamine calcium channel blocker. It suppresses SA node automaticity and AV node conduction, and also significantly suppresses cardiac contractility and causes coronary vasodilation.

Other classes of vasodilators include:

- ACE inhibitors
- Angiotensin II blockers
- Phosphodiesterase inhibitors
- α antagonists
- β agonists

These medications are indicated for a variety of conditions including hypertension, heart failure, angina, and peripheral vascular disease. Perioperatively, vasodilators may be indicated to manipulate and optimize cardiac performance or induce hypotension as desired for surgical procedures.

Refs: Brunton LL, Chabner BA, Knollman BC. *Goodman & Gilman's the Pharmacological Basis of Therapeutics.* 12th ed. New York, NY: McGraw Hill; 2011.

Katzung BG, Masters SB, Trevor AJ. *Basic and Clinical Pharmacology.* 12th ed. (LANGE Basic series). New York, NY: McGraw Hill; 2012.

7. A patient with hypertension is treated with an ACE inhibitor. Unfortunately, the patient develops angioedema, and the medication is discontinued. Which of the following effects of ACE inhibitors is considered a likely cause of the angioedema?

(A) decreased renin

(B) inhibition of AT_1 receptors

(C) activation of AT_2 receptors

(D) increased angiotensin II

(E) **increased bradykinin**

ACE inhibitors cause increased levels of bradykinin, which is thought to be a possible mechanism for ACE inhibitor induced angioedema.

ACE inhibitors are involved in the renin-angiotensin system (RAS). Renin, released by renal juxtaglomerular cells, cleaves angiotensinogen to form AngI. Angiotensin-converting enzyme (ACE) cleaves AngI and forms AngII. AngII is the active form that acts on angiotensin receptors (AT_1 and AT_2). AT_1 activation causes vasoconstriction of vascular smooth muscle and increased blood pressure.

ACE is a nonspecific enzyme and is also known as kininase II, which is involved in the inactivation of bradykinin. Bradykinin, a vasodilator, may be formed from a variety of pro-inflammatory reactions such as tissue damage or allergy.

The actions of ACE inhibitors include:

- reduced levels of AngII
- increased levels of bradykinin
- increased renin release (by interfering with AngII feedback inhibition)

ACE inhibitors do not interact with AT_1 or AT_2 receptors. In contrast, angiotensin receptor blockers (ARBs) are competitive inhibitors of the AT_1 receptor.

Ref: Brunton LL, Chabner BA, Knollman BC. *Goodman & Gilman's the Pharmacological Basis of Therapeutics.* 12th ed. New York, NY: McGraw Hill; 2011.

8. A hardworking anesthesiology resident rarely, if ever, is relieved from the operating room and unfortunately, over the course of many months, develops an electrolyte imbalance. The resident's electrocardiogram shows prolonged PR interval, prolonged QRS interval, and peaked T waves. Which of the following electrolytes is abnormal?

(A) Ca^{2+}
(B) K^+
(C) Mg^{2+}
(D) PO_4^{2-}
(E) Na^+

Inadequate intake of fluids and nutrients may result in a variety of metabolic disturbances:

Hyperkalemia may occur due to renal failure. **Hyperkalemia is associated with ECG changes including prolonged PR interval, prolonged QRS interval, peaked T waves, conduction blocks, ventricular fibrillation, and asystole.**

Hypokalemia may occur due to limited potassium intake. It is associated with ECG changes including prolonged PR interval, T-wave inversion, ST-depression, prominent U waves, prolonged QT interval, increased ectopy, and supraventricular and ventricular arrhythmias.

Hypocalcemia may occur due to vitamin D deficiency. Hypocalcemia is associated with neuromuscular irritability (tetany) and cardiovascular abnormalities including hypotension, heart failure, and ECG changes: bradycardia, prolonged QT interval, and T wave inversion.

Hypomagnesemia may occur due to limited magnesium intake. Hypomagnesemia is associated with hypokalemia, hypocalcemia, and hyponatremia. The ECG changes associated with hypomagnesemia are the same as with hypokalemia, including prolonged QT interval, prolonged QRS interval, and prominent U waves.

Hypernatremia may occur due to limited access to water and typically presents with thirst and neurologic symptoms such as lethargy, weakness, tremor, hyperreflexia, coma, and seizures.

Hypophosphatemia may occur due to limited phosphate intake. Severe hypophosphatemia may present with neurologic symptoms such as weakness, tremors, seizures, and coma. Other effects include muscle weakness, cardiomyopathy, and respiratory failure.

Ref: Hall JB, Schmidt GA, Kress JP. *Principles of Critical Care.* 4th ed. New York, NY: McGraw Hill; 2015.

9. A patient with sepsis is placed on an infusion of norepinephrine to maintain mean arterial pressure (MAP) of at least 65 mm Hg. As per the surviving sepsis guidelines, the addition of which of the following vasopressors may help to raise MAP and allow the norepinephrine infusion to be decreased?

(A) epinephrine
(B) dopamine
(C) dobutamine
(D) vasopressin
(E) phenylephrine

For a patient with septic shock, the addition of vasopressin to an infusion of norepinephrine may help maintain MAP and allow the norepinephrine infusion to be decreased.

Vasopressin is a peptide hormone involved in water conservation and regulation of blood volume and blood pressure. A potent vasoconstrictor at the V_1 receptor, vasopressin is released during periods of hypovolemia or hypotension. However, patients with septic shock (a form of vasodilatory shock) have a relative deficiency of vasopressin. The surviving sepsis guidelines make the following vasopressor recommendations for patients with septic shock:

- norepinephrine is the first-choice vasopressor
- epinephrine may be added or substituted for norepinephrine to maintain MAP of 65 mm Hg
- vasopressin (up to 0.03 U/min) may be added to norepinephrine to help raise MAP or reduce norepinephrine infusion. (The VASST trial compared norepinephrine to norepinephrine and vasopressin and found no difference in outcome.)

Dopamine and phenylephrine are not recommended as first-line therapies except for selected patients (e.g., dopamine may be considered for patients with relative bradycardia and low risk of tachyarrhythmia; phenylephrine may be considered for patients for who norepinephrine causes significant arrhythmia, or in whom cardiac output is elevated and blood pressure is low). For patients with septic shock and low cardiac output, dobutamine may be added to as a first-choice inotrope.

Refs: Dellinger RP, Levy MM, Rhodes A, et al. Surviving sepsis campaign: international guidelines for management of severe sepsis and septic shock: 2012. *Crit Care Med.* 2013;41(2):580–637.

Brunton LL, Chabner BA, Knollman BC. *Goodman & Gilman's the Pharmacological Basis of Therapeutics.* 12th ed. New York, NY: McGraw Hill; 2011.

10. Which of the following statements regarding beta-$_2$ (β_2) agonists is TRUE?

    (A) Inhalation of albuterol via a metered-dose inhaler typically results in 50%–60% of the drug deposited in the lungs.

    (B) Compared to short-acting β_2-agonists (SABAs), long-acting β_2-agonists (LABAs) are more lipid soluble.

    (C) Binding of β_2-agonists to the pulmonary epithelial membrane receptor leads to a decrease in cyclic AMP.

    (D) β_2-agonists are ineffective when administered orally.

    (E) Side effects include hyperkalemia.

β_2-agonists are the first-line bronchodilator therapy due to their prompt onset, efficacy, and relative scarcity of side effects when used in commonly prescribed doses. These drugs can be administered via several routes, such as intravenous and oral, but the inhaled route is usually preferable. Nebulizers provide the best delivery of inhaled drug to the airways; metered-dose inhalers typically lose most of the dose to the mouth and pharynx, and only 10–20% actually reaches the airways. The pharmacology of β_2-agonists is well described and involves the activation of adenylyl cyclase via a stimulatory G protein, leading to an increase in cyclic AMP. This triggers a lowering of the intracellular calcium concentration, which relaxes the bronchial smooth muscle.

Side effects of β_2-agonists include muscle tremor due to stimulation of β_2 receptors in skeletal muscle, palpitations due to stimulation of atrial β_2 receptors, and hypokalemia due to the driving of potassium ions into skeletal muscle caused by increased pancreatic secretion of insulin (remember: β_2-agonists are a specific therapy for hyperkalemia). The reversal of hypoxic pulmonary vasoconstriction due to β_2-agonists can sometimes lead to a small reduction in arterial oxygen tension due to vasodilation of blood vessels in poorly ventilated areas of the lung.

LABAs are more lipid soluble and therefore are have a longer duration of effect. LABAs are often combined with a similarly long-acting corticosteroid for their synergistic actions (e.g., fluticasone/salmeterol or Advair).

Ref: Brunton LL, Chabner BA, Knollman BC. *Goodman & Gilman's the Pharmacological Basis of Therapeutics*. 12th ed. New York, NY: McGraw Hill; 2011.

11. Which of the following statements regarding nebulized ipratropium is TRUE?

    (A) Ipratropium is slightly more effective in asthma than in COPD.

    (B) Ipratropium is only available in a nebulized form.

    (C) Ipratropium has no impact on mucociliary clearance.

    (D) Due to its pharmacology, ipratropium cannot be co-administered together with a β_2-agonist.

    (E) Activity is maximal at 2–3 hours after inhalation.

Ipratropium bromide is a muscarinic cholinergic antagonist that blocks the receptor in the bronchial smooth muscle and epithelium, thereby reducing the bronchoconstricting effects of increased vagal or parasympathetic tone. Ipratropium typically is not a first-line therapy in asthma due to its delayed onset of action (maximal by 30–60 minutes and lasting 6–8 hours), as well as its inferior efficacy in treating bronchospasm compared to β_2-agonists. However, in COPD, it may be equally effective or even superior to β_2-agonists, since vagal tone is frequently the only modifiable factor in this disease. Ipratropium has little effect on normal airways.

Ipratropium can be delivered via nebulizer or metered-dose inhaler, where it is frequently combined with a β_2-agonist (e.g., Combivent). Side effects are minimal, since there is little systemic activity. Notably, even though increased cholinergic activity results in increased mucus production, antagonism of pulmonary cholinergic receptors by ipratropium does not have any appreciable effect on decreasing mucus production.

Ref: Brunton LL, Chabner BA, Knollman BC. *Goodman & Gilman's the Pharmacological Basis of Therapeutics*. 12th ed. New York, NY: McGraw Hill; 2011.

DIRECTIONS: For each of the numbered phrases or statements below, select the ONE lettered heading that is most closely associated with it. Each lettered heading may be selected once, more than once, or not at all.

    (A) albuterol

    (B) antihistamines

    (C) anti-IgE receptor therapy

    (D) corticosteroids

    (E) cromolyn

    (F) dextromethorphan

    (G) magnesium sulfate

(H) methylxanthines

(I) leukotriene antagonists

(J) phosphodiesterase inhibitors

12. Side effects include osteoporosis and cataracts.

(D) corticosteroids

Steroids are a mainstay of therapy for moderate to severe asthma, and in patients with mild asthma who are taking β_2-agonists more than twice weekly. In contrast, the benefit in COPD is far less impressive, with no apparent short-term anti-inflammatory effect and no effect on the progression of the disease. Steroids do appear to reduce the number of COPD exacerbations in severe disease. Corticosteroids are frequently combined with either an inhaled β_2-agonist or an inhaled anticholinergic to provide additive or synergistic therapy. There are multiple proposed mechanisms of action (Figure 18-1), but the primary value is in reducing inflammation in the bronchial tissue. A limiting factor in the use of corticosteroids is the lengthy list of often serious side effects, especially with high and/or prolonged dosing. These adverse effects include adrenal insufficiency, easy bruising, osteoporosis, hypertension, peptic ulceration, glucose intolerance/diabetes, cataracts, psychosis, and increased susceptibility to infection.

Ref: Brunton LL, Chabner BA, Knollman BC. *Goodman & Gilman's the Pharmacological Basis of Therapeutics*. 12th ed. New York, NY: McGraw Hill; 2011.

13. A second-line anti-inflammatory agent that blocks the arachidonic acid pathway.

(I) Leukotriene antagonists

Leukotrienes are a type of inflammatory mediator produced primarily in mast cells and basophils. The initial step is the conversion of membrane phospholipids to arachidonic acid, which is then oxidized by 5-lipoxygenase to one of several leukotriene subtypes. These act both to sustain inflammatory reactions by cell signaling and to cause bronchial constriction directly.

Anti-leukotriene drugs (e.g., montelukast, zafirlukast) are taken orally, and inhibit bronchoconstriction caused by a variety of stimuli such as cold air, allergens,

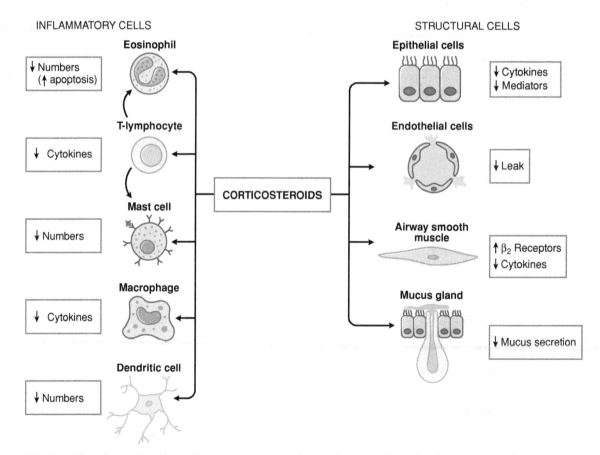

FIG. 18-1. Effect of corticosteroids on inflammatory and structural cells in the airways. (Reproduced with permission from Brunton LL, Chabner BA, Knollman BC. *Goodman & Gilman's the Pharmacological Basis of Therapeutics*. 12th ed. New York, NY: McGraw Hill; 2011.)

exercise, and aspirin (in aspirin-sensitive individuals). They have been shown to reduce the amount of β_2-agonist medication required in asthma, but are not as effective as inhaled corticosteroids or β_2-agonists alone. Therefore, they should be considered second-line therapy.

Ref: Brunton LL, Chabner BA, Knollman BC. *Goodman & Gilman's the Pharmacological Basis of Therapeutics*. 12th ed. New York, NY: McGraw Hill; 2011.

14. An injectable medication indicated for severe asthma that reduces corticosteroid requirements.

(C) anti-IgE receptor therapy

Omalizumab is a monoclonal antibody directed against IgE receptors on mast cells. By blocking these receptors, it prevents their activation by allergens and the subsequent release of inflammatory mediators. Most useful in severe asthma, the antibody is injected subcutaneously 1–2 times per month, and has been shown to reduce both the amount of systemic and inhaled steroids as well as the number of acute asthma exacerbations. Cost is a limiting factor, and the therapy is usually reserved for those patients who are poorly controlled on maximal β_2-agonist and corticosteroid regimens.

Ref: Brunton LL, Chabner BA, Knollman BC. *Goodman & Gilman's the Pharmacological Basis of Therapeutics*. 12th ed. New York, NY: McGraw Hill; 2011.

CHAPTER 19

Hematologic and Renal Pharmacology

DIRECTIONS: For questions 1–3, each group of items below consists of lettered headings followed by a list of numbered phrases or statements. For each numbered phrase or statement, select the ONE lettered heading or component that is most closely associated with it and fill in the circle containing the corresponding letter on the answer sheet. Each lettered heading or component may be selected once, more than once, or not at all.

(A) aspirin

(B) abciximab

(C) clopidogrel

(D) dabigatran

(E) enoxaparin

(F) fondaparinux

(G) hirudin

(H) rivaroxaban

(I) warfarin

(J) unfractionated heparin

1. An orally administered direct thrombin inhibitor.

2. An intravenous agent that inhibits platelet aggregation by binding to the glycoprotein IIb/IIIa receptor.

3. An orally administered direct inhibitor of factor Xa.

4. Compared to unfractionated heparin (UFH), low-molecular-weight heparin (LMWH) has all of the following advantages EXCEPT:

(A) Greater bioavailability when given by subcutaneous injection.

(B) The anticoagulant response is highly correlated to body weight.

(C) Significantly less likely to develop heparin-induced thrombocytopenia.

(D) Duration of action is shorter, permitting easier titration to effect.

(E) Can be safely used in the outpatient setting.

5. Which of the following is MOST accurate regarding interactions between warfarin and other drugs?

(A) Barbiturate use results in a decreased dose requirement of warfarin.

(B) Metronidazole use results in a significant increase in plasma concentrations of warfarin.

(C) Non-selective NSAIDs are contraindicated during warfarin use.

(D) Amiodarone may be used safely with warfarin.

(E) Phenytoin use results in a decreased dose requirement of warfarin.

6. Which of the following statements regarding the monitoring of the effect of anticoagulant drugs is LEAST accurate?

   (A) The effect of clopidogrel can be quantified by PT/INR.

   (B) Patients taking warfarin should be maintained at an INR between 2 and 3 for most indications.

   (C) Patients receiving a heparin infusion should be monitored using the partial thromboplastin time.

   (D) Monitoring of anti-factor Xa levels is recommended when prescribing enoxaparin in pregnant patients.

   (E) There is no reliable means by which to monitor the effect of the direct thrombin inhibitor dabigatran.

7. A patient has been receiving subcutaneous heparin for 5 days while on the ward. Which of the following tests should be ordered prior to placing a thoracic epidural for a colectomy?

   (A) prothrombin time (PT)

   (B) partial thromboplastin time (PTT)

   (C) international normalized ratio (INR)

   (D) fibrinogen level

   (E) complete blood count

8. Which of the following BEST describes the main toxicity of clopidogrel?

   (A) renal failure

   (B) thrombotic thrombocytopenic purpura (TTP)

   (C) neutropenia

   (D) bleeding

   (E) rash

9. Which of the following statements regarding acute normovolemic hemodilution (ANH) is LEAST correct?

   (A) ANH is indicated for cases where expected blood loss is >2 units.

   (B) Collected blood may be stored at room temperature for up to 4 hours before refrigeration is required.

   (C) Some Jehovah's Witnesses will accept blood collected via ANH.

   (D) Tissue perfusion is increased due to a reduction in blood viscosity.

   (E) The efficacy of ANH is unproven.

10. Which of the following is LEAST likely to be a complication related to intraoperative blood salvage?

    (A) air embolism

    (B) infection

    (C) anaphylaxis

    (D) fat embolism

    (E) disseminated intravascular coagulation (DIC)

11. Which of the following statements regarding the use of erythropoietin to treat preoperative anemia is LEAST accurate?

    (A) Erythropoietin acts on peritubular cells of the kidney.

    (B) The usual dosing schedule is three weekly doses leading up to surgery, plus a fourth dose on the day of surgery.

    (C) Iron supplementation is required for maximal efficacy.

    (D) Erythropoietin minimizes perioperative exposure to allogeneic blood transfusion in major orthopedic and cardiac surgical patients.

    (E) Erythropoietin is associated with increased risk of deep venous thrombosis.

12. Which of the following statements regarding the toxicity of immunosuppressive therapies for graft-versus-host disease is LEAST accurate?

    (A) Corticosteroid toxicities include aseptic vascular necrosis, hypertension and osteoporosis.

    (B) Methotrexate toxicities include hepatotoxicity and renal injury.

    (C) Cyclosporine toxicities include renal injury and elevated bilirubin.

    (D) Antithymocyte globulin toxicities include cardiomyopathy and lung injury.

    (E) Hydroxychloroquine toxicities include visual disturbances.

13. In the kidney, hydrochlorothiazide and other thiazide diuretics act as inhibitors at which of the following sites?

    (A) Na^+-K^+-$2Cl^-$ symport
    (B) Na^+-Cl^- symport
    (C) renal epithelial Na^+ channels
    (D) mineralocorticoid receptors
    (E) nonspecific cation channels

14. Which of the following diuretics is considered a K^+-sparing diuretic?

    (A) triamterene
    (B) hydrochlorothiazide
    (C) furosemide
    (D) mannitol
    (E) acetazolamide

15. Chronic administration of furosemide will result in **decreased** renal excretion of which of the following?

    (A) sodium
    (B) chloride
    (C) bicarbonate
    (D) potassium
    (E) uric acid

16. After acute administration of a diuretic, a patient notes tinnitus and hearing impairment. Which of the following diuretics is most likely to cause ototoxicity?

    (A) amiloride
    (B) acetazolamide
    (C) hydrochlorothiazide
    (D) furosemide
    (E) mannitol

17. A patient at risk of perioperative acute kidney injury (AKI) is administered an infusion of low-dose dopamine (1–3 mcg/kg/min). Theoretically, what is the potential benefit of using dopamine for renal protection?

    (A) D_1 receptor mediated increase in mean blood pressure and heart rate
    (B) D_2 receptor mediated natriuresis
    (C) D_1 receptor mediated diuresis
    (D) D_1 receptor mediated activation of Na^+-H^+ exchanger in distal convoluted tubule
    (E) D_2 receptor mediated renal vasodilatation

Answers and Explanations: Hematologic and Renal Pharmacology

DIRECTIONS: For questions 1–3, each group of items below consists of lettered headings followed by a list of numbered phrases or statements. For each numbered phrase or statement, select the ONE lettered heading or component that is most closely associated with it and fill in the circle containing the corresponding letter on the answer sheet. Each lettered heading or component may be selected once, more than once, or not at all.

(A) aspirin

(B) abciximab

(C) clopidogrel

(D) dabigatran

(E) enoxaparin

(F) fondaparinux

(G) hirudin

(H) rivaroxaban

(I) warfarin

(J) unfractionated heparin

1. An orally administered direct thrombin inhibitor.

(D) dabigatran

The clotting cascade begins with an injury to the vessel wall, exposing tissue factor (TF) to the circulating blood (Figure 19-1). Factor VIIa and TF combine to form a complex that activates factor X. This can occur either directly, or indirectly by activation of factor IX. Factor Xa catalyzed the conversion of prothrombin to thrombin, which then converts soluble fibrinogen into insoluble fibrin strands. Lastly, these strands are cross-linked by factor XIII to form a blood clot.

Since the final common pathway to fibrin generation involves thrombin, this serine protease has become a target for anticoagulant drugs. These include intravenous inhibitors of thrombin such as recombinant hirudin (derived from the salivary gland of medicinal leeches), bivalirudin, and argatroban, as well as the

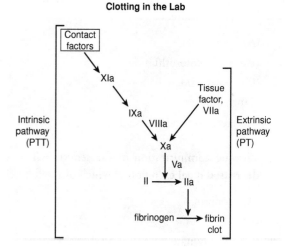

Clotting in the Lab

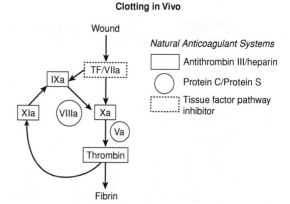

Clotting in Vivo

Natural Anticoagulant Systems

☐ Antithrombin III/heparin

◯ Protein C/Protein S

⬚ Tissue factor pathway inhibitor

FIG. 19-1. A model of blood coagulation. With tissue factor (TF), factor VII forms an activated complex (VIIa-TF) that catalyzes the activation of factor IX to factor IXa. Activated factor XIa also catalyzes this reaction. Tissue factor pathway inhibitor (TFPI) inhibits the catalytic action of the VIIa-TF complex. The cascade proceeds as shown, resulting ultimately in the conversion of fibrinogen to fibrin, an essential component of a functional clot. The two major anticoagulant drugs, heparin and warfarin, have very different actions. Heparin, acting in the blood, directly activates anticlotting factors, specifically antithrombin, which inactivates the factors enclosed in rectangles. Warfarin, acting in the liver, inhibits the synthesis of the factors enclosed in circles. Proteins C and S exert anticlotting effects by inactivating activated factors Va and VIIIa. (From: Katzung BG, Masters SB, Trevor AJ. *Basic and Clinical Pharmacology*. 12th ed. (LANGE Basic series). New York, NY: McGraw Hill; 2012.)

orally administered thrombin inhibitor dabigatran (trade name Pradaxa). Unlike heparin, which can only inactivate free thrombin, these drugs can inactivate fibrin-bound thrombin. Dabigatran is used primarily for the prevention of stroke in atrial fibrillation and for venous thromboembolism prophylaxis in patients undergoing total joint replacement.

While the half-life of dabigatran is relatively short (healthy patients: 12–17 hrs), there is no reliable method by which to monitor the effect of the drug (e.g. PTT, INR). In addition, reversal of the drug effect is challenging and until recently, there was no antidote. In late 2015, the FDA approved a monoclonal antibody (idarucizumab) which has been shown to reverse the anticoagulant effect within minutes. While apparently effective, the high cost of this agent may limit its widespread use.

Ref: Katzung BG, Masters SB, Trevor AJ. *Basic and Clinical Pharmacology.* 12th ed. (LANGE Basic series). New York, NY: McGraw Hill; 2012.

2. An intravenous agent that inhibits platelet aggregation by binding to the glycoprotein IIb/IIIa receptor.

(B) abciximab

Abciximab is an intravenous glycoprotein IIb/IIIa receptor antagonist primarily used during percutaneous coronary interventions such as angioplasty and/or stenting. The onset is rapid, and platelet aggregation is reduced to less than 20% of baseline within 10 minutes of commencement of infusion. The plasma elimination half-life is approximately 30 minutes, but the time to normal function of platelets is usually 24–48 hours. Conversely, platelet function returns to normal much faster (4–8 hours) after discontinuing infusion of the other two intravenous GPIIb/IIIa inhibitors, tirofiban and eptifibatide. The rapid onset and offset of these intravenous antiplatelet agents distinguish them from oral antiplatelet medications.

The GPIIb/IIIa receptor functions mainly as a receptor for fibrinogen, and to a lesser extent vitronectin, von Willebrand factor, and fibronectin. Since each molecule of fibrinogen can bind two GPIIb/IIIa receptors, this leads to cross-linking of platelets. There are approximately 50,000–80,000 GPIIb/IIIa receptors on the surface of each platelet.

Ref: Katzung BG, Masters SB, Trevor AJ. *Basic and Clinical Pharmacology.* 12th ed. (LANGE Basic series). New York, NY: McGraw Hill; 2012.

3. An orally administered direct inhibitor of factor Xa.

(H) rivaroxaban

The conversion of factor X to factor Xa is the first step common to both intrinsic and extrinsic coagulation pathways. Two commonly used direct inhibitors of factor Xa include fondaparinux and rivaroxaban. In general, both of these drugs have a rapid onset, with a peak anticoagulant effect within 2–4 hours, as well as stable pharmacokinetics that result in a predictable effect profile. Fondaparinux is a synthetic heparin pentasaccharide that is administered subcutaneously, and therefore has limited appeal as a long-term outpatient therapy.

Rivaroxaban is an oral anti-factor Xa drug used for stroke prevention in atrial fibrillation and thromboprophylaxis following total joint replacement. It inhibits both free factor Xa and factor Xa bound to factor Va in the prothrombinase complex. While its effects generally last approximately 8–2 hours, factor Xa activity may not return to normal until 24 hours after the last dose. There is no antidote to rivaroxaban currently available to reverse this effect, and major bleeding episodes can be complicated by this.

Ref: Katzung BG, Masters SB, Trevor AJ. *Basic and Clinical Pharmacology.* 12th ed. (LANGE Basic series). New York, NY: McGraw Hill; 2012.

4. Compared to unfractionated heparin (UFH), low-molecular-weight heparin (LMWH) has all of the following advantages EXCEPT:

(A) Greater bioavailability when given by subcutaneous injection.

(B) The anticoagulant response is highly correlated to body weight.

(C) Significantly less likely to develop heparin-induced thrombocytopenia.

(D) Duration of action is shorter, permitting easier titration to effect.

(E) Can be safely used in the outpatient setting.

Heparins exert their effect by binding with circulating antithrombin and inducing a conformational change that exposes the active site for binding with clotting factor proteases (thrombin, factor IXa and factor Xa). Normally the inhibition of these proteases by antithrombin is a slow reaction; heparin accelerates the rate 1,000-fold. LMWH have been shown to be as effective as UFH for several indications, such as prevention and treatment of venous thromboembolism. Unfractionated heparin contains heparin molecules of varying sizes, ranging from 5,000 to 30,000 Daltons. Only one third of all molecules in UFH are estimated to be capable of exerting the anticoagulant effect. However, UFH is active on all three coagulation factors. In contrast, LMWHs inactivate factor Xa, with a much more limited effect on thrombin.

Purported advantages to LMWH over UFH include:

- greater bioavailability than UFH when administered subcutaneously

- an anticoagulant response that correlates well with body weight; this allows for the prescription of a fixed dose

- a prolonged duration of effect due to reduced binding to macrophages and endothelial cells, allowing for dosing every 12–24 hours

- no need for laboratory monitoring, due to stable and predictable pharmacokinetics (as well as the poor correlation between anti-Xa activity and clinical bleeding)

- fewer side effects such as heparin-induced thrombocytopenia or osteoclast-mediated osteoporosis

- ease and safety of administration at home

One disadvantage of LMWH is that reversal is incomplete with protamine. Protamine is relatively effective in neutralizing the antithrombin activity, but much less effective at reversing the anti-factor Xa activity. No other reversal agent exists for use with LMWH.

Ref: Katzung BG, Masters SB, Trevor AJ. *Basic and Clinical Pharmacology*. 12th ed. (LANGE Basic series). New York, NY: McGraw Hill; 2012.

5. Which of the following is MOST accurate regarding interactions between warfarin and other drugs?

    (A) Barbiturate use results in a decreased dose requirement of warfarin.

    (B) Metronidazole use results in a significant increase in plasma concentrations of warfarin.

    (C) Non-selective NSAIDs are contraindicated during warfarin use.

    (D) Amiodarone may be used safely with warfarin.

    (E) Phenytoin use results in a decreased dose requirement of warfarin.

Barbiturates are cytochrome P450 isoenzyme inducers. As such, they increase the metabolism of warfarin and decrease the PT/INR. Dosage increases of 30% to

60% are frequently required to maintain adequate anticoagulation following barbiturate initiation.

Similarly, phenytoin induces a number of CYP isoenzymes, resulting in an accelerated rate of metabolism and a requirement for dosage increase. However, this effect is initially masked by a transient increase in warfarin effect that may be caused by displacement of warfarin from protein-binding sites by phenytoin. Eventually, these are overcome by the enzymatic induction effects.

Metronidazole is an inhibitor of CYP2C9, the principal enzyme responsible for warfarin metabolism. This has been shown to result in a significant increase in the half-life and effect of the S-isomer of racemic warfarin (R-isomer pharmacokinetic and pharmacodynamic effects were unchanged). Increases in the prothrombin time of up to 10-fold and multiple reports of an increased prevalence of serious hemorrhage have been documented. Amiodarone also likely inhibits one or more of the enzymes that metabolize warfarin, and its co-administration has been shown to cause a delayed onset (a week or more) as well as an effect that may last for several weeks following cessation of amiodarone.

Most studies have shown little to no effect of non-selective NSAIDs on warfarin effect, although there are scattered reports of minor increases in the prothrombin time or cases of minor bleeding. While not contraindicated, care should be taken when prescribing drugs that have an effect on platelet function while on warfarin.

Ref: Katzung BG, Masters SB, Trevor AJ. *Basic and Clinical Pharmacology*. 12th ed. (LANGE Basic series). New York, NY: McGraw Hill; 2012.

6. Which of the following statements regarding the monitoring of the effect of anticoagulant drugs is LEAST accurate?

    (A) The effect of clopidogrel can be quantified by PT/INR.

    (B) Patients taking warfarin should be maintained at an INR between 2 and 3 for most indications.

    (C) Patients receiving a heparin infusion should be monitored using the partial thromboplastin time.

    (D) Monitoring of anti-factor Xa levels is recommended when prescribing enoxaparin in pregnant patients.

    (E) There is no reliable means by which to monitor the effect of the direct thrombin inhibitor dabigatran.

Clopidogrel as well as prasugrel and ticlopidine reduce platelet aggregation by binding to P2Y12 receptors on the platelet surface, thereby inhibiting ADP-induced stimulation of GPIIb/IIIa receptors. Standard tests of coagulation (PT/PTT/INR) are not affected by these drugs. There are several laboratory and point-of-care tests that can determine the degree of platelet aggregation or P2Y12 receptor inhibition (e.g., the VerifyNow P2Y12 assay and Multiplate Analyzer). While these have been mostly the subject of clinical trials, their use in daily decision making is growing.

During warfarin therapy, INR should be increased by 2–3 times unless specifically indicated (e.g., caged ball or disk mechanical valves should be maintained at a range of 2.5–3.5). There is little therapeutic benefit to increasing the INR beyond 3.5–4, and these increases are associated with increased risk of bleeding.

Unfractionated heparin infusions should be monitored regularly and titrated to effect using the partial thromboplastin time (PTT). In contrast, low molecular weight heparins (LMWHs) have predictable pharmacokinetics and pharmacodynamics, and are typically not monitored. Exceptions to this include obese patients, pregnant patients, and those with renal impairment, mainly due to altered pharmacokinetics. Pregnant women have an increased volume of distribution and an increased renal clearance of LMWH compared to nonpregnant women, which results in lower peak anti-factor Xa activity levels. The peak anti-factor Xa levels also tend to occur later after injection (i.e., 4 hours versus 2 hours).

The direct thrombin inhibitors have no means of monitoring activity.

Ref: Katzung BG, Masters SB, Trevor AJ. *Basic and Clinical Pharmacology*. 12th ed. (LANGE Basic series). New York, NY: McGraw Hill; 2012.

7. A patient has been receiving subcutaneous heparin for 5 days while on the ward. Which of the following tests should be ordered prior to placing a thoracic epidural for a colectomy?

    (A) prothrombin time (PT)
    (B) partial thromboplastin time (PTT)
    (C) international normalized ratio (INR)
    (D) fibrinogen level
    (E) **complete blood count**

Heparin-induced thrombocytopenia (HIT) is a disorder that occurs in 15–40% of patients who are treated with heparin for 4 days or longer. Type I HIT is a milder, reversible fall in platelet count. Type II is more serious and relates to an immune-mediated destruction of platelets by the formation of antibodies against the heparin-platelet factor 4 complex. This typically leads to a fall in the platelet count >50%. HIT is most frequent in female surgical patients receiving unfractionated (vs. LMW) heparin. Type II HIT is also associated with venous or arterial thrombosis, perhaps due to release of procoagulants from activated platelets. Any patient who has been receiving heparin for longer than 3 days should be screened for HIT with a platelet count (i.e., CBC) prior to instrumentation of the neuraxial space.

Ref: Katzung BG, Masters SB, Trevor AJ. *Basic and Clinical Pharmacology*. 12th ed. (LANGE Basic series). New York, NY: McGraw Hill; 2012.

8. Which of the following BEST describes the main toxicity of clopidogrel?

    (A) renal failure
    (B) thrombotic thrombocytopenic purpura (TTP)
    (C) neutropenia
    (D) **bleeding**
    (E) rash

Bleeding is the most common and the most serious adverse effect of clopidogrel use. Minor bleeding episodes occur in 5% of patients, while major bleeding episodes occur in a further 4%. Gastrointestinal bleeding occurs in 2%. Clopidogrel use is contraindicated in patients with active pathological (i.e., not surgical) bleeding or intracranial hemorrhage. Risk factors for bleeding while taking clopidogrel include age over 74 years, recent bleeding episodes or surgery, weight <60 kg, and concomitant use of drugs that impair coagulation or platelet effect (e.g., heparin, warfarin).

TTP cases, some fatal, have been reported, but are rare. Rash is fairly uncommon (4%) and is usually self-limiting and mild. Neutropenia is very rare and is a side effect seen more commonly with the older thienopyridine drug, ticlopidine, with an incidence of 1%.

Clopidogrel's antiplatelet effect lasts approximately 7–10 days. Discontinuation of these medications prior to surgery can be a complicated clinical decision involving the weighing of risk-benefit, especially if the indication for clopidogrel is for prevention of coronary thrombosis following percutaneous stenting. Multidisciplinary discussion with anesthesiology, cardiology, and surgery is warranted in these cases. The American Society of Regional Anesthesia and Pain Medicine Consensus Guidelines regarding regional anesthesia and antithrombotic therapy suggests a delay of 7 days after discontinuation of clopidogrel therapy before instrumenting the neuraxis. However, there are reports of the use of point-of-care testing (e.g., VerifyNow P2Y12 assay) to gauge the degree of inhibition of P2Y12 receptors and aid decision making in those emergency cases where practitioners wish to perform a neuraxial anesthetic.

Ref: Katzung BG, Masters SB, Trevor AJ. *Basic and Clinical Pharmacology*. 12th ed. (LANGE Basic series). New York, NY: McGraw Hill; 2012.

9. Which of the following statements regarding acute normovolemic hemodilution (ANH) is LEAST correct?

    (A) ANH is indicated for cases where expected blood loss is >2 units.

    (B) Collected blood may be stored at room temperature for up to 4 hours before refrigeration is required.

    (C) Some Jehovah's Witnesses will accept blood collected via ANH.

    (D) Tissue perfusion is increased due to a reduction in blood viscosity.

    (E) The efficacy of ANH is unproven.

The principle of ANH is to remove fresh whole blood from the patient prior to the commencement of surgery, while maintaining blood volume with crystalloid or colloid, so that blood lost during the procedure is of a lower hemoglobin concentration. Once the major blood loss has occurred, the patient's blood can then be transfused to elevate the final hemoglobin concentration.

ANH is typically considered in young, healthy patients with good initial hemoglobin concentration (>12 g/dL), who are expected to lose two or more units of blood (about 900–1,000 ml). Some Jehovah's Witnesses will agree to ANH if the blood remains in a closed-circuit system. Contraindications include patients with cardiac disease who may not tolerate the induced anemia, those with impaired renal function (since large amounts of fluid will need to be filtered), baseline hemoglobin <12 g/dL, or technical problems such as lack of appropriate vascular access.

The volume of blood that can be drawn will vary depending on the patient's initial blood volume, the type of procedure, and the anticipated surgical blood loss. Many anesthesiologists aim to reduce the hemoglobin to a concentration of 8–9 g/dL before surgery begins. A simple calculation can be used to determine the amount of blood that should be removed to achieve a target hemoglobin:

$$V = EBV \times (Hb_{init} - Hb_{desired}) \div Hb_{average}$$

where EBV is estimated blood volume, Hb_{init} is the initial hemoglobin concentration, $Hb_{desired}$ is the desired hemoglobin concentration, and $Hb_{average}$ is the average of the initial and the desired. Blood is obtained by connecting standard blood collection tubing to a large vein or a peripheral artery and allowing standard blood bags containing anticoagulant to fill. These are then labeled, numbered, and weighed. According to the AABB (formerly the American Association of Blood Banks), blood can stored at room temperature in the operating room for 8 hours; if not used within that time, it can be stored at 1–6°C for 24 hours. The blood should be returned in the reverse order it was collected, so that the first bag, with the highest number of red cells, platelets, and coagulation factors, is given last.

While arterial oxygen content is reduced, compensatory hemodynamic changes occur. The reduced viscosity decreases systemic vascular resistance and improves venous return to the heart by enhanced peripheral venous flow. The increased preload and decreased afterload increase the stroke volume and the cardiac output.

A purported advantage of ANH is reduction of exposure to allogeneic blood with its host of potential risks. However, despite its theoretical attractiveness as a technique, there is little evidence supporting its efficacy. A 2004 meta-analysis concluded that the efficacy is likely to be small if at all present, and that bleeding and allogeneic blood requirements are only mildly reduced.

Ref: Longnecker DE, Brown DL, Newman MF, Zapol WM. *Anesthesiology*. 2nd ed. New York, NY: McGraw Hill; 2012.

10. Which of the following is LEAST likely to be a complication related to intraoperative blood salvage?

    (A) air embolism

    (B) infection

    (C) anaphylaxis

    (D) fat embolism

    (E) disseminated intravascular coagulation (DIC)

Intraoperative blood salvage (IBS) is a procedure whereby shed blood is collected, anticoagulated, centrifuged, washed, and then re-suspended in saline to provide bags of autologous cells with a hematocrit of approximately 50–70%. IBS reduces the requirements for allogeneic transfusion by 40% with a good safety profile. It is indicated for a wide variety of surgical procedures, and contraindications are few. These include the surgical use of collagen hemostatic agents, betadine or hydrogen peroxide, and blood-borne infections that could endanger the health care workers if the IBS apparatus malfunctioned.

Three other situations (malignancy, bacteremia, and obstetrics) have been cited as contraindications, but all three are controversial and should be decided on a case-by-base basis. Concern regarding hematogenous seeding of cancer cells during surgery for malignancy has largely been shown to be unwarranted, as the evidence shows no greater risk for recurrence in urologic cancer surgery. Similarly, there is no evidence that amniotic fluid embolus rates are higher when IBS is used than when it is not. In both situations, the use of a leukodepletion filter is advocated to filter out cells and debris. IBS use during surgery on infected/contaminated tissue is also controversial, but appears to be safe, provided the area is thoroughly irrigated beforehand and prophylactic antibiotics are used.

Complications include:

- air embolism (prevented by using in-line air detectors)
- fat embolism (prevented by washing and using a microaggregate filter for infusion)
- infection (prevented by using prophylactic antibiotics and avoiding aspirating grossly contaminated sites)
- coagulopathy (prevented by washing the salvaged blood)
- "salvaged blood syndrome." This refers to the development of DIC and/or increased capillary permeability in the lungs (ARDS) or periphery (peripheral edema) after transfusion of washed cells. It may be caused by activation of platelets (DIC) and white blood cells (capillary leak) during salvage (prevented by using citrate as the anticoagulant, rather than heparin).

Anaphylaxis is not a typical complication of IBS, but is more common in allogeneic blood transfusion.

Ref: Kuppurao L, Wee M. Perioperative Cell Salvage. *Contin Educ Anaesth Crit Care Pain.* 2010;10(4):104–108.

11. Which of the following statements regarding the use of erythropoietin to treat preoperative anemia is LEAST accurate?

(A) Erythropoietin acts on peritubular cells of the kidney.

(B) The usual dosing schedule is three weekly doses leading up to surgery, plus a fourth dose on the day of surgery.

(C) Iron supplementation is required for maximal efficacy.

(D) Erythropoietin minimizes perioperative exposure to allogeneic blood transfusion in major orthopedic and cardiac surgical patients.

(E) Erythropoietin is associated with increased risk of deep venous thrombosis.

Erythropoietin (EPO) is a glycoprotein growth factor that is produced by the peritubular cells of the kidney in response to hypoxia. It is the primary trigger for erythropoiesis, acting on the bone marrow to stimulate red cell production. Recombinant human EPO is used in chronic renal failure, as well as in the preoperative setting in those patients who are anemic and undergoing preoperative autologous donation. EPO is also used for those patients who are anemic and will not accept a blood transfusion for religious reasons.

The administration of iron (oral or parenteral) with EPO maximizes the gains in red cell mass. One systematic review and several randomized controlled trials have demonstrated that EPO is associated with significant reductions in perioperative allogeneic blood transfusion compared with placebo or preoperative autologous donation. However, patients undergoing spinal surgery with pneumatic compression devices were more likely to develop deep venous thromboses if they received EPO than if they received placebo. In 2007, the FDA required manufacturers of erythropoiesis-stimulating agents such as EPO to carry a black box warning specifying the increased risk of deep venous thrombosis, and encouraging the use of thromboprophylaxis in surgical populations receiving these drugs.

Ref: Kumar A. Perioperative management of anemia: limits of blood transfusion and alternatives to it. *Cleve Clin J Med.* 2009;76(Suppl 4):S112–S118.

12. Which of the following statements regarding the toxicity of immunosuppressive therapies for graft-versus-host disease is LEAST accurate?

   (A) Corticosteroid toxicities include aseptic vascular necrosis, hypertension and osteoporosis.

   (B) Methotrexate toxicities include hepatotoxicity and renal injury.

   (C) Cyclosporine toxicities include renal injury and elevated bilirubin.

   (D) Antithymocyte globulin toxicities include cardiomyopathy and lung injury.

   (E) Hydroxychloroquine toxicities include visual disturbances.

Graft-versus-host disease (GVHD) occurs when T cells from donor blood or bone marrow are engrafted and become activated in the presence of host ("foreign") antigen. Typically the host is immuno-incompetent, although immunocompetent hosts can suffer GVHD as well. The graft begins to produce and secrete various inflammatory cytokines. This leads to tissue damage of the host, particularly in the liver, skin, mucosa, and gastrointestinal system. Posttransfusion GVHD carries a mortality of >90%, most of these a direct result of aplastic bone marrow. Since leukocyte reduction is not 100% successful in filtering lymphocytes, irradiation of blood is indicated in high-risk patients.

Immunosuppressive and antirejection drugs are often targeted at components of the cell-mediated immunologic system (e.g., T lymphocytes). Several pharmacologic therapies are used for both prevention and treatment of graft-versus-host disease, and are summarized in Table 19-1.

Ref: Longnecker DE, Brown DL, Newman MF, Zapol WM. *Anesthesiology.* 2nd ed. New York, NY: McGraw Hill; 2012.

13. In the kidney, hydrochlorothiazide and other thiazide diuretics act as inhibitors at which of the following sites?

   (A) Na^+-K^+-$2Cl^-$ symport

   (B) Na^+-Cl^- symport

   (C) renal epithelial Na^+ channels

   (D) mineralocorticoid receptors

   (E) nonspecific cation channels

Hydrochlorothiazide and other thiazide diuretics are inhibitors of Na^+-Cl^- symport. The predominant site of action is the distal convoluted tubule (DCT). Urinary excretion of sodium, potassium, and chloride is increased. Note that thiazide diuretics are relatively weak, as most sodium reabsorption (~90%) occurs proximal to the DCT. Other classes of diuretics include:

- Inhibitors of carbonic anhydrase (e.g., acetazolamide)—primary site of action is the proximal convoluted tubule. This prevents reabsorption of HCO_3^-, leading to alkalinization of urine and increased renal excretion of bicarbonate, phosphate, potassium, and sodium.

- Osmotic diuretics (e.g., mannitol) act to increase the osmolality of tubular fluid. Loop of Henle is the primary site of action. Mechanism of action is increased water extraction and decreased medullary tonicity (by increasing renal blood flow). This results in increased excretion of most electrolytes.

- Inhibitors of Na^+-K^+-$2Cl^-$ symport (e.g., loop diuretics such as furosemide) inhibit the Na^+-K^+-$2Cl^-$ symporter in the thick ascending limb of the loop of Henle. Urinary excretion of water and most electrolytes is increased, particularly sodium, chloride, calcium, and magnesium.

- Inhibitors of renal epithelial Na^+ channels (e.g., potassium-sparing diuretics such as triamterene and amiloride) act in the distal tubule and collecting duct to increase sodium excretion. Blockade of sodium

TABLE 19-1. Common pharmacologic options for prevention and treatment of graft-versus-host disease.

Immunosuppressive drug	Mechanism of action	Serious toxicities
Corticosteroids	Unclear; may be suppression of pro-inflammatory cytokines	Infection, hyperglycemia, Cushing's syndrome, psychosis, myopathy, avascular necrosis, osteoporosis
Methotrexate	Antimetabolite; inhibits dihydrofolate reductase, leading to impaired purine and thymidylate synthesis	Hepatotoxicity, lung injury, myelosuppression, renal tubular injury
Cyclosporine and tacrolimus	Interrupts T-cell signaling	Renal injury, hyperbilirubinemia
Sirolimus	Interrupts T-cell signaling	Elevated liver function tests, diarrhea
Mycophenolate	Blocks purine synthesis	Neutropenia
Antithymocyte globulin	Immunologic destruction of leukocytes	Serum sickness
Hydroxychloroquine	Interferes with antigen presentation	Visual disturbances (difficulty with accommodation, blurred vision, photophobia, retinopathy)

channels also results in membrane hyperpolarization and decreased excretion of other cations such as K^+, H^+, Ca^{2+}, Mg^{2+}.

- Antagonists of mineralocorticoid receptors (e.g., potassium-sparing diuretics such as spironolactone) act via mineralocorticoid receptors in the distal tubule and collecting duct. Results are similar to triamterene and amiloride, in that urinary sodium excretion increases while membrane hyperpolarization decreases excretion of other cations such as K^+, H^+, Ca^{2+}, Mg^{2+}.

- Inhibitors of nonspecific cation channels (e.g., natriuretic peptides such as nesiritide) act at the inner medullary collecting duct to decrease sodium reabsorption.

Ref: Brunton LL, Chabner BA, Knollman BC. *Goodman & Gilman's the Pharmacological Basis of Therapeutics.* 12th ed. New York, NY: McGraw Hill; 2011.

14. Which of the following diuretics is considered a K^+-sparing diuretic?

(A) **triamterene**

(B) hydrochlorothiazide

(C) furosemide

(D) mannitol

(E) acetazolamide

Triamterene is an example of a potassium-sparing diuretic. Both triamterene and amiloride are examples of diuretics that inhibit renal epithelial sodium channels. The site of action for these drugs are sodium channels on the luminal membrane of principal cells in the distal tubule and collecting duct. Usually, the epithelial sodium channel is a conduit for sodium reabsorption, the gradient for which is set up by the Na-K-ATPase on the basolateral membrane of the principal cell. Blockage of the sodium channel by triamterene decreases the electrochemical gradient for potassium (and other cation) excretion. Mineralocorticoid receptor antagonists (e.g., spironolactone) are another class of potassium-sparing diuretics. In general, mineralocorticoids such as aldosterone have a variety of intracellular actions that promote sodium reabsorption. Blockage of the mineralocorticoid receptor decreases sodium reabsorption and, much like triamterene, alters the intracellular electrochemical gradient such that potassium (and other cation) excretion is decreased.

Ref: Brunton LL, Chabner BA, Knollman BC. *Goodman & Gilman's the Pharmacological Basis of Therapeutics.* 12th ed. New York, NY: McGraw Hill; 2011.

15. Chronic administration of furosemide will result in **decreased** renal excretion of which of the following?

(A) sodium

(B) chloride

(C) bicarbonate

(D) potassium

(E) **uric acid**

In general, loop diuretics such as furosemide will increase urinary excretion of Na^+, Cl^-, Ca^+, Mg^+, and H^+. These effects are due to inhibition of Na^+-K^+-$2Cl^-$ symport in the thick ascending limb of the loop of Henle. It is important to note that loop diuretics may also have additional effects. Furosemide also inhibits carbonic anhydrase, resulting in increased urinary excretion of HCO_3^- and phosphate. Acute administration of loop diuretics will increase uric acid excretion while **chronic administration of loop diuretics will decrease uric acid excretion**. This decrease in uric acid excretion may be due to changes in uric acid handling in the proximal convoluted tubule.

Ref: Brunton LL, Chabner BA, Knollman BC. *Goodman & Gilman's the Pharmacological Basis of Therapeutics.* 12th ed. New York, NY: McGraw Hill; 2011.

16. After acute administration of a diuretic, a patient notes tinnitus and hearing impairment. Which of the following diuretics is most likely to cause ototoxicity?

(A) amiloride

(B) acetazolamide

(C) hydrochlorothiazide

(D) **furosemide**

(E) mannitol

Furosemide and other loop diuretics, particularly after rapid intravenous administration, may cause ototoxicity (tinnitus, vertigo, hearing impairment, and even deafness). Other side effects of loop diuretics include hyperuricemia and gout; hyperglycemia; increased plasma levels of cholesterol, triglycerides, and low-density lipoprotein; and bone marrow depression. Amiloride (and other potassium-sparing diuretics) may cause significant hyperkalemia.

Other side effects may include nausea, vomiting, and headache. Carbonic anhydrase inhibitors (e.g., acetazolamide) are sulfonamide derivatives and may be associated with bone marrow depression and allergic hypersensitivity. Other side effects include precipitation of calcium phosphate salts leading to ureteral colic and aggravating metabolic or respiratory acidosis. Thiazide diuretics may rarely cause neurologic symptoms such as headache, paresthesias, or vertigo. They may also cause gastrointestinal symptoms such as nausea, vomiting, cholecystitis, and pancreatitis. Osmotic diuretics such as mannitol expand the volume of the extracellular compartment. In patients with cardiac dysfunction this may precipitate pulmonary edema. Other side effects of mannitol may include nausea, vomiting, and headache.

Ref: Brunton LL, Chabner BA, Knollman BC. *Goodman & Gilman's the Pharmacological Basis of Therapeutics.* 12th ed. New York, NY: McGraw Hill; 2011.

17. A patient at risk of perioperative acute kidney injury (AKI) is administered an infusion of low-dose dopamine (1–3 mcg/kg/min). Theoretically, what is the potential benefit of using dopamine for renal protection?

    (A) D_1 receptor mediated increase in mean blood pressure and heart rate

    (B) D_2 receptor mediated natriuresis

    (C) D_1 receptor mediated diuresis

    (D) D_1 receptor mediated activation of Na^+-H^+ exchanger in distal convoluted tubule

    (E) D_2 receptor mediated renal vasodilatation

Low-dose dopamine (1–3 mcg/kg/min) will cause a D_1 receptor mediated diuresis and increase in urine output. Theoretically, low-dose dopamine acts specifically on dopaminergic receptors, while at higher doses the α- and β-adrenergic receptor effects of dopamine predominate. The dopaminergic effects in the kidneys are mediated by the D_1 receptor, which causes vasodilation of renal vasculature. Renal vasodilation leads to an increase in renal blood flow and glomerular filtration rate. D_1 receptor activation also increases cAMP levels in epithelial cells of the proximal convoluted tubule and medullary thick ascending limb of the loop of Henle. This inhibits Na^+-H^+ exchange and the Na^+-K^+- ATPase, resulting in both natriuresis and diuresis. Although dopamine can increase renal blood flow and urine output, it has NOT proven efficacious in the treatment or prevention of acute kidney injury (AKI). In general, the α1- and β1-adrenergic receptor effects of progressively higher concentrations of dopamine will increase heart rate and mean blood pressure, while systemic vascular resistance will initially decrease (β1-adrenergic receptor activation predominates) and then increase (α1-adrenergic receptor activation predominates). The difficulty in predicting the hemodynamic or renal effects of any particular dose of dopamine are due to the complex pharmacokinetics of dopamine (as cardiac output increases, dopamine alters its own metabolism), resulting in wide inter-individual plasma concentrations of dopamine for any given infusion rate, meaning what is low-dose dopamine for one patient may not be so for another patient.

Refs: Brunton LL, Chabner BA, Knollman BC. *Goodman & Gilman's the Pharmacological Basis of Therapeutics.* 12th ed. New York, NY: McGraw Hill; 2011.

Johnson KB. *Clinical Pharmacology for Anesthesiology.* 1st ed. New York, NY: McGraw Hill; 2015.

Hussain T, Lokhandwala MF. Renal dopamine receptor function in hypertension. *Hypertension.* 1998;32: 187–197.

MacGregor DA, Smith TE, Prielipp RC, et al. Pharmacokinetics of dopamine in healthy male subjects. *Anesthesiology.* 2000;92(2):338–346.

PART 3

Physics, Equipment, Monitors, and Mathematics

CHAPTER 20

Physics

1. Which of the following most closely represents the equivalent of 10 cm H_2O?

   (A) 1.47 psi
   (B) 97 mbar
   (C) 7.4 mm Hg
   (D) 0.1 kPa
   (E) 0.5 atm

2. Which of the following best prevents the inadvertent connection of the wrong gas cylinder to the anesthesia machine?

   (A) the Diameter Index Safety System
   (B) the Pin Index Safety System
   (C) yokes that are specifically sized for each type of gas
   (D) Department of Transport markings on cylinders
   (E) color-coding of cylinders

3. You are delivering sedation at a remote site within the hospital using an E-cylinder of oxygen at 5 L/min. The pressure gauge reads 500 psi. How much longer will the tank last approximately?

   (A) 33 minutes
   (B) 66 minutes
   (C) 99 minutes
   (D) 120 minutes
   (E) 150 minutes

4. The pressure gauge of an E-cylinder containing nitrous oxide reads 745 psi. What volume of nitrous oxide is left in the tank?

   (A) 330 L
   (B) 660 L
   (C) 1,590 L
   (D) 2,000 L
   (E) unable to determine with this information

5. Which of the following best describes the purpose of the oxygen cylinder regulator in the anesthesia machine?

   (A) allow gas flow to commence when the valve is turned counterclockwise
   (B) prevent contamination of the cylinder with nitrous oxide
   (C) converts the upstream pressure of 2,200 psi to a downstream pressure of 45 psi
   (D) prevents a hypoxic mixture from being delivered
   (E) provides oxygen to drive the bellows

6. In the middle of a long case, the arterial blood pressure transducer falls from its mount and is now hanging 30 cm below its original position. What is the result of this on the blood pressure values shown on the monitor?

   (A) Arterial blood pressure will be underestimated by approximately 30 mm Hg.
   (B) Arterial blood pressure will be overestimated by approximately 30 mm Hg.
   (C) Arterial blood pressure will be underestimated by approximately 20 mm Hg.
   (D) Arterial blood pressure will be overestimated by approximately 20 mm Hg.
   (E) There will be no net effect since the transducer is zeroed to atmospheric pressure.

7. A patient with tracheal tumor is prescribed a mixture of oxygen and helium (heliox) in the critical care unit. Which property of this gas mixture improves the flow within the large airways?

    (A) temperature
    (B) density
    (C) viscosity
    (D) kinetic energy
    (E) miscibility

8. A patient presents to the operating room in hemorrhagic shock from a motor vehicle accident. In considering how best to resuscitate the patient, which of the following single physical properties will best permit the most rapid administration of fluids and blood?

    (A) the length of the intravenous cannula
    (B) the diameter of the intravenous cannula
    (C) the density of the fluid solution
    (D) the viscosity of the fluid solution
    (E) the pressure differential between the IV bag and the vein

9. Which of the following increases the likelihood that flow in a tube will be turbulent, and not laminar?

    (A) low velocity
    (B) narrow diameter tubes
    (C) decreased density of fluids
    (D) decreased viscosity of fluids
    (E) increased temperature of fluids

10. In designing the gas-specific tapered glass tubes (Thorpe tubes) used in variable orifice flowmeters, which of the following factors must be taken into account to ensure precise measurements at all flow rates?

    (A) the density of the gas
    (B) the viscosity of the gas
    (C) both the density and the viscosity of the gas
    (D) neither the density nor the viscosity of the gas
    (E) the solubility coefficient of the gas

11. An ultrasound transducer is placed over the radial aspect of the wrist in order to locate the radial artery. The color Doppler function is activated, but no color is seen on the grayscale screen. Which of the following is the most likely explanation for this?

    (A) The ultrasound transducer is not correctly positioned on the patient.
    (B) The patient has an insufficient arterial blood pressure.
    (C) The ultrasound beam is directed (insonated) at an angle of 90 degrees with respect to the artery.
    (D) The gain on the color Doppler function is incorrectly set.
    (E) A Doppler shift should not be expected in the radial artery.

12. All of the following affect the rate of diffusion of gases across a membrane EXCEPT:

    (A) molecular size
    (B) partial pressure gradient
    (C) solubility coefficient of the gas
    (D) viscosity of the gas
    (E) membrane thickness

13. Which of the following statements regarding solubility of gases is TRUE?

    (A) At constant temperature, the amount of gas dissolved in liquid is inversely proportional to the partial pressure of the gas next to it.
    (B) Solubility of gases is increased with lower temperatures.
    (C) Solubility is increased with lower atmospheric pressures.
    (D) Solubility of a gas is a negligible factor in the diffusion rate across the alveolar-capillary interface.
    (E) The solubility of a volatile agent in olive oil is directly proportional to its minimum alveolar concentration (MAC).

14. Which of the following inhalational agents has the LOWEST blood/gas partition coefficient?

    (A) desflurane
    (B) halothane
    (C) isoflurane
    (D) nitrous oxide
    (E) sevoflurane

15. A gas that is 100% saturated with water vapor is heated by 5°C. Which of the following statements concerning the humidity is true?

    (A) the relative humidity of the gas increases
    (B) the relative humidity of the gas decreases
    (C) the absolute humidity of the gas increases
    (D) the absolute humidity of the gas decreases
    (E) water condenses in the breathing circuit

16. Critical temperature is best defined by which of the following?

    (A) the boiling point of a substance minus the melting point
    (B) the temperature above which proteins denature
    (C) the temperature above which no amount of pressure can convert a gas to liquid
    (D) the temperature at which spontaneous cardiac activity stops
    (E) the temperature at which, if dantrolene is not administered, malignant hyperthermia is 95% lethal

17. Critical pressure is best defined by which of the following?

    (A) the pressure at which a substance begins to melt
    (B) the pressure at which a substance begins to boil
    (C) the pressure at which a substance condenses at 100% relative humidity
    (D) the pressure required to liquefy a gas at its critical temperature
    (E) the pressure required to sublimate a solid at room temperature

18. A syringe with a known volume of gas is compressed to half of its volume while attached to a pressure transducer. The pressure rises from 20 mm Hg to 40 mm Hg (Figure 20-4). This is an example of which of the following laws?

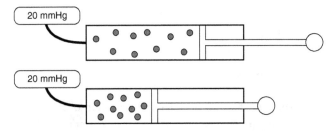

FIG. 20-4. A volume of gas compressed to half of its original volume.

    (A) Henry's Law
    (B) Dalton's Law
    (C) Boyle's Law
    (D) Avogadro's Law
    (E) Pascal's Law

19. You are giving anesthesia in Denver (atmospheric pressure: 630 mm Hg). Your fresh gas mix is 50% air and 50% oxygen. What is the approximate partial pressure of oxygen delivered to the patient (assuming dry gas with no water vapor pressure)?

    (A) 100 mm Hg
    (B) 130 mm Hg
    (C) 315 mm Hg
    (D) 380 mm Hg
    (E) unable to calculate with this information

20. A patient is being mechanically ventilated in a critical care unit in San Diego (sea level). He is receiving an FiO_2 of 30%. A recent arterial blood gas shows the following: pH 7.31, $PaCO_2$ 50 mm Hg, PaO_2 133 mm Hg, HCO_3^- 19 mmol/L. Which of the following answers best represents the patient's alveolar-arterial (A-a) gradient?

    (A) 5 mm Hg
    (B) 8 mm Hg
    (C) 12 mm Hg
    (D) 18 mm Hg
    (E) 24 mm Hg

21. At a constant temperature, the amount of gas dissolved in a liquid is directly proportional to the partial pressure of the gas in contact with the liquid. This statement is best described as:

    (A) Pascal's law
    (B) Henry's law
    (C) Boyle's law
    (D) Dalton's law
    (E) Avogadro's law

22. The rate at which alveolar concentration of anesthetic agent rises to meet the inspired concentration (FA/FI) is primarily determined by which pair of factors?

    (A) cardiac output and blood solubility
    (B) blood solubility and inspired concentration
    (C) cardiac output and inspired concentration
    (D) minute ventilation and inspired concentration
    (E) cardiac output and minute ventilation

23. Which of the following combination of factors serves to INCREASE the uptake of anesthetic agent from the alveoli, where P_A-P_V is the alveolar-to-venous partial pressure difference?

    (A) increased solubility; increased cardiac output; increased P_A-P_V
    (B) increased solubility; decreased cardiac output; decreased P_A-P_V
    (C) decreased solubility; decreased cardiac output; increased P_A-P_V
    (D) decreased solubility; decreased cardiac output; decreased P_A-P_V
    (E) decreased solubility; increased cardiac output; increased P_A-P_V

24. A general anesthetic is being administered in a healthy patient for bunion surgery. After 60 minutes of breathing 2% sevoflurane with a fresh gas flow of 2 L/min, which of the following best represents the partial pressures of sevoflurane found at different locations, from highest to lowest?

    (A) Brain > Muscle > Fat > Circuit
    (B) Brain > Circuit > Muscle > Fat
    (C) Circuit > Brain > Muscle > Fat
    (D) Circuit > Muscle > Brain > Fat
    (E) Circuit > Muscle > Fat > Brain

25. The concentration of an inhaled anesthetic is increased by a factor of 5. The resulting alveolar concentration is increased by a factor of over 6. This is an example of:

    (A) concentration effect
    (B) second gas effect
    (C) solubility effect
    (D) ventilation effect
    (E) blood:gas partition effect

26. The increase in alveolar concentration of a volatile agent when nitrous oxide is used as a carrier gas is termed:

    (A) concentrating effect
    (B) replenishment effect
    (C) second gas effect
    (D) capillary uptake effect
    (E) ventilation effect

27. A trauma patient has a small (75 mL) unrecognized pneumothorax. Following intravenous induction of anesthesia, she is maintained with desflurane in 50:50 oxygen:nitrous oxide. After 30 minutes (at steady state), the volume of the pneumothorax will be:

    (A) 25 mL
    (B) 50 mL
    (C) 75 mL
    (D) 150 mL
    (E) 225 mL

Answers and Explanations: Physics

1. Which of the following most closely represents the equivalent of 10 cm H_2O?

   (A) 1.47 psi
   (B) 97 mbar
   (C) 7.4 mm Hg
   (D) 0.1 kPa
   (E) 0.5 atm

Pressure is the ratio of force to the area over which it is applied. While the SI unit for force is the pascal (Pa), which is equal to 1 newton per square meter, other traditional non-SI units are commonly used, especially in the United States. For example, in anesthetic practice, pounds per square inch (psi) is used to describe cylinder and pipeline pressures. Pressure is commonly described by its ability to displace a column of fluid; for instance, millimeters of mercury (mm Hg) are used for pressures within body systems (e.g., arterial blood pressure, intracranial pressure, tissue compartment pressure). The use of centimeters of water (cm H_2O) is typically confined to measurement of airway pressure. However, the reporting of central venous pressures using water manometry in cm H_2O is still relatively common practice and a frequent source of confusion for trainees. The use of electronic pressure transducers is now almost universal for CVP monitoring, and these values are reported in mm Hg. Millibar and atmosphere units are not typically used in clinical medicine. A conversion table is presented in Table 20-1.

TABLE 20-1. **Approximate conversions between SI (kPa) and other common units of pressure measurement.**

kPa	cm H_2O	mm Hg	mbar	psi	atm
1	10	7.4	9.7	0.147	0.01

Ref: Middleton B, Phillips J, Thomas R, Stacey S. *Physics in Anesthesia.* 1st ed. Banbury, UK: Scion Publishing; 2012.

2. Which of the following best prevents the inadvertent connection of the wrong gas cylinder to the anesthesia machine?

   (A) the Diameter Index Safety System
   (B) the Pin Index Safety System
   (C) yokes that are specifically sized for each type of gas
   (D) Department of Transport markings on cylinders
   (E) color-coding of cylinders

Connection of the wrong cylinder of gas to the oxygen yoke of an anesthesia machine presents a serious and avoidable hazard. Color-coding of cylinders was an early strategy to prevent this, although it did not prevent human error. Moreover, the US convention for color-coding oxygen and air differs from the international convention (Table 20-2). Since E-cylinders are uniform in size regardless of the gas inside, the yokes must be as well. The Department of Transport does stamp markings permanently onto the shoulder of each cylinder, but they relate to the service pressure at a standard temperature, the manufacturer, and the serial number, rather than the composition of the gas inside.

TABLE 20-2. **Color coding for medical gas cylinders.**[a]

Gas cylinder	US convention	International convention
Oxygen	Green	White
Carbon dioxide	Gray	Gray
Nitrous oxide	Blue	Blue
Helium	Brown	Brown
Nitrogen	Black	Black
Air	Yellow	White and black checkered

[a]On your next break from studying, look up the 1947 movie "Green for Danger" starring Alistair Sim, who plays a detective trying to solve a string of operating room deaths. Spoiler alert: the title of the film refers in part to the medical gas cylinders used and a deliberate act of sabotage.

The Pin Index Safety System consists of a series of two holes on the cylinder valve apparatus just below the gas outlet port. Specific pin configurations exist for each gas, including cylinders containing mixed gases such as helium-oxygen and N_2O-oxygen. The pins on

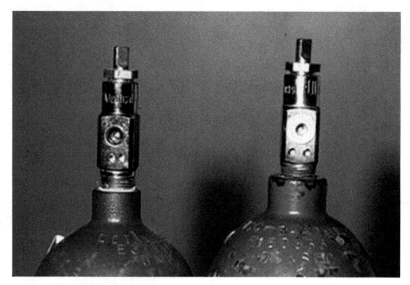

FIG. 20-1. Pin-indexed safety system for a nitrous oxide tank (*left*) and an oxygen tank (*right*). Note different pin arrangements for each tank. (Reproduced with permission from Longnecker DE, Brown DL, Newman MF, Zapol WM. *Anesthesiology*. 2nd ed. New York, NY: McGraw Hill; 2012.)

the yoke align with the holes drilled in the valve in such a way that erroneous connection of a different gas is not possible (Figure 20-1). An exception to this is a case of damage (either accidental or deliberate) to the pins in the yoke; without the correct number and alignment of pins, the yoke may accept different types of cylinders.

The Diameter Index Safety System is a similar concept, but relates to pipeline hoses. Each type of gas hose has a specific nipple design with two concentric shoulders of differing diameters; these are accepted securely only into the bodies of the appropriate port on the machine and the wall.

Ref: Dorsch JA, Dorsch SE. *Understanding Anesthesia Equipment*. 5th ed. Philadelphia, PA: Lippincott Williams & Wilkins; 2008.

3. You are delivering sedation at a remote site within the hospital using an E-cylinder of oxygen at 5 L/min. The pressure gauge reads 500 psi. How much longer will the tank last approximately?

    (A) **33 minutes**
    (B) 66 minutes
    (C) 99 minutes
    (D) 120 minutes
    (E) 150 minutes

When full at room temperature, an E-cylinder of oxygen has a capacity of 660 L and a pressure of approximately 2,000 psi (range typically 1,900–2,200 psi). Oxygen exists only as a gas at ambient temperature, so

we can calculate the remaining volume knowing that the pressure and volume will decrease proportionally. 500 psi is 25% of 2,000 psi, and so there should be 0.25×660 L in the tank, or 165 L. At a rate of 5 L/min, this will be used up in 33 minutes.

Ref: Dorsch JA, Dorsch SE. *Understanding Anesthesia Equipment*. 5th ed. Philadelphia, PA: Lippincott Williams & Wilkins; 2008.

4. The pressure gauge of an E-cylinder containing nitrous oxide reads 745 psi. What volume of nitrous oxide is left in the tank?

    (A) 330 L
    (B) 660 L
    (C) 1,590 L
    (D) 2,000 L
    (E) **unable to determine with this information**

The critical temperature of a gas is defined as the temperature above which no amount of pressurization can convert it to a liquid. For example, the critical temperature of oxygen is −118°C, meaning that in order to have a tank of liquid oxygen, it must be cooled to or below −118°C. In contrast, the critical temperature for nitrous oxide is considerably higher, at +36.5°C. Therefore, in a full, pressurized E-cylinder of nitrous oxide, there exists some liquid and some vapor, with a capacity of 1,590 L and a pressure of 745 psi. As long as there is some liquid phase in the tank, the pressure exerted by the vaporized portion will remain at 745 psi.

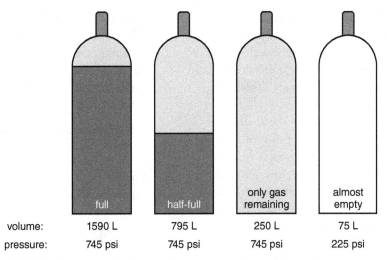

FIG. 20-2. Comparison of volumes and pressures in nitrous oxide cylinders.

Only when the liquid is fully evaporated will the volume of gas remaining start to decline proportionally to pressure. This usually begins to occur with approximately 250 L of gas left (Figure 20-2).

If it is necessary to estimate the remaining volume while some nitrous oxide still exists as liquid, weighing the cylinder and comparing against the tare weight (empty cylinder weight) should give a rough estimate of the remaining weight of the liquid N_2O. Avogadro's law can be applied, knowing that 1 mole of N_2O (i.e., 44 g) will occupy 22.4 L at standard temperature and pressure. For example:

- assume the calculated difference between actual weight and tare weight is 1.65 kg, or 1650 g
- 1650 g/44 g/mol = 37.5 mol
- 37.5 mol × 22.4 L of gas/mol = 840 L of nitrous oxide left in the tank

Ref: Dorsch JA, Dorsch SE. *Understanding Anesthesia Equipment.* 5th ed. Philadelphia, PA: Lippincott Williams & Wilkins; 2008.

5. Which of the following best describes the purpose of the oxygen cylinder regulator in the anesthesia machine?

(A) allow gas flow to commence when the valve is turned counterclockwise

(B) prevent contamination of the cylinder with nitrous oxide

(C) **converts the upstream pressure of 2,200 psi to a downstream pressure of 45 psi**

(D) prevents a hypoxic mixture from being delivered

(E) provides oxygen to drive the bellows

The regulators placed just after the cylinder gas enters the machine adjusts the incoming pressure of up to 2,200 psi to between 45 and 47 psi. There is also a similar regulator for nitrous oxide, adjusting the incoming pressure of up to 745 psi to 45 psi. This adjustment to slightly less than pipeline pressure (50 psi) also prevents inadvertent depletion of cylinder gas when the E-cylinder is left open, as the higher pipeline pressure keeps the regulator shut.

Ref: Butterworth JF IV, Mackey DC, Wasnick JD. *Morgan & Mikhail's Clinical Anesthesiology.* 5th ed. New York, NY: McGraw Hill; 2013.

6. In the middle of a long case, the arterial blood pressure transducer falls from its mount and is now hanging 30 cm below its original position. What is the result of this on the blood pressure values shown on the monitor?

(A) Arterial blood pressure will be underestimated by approximately 30 mm Hg.

(B) Arterial blood pressure will be overestimated by approximately 30 mm Hg.

(C) Arterial blood pressure will be underestimated by approximately 20 mm Hg.

(D) **Arterial blood pressure will be overestimated by approximately 20 mm Hg.**

(E) There will be no net effect since the transducer is zeroed to atmospheric pressure.

Invasive intravascular monitoring lines are connected via a continuous column of saline to a pressure transducer, which converts mechanical energy into electrical energy. Modern transducers have a flexible diaphragm across which an electrical current is applied. As pressure is applied to the diaphragm, it stretches, and the electrical resistance changes. The altered electrical output from the system is interpreted by the monitor and a pressure waveform displayed graphically. This is an example of a strain gauge.

Transducers measure the pressure in the line relative to the original pressure detected. For this reason, it is necessary to calibrate or zero the transducer to atmospheric pressure ("room air") before use. Since the column of fluid between the transducer and the patient is subject to gravitational forces, any change in the relative height will affect the interpretation of the values. For example, lowering the bed while keeping the transducer at the same level on the IV pole will result in less pressure transmitted to the diaphragm, and an underestimation of BP. Similarly, a transducer that accidentally dangles below the level of the patient will be exposed to a longer vertical column of fluid, and BP will be overestimated. In this case, 30 cm of water is roughly equivalent to 20 mm Hg (10 cm H_2O = 7.4 mm Hg).

This property can be used deliberately in certain monitoring instances. For example, while for most cases monitoring at the level of the heart is desired, in many neurosurgical procedures it is useful to know the arterial pressure at the circle of Willis, so that brain perfusion can be ensured. The height of the transducer is adjusted to that of the base of the skull in these cases.

Ref: Middleton B, Phillips J, Thomas R, Stacey S. *Physics in Anesthesia.* 1st ed. Banbury, UK: Scion Publishing; 2012.

7. A patient with tracheal tumor is prescribed a mixture of oxygen and helium (heliox) in the critical care unit. Which property of this gas mixture improves the flow within the large airways?

   (A) temperature

   (B) density

   (C) viscosity

   (D) kinetic energy

   (E) miscibility

In patients with upper airway obstruction, flow is turbulent and dependent on the density of the gas. Thus, for a given pressure gradient (i.e., when the patient inspires), a gas with a lower density will achieve higher flow rates around the obstruction. Heliox is a mixture of helium and oxygen (usually 79% helium to 21% oxygen). By replacing the nitrogen in air with the much less dense helium, the flow rates achieved with heliox are much higher, and a reduction in the work of breathing can be achieved. This effect is less beneficial for conditions where small airway obstruction predominates such as COPD or asthma, as flow is likely to be laminar.

Ref: Middleton B, Phillips J, Thomas R, Stacey S. *Physics in Anesthesia.* 1st ed. Banbury, UK: Scion Publishing; 2012.

8. A patient presents to the operating room in hemorrhagic shock from a motor vehicle accident. In considering how best to resuscitate the patient, which of the following single physical properties will best permit the most rapid administration of fluids and blood?

   (A) the length of the intravenous cannula

   (B) the diameter of the intravenous cannula

   (C) the density of the fluid solution

   (D) the viscosity of the fluid solution

   (E) the pressure differential between the IV bag and the vein

IV cannulae can be assumed to have laminar flow, as they have a relatively small diameter. Flow rates during laminar flow are NOT dependent on density (as turbulent flow is), but instead are influenced by the length and diameter of the tube, the pressure head, and the viscosity of solution, as given by the Hagan-Poiseuille equation:

$$\text{Flow (Q)} = (\pi \, \Delta P \, r^4)/(8\eta l)$$

where ΔP = pressure differential, η = viscosity, l = length of tube, r = radius of tube.

Note that a doubling of the pressure head or a halving of the tube length produces a doubling of the flow rate; in contrast, a doubling of the radius results in a flow rate 16 times higher. It is for this reason that during resuscitation, short large-bore IV cannulae are preferred over long, narrower gauge central lines.

Ref: Middleton B, Phillips J, Thomas R, Stacey S. *Physics in Anesthesia.* 1st ed. Banbury, UK: Scion Publishing; 2012.

9. Which of the following increases the likelihood that flow in a tube will be turbulent, and not laminar?

   (A) low velocity

   (B) narrow diameter tubes

   (C) decreased density of fluids

   (D) decreased viscosity of fluids

   (E) increased temperature of fluids

Flow in a tube can be either laminar or turbulent. Laminar flow describes an ordered pattern where all the molecules are moving in layers (or "laminae") of straight lines down the tube. Flow rates in laminar flow are fastest in the center and slowest at the periphery (Figure 20-3). Turbulent flow is characterized by disorganized movement and the presence of eddy currents within the tube. These eddy currents interfere with forward movement of molecules and increase the energy input required to achieve a given flow rate. In laminar flow, the flow rate is directly proportional to the pressure gradient; in turbulent flow, the flow rate is proportional to the square root of the pressure gradient. In other words, the amount of pressure required to squeeze fluid through an IV cannula using a pressure bag is doubled when flow turns from laminar to turbulent.

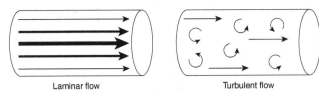

FIG. 20-3. Laminar and turbulent flow within tubes.

A number of factors influence the likelihood of flow becoming turbulent:

- increased velocity
- increased tube diameter
- increased fluid density (NB: increases in temperature decrease fluid density)
- decreased fluid viscosity

These factors can be put together in what is termed the Reynolds number:

$$\text{Reynolds number} = (v\, \rho\, d)/\eta$$

where v = velocity, ρ = density, d = diameter, η = viscosity.

In general, when the Reynolds number < 2,000, there is laminar flow. When the Reynolds number is > 4,000, there is turbulent flow. A Reynolds number between 2,000 and 4,000 is likely to have transitional flow (a mixture of laminar and turbulent).

Ref: Middleton B, Phillips J, Thomas R, Stacey S. *Physics in Anesthesia.* 1st ed. Banbury, UK: Scion Publishing; 2012.

10. In designing the gas-specific tapered glass tubes (Thorpe tubes) used in variable orifice flowmeters, which of the following factors must be taken into account to ensure precise measurements at all flow rates?

(A) the density of the gas
(B) the viscosity of the gas
(C) both the density and the viscosity of the gas
(D) neither the density nor the viscosity of the gas
(E) the solubility coefficient of the gas

Variable orifice flowmeters consist of a tapered glass (Thorpe) tube and an indicator ball, bobbin, or float that is suspended within the tube by the balance of two forces: gravity and the upward force of gas flow that can be adjusted by the operator. At the bottom of the tube, where the diameter is small, just a small amount of gas flow is required to push the bobbin up and allow flow around it. This flow is laminar in nature. As the control knob is turned and more flow is allowed into the tube, the bobbin rises into the increasingly wider tube until a point is reached where the increased velocity and diameter of the tube create turbulent flow conditions. Therefore, both the density (at turbulent flow) and viscosity (both turbulent and laminar flow) play a role in exactly how high the bobbin will float, and Thorpe tubes must be manufactured specifically for these parameters.

Ref: Middleton B, Phillips J, Thomas R, Stacey S. *Physics in Anesthesia.* 1st ed. Banbury, UK: Scion Publishing; 2012.

11. An ultrasound transducer is placed over the radial aspect of the wrist in order to locate the radial artery. The color Doppler function is activated, but no color is seen on the grayscale screen. Which of the following is the most likely explanation for this?

(A) The ultrasound transducer is not correctly positioned on the patient.
(B) The patient has an insufficient arterial blood pressure.
(C) The ultrasound beam is directed (insonated) at an angle of 90 degrees with respect to the artery.
(D) The gain on the color Doppler function is incorrectly set.
(E) A Doppler shift should not be expected in the radial artery.

The Doppler effect refers to the apparent change in the frequency of a wave when it is reflected back from a moving surface. This is heard every day when an ambulance, traveling toward you, appears to emit a siren with an increasing pitch. After passing, the pitch appears to decrease, although of course the pitch never changed in reality.

In ultrasound physics, a sound beam reflected off of a moving target (e.g., blood cells) will experience a Doppler shift, or change in frequency. This can be graphically represented in a number of ways by modern ultrasound machines. One of the most useful for clinical medicine is color Doppler, where varying velocities will be displayed as shades of red or blue. Targets moving toward the transducer will have a positive Doppler shift, and conventionally appear as shades of red; those that move away appear as blue ("BART: blue away, red towards"). The lighter the shade of blue or red, the higher the velocity.

A common error when attempting to use color Doppler is to insonate the transducer at 90 degrees to the vessel. This results in blood cells that travel neither toward nor away from the beam path, but rather travel parallel to the transducer surface. Tilting the transducer in either direction (i.e., proximally or distally) usually corrects this.

Ref: Middleton B, Phillips J, Thomas R, Stacey S. *Physics in Anesthesia*. 1st ed. Banbury, UK: Scion Publishing; 2012.

12. All of the following affect the rate of diffusion of gases across a membrane EXCEPT:

   (A) molecular size
   (B) partial pressure gradient
   (C) solubility coefficient of the gas
   (D) viscosity of the gas
   (E) membrane thickness

Diffusion is the random thermal motion of molecules (primarily gases and liquids), which results in the net transfer of molecules from a region of high concentration to low concentration. There are three broad determinants of gas diffusion:

- physicochemical characteristics of the gas (molecular weight, solubility)
- partial pressure gradient
- membrane characteristics (area, thickness)

They interact as described in Fick's Law of diffusion:

$$V_{gas} = \frac{A \times D \times (P_1 - P_2)}{T}$$

where V_{gas} = volume of gas diffusing through the tissue barrier per time (mL/min).

- A = surface area of the barrier

- D = diffusion coefficient (diffusivity) of the particular gas
- $(P_1 - P_2)$ = partial pressure difference across the gas barrier
- T = thickness of the barrier

The most important diffusion barrier in the body is the alveolar-capillary interface. Its surface area is approximately 70 m² in an adult. However, this may change as capillaries are recruited, as in the case of exercise, or if they are de-recruited, as in the case of hypotension or excessive PEEP. The thickness of this barrier is negligible (0.2–0.5 mm) unless disease processes such as fibrosis of pulmonary edema occur.

The term D, or diffusion constant, is directly proportional to solubility and inversely proportional to the square root of its molecular weight:

$$D \propto \frac{\text{solubility}}{\sqrt{MW}}$$

In other words, the heavier the gas, the longer it takes to diffuse, because lighter molecules travel faster and collide more frequently. The more soluble the gas in the barrier tissue, the faster the rate of diffusion. An example is carbon dioxide, which is 24 times more soluble in water than oxygen is, and therefore diffuses 20 times faster through the alveolar-capillary membrane than does oxygen. For this reason, patients are much more likely to develop problems with oxygenation than with hypercarbia when diffusion impairment occurs.

Ref: Levitzky MG. *Pulmonary Physiology*. 8th ed. New York, NY: McGraw Hill; 2013.

13. Which of the following statements regarding solubility of gases is TRUE?

   (A) At constant temperature, the amount of gas dissolved in liquid is inversely proportional to the partial pressure of the gas next to it.
   (B) Solubility of gases is increased with lower temperatures.
   (C) Solubility is increased with lower atmospheric pressures.
   (D) Solubility of a gas is a negligible factor in the diffusion rate across the alveolar-capillary interface.
   (E) The solubility of a volatile agent in olive oil is directly proportional to its minimum alveolar concentration (MAC).

Henry's Law states that for a constant temperature, the amount of a given gas that dissolves in a given type and volume of liquid is directly (not inversely) proportional to the partial pressure of that gas in equilibrium with that liquid. At equilibrium, there will be the same number of molecules existing in the gaseous phase and in the dissolved phase, both exerting the same kinetic energy.

Solubility of gases increases as temperature drops. Conversely, at higher temperatures, gases are more active and have more energy with which to escape from solution. This is why on opening a room-temperature can of carbonated soda will result in more bubbles of carbon dioxide escaping than a very cold can; the solubility of the gas is decreased. Likewise, rapidly warming cold blood from the blood bank often results in bubbles in solution as various gases decrease in solubility; for this reason, fluid warmers must always have a "bubble trap."

If the system is depressurized, the solubility decreases and gas will again come out of solution. The most dramatic example of this is deep-water divers who experience decompression sickness, or the "bends," when nitrogen bubbles form in the blood and tissues.

Solubility is a very important factor in diffusion rate across the alveolar-capillary membrane, as it is directly proportional to the diffusion constant in Fick's Law.

The oil:gas partition coefficient is proportional to potency and inversely proportional to MAC.

Ref: Middleton B, Phillips J, Thomas R, Stacey S. *Physics in Anesthesia.* 1st ed. Banbury, UK: Scion Publishing; 2012.

14. Which of the following inhalational agents has the LOWEST blood/gas partition coefficient?

   (A) desflurane
   (B) halothane
   (C) isoflurane
   (D) nitrous oxide
   (E) sevoflurane

Partition coefficients refer to the relative concentrations of a gas in each of two phases at steady state (i.e., when partial pressures are at equilibrium) (Table 20-3). For example, the blood:gas partition coefficient for desflurane is 0.42. At steady state, a given volume of blood has 0.42 times as much desflurane as gas in the alveoli. Bear in mind that the partial pressures are the same, even though the amount of anesthetic is different in the two phases. Blood has a much greater affinity for a soluble gas such as halothane than relatively insoluble gases like desflurane or nitrous oxide. With a blood:gas partition coefficient of 2.4, there will be over 5 times as

TABLE 20-3. Partition coefficients of volatile anesthetics at 37°C.[a]

Agent	Blood/ gas	Brain/ blood	Muscle/ blood	Fat/ blood
Nitrous oxide	0.47	1.1	1.2	2.3
Halothane	2.4	2.9	3.5	60
Isoflurane	1.4	2.6	4.0	45
Desflurane	0.42	1.3	2.0	27
Sevoflurane	0.65	1.7	3.1	48

[a]These values are averages derived from multiple studies and should be used for comparison purposes, not as exact numbers.
From: Butterworth JF IV, Mackey DC, Wasnick JD. *Morgan and Mikhail's Clinical Anesthesiology.* 5th ed. New York, NY: McGraw Hill; 2013.

much halothane than desflurane dissolved at steady state to ensure equal partial pressures in both phases.

Anesthetic agents with a low blood/gas solubility coefficient act more rapidly than highly soluble agents. This is often a difficult concept to understand. The more soluble the agent, the more is taken up by the blood and dissolved (i.e., "held on" by the blood). The volume of agent transferred from alveoli to blood may be *initially* greater because it has an affinity for that blood, but this occurs at the expense of a *resulting* lower partial pressure such that the partial pressure gradient drops. At the conclusion of anesthesia, poorly soluble agents leave the blood quickly and, provided ventilation is adequate, create a partial pressure gradient in favor of rapid transfer of agent out of the blood. A day-to-day analogy might be this: picture two glasses of a carbonated beverage, where one is ice-cold and one is room temperature. The solubility of the cold drink is greater, and it will take substantially longer for the bubbles to come out of the solution and for the drink to go flat, compared with the warm drink. Picture the blood as the soda (if you can stomach this distasteful image), and the gas just above the fluid as the brain or alveoli. Insoluble gases tend to reach equilibrium faster with tissues/alveoli because they are simply forced out of the solution much more easily.

15. A gas that is 100% saturated with water vapor is heated by 5°C. Which of the following statements concerning the humidity is true?

   (A) the relative humidity of the gas increases
   (B) the relative humidity of the gas decreases
   (C) the absolute humidity of the gas increases
   (D) the absolute humidity of the gas decreases
   (E) water condenses in the breathing circuit

Humidity is defined as the amount of water vapor in a gas. *Absolute* humidity is the mass of water vapor in a certain volume of gas. In contrast, *relative* humidity is the percent saturation, or the amount of water vapor at a particular temperature expressed as a percentage of the total capacity for water vapor.

If a gas that is saturated (100% relative humidity) is heated, its capacity for holding more water vapor increases, and so the relative humidity starts to drop as the gas expands. Because the absolute amount of water molecules remains the same, absolute humidity does not increase or decrease. Conversely, saturated gas that is cooled becomes oversaturated with water vapor and water begins to condense on the surface of the breathing circuit.

The water vapor pressure is a term describing the partial pressure of water vapor in a gas mixture. At body temperature, this pressure is 47 mm Hg. This becomes useful when using the alveolar gas equation: $PaO_2 = FiO_2 (P_{atm}-47 \text{ mm Hg}) \times PaCO_2/0.8$.

Ref: Dorsch JA, Dorsch SE. *Understanding Anesthesia Equipment.* 5th ed. Philadelphia, PA: Lippincott Williams & Wilkins; 2008.

16. Critical temperature is best defined by which of the following?

(A) the boiling point of a substance minus the melting point

(B) the temperature above which proteins denature

(C) the temperature above which no amount of pressure can convert a gas to liquid

(D) the temperature at which spontaneous cardiac activity stops

(E) the temperature at which, if dantrolene is not administered, malignant hyperthermia is 95% lethal

Gases can be converted to a liquid state with sufficient pressure at a certain temperature. In general, the higher the temperature, the more kinetic energy in the substance, and the more likely it is to remain as a gas. Every substance has a critical temperature (see examples in Table 2-4). The critical temperature for oxygen is −118°C, meaning that at room temperature, a cylinder of oxygen will always be in gaseous form. In contrast, the critical temperature for nitrous oxide is considerably higher, at +36.5°C. Therefore, in a full, pressurized E-cylinder of nitrous oxide, there exists some liquid and some gas.

Ref: Dorsch JA, Dorsch SE. *Understanding Anesthesia Equipment.* 5th ed. Philadelphia, PA: Lippincott Williams & Wilkins; 2008.

17. Critical pressure is best defined by which of the following?

(A) the pressure at which a substance begins to melt

(B) the pressure at which a substance begins to boil

(C) the pressure at which a substance condenses at 100% relative humidity

(D) the pressure required to liquefy a gas at its critical temperature

(E) the pressure required to sublimate a solid at room temperature

Even at its critical temperature (above which *no* amount of pressure can liquefy a gas), gases often require a substantial pressure to be converted to a liquid. For example, the critical temperature for oxygen is −118°C. The critical pressure for oxygen is 49.7 atm.

A vacuum-insulated evaporator is a specialized container to store liquid oxygen. Designed like a Thermos, it has two layers with a near-vacuum in the middle, and are maintained at −170°C, well below critical temperature. As such, it is only necessary to pressurize the container to about 10.5 atm.

Ref: Middleton B, Phillips J, Thomas R, Stacey S. *Physics in Anesthesia.* 1st ed. Banbury, UK: Scion Publishing; 2012.

18. A syringe with a known volume of gas is compressed to half of its volume while attached to a pressure transducer. The pressure rises from 20 mm Hg to 40 mm Hg (Figure 20-4). This is an example of which of the following laws?

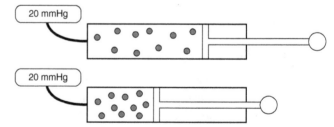

FIG. 20-4. A volume of gas compressed to half of its original volume.

(A) Henry's Law

(B) Dalton's Law

(C) Boyle's Law

(D) Avogadro's Law

(E) Pascal's Law

Boyle's Law states that at a constant temperature the volume of a confined ideal gas varies inversely with its pressure. Mathematically, this is represented as:

$$P_1 \times V_1 = P_2 \times V_2,$$

where P = pressure and V = volume.

An example of Boyle's Law is the calculation of the volume of an E-cylinder of oxygen. It is known that these are designed to produce 660 L of oxygen at 1 atmosphere (14.7 psi), and that its pressure when full is roughly 2,000 psi. Substituting, we get:

$$P_1 \times V_1 = P_2 \times V_2$$
$$14.7 \text{ psi} \times 660 \text{ L} = 2{,}000 \text{ psi} \times \underline{\hspace{1cm}} \text{ L}$$
$$V_2 = 4.8 \text{ L}$$

This value is known as the "water capacity" of the cylinder (e.g., as if you simply filled it with a noncompressible liquid such as water).

Ref: Middleton B, Phillips J, Thomas R, Stacey S. *Physics in Anesthesia.* 1st ed. Banbury, UK: Scion Publishing; 2012.

19. You are giving anesthesia in Denver (atmospheric pressure: 630 mm Hg). Your fresh gas mix is 50% air and 50% oxygen. What is the approximate partial pressure of oxygen delivered to the patient (assuming dry gas with no water vapor pressure)?

(A) 100 mm Hg

(B) 130 mm Hg

(C) 315 mm Hg

(D) 380 mm Hg

(E) unable to calculate with this information

Dalton's Law of partial pressures states that the total pressure exerted by a gas mixture is the sum of all of the component partial pressures ($P_{total} = P_a + P_b + P_c +$ etc.). Knowing that the total pressure is 1 atmosphere (which in Denver is lower than typical sea-level pressure of 760 mm Hg), the calculation can be made by first estimating the fractional concentration of oxygen (50% + 0.21 × 50% = 60.5%). 630 mm Hg × 60.5 = 381 mm Hg.

Ref: Middleton B, Phillips J, Thomas R, Stacey S. *Physics in Anesthesia.* 1st ed. Banbury, UK: Scion Publishing; 2012.

20. A patient is being mechanically ventilated in a critical care unit in San Diego (sea level). He is receiving an FiO_2 of 30%. A recent arterial blood gas shows the following: pH 7.31, $PaCO_2$ 50 mm Hg, PaO_2 133 mm Hg, HCO_3^-

19 mmol/L. Which of the following answers best represents the patient's alveolar-arterial (A-a) gradient?

(A) 5 mm Hg

(B) 8 mm Hg

(C) 12 mm Hg

(D) 18 mm Hg

(E) 24 mm Hg

This is easily solvable using the alveolar gas equation:

$$P_AO_2 = FiO_2 (P_{atm} - P_{H_2O}) - PaCO_2/0.8$$

where P_{atm} = barometric pressure (760 mm Hg at sea level).

P_{H_2O} = water vapor pressure (47 mm Hg at 37°C)

Substituting for the variables, we get:

$$P_AO_2 = 0.3 \times (760 - 47) \times (50/0.8)$$
$$P_AO_2 = 151.4 \text{ mm Hg}$$

Subtracting the measured PaO_2 from the P_AO_2 we get:

$$151.4 \text{ mm Hg} - 133 \text{ mm Hg} = 18.4 \text{ mm Hg}$$

Ref: Middleton B, Phillips J, Thomas R, Stacey S. *Physics in Anesthesia.* 1st ed. Banbury, UK: Scion Publishing; 2012.

21. At a constant temperature, the amount of gas dissolved in a liquid is directly proportional to the partial pressure of the gas in contact with the liquid. This statement is best described as:

(A) Pascal's law

(B) Henry's law

(C) Boyle's law

(D) Dalton's law

(E) Avogadro's law

Henry's law states that at a constant temperature, the amount of a gas dissolved in a liquid is proportional to the partial pressure of the gas in contact with the liquid. For a given combination of various gases, liquids, and temperatures there is a unique solubility coefficient or constant. At higher temperatures a gas will be less soluble in a liquid (given a constant pressure).

Volatile anesthetics exert their effect proportional to the partial pressure of the agent in the blood. In other words, the greater the partial pressure, the greater the anesthetic effect. As per Henry's law, the partial pressure of anesthetic agent dissolved in the blood is proportional to the partial pressure exerted by the anesthetic vapor in the alveoli. Working backwards, Dalton's law states that the partial pressure exerted by the anesthetic vapor in the alveoli is independent of the other gases present. As such, the only factors that alter the pressure exerted by the anesthetic vapor are the vapor pressure itself and the amount of agent delivered to the alveoli per unit volume (i.e., concentration of the agent).

Ref: Middleton B, Phillips J, Thomas R, Stacey S. *Physics in Anesthesia.* 1st ed. Banbury, UK: Scion Publishing; 2012.

22. The rate at which alveolar concentration of anesthetic agent rises to meet the inspired concentration (FA/FI) is primarily determined by which pair of factors?

   (A) cardiac output and blood solubility
   (B) blood solubility and inspired concentration
   (C) cardiac output and inspired concentration
   (D) **minute ventilation and inspired concentration**
   (E) cardiac output and minute ventilation

The rate of rise of the alveolar concentration relative to the inspired concentration (FA/FI) is primarily determined by two factors: the inspired concentration (i.e., the concentration delivered to the respiratory system) and the minute ventilation. Therefore, both an increase in the dial concentration on the vaporizer and hyperventilation will serve to bring the FA into equilibrium with FI more rapidly (Figure 20-5).

At the same time, anesthetic is being taken up by the pulmonary vasculature, which works against the increase in FA. The three factors that determine uptake of agent are solubility, cardiac output, and the difference between the partial pressure of anesthetic agent in the alveolus and that in the mixed venous blood. Thus, these factors do play a role in determining FA/FI, but far less than the inspired concentration and minute ventilation.

23. Which of the following combination of factors serves to INCREASE the uptake of anesthetic agent from the alveoli, where P_A-P_V is the alveolar-to-venous partial pressure difference?

   (A) **increased solubility; increased cardiac output; increased P_A-P_V**
   (B) increased solubility; decreased cardiac output; decreased P_A-P_V
   (C) decreased solubility; decreased cardiac output; increased P_A-P_V
   (D) decreased solubility; decreased cardiac output; decreased P_A-P_V
   (E) decreased solubility; increased cardiac output; increased P_A-P_V

Uptake is the product of three factors: solubility, cardiac output, and alveolar-to-venous partial pressure difference (P_A-P_V).

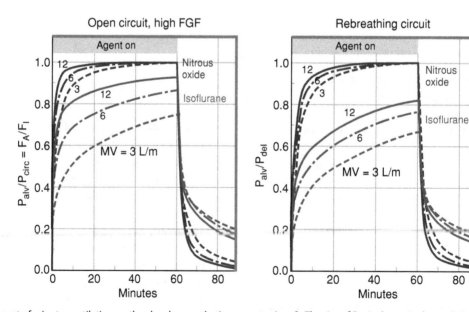

FIG. 20-5. The impact of minute ventilation on the alveolar anesthetic concentration. **A.** The rise of P_{alv} is shown in the traditional manner, normalized to inspired concentration (P_{circ}), which is constant only with very high fresh gas flows (FGFs) and no rebreathing. Increased minute ventilation (MV) accelerates the rise of P_{alv} and increases clearance after delivery stops. **B.** P_{alv} is shown normalized to the constant delivered anesthetic concentration. This illustration better reflects the rise of P_{alv} during a typical induction when rebreathing occurs (FGF = 6 L/min). (Reproduced with permission from Longnecker DE, Brown DL, Newman MF, Zapol WM. *Anesthesiology.* 2nd ed. New York, NY: McGraw Hill; 2012.)

Solubility (also termed partition coefficient) refers to the relative affinity of an anesthetic agent for one of two phases at equilibrium. For example, the blood:gas partition coefficient for desflurane is 0.45. This means that when the *partial pressures* of desflurane are equal across the alveolar-capillary membrane, there is 0.45 times the number of desflurane molecules in the alveolus (i.e., for every 100 molecules of gas in the alveolus, there are 45 in the blood). Examples of blood:gas partition coefficients for commonly used anesthetic agents are shown in Table 20-4. A larger blood:gas coefficient means the uptake is increased (the gas is more soluble), thereby lowering the FA/FI ratio.

TABLE 20-4. Blood gas partition coefficients at 37°C.

Anesthetic agent	Blood:gas partition coefficient
Desflurane	0.45
Nitrous oxide	0.47
Sevoflurane	0.65
Isoflurane	1.4
Halothane	2.5
Diethyl ether	12

Increased pulmonary blood flow (cardiac output) results in greater uptake of anesthetic agent and lowers the FA/FI ratio. On the other hand, a decreased cardiac output allows for more time for equilibration between capillary and alveolus; in this case, the reduced concentration gradient reduces uptake. This effect is more pronounced for the more soluble agents.

Similarly, if the blood returning to the lungs has a low concentration of anesthetic molecules, the concentration gradient will be high, increasing uptake. Conversely, mixed venous blood saturated with anesthetic results in a low-concentration gradient from alveolus to blood, and uptake will be relatively poor.

Ref: Longnecker DE, Brown DL, Newman MF, Zapol WM. *Anesthesiology.* 2nd ed. New York, NY: McGraw Hill; 2012.

24. A general anesthetic is being administered in a healthy patient for bunion surgery. After 60 minutes of breathing 2% sevoflurane with a fresh gas flow of 2 L/min, which of the following best represents the partial pressures of sevoflurane found at different locations, from highest to lowest?

(A) Brain > Muscle > Fat > Circuit

(B) Brain > Circuit > Muscle > Fat

(C) Circuit > Brain > Muscle > Fat

(D) Circuit > Muscle > Brain > Fat

(E) Circuit > Muscle > Fat > Brain

Pulmonary capillary blood rapidly equilibrates with alveolar partial pressures, so that blood entering the pulmonary veins and the left atrium should have a partial pressure close to that of the alveolus (P_{alv}). The extent to which anesthetic is delivered to different tissues depends on the proportion of blood flow to that tissue, its anatomic volume, and the tissue-blood partition coefficient. For example, the vessel-rich group, composed primarily of the heart, brain, spinal cord, liver, and kidney and endocrine glands, accounts for approximately 10% of body mass and yet receives about 70% of the cardiac output. Hence, tissues in this group equilibrate with P_{alv} quickly (Figure 20-6).

On the other hand, muscle accounts for approximately 50% of body mass, but only 20% of cardiac output (at rest). As a result, the anesthetic partial pressures in this tissue rise more slowly, reaching equilibrium in approximately 2–4 hours. Following equilibration with the muscle group, fat become the only effective depot for anesthetic. Fat represents about 20% of body mass and receives <10% of cardiac output. Most volatile agents partition very easily into fat: the partition coefficients are typically in the range of 25–50,

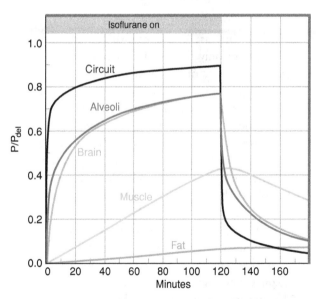

FIG. 20-6. Uptake of anesthetics into different tissues. The partial pressure of isoflurane in different tissue beds is depicted during induction with fresh gas flow (FGF) = 6 L/min, $\dot{V}$ = 5 L/min, and $\dot{Q}$ = 5 L/min. Note that the isoflurane partial pressure in highly perfused tissues (brain) closely matches that in alveoli except when P_{alv} is changing very rapidly. Also note that the partial pressure of anesthetic in fat continues to rise after discontinuing isoflurane delivery, as long as P_{alv} is greater than P_{fat}. $\dot{V}$, minute alveolar ventilation; $\dot{Q}$, cardiac output. (Reproduced with permission from Longnecker DE, Brown DL, Newman MF, Zapol WM. *Anesthesiology.* 2nd ed. New York, NY: McGraw Hill; 2012.)

compared with 1–3 for muscle. As such, it is difficult to reach steady-state partial pressures in typical clinical practice, with the equilibrium half-time for sevoflurane being approximately 30 hours. The final group is the vessel-poor group, composed of bone, tendon, ligament, and cartilage, which has negligible uptake of anesthetic due to its minimal overall perfusion.

It should be clear that if the dial setting for inhaled concentration has not decreased since the commencement of the anesthetic, the partial pressure in the circuit will always be higher than in any other tissue. This of course changes when the dial is turned down or off, and the partial pressure in the inspiratory limb of the circuit approaches or equals zero.

Ref: Longnecker DE, Brown DL, Newman MF, Zapol WM. *Anesthesiology.* 2nd ed. New York, NY: McGraw Hill; 2012.

25. The concentration of an inhaled anesthetic is increased by a factor of 5. The resulting alveolar concentration is increased by a factor of over 6. This is an example of:

(A) concentration effect
(B) second gas effect
(C) solubility effect
(D) ventilation effect
(E) blood:gas partition effect

The concentration effect describes the manner in which an increase in the inspired concentration will increase not only the alveolar concentration of a gas but also the rate of rise of that concentration. It has two components: the confusingly termed *concentrating* effect and the *augmented inflow effect.*

Consider a situation where an anesthetic is being administered at a concentration of 10% (i.e., 10 parts anesthetic and 90 parts other gas such as air). If 50% of the anesthetic gas is taken up by the pulmonary capillary blood, that would leave half of its original volume, or 5 parts, in the alveolus. The resulting alveolar concentration of anesthetic would then be 5 divided by the total number of gas parts (5 + 90), or 5/95 = 5.3%.

If that same gas is then administered at 50% inspired concentration (or 5 times its concentration in the previous example), a different story emerges. When 50% of that alveolar anesthetic volume is absorbed by the blood, this leaves 25 parts in 75, or 33%. This increased alveolar concentration is not surprising. However, calculation of the ratios between the two examples reveals that while the inspired concentrations differed by a factor of 5 (10% vs. 50%),

the alveolar concentrations differed by a factor of 6.2 (33%/5.3% = 6.2). This phenomenon is the concentrating effect.

The other effect contributing to the concentration effect is the augmented inflow effect. Using the first example above, the 5 parts of absorbed gas must be replaced to avoid collapse of the alveolus. As 5 parts of the original 10% mixture enters the alveolus, the alveolar concentration becomes 5.5% (5 + 0.5/90 + 4.5). By way of contrast, in the second example, replacement of the 25 parts of anesthetic gas with the 50% gas mixture leads to an alveolar concentration of 37.5% (25 + 12.5/50 + 12.5). This equates to a 6.8-fold greater alveolar concentration (37.5/5.5) with augmented inflow compared to concentrating effect alone when the inspired concentration is quintupled.

Ref: Butterworth JF IV, Mackey DC, Wasnick JD. *Morgan & Mikhail's Clinical Anesthesiology.* 5th ed. New York, NY: McGraw Hill; 2013.

26. The increase in alveolar concentration of a volatile agent when nitrous oxide is used as a carrier gas is termed:

(A) concentrating effect
(B) replenishment effect
(C) second gas effect
(D) capillary uptake effect
(E) ventilation effect

The second gas effect is a phenomenon observed when the absorption of nitrous oxide by the pulmonary capillaries increases the alveolar concentration of a "second" gas. The second gas is almost always a volatile inhalational agent. The second gas effect is explained graphically in Figure 20-7.

Ref: Butterworth JF IV, Mackey DC, Wasnick JD. *Morgan & Mikhail's Clinical Anesthesiology.* 5th ed. New York, NY: McGraw Hill; 2013.

27. A trauma patient has a small (75 mL) unrecognized pneumothorax. Following intravenous induction of anesthesia, she is maintained with desflurane in 50:50 oxygen:nitrous oxide. After 30 minutes (at steady state), the volume of the pneumothorax will be:

(A) 25 mL
(B) 50 mL
(C) 75 mL
(D) 150 mL
(E) 225 mL

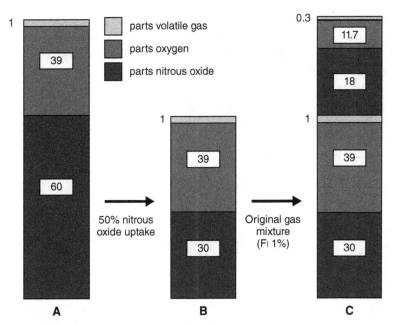

FIG. 20-7. The second gas effect. **(A)** The first breath, consisting of 60% N₂O, 39% O₂ and 1% volatile gas. If 50% of the nitrous oxide were absorbed by the blood (ignoring uptake of the volatile agent), the resulting alveolar concentration of the volatile would be 1 part in 70, or 1.4% **(B)**. In the subsequent breath **(C)**, 30 parts of the original mixture flow into the alveolus, resulting in an additional 1% of 30 parts anesthetic, or 0.3%. Therefore, the total concentration at the end of the second breath would be 1.3%.

Nitrous oxide is roughly 35 times more soluble than nitrogen in blood. Since airspaces (such as venous air emboli, pneumothoraces, or the middle ear) contain mostly nitrogen, any nitrous oxide in the bloodstream will equilibrate very quickly while the nitrogen remains more or less trapped. As a result, the volume of the airspace will increase in proportion to the partial pressure of nitrous oxide. If the space is highly compliant, then only the volume changes; however, if it is a poorly compliant space with little room for volume change (e.g., the middle ear), the pressure will begin to increase as the volume remains the same.

Figure 20-8 illustrates the principle of volume expansion with nitrous oxide. If we assume that the bubble has a high compliance and can expand easily, the total pressure in the bubble will remain at 1 atmosphere. The new volume at steady-state nitrous oxide inhalation can be calculated by:

$$\text{New volume} = \text{original volume} \times (1 \div \text{partial pressure of } \textit{nitrogen})$$

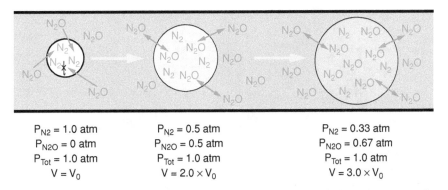

FIG. 20-8. Expansion of venous air emboli by nitrous oxide. Nitrous oxide (N₂O) enters air pockets far faster than nitrogen leaves (because of low blood nitrogen-carrying capacity), causing airspace expansion. Expansion continues until the partial pressure of N₂O inside the air bubble matches that in surrounding blood. Thus, at 50% N₂O (P_{N2O} = 0.5 atm), air emboli can double in volume, and at 67% N₂O (P_{N2O} = 0.67 atm), they can triple in volume. Expansion of small venous air emboli can lead to occlusion of pulmonary capillaries, compromising both blood flow and gas exchange. (Reproduced with permission from Longnecker DE, Brown DL, Newman MF, Zapol WM. *Anesthesiology.* 2nd ed. New York, NY: McGraw Hill; 2012.)

With a partial pressure of nitrous oxide of 0.5 atm, the remaining partial pressure of nitrogen is 0.5 atm, and the bubble will expand to *twice* its original volume (with equal volumes of each gas). With a partial pressure of nitrous oxide of 0.67 atm, the partial pressure of nitrogen will be 0.33, and the bubble will triple in size. If 75% nitrous oxide is used, the bubble will quadruple in size.

This can be a significant clinical problem in a number of scenarios, including venous or arterial air emboli, pneumothorax, intestinal obstruction, pneumocephalus, pulmonary bullae or cysts, intraocular gas bubbles, and tympanic membrane grafting.

Ref: Longnecker DE, Brown DL, Newman MF, Zapol WM. *Anesthesiology*. 2nd ed. New York, NY: McGraw Hill; 2012.

CHAPTER 21

The Anesthesia Machine and Ventilators

1. You are planning on intubating a patient in respiratory distress with a 7.0 mm internal diameter standard endotracheal tube. In order to decrease the resistance associated with the tube during the anticipated prolonged mechanical ventilation, the most efficient maneuver is to:

   (A) cut the tube by 4 cm to decrease its length
   (B) use an 8.0 mm rather than 7.0 mm internal diameter endotracheal tube
   (C) lubricate the inside of the tube with silicone spray
   (D) warm the tube in a jug of hot water prior to insertion
   (E) position the tube so the cuff is immediately below the vocal cords

2. Rebreathing of expired gas occurs when:

   (A) carbon dioxide absorbent is 50% saturated
   (B) carbon dioxide absorbent is 97% saturated
   (C) fresh gas flow is less than minute ventilation
   (D) the I:E ratio is 1:3
   (E) auto-PEEP exceeds 10 cm H_2O

3. Which of the following factors is most likely to lead to a discrepancy between delivered and inspired concentrations of anesthetics?

   (A) the use of soda lime versus Baralyme
   (B) the use of sevoflurane at low concentrations
   (C) the use of nitrous oxide in the inspired fresh gas
   (D) air dilution
   (E) hypercarbia

4. Which of the following statements regarding humidification of airway gases using heat and moisture exchangers (HMEs) is TRUE?

   (A) Adult HMEs increase dead space by less than 10 mL.
   (B) Low tidal volumes decrease the effective humidification of the gases.
   (C) HMEs decrease the incidence of ventilator associated pneumonia in critically ill patients.
   (D) Life-threatening airway blockage may occur with HMEs.
   (E) HMEs increase the resistance to airflow by approximately 15–20%.

5. The specific heats of various compounds are listed below in Table 21-1. In order to make a piece of monitoring equipment least susceptible to temperature changes, which material would be best suited to use in its manufacture?

TABLE 21-1. **Specific heats of selected materials.**

Material	Specific heat (cal/g/°C)
Copper	0.09
Aluminum	0.214
Glass	0.16
Steel	0.107
Lead	0.03

   (A) copper
   (B) aluminum
   (C) glass
   (D) steel
   (E) lead

6. A right-angle elbow connector is shown in Figure 21-1. What are the outer diameters of the ends marked A and B?

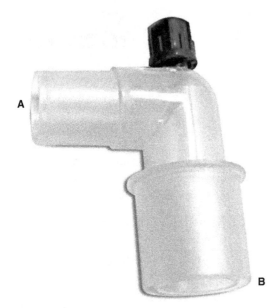

FIG. 21-1. A right-angle elbow connector.

(A)   A = 11 mm; B = 15 mm
(B)   A = 11 mm; B = 22 mm
(C)   A = 11 mm; B = 25 mm
(D)   A = 15 mm; B = 22 mm
(E)   A = 19 mm; B = 30 mm

7. Which of the following is a required standard of all endotracheal tubes?

(A)   tube size in external diameter (OD) marked in millimeters
(B)   a radius of curvature of 5–8 cm
(C)   cross-sectional shape that is circular or oval
(D)   a bevel angle of 24 to 30 degrees
(E)   the area of the Murphy eye be <80% of cross-sectional area

8. A 2-L rubber reservoir bag is filled with 8 L of air in a closed system. The resulting peak pressure would most likely be:

(A)   10 cm H_2O
(B)   20 cm H_2O
(C)   50 cm H_2O
(D)   70 cm H_2O
(E)   0 . . . the bag exploded long before 8 L was reached

9. Which of the following features distinguishes the ProSeal™ laryngeal mask airway (LMA) from the LMA Classic™?

(A)   higher intracuff pressures
(B)   lower airway seal pressures
(C)   a preformed curve in the shaft
(D)   integral bite block
(E)   the ability to ventilate using positive pressure

10. What is the largest size endotracheal tube that can be passed through a size 4 Classic or Unique laryngeal mask airway (LMA)?

(A)   5.5 mm ID
(B)   6.0 mm ID
(C)   6.5 mm ID
(D)   7.0 mm ID
(E)   7.5 mm ID

11. You are administering anesthesia in the interventional radiology suite with a . . . um . . . "vintage" anesthesia machine (okay, it's old). The ventilator is equipped with hanging bellows. The potential hazard of this style of bellows is:

(A)   the bellows will not inflate during a power failure
(B)   the bellows may fail to inflate if there is a leak in the system
(C)   the bellows may fill during exhalation even if the circuit is disconnected
(D)   the bellows cannot deliver very high flow rates
(E)   the bellows are typically made of cheap material

12. An anesthetic is being delivered in New York City (sea level). If the partial pressure of sevoflurane in the alveolus is 13 mm Hg, what is the concentration of sevoflurane?

(A)   0.5%
(B)   1.1%
(C)   1.7%
(D)   2%
(E)   2.3%

13. Which of the following is NOT a characteristic of modern vaporizers?

    (A) agent specificity
    (B) temperature compensation
    (C) variable bypass
    (D) in-circuit placement
    (E) flow over design

14. Which of the following is NOT a safety standard mandated by the American Society of Testing and Materials (ASTM) regarding the manufacture and function of vaporizers?

    (A) All vaporizer control knobs must open counterclockwise.
    (B) Either the maximum and minimum fillings levels or the actual usable volume must be displayed.
    (C) The vaporizer must be designed so that it cannot be overfilled when in the normal operating position.
    (D) A system that prevents gas from passing through the vaporizing chamber of one vaporizer and then through that of another must be provided.
    (E) The vaporizer must be designed so that tilting does not affect the output.

15. Intermittent back pressure in the breathing circuit is most likely to result in increased concentrations of volatile anesthetic delivered to the patient when which of the following is present?

    (A) a check valve downstream from the vaporizer
    (B) spontaneous ventilation
    (C) low carrier gas flow rates
    (D) high volatile anesthetic agent levels in the vaporizing chamber
    (E) a short and/or wide-diameter input tube to the vaporizing chamber

16. The bimetallic strip found in many modern vaporizers is designed to prevent the incorrect delivery of volatile anesthetic by which of the following mechanisms?

    (A) temperature compensation
    (B) overfill protection
    (C) prevents filling with an incorrect agent
    (D) ensures only one vaporizer dial can be in the ON position
    (E) prevents volatile agent from reaching bypass chamber if tipped

17. A sevoflurane vaporizer is accidentally filled with isoflurane. Which of the following is MOST likely to be true?

    (A) The vapor output will be higher than the reading on the dial.
    (B) No change will be required in the concentration of volatile.
    (C) The vapor output will be lower than the reading on the dial.
    (D) The gas should be treated as if it is sevoflurane.
    (E) The mixture can be determined by smelling the gas.

18. Which of the following is a design feature of the Ohmeda Tec 6 vaporizer?

    (A) variable bypass
    (B) flow-over
    (C) in-circuit
    (D) gas/vapor blender
    (E) agent nonspecific (may be used with several agents)

19. A patient is receiving anesthesia in Taos, NM (barometric pressure 594 mm Hg). The sevoflurane vaporizer dial is set to 2% (1 MAC). Which one of the following is true regarding the effect of altitude on the vaporizer and its effect on the patient?

    (A) The dial concentration should be increased by 50%.
    (B) The dial concentration should be increased by 25%.
    (C) The dial concentration should remain the same.
    (D) The dial concentration should be decreased by 33%.
    (E) The dial concentration should be decreased by 25%.

20. Which of the following represents the preferred arrangement of components in a circle breathing system?

    (A) The reservoir bag is placed between the expiratory valve and the carbon dioxide absorber.

    (B) Unidirectional valves are placed within the Y-piece of the circuit to be as close as possible to the patient.

    (C) The fresh gas inlet is positioned between the inspiratory valve and the patient.

    (D) The adjustable pressure limiting (APL) valve is positioned downstream from the carbon dioxide absorber.

    (E) The reservoir bag is placed on the opposite side of the APL valve to decrease wasted gas.

21. Which one of the following is NOT a proposed advantage of low-flow anesthesia using a circle circuit breathing system?

    (A) reduced cost

    (B) reduced atmospheric pollution from greenhouse and ozone-depleting gases

    (C) reduced operating room pollution

    (D) improved heat and humidity conservation

    (E) improved correlation between delivered and end-tidal concentrations of gases

22. In order to minimize rebreathing of exhaled carbon dioxide using a Mapleson A breathing system in a spontaneously breathing patient, what is the minimum fresh gas flow required?

    (A) equal to 75% of minute ventilation

    (B) equal to minute ventilation

    (C) 2× minute ventilation

    (D) 3× minute ventilation

    (E) impossible to predict

23. Your co-resident suggests a trial of T-piece ventilation for a patient in the ICU. Not to be outdone in front of the team, you respond by casually saying, "Oh, so what you'd like is ...":

    (A) "a Mapleson B"

    (B) "a Mapleson C"

    (C) "a Mapleson E"

    (D) "a Mapleson F"

    (E) "a Mapleson G"

24. Which of the following is a feature of the self-reinflating resuscitation bag device?

    (A) requires a pressurized gas supply to work

    (B) a 22-mm male/15-mm female connector for the airway device (LMA, mask, etc.)

    (C) an oxygen inlet with a two-way valve

    (D) a valve to prevent air entrainment into the bag

    (E) can only provide approximately 50% FiO_2

25. Soda lime is a mixture of:

    (A) $Ca(OH)_2$ and $NaOH$

    (B) $CaCO_3$ and $NaOH$

    (C) $NaOH$ and KOH

    (D) Na_2CO_3 and KOH

    (E) Na_2CO_3 and $NaOH$

26. Baffles in the carbon dioxide absorber function to:

    (A) prevent caking of absorbent dust in the exhaust tubing

    (B) catch water droplets that condense in the absorbent

    (C) channel airflow to the center of the absorber

    (D) evenly distribute heat within the absorbent

    (E) prevent evaporation of indicator dye from the absorbent granules

27. Which of the following devices provides a constant FiO$_2$ that is independent of a patient's peak inspiratory flow?

(A) nasal cannulae

(B) simple face mask

(C) partial rebreather mask

(D) Venturi mask

(E) manual resuscitator (self-inflating bag-valve-mask)

28. Which of the following statements regarding waste gas scavenging systems is TRUE?

(A) The standard fitting size for scavenging tubing is 22 mm.

(B) A negative pressure valve is not required with a closed scavenging system.

(C) Open scavenging systems may be active or passive.

(D) A reservoir chamber or bag is required with closed scavenging systems.

(E) If the scavenging reservoir bag is constantly collapsed, suction flow should be increased.

29. In Datex-Ohmeda machines, the Link-25 system serves to:

(A) electronically connect the gas flow data to the monitor

(B) prevent more than one vaporizer from being turned on at a time

(C) shut off pipeline flow of nitrous oxide in the event of low oxygen pressure

(D) permit only certain proportions of nitrous oxide and oxygen using the flow control knobs

(E) activate the oxygen flush mechanism

30. Which of the following sequence of flowmeter tubes would be MOST likely to prevent a hypoxic mixture in the event of a crack in the air flowmeter tube (from left to right)?

(A) oxygen, air, nitrous oxide

(B) oxygen, nitrous oxide, air

(C) nitrous oxide, oxygen, air

(D) air, oxygen, nitrous oxide

(E) air, nitrous oxide, oxygen

31. Which of the following is NOT an example of an ergonomic feature of the anesthesia workstation?

(A) standardization of workstation dimensions and arrangements between manufacturers

(B) wheel protectors to push cords away

(C) patient attachments (e.g., suction, breathing circuits) mounted on the right-hand side of the workstation

(D) suction canister height below the level of the surgical table

(E) electrical and gas outlets mounted on booms over or near the workstation

32. In the diagram below, the waveforms in column A are representative of which type of ventilation?

    (A) pressure-controlled ventilation

    (B) volume-controlled ventilation

    (C) flow-controlled ventilation

    (D) high-frequency oscillatory ventilation

    (E) interpulmonary percussive ventilation

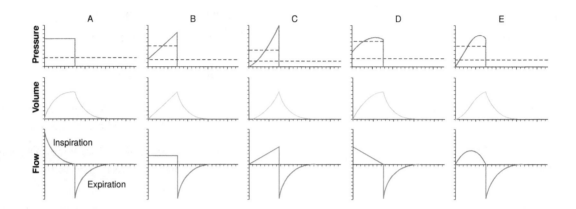

DIRECTIONS: For questions 33–37, each group of items below consists of lettered headings followed by a list of numbered phrases or statements. For each numbered phrase or statement, select the ONE lettered heading or component that is most closely associated with it. Each lettered heading or component may be selected once, more than once, or not at all.

    (A) assist-control

    (B) pressure-control

    (C) volume-control

    (D) periodic sigh

    (E) high-frequency ventilation

    (F) intermittent mandatory ventilation (IMV)

    (G) synchronized intermittent mandatory ventilation (SIMV)

    (H) pressure support

    (I) biphasic positive airway pressure (BIPAP)

33. Which ventilator mode delivers the same tidal volume during every inspiration, regardless of whether initiated by patient or ventilator?

34. Which ventilator mode allows the patient to breathe spontaneously, without support, between machine-cycled breaths, which are delivered regardless of respiratory timing?

35. Which ventilator mode provides partial ventilator support to patients with preserved respiratory drive by increasing the pressure at the airway above the expiratory pressure in response to an inspiratory effort?

36. Which ventilator mode is a form of airway pressure release ventilation (APRV)?

37. Which ventilator mode is flow-controlled and time-cycled?

38. With respect to ventilator phase variables, the inspiratory phase ends when either a preset pressure, volume, flow, or time is reached. This preset variable that ends inspiration is referred to as the:

    (A) trigger variable

    (B) target variable

    (C) cycle variable

    (D) baseline variable

    (E) limit variable

39. Which of the following will cause an increase in peak inspiratory pressure (PIP) without a change in plateau pressure?

   (A) increased tidal volume
   (B) pulmonary edema
   (C) ascites
   (D) endobronchial intubation
   (E) bronchospasm

40. Which of the following conditions will alter a static pressure-volume (PV) curve?

   (A) pulmonary embolus
   (B) mucous plugging
   (C) bronchospasm
   (D) endotracheal cuff herniation
   (E) tension pneumothorax

41. The diagram in below shows an inspiratory and expiratory pressure-volume (PV) curve for an intubated and ventilated patient with an acute lung injury (ALI). In order to maintain alveolar recruitment and minimize the risk of alveolar overdistention, at what point should positive end-expiratory pressure (PEEP) be set?

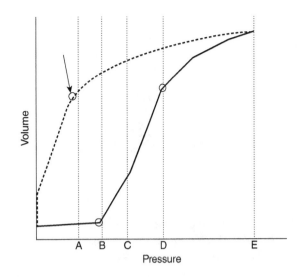

   (A) A
   (B) B
   (C) C
   (D) D
   (E) E

42. Which of the following methods is the best to detect postoperative apnea in a nonintubated patient?

   (A) pulse oximeter
   (B) nasal-oral airflow system
   (C) electrocardiographic transthoracic impedance system
   (D) respiratory inductive plethysmography
   (E) photoplethysmography

Answers and Explanations: The Anesthesia Machine and Ventilators

1. You are planning on intubating a patient in respiratory distress with a 7.0 mm internal diameter standard endotracheal tube. In order to decrease the resistance associated with the tube during the anticipated prolonged mechanical ventilation, the most efficient maneuver is to:

   (A) cut the tube by 4 cm to decrease its length
   (B) **use an 8.0 mm rather than 7.0 mm internal diameter endotracheal tube**
   (C) lubricate the inside of the tube with silicone spray
   (D) warm the tube in a jug of hot water prior to insertion
   (E) position the tube so the cuff is immediately below the vocal cords

Assuming that flow is laminar in an endotracheal tube (an assumption that is NOT correct in the presence of kinks, secretions, sharp bends with RAE tubes, or very high gas flows), resistance is proportional to the length of the tube and viscosity of the gas, and inversely proportional to the radius of the internal diameter to the 4th power. Cutting the tube is a maneuver that is sometimes performed in an effort to reduce the resistance to airflow, or to prevent the external portion of the tube from becoming kinked due to traction from the circuit. However, given that most endotracheal tubes are approximately 30 cm long, a reduction in length of 4 cm only provides about 15% less resistance. In contrast, increasing the internal *radius* by 0.5 mm (from 3.5 mm to 4 mm), the resistance is reduced by over 40%.

Large tubes also improve pulmonary toilet during mechanical ventilation by allowing for improved suctioning of secretions and improved work of breathing during weaning off ventilation. It has been advocated by some that during anesthesia, a size 6.0 mm to 7.0 mm is appropriate, whereas 7.5 mm to 8.5 mm is preferred during long-term ventilation in the critical care unit (0.5–1.0 mm smaller for nasal intubation).

Lubrication with silicone spray, warming, or altering position within the trachea is not effective at reducing resistance to airflow.

Ref: Tobin MJ. *Principles and practice of mechanical ventilation*, 3rd ed. New York, NY: McGraw Hill; 2013.

2. Rebreathing of expired gas occurs when:

   (A) carbon dioxide absorbent is 50% saturated
   (B) carbon dioxide absorbent is 97% saturated
   (C) **fresh gas flow is less than minute ventilation**
   (D) the I:E ratio is 1:3
   (E) auto-PEEP exceeds 10 cm H_2O

Rebreathing is defined as the inhalation of previously expired gases. While there is a tendency to associate rebreathing with carbon dioxide specifically, this is not technically correct, as it is possible to rebreathe without inhaling any carbon dioxide. The amount of rebreathing that takes place depends on the fresh gas flow, the amount of mechanical (apparatus) dead space, and the type of breathing system. The higher the fresh gas flow, the less rebreathing will occur, depending on the type of breathing system (circle vs. Mapleson A, B, C, etc.). In general, if fresh gas flow is less than minute ventilation, some rebreathing of exhaled gas must occur (assuming no air dilution).

Ref: Dorsch JA, Dorsch SE. *Understanding anesthesia equipment*, 5th ed. Philadelphia, PA: Lippincott Williams & Wilkins; 2008.

3. Which of the following factors is most likely to lead to a discrepancy between delivered and inspired concentrations of anesthetics?

   (A) the use of soda lime versus Baralyme
   (B) the use of sevoflurane at low concentrations
   (C) the use of nitrous oxide in the inspired fresh gas
   (D) air dilution
   (E) hypercarbia

The inspired composition of gas may not always reflect what is set on the anesthesia machine, for a variety of reasons. Rebreathing is a principal cause; the more the fraction of rebreathed gas, the less the inspired gas will precisely match what is delivered into the breathing system. Air dilution is possible if the fresh gas supplied is less than tidal volume during spontaneous respiration. In this case, inspiration may draw in ambient air if the inspiratory limb is open to the atmosphere or if there is a leak. Dilution creates a positive feedback loop, whereby diluted anesthetic concentrations result in a lighter plane of anesthesia, which causes increases in minute ventilation and an increased rate of air dilution. On the other hand, gas may be forced out of the system during positive pressure ventilation if leaks are present; the amount of gas lost is dependent on the location and size of the leak, as well as the compliance of the breathing system and the patient. Anesthetic agents may also be adsorbed and released by the components of the breathing circuit. Following a long anesthetic, the breathing circuit may act as a reservoir for volatile agent, prolonging the emergence even when the vaporizer has been shut off for a period of time.

Ref: Dorsch JA, Dorsch SE. *Understanding anesthesia equipment,* 5th ed. Philadelphia, PA: Lippincott Williams & Wilkins; 2008.

4. Which of the following statements regarding humidification of airway gases using heat and moisture exchangers (HMEs) is TRUE?

   (A) Adult HMEs increase dead space by less than 10 mL.
   (B) Low tidal volumes decrease the effective humidification of the gases.
   (C) HMEs decrease the incidence of ventilator associated pneumonia in critically ill patients.
   (D) Life-threatening airway blockage may occur with HMEs.
   (E) HMEs increase the resistance to airflow by approximately 15–20%.

Medical gases passing through the anesthesia machine (or mechanical ventilator in the critical care unit) are devoid of moisture in order to prevent corrosion or condensation in regulators and valves. Endotracheal tubes and supraglottic airway devices bypass the oral/nasal respiratory tract where humidification and warming normally occur, so that the tracheobronchial mucosa is made to assume those roles. This has predictably deleterious effects, especially over prolonged periods of time, as the mucosa dries and cools: secretions thicken, surfactant activity is impaired, mucociliary function is reduced, and the mucosa becomes more prone to bronchoconstriction. Over time, mucus plugging, atelectasis, increased airway pressures, and pneumonia may occur.

Humidification of airway gases is an important priority in long cases in order to prevent these changes. Some patients may be candidates for *active* heating and humidification of the gases in the circuit limbs using a heated humidifier (e.g., patients with hypothermia, severe bronchopleural fistula, or severe respiratory acidosis). These devices are inserted into the inspiratory limb of the circuit and function by allowing fresh gas to pass over heated water, achieving near-physiologic values of absolute humidity (44 mg H_2O/L). However, the vast majority of patients undergoing mechanical ventilation in the operating room or critical care unit achieve good results with heat and moisture exchangers (HMEs). HMEs are constructed of a plastic casing and an insert made of foam or paper treated with a moisture-retaining chemical. As warm, saturated gas passes through this material on exhalation, the HME cools it slightly, causing condensation on the patient's side of the apparatus. Fresh gas entering from the other side during inhalation takes up some of the condensed water and is warmed. These simple devices are inexpensive, easy to use, reliable, and, in contrast to heated humidifiers, do not require water or a source of power. The main drawback to the use of HMEs compared to heated humidifiers is that the value of absolute humidity delivered is limited: only about 60–80% of normal absolute humidity can be retained (approximately 25–35 mg H_2O/L), although there is no evidence that this impacts outcomes.

HMEs do increase dead space, and depending on the model this may amount to 30–100 mL for adult versions. Specialized neonatal and pediatric HME are designed to reduce dead space to 2–3 mL. Nevertheless, small increases in tidal volume may be required to maintain $PaCO_2$ and pH. In spontaneously breathing patients, there is only a marginal increase in airway resistance; the addition of a small amount of CPAP (5–10 cm H_2O) should be considered in these cases. The faster the rate of gas flow through the HME, the less effective it is at exchanging heat and moisture. High fresh gas flows and higher tidal volumes are less effective than lower flows and smaller tidal volumes.

There is no evidence that HMEs decrease the incidence of ventilator-associated pneumonia (VAP) in critically ill patients. Some HMEs are coated with the bacteriocidal compound and most are efficient microbial filters; however, the pathogenesis of VAP is related primarily to silent aspiration of regurgitated gastric contents, not the contamination of the breathing circuit.

HMEs can become obstructed due to blood, secretions, sputum, and nebulized bronchodilators, causing hypoxia and increased airway pressures. In addition, airway obstruction due to dislodgment of paper inserts has been reported. Removal and replacement of the HME must be on the troubleshooting checklist for increased airway pressures.

Fun fact: HMEs are also known as "Swedish noses"—a much more playful name. Next time you're bored in a case, test your anesthesia tech's historical name knowledge by overhead-paging for a Swedish nose.

Ref: Tobin MJ. *Principles and Practice of Mechanical Ventilation*, 3rd ed. New York, NY: McGraw Hill; 2013.

5. The specific heats of various compounds are listed below in Table 21-1. In order to make a piece of monitoring equipment least susceptible to temperature changes, which material would be best suited to use in its manufacture?

TABLE 21-1. Specific heats of selected materials.

Material	Specific heat (cal/g/°C)
Copper	0.09
Aluminum	0.214
Glass	0.16
Steel	0.107
Lead	0.03

   (A) copper
   (B) aluminum
   (C) glass
   (D) steel
   (E) lead

Specific heat is defined as the quantity of heat required to raise the temperature of 1 g of a particular substance

1°C. Materials with higher specific heats require more heat to raise the temperature of a given quantity of that substance. A substance with a high specific heat will change temperature more slowly and will provide a more stable temperature than a substance with a low specific heat. In the above example, aluminum has the highest specific heat of the compounds listed, and will be the slowest to respond to fluctuations in temperature. In real-life manufacturing of devices such as vaporizers, other factors have to be considered such as the conductivity and strength of the material.

Ref: Dorsch JA, Dorsch SE. *Understanding Anesthesia Equipment*, 5th ed. Philadelphia: Lippincott Williams & Wilkins; 2008.

6. A right-angle elbow connector is shown in Figure 21-1. What are the outer diameters of the ends marked A and B?

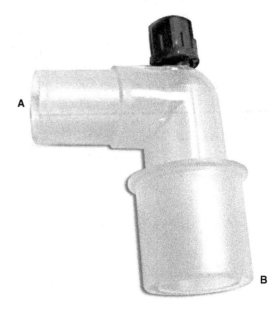

FIG. 21-1. A right-angle elbow connector.

   (A) A = 11 mm; B = 15 mm
   (B) A = 11 mm; B = 22 mm
   (C) A = 11 mm; B = 25 mm
   (D) A = 15 mm; B = 22 mm
   (E) A = 19 mm; B = 30 mm

Breathing systems are standardized by the American Society for Testing and Materials (ASTM) in order to reduce disconnection and improve safety, and are described in terms of diameter and whether it is a male or female fitting. All connectors in an adult breathing system are either 15 mm or 22 mm in diameter. Hoses and connectors are all built with a very slight taper so that a firm push and twist will provide a tight connection.

Starting from the outside of the machine and moving toward the patient, the inspiratory and expiratory ports on the absorber are the 22-mm male, designed to accommodate the 22-mm female ends of the breathing tubes of the circuit. Some machines have a 22-mm male/15-mm female coaxial inspiratory/expiratory port design to allow for the attachment of special 15-mm male pediatric hose connections. On the other end of the circuit, Y-pieces have two 22-mm male connectors for the breathing hoses and one 15-mm female/22-mm male coaxial connector that allows for connection directly to a either a face mask or an endotracheal tube. Face masks always have a female 22-mm connector, and endotracheal tubes always have a male 15-mm connector.

The elbow connector is similar to the Y-piece. In Figure 21-1, the proximal end (A) is a 15-mm male fitting. It can be seen that the distal end has two concentric rings, making up the 15-mm female and 22-mm male coaxial fitting permitting attachment to either mask or endotracheal tube.

Ref: Dorsch JA, Dorsch SE. *Understanding Anesthesia Equipment*, 5th ed. Philadelphia: Lippincott Williams & Wilkins; 2008.

7. Which of the following is a required standard of all endotracheal tubes?

(A) tube size in external diameter (OD) marked in millimeters

(B) a radius of curvature of 5–8 cm

(C) cross-sectional shape that is circular or oval

(D) a bevel angle of 24 to 30 degrees

(E) the area of the Murphy eye be <80% of cross-sectional area

The American Society for Testing and Materials (ASTM) standards for tube design require that endotracheal tubes conform to the following:

- The radius of curvature is 12–16 cm. (Imagine the curve of the tube continuing on to make a complete circle. The radius of that circle should be 12–16 cm.)
- Cross-sectional shape should be circular. Oval or elliptical shapes are more likely to kink.
- Bevel angle is an acute angle of 38 ± 8 degrees, and the opening of the bevel should face left.

- The Murphy eye is a hole on the opposite side to the bevel that permits gas exchange if the main opening is blocked for some reason. The Murphy eye should not be too large (<80% of cross-sectional area) in order to avoid passage through by fiberoptic scopes, tube exchangers, etc.
- The following markings should appear on the tube: the word *oral* or *nasal* or *oral/nasal*; tube size in internal diameter (ID) in millimeters; the outside diameter for size 6 and smaller tubes; depth markings starting at the patient end; a radiopaque marker at the patient end or along the length of the tube; the name or trademark of the manufacturer; and the notation *F-29* or *Z-79* or *IT*, which indicates the tube has passed a toxicity test.

Ref: Dorsch JA, Dorsch SE. *Understanding Anesthesia Equipment*, 5th ed. Philadelphia: Lippincott Williams & Wilkins; 2008.

8. A 2-L rubber reservoir bag is filled with 8 L of air in a closed system. The resulting peak pressure would most likely be:

(A) 10 cm H_2O

(B) 20 cm H_2O

(C) 50 cm H_2O

(D) 70 cm H_2O

(E) 0 . . . the bag exploded long before 8 L was reached

Reservoir bags perform several important functions. They act first and foremost as a storage container during the exhalation phase so that a volume of gas is available to draw upon during inspiration. This permits rebreathing of exhaled gas, minimizing waste and preventing air dilution. The bag is also a means for the anesthesiologist to manually ventilate the patient, and acts as a monitor of a patient's respirations. Extremely small changes in bag volume can be detected by tactile sensation, which is the origin of the old phrase, "the educated hand of the anesthesiologist."

Since reservoir bags are usually made of rubber or neoprene, and are very compliant, they also serve to protect the patient from excessive airway pressures. As volume increases beyond its natural capacity, the pressure begins to rise in the bag (and the system) up to approximately 50–60 cm H_2O. After this point the pressure reaches a plateau, and in fact decreases slightly as more volume is added. The ASTM standard for reservoir bags requires that for bags 2 L or greater the pressure should be greater than 35 cm H_2O and less than 60 cm H_2O when the bag is expanded to 4 times its size. The high pressure limit of 60 cm H_2O may be exceeded when using brand-new bags; overinflating or stretching a new bag before using it may improve its compliance and keep the peak pressures within the acceptable range.

Ref: Dorsch JA, Dorsch SE. *Understanding Anesthesia Equipment*, 5th ed. Philadelphia: Lippincott Williams & Wilkins; 2008.

9. Which of the following features distinguishes the ProSeal™ laryngeal mask airway (LMA) from the LMA Classic™?

(A) higher intracuff pressures

(B) lower airway seal pressures

(C) a preformed curve in the shaft

(D) **integral bite block**

(E) the ability to ventilate using positive pressure

Laryngeal mask airways (LMAs) are extraglottic devices that incorporate a wide-bore tube connected to an oval inflatable cuff that seals around the larynx. Advocates of LMAs over endotracheal tubes argue that these devices are easily placed, and are associated with reduced sympathetic stimulation upon insertion, reduced anesthetic requirements for airway tolerance, and a lower frequency of coughing, sore throat and hypoxemia during emergence. Since its invention in 1981, several different subtypes have been manufactured:

- LMA Classic™: The original, reusable LMA. Tube plus cuff.
- LMA ProSeal™ (PLMA): A second-generation version of the Classic that features a softer, larger oval laryngeal cuff as well as a posterior cuff that improves the seal with lower intracuff pressures but higher airway seal pressures. It also features a drainage tube at the tip of the PLMA bowl that sits in the upper esophagus, providing a pathway for passive egress of gastric contents, or the insertion of a <18 French gastric tube to decompress the stomach. The drainage tube is also used when performing the PLMA insertion by inserting a tracheal introducer through this channel and directing it under direct laryngoscopy into the esophagus, ensuring proper placement. The shaft of the PLMA is wire reinforced and flexible—a separate metal introducer is provided to temporarily shape the shaft into a curved shape, facilitating placement. The PLMA

also has a built-in bite block so that the shaft cannot be occluded.

- LMA Fastrach™ (intubating LMA or ILMA): This device has a similar cuffed bowl but a rigid, curved shaft attached to a flanged handle for easy insertion. The device comes with a special wire-reinforced endotracheal tube that can be passed through the ILMA shaft. At the junction of the shaft and the bowl is a levered epiglottis-lifting bar. Gently pushing the tube past this bar should result in the tube entering the trachea. The ILMA can then be removed and the endotracheal tube left in place.
- LMA Flexible™: This is a simple, wire-reinforced LMA with a narrower shaft that make it suitable for head and neck procedures.
- LMA Unique™: Same as the Classic, just disposable.
- LMA Supreme™: A single-use LMA that combines features of the ILMA and the PLMA. It has a preformed curve to the shaft for easy insertion, along with a drainage channel, bite block, and improved cuff design that allow for better seal than the Classic does.

All LMAs can be used during positive pressure ventilation. There has been some reluctance in the past to do so on the part of some clinicians for fear of gastric insufflation. However, it has been shown that oropharyngeal leak pressures are approximately 20 cm H_2O for the classic and unique LMA, and between 25 and 30 cm H_2O for the PLMA and Supreme.

Ref: Hung O, Murphy MF. *Management of the Difficult and Failed Airway*, 2nd ed. New York, NY: McGraw Hill; 2012.

10. What is the largest size endotracheal tube that can be passed through a size 4 Classic or Unique laryngeal mask airway (LMA)?

(A) 5.5 mm ID

(B) **6.0 mm ID**

(C) 6.5 mm ID

(D) 7.0 mm ID

(E) 7.5 mm ID

Standard endotracheal tubes can be passed through the Classic or Unique LMA devices, which can be extremely useful in an emergency airway situation in which ventilation is possible through the LMA, but not ideal, and laryngoscopy or intubation is impossible. It is possible to pass a size 6.0 tube through a size 3 or 4 LMA, and a size 7.0 tube through a size 5 LMA. Good lubrication of the tube is crucial for success in this endeavor. Unlike the intubating LMA (Fastrach), where the specialized endotracheal tube tends to be delivered to the glottis when advanced blindly, a standard tube passed through an LMA often requires a fiberoptic scope to be advanced through both lumens and into the trachea before the endotracheal tube is passed over it.

Ref: LMA International. Accessed July 10, 2016 from http://www.lmaco.com.

11. You are administering anesthesia in the interventional radiology suite with a…um…"vintage" anesthesia machine (okay, it's old). The ventilator is equipped with hanging bellows. The potential hazard of this style of bellows is:

(A) the bellows will not inflate during a power failure

(B) the bellows may fail to inflate if there is a leak in the system

(C) **the bellows may fill during exhalation even if the circuit is disconnected**

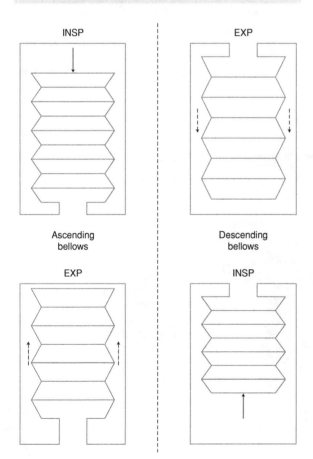

FIG. 21-2. Schematic of anesthesia machine bellows. *Left:* Ascending type; *right:* descending type. *Straight lined arrows* represent the direction of movement during inspiration; *dashed line arrows* represent the direction of movement during expiration. Exp, expiration; Insp, inspiration. (Reproduced with permission from Tobin MJ. *Principles and Practice of Mechanical Ventilation*, 3rd ed. New York, NY: McGraw Hill; 2013.)

(D) the bellows cannot deliver very high flow rates

(E) the bellows are typically made of cheap material

There are two arrangements of bellows in anesthesia machine ventilators, based on their behavior during *exhalation. Ascending* or *standing* bellows rise as they fill during exhalation; *descending* or *hanging* bellows fall as they fill during exhalation (Figure 21-2). In both cases the driving gas compresses the bellows during inspiration and they fill passively during the exhalation phase with pressure provided by the patient's lung and chest wall recoil. The danger with hanging bellows is that they may descend due to gravity even in the event of a major leak or circuit disconnection—they will appear to be working properly even though gas is not being delivered to the patient. Most modern machines have ascending bellows.

Ref: Longnecker DE, Brown DL, Newman MF, et al. *Anesthesiology*, 2nd ed. New York, NY: McGraw Hill; 2012.

12. An anesthetic is being delivered in New York City (sea level). If the partial pressure of sevoflurane in the alveolus is 13 mm Hg, what is the concentration of sevoflurane?

(A) 0.5%

(B) 1.1%

(C) **1.7%**

(D) 2%

(E) 2.3%

Vapor pressure is the pressure exerted by the gaseous molecules on the walls of a container in a closed system, for a given temperature. Within the closed container, as long as any amount of liquid remains, the vapor pressure will be the same. Vapor pressure increases with temperature (more molecules detach from the liquid phase and become vaporized), until the boiling point is reached. At this temperature, molecules no longer vaporize from just the surface of the liquid, but within the liquid itself, forming bubbles that rise to the top.

For any mixture of gases in a closed system, each gas exerts a pressure proportional to its own volume (Dalton's Law). Gases equilibrate to their respective partial pressures, so that at steady state, the alveolar partial pressure of a gas is equal to the blood partial pressure as well as the brain partial pressure. For convention in clinical practice, it is often convenient to communicate in terms of volumes percent, or concentration (the number of units of gas per 100 units of total gas). It is important to note that uptake and anesthetic depth are directly related to partial pressure, not concentration. In addition, a given partial pressure represents the same anesthetic potency under different barometric conditions; this is not the case with concentrations. The relationship between partial pressure and concentration is:

Volumes percent = partial pressure/total pressure

In the above example, the equation can be shown as:

Volumes percent = 13 mm Hg/760 mm Hg

(barometric pressure at sea level)

Volumes percent = 1.7%

Ref: Dorsch JA, Dorsch SE. *Understanding Anesthesia Equipment*, 5th ed. Philadelphia: Lippincott Williams & Wilkins; 2008.

13. Which of the following is NOT a characteristic of modern vaporizers?

   (A) agent specificity
   (B) temperature compensation
   (C) variable bypass
   (D) in-circuit placement
   (E) flow over design

Modern anesthesia vaporizers are agent specific, meaning that they are calibrated for one and only one

agent. If a vaporizer is filled with an agent not intended for it, an underdose or overdose of agent will result, depending on the specific combination. For that reason, safety features such as keyed bottles and adaptors as well as color-coding are now universal.

Carrier gas flows over the surface of the liquid volatile agent, rather than bubbling up through, as in the old copper kettle vaporizers. In addition, typical modern vaporizers are all variable bypass, meaning that turning the control knob splits the stream of fresh gas into bypass gas, which does not enter the vaporizing chamber, and carrier gas, which enters the chamber and becomes saturated with vapor (Figure 21-3).

Modern vaporizers are temperature compensated as well, providing consistent output of gas concentrations over a wide range of temperatures.

A very old type of vaporizer (e.g., Boyle's bottle) that are no longer used were inserted directly into the circle system. These were problematic for a number of reasons, primarily due to their flow dependence on anesthetic output.

Ref: Butterworth JF IV, Mackey DC, Wasnick JD. *Morgan & Mikhail's Clinical Anesthesiology*, 5th ed. New York, NY: McGraw Hill; 2013.

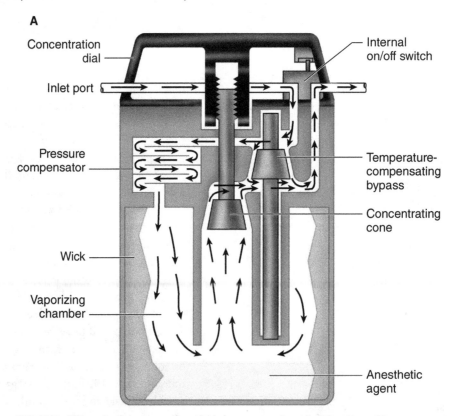

A

Concentration dial

Inlet port

Pressure compensator

Wick

Vaporizing chamber

Internal on/off switch

Temperature-compensating bypass

Concentrating cone

Anesthetic agent

FIG. 21-3. Schematic of agent-specific variable-bypass vaporizers. **A:** Dräger Vapor 19.n.

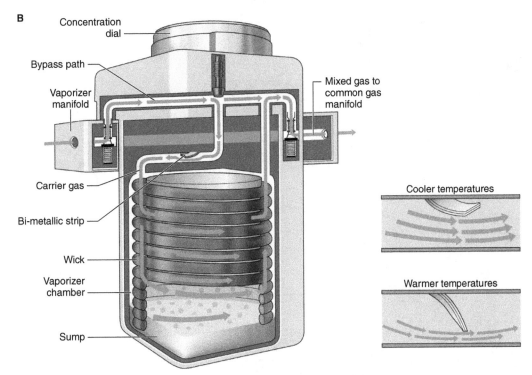

B

Concentration dial

Bypass path

Vaporizer manifold

Carrier gas

Bi-metallic strip

Wick

Vaporizer chamber

Sump

Mixed gas to common gas manifold

Cooler temperatures

Warmer temperatures

FIG. 21-3. *(continued)* **B**: Datex-Ohmeda Tec 7. (Reproduced with permission from Butterworth JF IV, Mackey DC, Wasnick JD. *Morgan & Mikhail's Clinical Anesthesiology*, 5th ed. New York, NY: McGraw Hill; 2013.)

14. Which of the following is NOT a safety standard mandated by the American Society of Testing and Materials (ASTM) regarding the manufacture and function of vaporizers?

(A) All vaporizer control knobs must open counterclockwise.

(B) Either the maximum and minimum fillings levels or the actual usable volume must be displayed.

(C) The vaporizer must be designed so that it cannot be overfilled when in the normal operating position.

(D) A system that prevents gas from passing through the vaporizing chamber of one vaporizer and then through that of another must be provided.

(E) **The vaporizer must be designed so that tilting does not affect the output.**

The ASTM does not mandate that vaporizer design must be able to function independent of position (i.e., tilting). However, the standard does state that the effects of variations in ambient temperature and pressure, tilting, back pressure, and input flow rate and gas mixture composition on performance be described in the accompanying documentation. If the vaporizer is tilted or tipped over, volatile agent may spill into the outlet or bypass. This may result in a high concentration of agent when first used. Vaporizers should always remain upright unless servicing. If a vaporizer is tipped more than 30–45 degrees away from vertical, the recommended course of action is to flush at high flow rates with a high concentration set on the dial; however, individual models vary, so it is best to consult the operator's manual to obtain precise guidance. There are two models of tippable vaporizers: the Drager Vapor 2000 (which has a dial setting marked "T" for transport) and the Ohmeda Aladin cassette vaporizer, which is essentially a portable sump and can be tipped in any direction.

All of the other options (A through D) are provisions in the ASTM anesthesia workstation standard. Side-fill rather than top-fill designs in modern vaporizers have virtually eliminated the problem of overfilling. Multiple vaporizers are prevented from being turned on simultaneously by the interlock system. This is a set of bars and pins behind the vaporizers that click into place when the control knob of one vaporizer is turned, thereby locking the other control knobs.

Ref: Dorsch JA, Dorsch SE. *Understanding Anesthesia Equipment*, 5th ed. Philadelphia: Lippincott Williams & Wilkins; 2008.

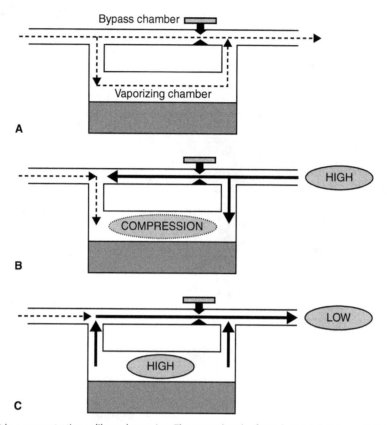

FIG. 21-4. The pumping effect in a concentration-calibrated vaporizer. The normal path of gas during exhalation is indicated in **(A)**. During inspiration **(B)**, high pressure forces gas back into both the bypass and vaporizing chambers. More gas enters the vaporizing chamber than the bypass chamber, since the former has a larger volume. At the same time, fresh gas flow from upstream continues to flow into the vaporizer and is largely shunted into the vaporizing chamber due to the increased pressure (and small volume) of the bypass chamber. The result is a compression of gas in the vaporizing chamber, which is saturated with vapor. Upon release of the downstream pressure on exhalation or decompression of the circuit **(C)**, the pressurized and saturated gas from the vaporizing chamber exits through both the input and output tubes, resulting in a concentration at the fresh gas outlet higher than that set on the dial.

15. Intermittent back pressure in the breathing circuit is most likely to result in increased concentrations of volatile anesthetic delivered to the patient when which of the following is present?

    (A) a check valve downstream from the vaporizer

    (B) spontaneous ventilation

    (C) **low carrier gas flow rates**

    (D) high volatile anesthetic agent levels in the vaporizing chamber

    (E) a short and/or wide-diameter input tube to the vaporizing chamber

Positive pressure generated during inspiration during assisted or controlled ventilation can be transmitted back to the vaporizer and result in increased concentrations of volatile agent being delivered to the common gas outlet. The reason for this relates to what is referred to as the pumping effect (Figure 21-4). The pumping effect is more pronounced during controlled or assisted ventilation, with low carrier gas flow rates, with low volumes of volatile agent in the vaporizing chamber, when pressure fluctuations are high and frequent, and when the dial setting is low. Modifications to older-style vaporizers that work to minimize this effect include decreasing the size of the vaporizing chamber (or increasing the size of the bypass) and increasing the length of the input tube (by making it a long spiral; see Figure 21-3). This latter improvement increases the dead space in the input tube so that even if pressurization of the vaporizing chamber occurs, there will be sufficient volume of gas in the input tube to reduce the likelihood of the saturated gas reaching the bypass chamber by this alternate route. Check valves at the vaporizer outlets also offer some protection, but they are not immune to some degree of the pumping effect.

Ref: Dorsch JA, Dorsch SE. *Understanding Anesthesia Equipment*, 5th ed. Philadelphia: Lippincott Williams & Wilkins; 2008.

16. The bimetallic strip found in many modern vaporizers is designed to prevent the incorrect delivery of volatile anesthetic by which of the following mechanisms?

    (A) temperature compensation
    (B) overfill protection
    (C) prevents filling with an incorrect agent
    (D) ensures only one vaporizer dial can be in the ON position
    (E) prevents volatile agent from reaching bypass chamber if tipped

As the liquid agent is vaporized, energy is lost in the form of heat. The liquid in the vaporizing chamber then cools, resulting in a decrease in the vapor pressure and a reduction in the amount of volatile gas molecules in the chamber. A bimetallic strip found in many vaporizers is simply two metals welded together that expand at different rates with changes in temperature, thereby bending and regulating the amount of carrier gas that enters the bypass chamber. For example, as the vaporizer cools, the bimetallic strip restricts the amount of gas entering the bypass chamber, forcing more gas into the vaporizing chamber to make up for the reduced saturated vapor pressure. Other methods of temperature compensation include the provision of an electric heater to maintain a constant temperature, and computerized thermocompensation.

Ref: Dorsch JA, Dorsch SE. *Understanding Anesthesia Equipment*, 5th ed. Philadelphia: Lippincott Williams & Wilkins; 2008.

17. A sevoflurane vaporizer is accidentally filled with isoflurane. Which of the following is MOST likely to be true?

    (A) the vapor output will be higher than the reading on the dial
    (B) no change will be required in the concentration of volatile
    (C) the vapor output will be lower than the reading on the dial
    (D) the gas should be treated as if it is sevoflurane
    (E) the mixture can be determined by smelling the gas

Modern vaporizers are agent specific. The clinical result of filling with the incorrect agent depends on the vapor pressure and potency of the agent. For example, the vapor pressure of sevoflurane is 160 mm Hg (at 20°C), whereas that of isoflurane is 240 mm Hg. Therefore, 33% more isoflurane vapor will be present in the vaporizing chamber than would be the case with sevoflurane.

Moreover, isoflurane is more potent (MAC of 1.2 vs. 2.0 for sevoflurane). In contrast, filling an isoflurane vaporizer with sevoflurane will lead to an underdosage. Vaporizers have agent-specific and color-coded keyed filling ports to prevent incorrect filling.

Ref: Butterworth JF IV, Mackey DC, Wasnick JD. *Morgan & Mikhail's Clinical Anesthesiology*, 5th ed. New York, NY: McGraw Hill; 2013.

18. Which of the following is a design feature of the Ohmeda Tec 6 vaporizer?

    (A) variable bypass
    (B) flow-over
    (C) in-circuit
    (D) gas/vapor blender
    (E) agent nonspecific (may be used with several agents)

The Tec 6 is a vaporizer designed specifically for use with desflurane. The boiling point of desflurane at sea level is only 23.5°C. Therefore, at room temperature, there is likely to be intermittent boiling, which, in a conventional variable bypass vaporizer, would lead to excessive agent delivery. At the same time, boiling requires energy, which draws heat out of the surrounding structures, cooling it down. This leads to a cooling of the agent and a decrease in saturated vapor pressure, with a resulting under-delivery of volatile agent.

To address these problems, the Tec 6 vaporizer utilizes a desflurane reservoir (sump) that is heated to well above the boiling point (39°C), creating a "pressure-cooker" of vapor at a pressure of approximately 2 atmospheres. Rather than shunt a proportion of fresh gas through the reservoir, the vaporizer injects this concentrated desflurane vapor directly into the fresh gas flow. The proportion of desflurane joining the fresh gas flow is dependent on both the dial concentration and the fresh gas flow rate, and is electronically controlled.

Ref: Butterworth JF IV, Mackey DC, Wasnick JD. *Morgan & Mikhail's Clinical Anesthesiology*, 5th ed. New York, NY: McGraw Hill; 2013.

19. A patient is receiving anesthesia in Taos, NM (barometric pressure 594 mm Hg). The sevoflurane vaporizer dial is set to 2% (1 MAC). Which one of the following is true regarding the effect of altitude on the vaporizer and its effect on the patient?

    (A) The dial concentration should be increased by 50%.
    (B) The dial concentration should be increased by 25%.

(C) **The dial concentration should remain the same.**

(D) The dial concentration should be decreased by 33%.

(E) The dial concentration should be decreased by 25%.

The effect of a volatile agent is determined only by its partial pressure in the tissues. Recall that:

Volumes percent = partial pressure/total pressure

Therefore, if sevoflurane were being delivered with a dialed concentration of 2% at sea level, the partial pressure of sevoflurane would be:

$$P_{partial} = 2\% \times 760 \text{ mm Hg} = 15.2 \text{ mm Hg}$$

Also remember that saturated vapor pressure is not affected by ambient pressure, so output from the vaporizer is unaffected. In Taos, the delivered concentration if 2% was dialed in would be calculated as follows (where alt = altitude):

Delivered concentration = Volumes percent$_{dialed}$
$\times$ (Pressure$_{sea\ level}$/Pressure$_{alt}$)

Delivered concentration = 2 × (760/594) = 2.56%

The concentration of volatile agent in the alveolus of the patient in Taos is therefore approximately 25% higher than at sea level. However, the partial pressure is exactly the same, because the ambient pressure in the alveolus is not 760 mm Hg, but 594 mm Hg. Therefore, the partial pressure of 2.56% sevoflurane in Taos is 15.2 mm Hg (2.56% × 594). For this reason, the clinical effect of altitude on a variable bypass vaporizer is negligible.

This is not the case for the Tec 6 vaporizer, which is pressurized to 2 atmospheres regardless of altitude. Therefore, while a 6% concentration of desflurane provides a partial pressure of 45.6 mm Hg at sea level (and provides approximately 1 MAC of effect), in Taos this partial pressure would only be 6% × 594, or 35.6 mm Hg. Therefore, an increase in the dial concentration of the Tec 6 vaporizer is required when anesthetizing a patient at altitude. The recommended adjustments relative to altitude can be found in the operator's manual.

Refs: Boumphrey S, Marshal N. Understanding vaporizers: continuing education in anaesthesia. *Critical Care & Pain* 2011;11:199–203.

Butterworth JF IV, Mackey DC, Wasnick JD. *Morgan & Mikhail's Clinical Anesthesiology*, 5th ed. New York, NY: McGraw Hill; 2013.

20. Which of the following represents the preferred arrangement of components in a circle breathing system?

(A) **The reservoir bag is placed between the expiratory valve and the carbon dioxide absorber.**

(B) Unidirectional valves are placed within the Y-piece of the circuit to be as close as possible to the patient.

(C) The fresh gas inlet is positioned between the inspiratory valve and the patient.

(D) The adjustable pressure limiting (APL) valve is positioned downstream from the carbon dioxide absorber.

(E) The reservoir bag is placed on the opposite side of the APL valve to decrease wasted gas.

The circle system is made up of hoses connecting two unidirectional valves (inspiratory and expiratory), an inlet for fresh gas flow, a reservoir bag, the adjustable pressure limiting (APL) valve, and the carbon dioxide absorber. It is possible to place these in several configurations relatively safely; however, for maximum efficiency, the arrangement shown in Figure 21-5 is preferred.

The fresh gas inlet should be placed between the absorber and the inspiratory valve. A position distal to the inspiratory valve would permit fresh gas to be pushed into the expiratory limb (bypassing the patient) and wasted during exhalation. The fresh gas inlet should not be placed between the expiratory valve and the absorber as this may lead to volatile anesthetics being absorbed and subsequently released by the absorbent crystals, prolonging emergence.

Unidirectional valves should be placed as close to the patient as is feasible to prevent backflow into the inspiratory limb if a leak develops in either of the valves. Valves should not be placed within the Y-piece, since attaching the Y-piece to the breathing tubes in the wrong orientation would prevent fresh gas from flowing to the patient.

Placing the APL valve between the expiratory valve and the absorber minimizes the venting of fresh gas and conserves absorption capacity.

The reservoir bag is best placed on the expiratory limb so that resistance to exhalation is low—the bag "catches" the exhaled volume as it quickly flows from the patient. Also, bag compression during assisted ventilation will vent excess expired gas through the APL valve, preventing unnecessary use of the absorbent.

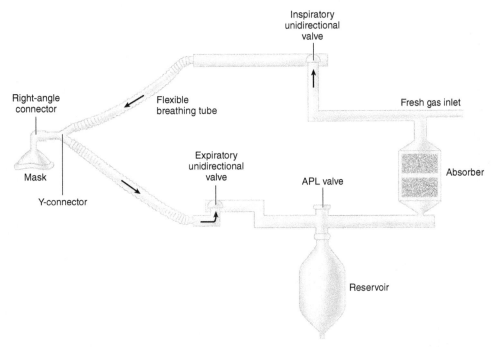

FIG. 21-5. A circle system. APL, adjustable pressure-limiting (valve). (Reproduced with permission from Butterworth JF IV, Mackey DC, Wasnick JD. *Morgan & Mikhail's Clinical Anesthesiology*, 5th ed. New York, NY: McGraw Hill; 2013.)

Ref: Butterworth JF IV, Mackey DC, Wasnick JD. *Morgan & Mikhail's Clinical Anesthesiology*, 5th ed. New York, NY: McGraw Hill; 2013.

21. Which one of the following is NOT a proposed advantage of low-flow anesthesia using a circle circuit breathing system?

(A) reduced cost

(B) reduced atmospheric pollution from greenhouse and ozone-depleting gases

(C) reduced operating room pollution

(D) improved heat and humidity conservation

(E) **improved correlation between delivered and end-tidal concentrations of gases**

Low-flow anesthesia is the practice of delivering low fresh gas flows to the circuit in an effort to increase economy, efficiency, and heat/humidity conservation. There is no one fresh gas flow rate that is universally accepted as the definition of "low-flow anesthesia"; some define it as less than 1 L/min, while others hold to a stricter 500 mL/min or less definition. In any case, this should be contrasted to the definition of "closed-circuit anesthesia" in which the only fresh gas entering the system is the same amount of oxygen being taken up by the patient (e.g., 200 mL/min). This is intellectually interesting and makes

for good old-school MCQ, but in reality this is never done outside a laboratory, since the hazards of such low oxygen flow rates far outweigh any benefits of closed-circuit anesthesia using modern equipment.

In contrast to high flow rates (let's say 2–4 L/min), low-flow anesthesia confers a number of advantages. Since far less mixed gas is being shunted out of the system via the APL valve, there are cost savings to be realized with the reduction of volatile agent used. This is more relevant with desflurane and sevoflurane than with isoflurane. By the same token, since less nitrous oxide and volatile agent are being expelled into the atmosphere, there is less environmental pollution. The fluorocarbon volatile agents as well as nitrous oxide attack the Earth's ozone layer; nitrous oxide is also a greenhouse gas. With modern scavenging equipment, the impact of low-flow anesthesia on operating room pollution is minimized, although leaks or improper face mask fit may result in increased exposure of operating room personnel to anesthetic gases.

Low-flow anesthesia reduces the washout of warmer, humid gas in the system with cold dry fresh gas, conserving heat and humidity. This is only really relevant if a heat-moisture exchanger is NOT being used.

The low flow rate has the principal disadvantage of a long time constant; in other words, in order to change the brain concentration of anesthetic agent, the

TABLE 21-2. Classification and characteristics of Mapleson circuits.

Mapleson class	Other names	Configuration[a]	Required fresh gas flows		Comments
			Spontaneous	Controlled	
A	Magill attachment	FGI → Breathing tube / APL valve / Breathing bag / Mask	Equal to minute ventilation (≈80 mL/kg/min)	Very high and difficult to predict	Poor choice during controlled ventilaton. Enclosed Magill system is a modification that improves efficiency. Coaxial Mapleson A (Lack breathing system) provides waste gas scavenging.
B		FGI / APL valve	2 × minute ventilation	2–2½ × minute ventilation	
C	Waters' to-and-Fro	FGI / APL valve	2 × minute ventilation	2–2½ × minute ventilation	
D	Bain circuit	APL valve / FGI	2–3 × minute ventilation	1–2 × minute ventilation	Bain coaxial modification: fresh gas tube inside breathing tube.
E	Ayre's T-piece	FGI	2–3 × minute ventilation	3 × minute ventilation (I:E·1:2)	Exhalation tubing should provide a larger volume than tidal volume to prevent rebreathing. Scavenging is difficult.
F	Jackson-Rees' modification	FGI / APL valve	2–3 × minute ventilation	2 × minute ventilation	A Mapleson E with a breathing bag connected to the end of the breathing tube to allow controlled ventilation and scavenging.

[a]FGI, fresh gas inlet; APL, adjustable pressure-limiting (value). (Reproduced with permission from Butterworth JF IV, Mackey DC, Wasnick JD. Morgan & Mikhail's Clinical Anesthesiology, 5th ed. New York, NY: McGraw Hill; 2013.)

duration of time between the change on the vaporizer setting and reaching that tissue concentration is prolonged. In addition, modern vaporizers are designed to be used at relatively high fresh gas flow rates, and the lower the fresh gas flow rate, the greater the disparity between what is set on the rotameters and vaporizer dial and what is in the alveolus. Obviously, if the end-tidal concentration needs to be adjusted quickly in response to changes in surgical stimulation, short intervals of high flow can rapidly bring the system to equilibrium before returning to the low-flow state.

Ref: Dorsch JA, Dorsch SE. *Understanding Anesthesia Equipment*, 5th ed. Philadelphia: Lippincott Williams & Wilkins; 2008.

22. In order to minimize rebreathing of exhaled carbon dioxide using a Mapleson A breathing system in a spontaneously breathing patient, what is the minimum fresh gas flow required?

(A) equal to 75% of minute ventilation

(B) equal to minute ventilation

(C) 2× minute ventilation

(D) 3× minute ventilation

(E) impossible to predict

Mapleson A? Good grief, here we go again with this Mapleson business. Here's the skinny on the ol' Mapleson family so that you can answer any (reasonable) question variation.

The Mapleson breathing systems (sometimes curiously called circuits) are a family of semi-open systems made up of many of the same pieces as a circle circuit (tubing, fresh gas inlet, reservoir bag, APL valve), but they conspicuously lack both unidirectional valves or carbon dioxide absorbent. Because there is no distinct separation of inspired and expired gases, some rebreathing can occur, which can be overcome principally by jacking up the fresh gas flow to wash out the tubing during the expiratory pause. If you ever get the chance to use any Mapleson circuit: (A) know that you can overcome all of its rebreathing potential by increasing gas flow; (B) do use EtCO$_2$ monitoring as the safest means of knowing where you stand with rebreathing carbon dioxide; and (C) please let us know how you time-traveled back several decades to find one. DeLorean?

There are six types, labeled A through F (Table 21-2). Some have eponymous names as well (e.g., A = Magill

attachment, D = Bain circuit). The arrangement of components determines its efficiency, defined as the amount of gas flow required to minimize or prevent rebreathing. Here is something you need to know: during spontaneous respiration, the Mapleson A is the most efficient, requiring a fresh gas flow equal to minute ventilation. Look at the picture in Table 21-2. Imagine what's happening during exhalation: as expired gas exits the patient, it meets the pressure head of fresh gas coming down the tube toward the patient. The result is alveolar gas being exhausted through the APL valve, with mostly fresh gas being available for the next breath. In contrast, during controlled ventilation, there is very low pressure in the tubing during exhalation and the expiratory pause, so alveolar gas is NOT shunted out the APL valve, but travels along the tubing and begins to fill the bag; at the beginning of the next breath, much of the tidal volume is previously exhaled alveolar gas. High and unpredictable flows are required to prevent rebreathing in this scenario. **For this reason, Mapleson A is considered most efficient for spontaneous breathing and least efficient for controlled breathing.**

The Mapleson D is the reverse situation, due to the switching of the position of the APL valve and fresh gas inlet. During exhalation, alveolar gases are pushed down the tubing and partially fill the breathing bag before being vented through the APL valve. Elimination of alveolar gas in the tubing must occur during the expiratory pause. During spontaneous breathing, the sinusoidal respiratory pattern results in very little expiratory pause, whereas during controlled ventilation there is a much greater pause, allowing for venting of alveolar gases and greater efficiency. Fresh gas flows of 1–2× minute ventilation are adequate during controlled ventilation, whereas spontaneous ventilation requires 2–3× minute ventilation.

Mapleson efficiency for spontaneous ventilation: A>D>C>B (*Mnemonic: "All Dogs Can Breathe." Dogs are spontaneous creatures, right?*)

Mapleson efficiency for controlled ventilation: D>B>C>A (*Mnemonic: "David Bolused Cis-Atracurium." You're gonna need controlled ventilation once Dave gives that muscle relaxant…*)

Ref: Butterworth JF IV, Mackey DC, Wasnick JD. *Morgan & Mikhail's Clinical Anesthesiology*, 5th ed. New York, NY: McGraw Hill; 2013.

23. Your co-resident suggests a trial of T-piece ventilation for a patient in the ICU. Not to be outdone in front of the team, you respond by casually saying, "Oh, so what you'd like is ...":

(A) "a Mapleson B"
(B) "a Mapleson C"
(C) "a Mapleson E"
(D) "a Mapleson F"
(E) "a Mapleson G"

The Mapleson E is also known as a "T-piece," as it is simply a T-connector with a fresh gas inlet on one side and a length of corrugated tubing that acts a reservoir on the other. It is not used so much for anesthesia these days, since it is difficult to scavenge waste gases, but is very useful for providing an enriched FiO_2 to patients who are intubated but breathing spontaneously (e.g., in the PACU or ICU); it is also a means to provide a trial of weaning in the intubated patient. The FiO_2 is dependent on the fresh gas flow, since with low flows air entrainment and rebreathing of carbon dioxide can occur. At flows greater than 3–5× minute ventilation, this is thought to be minimized.

Ref: Dorsch JA, Dorsch SE. *Understanding Anesthesia Equipment*, 5th ed. Philadelphia: Lippincott Williams & Wilkins; 2008.

24. Which of the following is a feature of the self-reinflating resuscitation bag device?

(A) requires a pressurized gas supply to work
(B) a 22-mm male/15-mm female connector for the airway device (LMA, mask, etc.)
(C) an oxygen inlet with a two-way valve

(D) a valve to prevent air entrainment into the bag
(E) can only provide approximately 50% FiO_2

The "resuscitator bag" is a ventilation device that is compact, portable, and, because the self-inflating bag maintains its shape, requires no source of pressurized gas to operate (Figure 21-6). The standard features common to these bags are:

- A 22-mm/15-mm patient connector that accommodates endotracheal tubes, face masks, and LMAs
- A two-way non-rebreathing (patient) valve. This valve opens during compression of the bag to force gas into the patient, and allows venting of expired gas to the ambient environment through ports in the valve. Air is not entrained through this valve during inspiration, and exhaled gas is prevented from re-entering the ventilation bag
- A self-inflating ventilation bag typically made of silicone or a styrene thermoplastic polymer that has rapid recoil after compression. Adult sizes are usually about 1500 mL, while smaller sizes exist for pediatric (500–650 mL) and infant (220–240 mL) use
- An oxygen inlet to fill the bag with high-flow (10–15 L/min) oxygen
- A reservoir bag that reduces the entrainment of air during re-expansion of the ventilation bag
- A one-way intake valve that provides gas for re-expansion from the reservoir bag. If the reservoir bag becomes empty or if the oxygen delivery fails for whatever reason, this valve permits the entrainment of room air, which is a safety measure so the ventilation bag will always reinflate.

Other features that some models incorporate include side ports on the neck to allow for end-tidal carbon dioxide monitoring, pressure manometers, PEEP

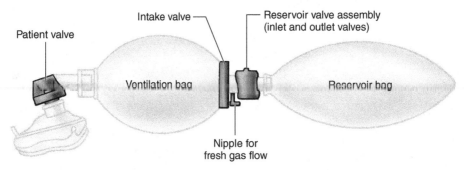

Patient valve

Intake valve

Reservoir valve assembly
(inlet and outlet valves)

Ventilation bag

Reservoir bag

Nipple for
fresh gas flow

FIG. 21-6. The Laerdal resuscitator. (Reproduced with permission from Laerdal Medical Corp.)

valves, and pressure or flow-limiting valves that prevent excessive airway pressures and barotrauma. With good mask fit and high (>10 L/min) oxygen flows, an FiO_2 >90% can be achieved provided that minute ventilation is not excessive.

Ref: Hung O, Murphy MF. *Management of the Difficult and Failed Airway*, 2nd ed. New York, NY: McGraw Hill; 2012.

25. Soda lime is a mixture of:

(A) **$Ca(OH)_2$ and NaOH**

(B) $CaCO_3$ and NaOH

(C) NaOH and KOH

(D) Na_2CO_3 and KOH

(E) Na_2CO_3 and NaOH

Soda lime is the most common absorbent material used in carbon dioxide absorbers, and is capable of absorbing up to 23 L of CO_2 per 100 g of absorbent. It is supplied in granules of varying sizes; when packed in the absorber canister, the space between the granules ("void space") is approximately 45%, which provides a good trade-off between airflow resistance and absorptive capacity. The vast majority of soda lime is calcium hydroxide (80%), with the remainder made up of sodium hydroxide, water, and a small amount of potassium hydroxide. The reactions that take place in the carbon dioxide "scrubbing" process are as follows:

$$CO_2 + H_2O \rightarrow H_2CO_3$$
$$H_2CO_3 + 2NaOH \rightarrow Na_2CO_3 + 2H_2O + heat$$
$$Na_2CO_3 + Ca(OH)_2 \rightarrow CaCO_3 + 2NaOH$$

Soda lime is manufactured with an indicator dye that changes color from white to purple when the pH drops, due to accumulation of hydrogen ions when the absorbent becomes exhausted. Canisters should be replenished when 50–70% of the absorbent turns color.

One of the potential hazards of soda lime is the degradation of sevoflurane and desflurane into compound A and carbon monoxide, respectively. A newer absorbent called Amsorb is made of calcium hydroxide and calcium chloride, and does not appear to degrade volatile anesthetics to any meaningful degree.

You may read about Baralyme; it is only of historical interest as it is no longer used. Baralyme was associated with reports of spontaneous fires, explosions, and melting of absorbent canisters when it became dessicated; temperatures as high as 400°C were reported in

some cases. The high fraction of potassium hydroxide (a strong base) in Baralyme was thought to be responsible for this.

Ref: Butterworth JF IV, Mackey DC, Wasnick JD. *Morgan & Mikhail's Clinical Anesthesiology*, 5th ed. New York, NY: McGraw Hill; 2013.

26. Baffles in the carbon dioxide absorber function to:

(A) prevent caking of absorbent dust in the exhaust tubing

(B) catch water droplets that condense in the absorbent

(C) **channel airflow to the center of the absorber**

(D) evenly distribute heat within the absorbent

(E) prevent evaporation of indicator dye from the absorbent granules

Gases entering the absorber canisters tend to flow down the periphery of the canisters, a tendency known as the "wall effect." If left unchecked, the granules on the outside of the containers will become exhausted far earlier than the central granules will. Since the outer granules are the visible ones, this would result in premature changing of the absorbent. Baffles are annular rings placed in the container housing that channel gas flow into the center, thereby ensuring more even distribution of gas.

Ref: Dorsch JA, Dorsch SE. *Understanding Anesthesia Equipment*, 5th ed. Philadelphia: Lippincott Williams & Wilkins; 2008.

27. Which of the following devices provides a constant FiO_2 that is independent of a patient's peak inspiratory flow?

(A) nasal cannulae

(B) simple face mask

(C) partial rebreather mask

(D) **Venturi mask**

(E) manual resuscitator (self-inflating bag-valve-mask)

The Venturi mask incorporates specifically designed plastic barrels that are inserted between the oxygen tubing and face mask. Using Bernoulli's principle, the shape and size of the side holes in each color-coded barrel permits the delivery of a precise FiO_2 by entraining a predictable amount of air. Venturi masks provide a fixed concentration of oxygen independent

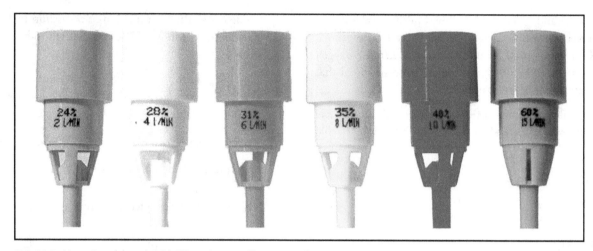

FIG. 21-7. Venturi mask barrels with FiO$_2$ and oxygen flow rate markings.

of the respiratory pattern of the patient. Barrels are available for the following FiO$_2$ settings: 24%, 28%, 31%, 35%, 40%, and 60% (Figure 21-7). Each barrel has the oxygen flow rate printed on it to indicate the appropriate oxygen flow rate.

Ref: Hagberg CA. *Benumof's Airway Management*, 2nd ed. Philadelphia, PA: Elsevier; 2007.

28. Which of the following statements regarding waste gas scavenging systems is TRUE?

(A) The standard fitting size for scavenging tubing is 22 mm.

(B) A negative pressure valve is not required with a closed scavenging system.

(C) Open scavenging systems may be active or passive.

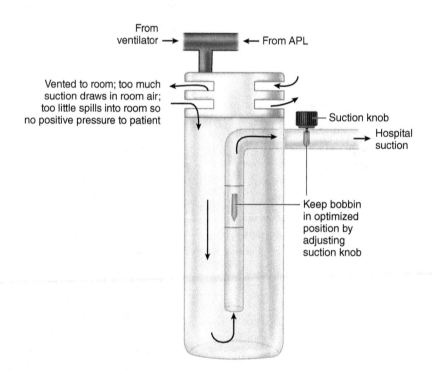

FIG. 21-8. Open interface scavenger system. APL, adjustable pressure-limiting. (Reproduced with permission from Rose G, McLarney JT. *Anesthesia equipment simplified*, 1st ed. New York, NY: McGraw Hill; 2014.)

(D) A reservoir chamber or bag is required with closed scavenging systems.

(E) If the scavenging reservoir bag is constantly collapsed, suction flow should be increased.

Waste gas scavenging assemblies divert excess gas outside the operating room to reduce contamination of the workspace and exposure of personnel to potentially hazardous anesthetic agents. While systems vary somewhat in design, they all contain (1) a relief valve through which gas exits the breathing circuit; (2) tubing that conducts the gas to the scavenging interface; (3) an interface that serves to regulate the pressure in the system; and (4) disposal tubing that vents the gas to the external atmosphere. The disposal tubing can be connected to suction (an active system) or simply allowed to passively vent to the outside world (passive system). Tubing in the scavenging system is always a different caliber (30 mm) than breathing system tubing (22 mm for adults, 15 mm for pediatric circuits) to prevent dangerous misconnections.

The scavenging interface may contain either an open or closed reservoir, which can be a container, a bag, or simply a section of tubing. Open interfaces are open to the atmosphere and contain no valves (Figure 21-8). In these systems gas is pushed passively into the reservoir in a pulsatile manner during the respiratory cycle. The disposal tubing, which opens into the reservoir, is always active in open systems to keep the reservoir from filling up and the leakage of waste gases in the operating room. The openings in the reservoir ensure that neither positive nor negative pressure is applied to the patient.

In a closed interface system, the connection to the atmosphere is through valves (Figure 21-9). Closed interfaces always contain a positive pressure relief valve, which is activated between 5 cm and 10 cm H_2O. This is critical if the scavenging system becomes blocked downstream to prevent pressure buildup. Negative pressure valves are only required if the disposal system is active to prevent excessive suction pressure from being transmitted to the breathing circuit. These kick in at −0.5 cm H_2O. Reservoirs are not necessarily required in closed systems; however, if a reservoir is present, the disposal system should be active. These are usually inflatable bags that look like the ventilation bag of the breathing circuit (they are often a different color for identification). The flow rate of the

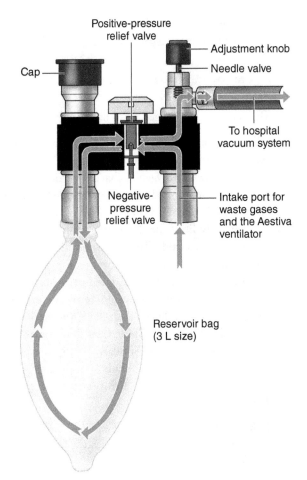

FIG. 21-9. Closed interface with active scavenging (Datex-Ohmeda).

disposal suction can be adjusted with a small valve so that the bag is partially filled. If it is constantly collapsed, too much suction is being applied to the interface, and suction flow should be decreased. If the bag is distended, flow should be increased.

Ref: Dorsch JA, Dorsch SE. *Understanding Anesthesia Equipment*, 5th ed. Philadelphia: Lippincott Williams & Wilkins; 2008.

29. In Datex-Ohmeda machines, the Link-25 system serves to:

(A) electronically connect the gas flow data to the monitor

(B) prevent more than one vaporizer from being turned on at a time

(C) shut off pipeline flow of nitrous oxide in the event of low oxygen pressure

(D) **permit only certain proportions of nitrous oxide and oxygen using the flow control knobs**

(E) activate the oxygen flush mechanism

All anesthesia machines have either a mechanical or electronic method of proportioning flow rates of nitrous oxide and oxygen so that a hypoxic gas mixture may not be delivered. In the Datex-Ohmeda machines, the Link-25 system is a chain-and-sprocket system that mechanically links the flowmeter knobs of both oxygen and nitrous oxide. The sprocket of the oxygen flow control has 29 teeth, and the sprocket for nitrous oxide has 14 teeth. If an operator attempts to increase the nitrous oxide flow that would result in a ratio of oxygen:nitrous oxide less than 25%, the teeth engage and mechanically turn the oxygen flow control knob to maintain this ratio. Similarly, if nitrous oxide is flowing and the oxygen knob is turned down, the chain will engage to protect this ratio and the nitrous flow will begin to drop.

Ref: Dorsch JA, Dorsch SE. *Understanding Anesthesia Equipment*, 5th ed. Philadelphia: Lippincott Williams & Wilkins; 2008.

30. Which of the following sequence of flowmeter tubes would be MOST likely to prevent a hypoxic mixture in the event of a crack in the air flowmeter tube (from left to right)?

(A) oxygen, air, nitrous oxide

(B) oxygen, nitrous oxide, air

(C) nitrous oxide, oxygen, air

(D) air, oxygen, nitrous oxide

(E) **air, nitrous oxide, oxygen**

Carrier gas flows through the flowmeters and into a common manifold, where it is delivered (by convention) out the right hand side to the vaporizers. If oxygen is placed in any position but the rightmost with respect to nitrous oxide and air, the risk for a hypoxic mixture exists when any tube has a crack in it (Figure 21-10).

Ref: Dorsch JA, Dorsch SE. *Understanding Anesthesia Equipment*, 5th ed. Philadelphia: Lippincott Williams & Wilkins; 2008.

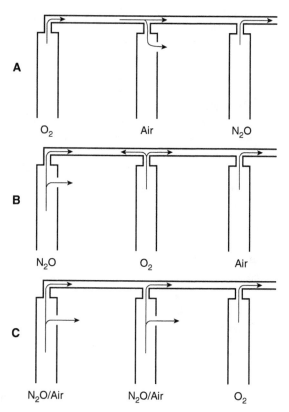

FIG. 21-10. Sequence of flowmeters on a three-gas machine. **(A)** and **(B)** represent unsafe sequences, as oxygen may flow to the cracked tubes due to pressure differentials. In sequence **(C)**, it is unlikely that oxygen would flow retrograde to the cracked tubes, as it is the last gas in the manifold and there should be no resistance to flow distally. Note that a cracked *oxygen* tube in any position may result in hypoxia.

31. Which of the following is NOT an example of an ergonomic feature of the anesthesia workstation?

(A) standardization of workstation dimensions and arrangements between manufacturers

(B) wheel protectors to push cords away

(C) **patient attachments (e.g., suction, breathing circuits) mounted on the right-hand side of the workstation**

(D) suction canister height below the level of the surgical table

(E) electrical and gas outlets mounted on booms over or near the workstation

Ergonomics is the study of people's efficiency in their working environment. Poor ergonomics in a highly complex environment such as the operating room leads to fatigue, injuries, reductions in productivity, and medical errors. The anesthesia workstation incorporates a number of features that leads to improvements in efficiency and reductions in stress, fatigue, and errors.

Machine design is generally consistent between manufacturers with respect to dimensions and layout of the various elements. Patient attachments such as suction, breathing circuit, and monitors are all positioned on the left side of the machine by convention; as such, the best place for the machine to rest is on the right side of the surgical table at the head, so that the cords and tubing are not stretched over a long distance. The suction canister should be below the height of the surgical table to reduce the effect of hydrostatic pressure. Electrical, compressed gas, and phone cords should not cross spaces where personnel are expected to walk to reduce tripping hazard; ideally these are located above the workstation on a special boom. Wheel protectors prevent the anesthesia machine from running over cords or getting stuck.

A practitioner sitting or standing in the anesthesia "cockpit" should be able to reach the flowmeters, vaporizers, suction, monitors, electronic patient record, and other important controls without much effort or turning. Temperature and lighting should be adjustable to meet the needs of the patient as well as the operating room personnel. Loud noise can be a distraction and prevent audible alarms from being noticed.

Ref: Leob R, Berguer R. Ergonomics and workflow. In: Block FE, Helfman S, Eds. *American Society of Anesthesiologists Operating Room Design Manual.* Accessed from https://www.asahq.org/resources/resources-from-asa-committees/operating-room-design-manual.

32. In the diagram below, the waveforms in column A are representative of which type of ventilation?

(A) pressure-controlled ventilation

(B) volume-controlled ventilation

(C) flow-controlled ventilation

(D) high-frequency oscillatory ventilation

(E) interpulmonary percussive ventilation

The rectangular pressure wave in column A is indicative that pressure is the independent variable (i.e., pressure controlled ventilation). The "equation of motion for the respiratory system" describes the relationship of pressure, volume, and flow for inspiration and expiration:

$$P_{TR} = P_E + P_R$$

Given that P_{TR} = transrespiratory pressure (= pressure generated by both the ventilator and respiratory muscles); P_E = elastic recoil pressure (= elastance × volume); and P_R = resistive pressure (= resistance × flow), the formula becomes:

$$P_{ventilator} + P_{muscles} = (E \times volume) + (R \times flow)$$

As this formula indicates, only one variable (pressure, volume, or flow) can control a breath at one time. Determining this "control variable" serves as a basis for classifying ventilators. Note, because volume and flow are inverse functions of each other, ventilators are typically classified as either volume-controlled (both volume and flow are controlled) or pressure-controlled. There are exceptions to this classification: interpulmonary percussive ventilation and high-frequency oscillatory ventilation control neither volume, pressure, nor flow and are time controlled (as only the duration of the flow pulses are controlled).

Refs: Tobin MJ. *Principles and Practice of Mechanical Ventilation,* 3rd ed. New York, NY: McGraw Hill; 2013.

Miller RD. *Miller's Anesthesia,* 8th ed. Philadelphia, PA: Elsevier; 2015.

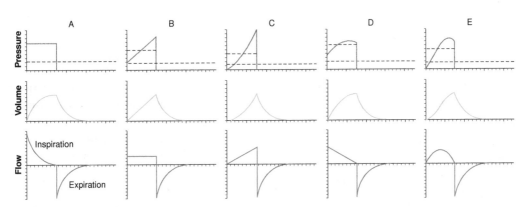

FIG. 21-11. This figure illustrates the distinction between the terms target and cycle. **A.** Inspiration is pressure-targeted and time-cycled. **B.** Flow is targeted, but volume is not, and inspiration is volume-cycled. **C.** Both volume and flow are targeted, and inspiration is time-cycled. (Modified from Tobin MJ: *Principles and practice of mechanical ventilation,* 3rd Ed. New York, NY: McGraw Hill; 2013.)

DIRECTIONS: For questions 33–37, each group of items below consists of lettered headings followed by a list of numbered phrases or statements. For each numbered phrase or statement, select the ONE lettered heading or component that is most closely associated with it. Each lettered heading or component may be selected once, more than once, or not at all.

(A)   assist-control

(B)   pressure-control

(C)   volume-control

(D)   periodic sigh

(E)   high-frequency ventilation

(F)   intermittent mandatory ventilation (IMV)

(G)   synchronized intermittent mandatory ventilation (SIMV)

(H)   pressure support

(I)   biphasic positive airway pressure (BIPAP)

33.   Which ventilator mode delivers the same tidal volume during every inspiration, regardless of whether initiated by patient or ventilator?

(A)   assist-control

Ventilators may control either volume or pressure and can use three different sequences for breathing: continuous spontaneous ventilation, intermittent mandatory ventilation, or continuous mandatory ventilation. This means there are five main types of ventilation:

1)   Volume-control, continuous mandatory ventilation

2)   Volume-control, intermittent mandatory ventilation

3)   Pressure-control, continuous mandatory ventilation

4)   Pressure-control, intermittent mandatory ventilation

5)   Pressure-control, continuous spontaneous ventilation

Either the patient or ventilator may trigger breaths in assist-control ventilation. When triggered, the ventilator delivers a preset tidal volume. Assist control is a form of volume-control, intermittent mandatory ventilation. In assist-control ventilation, the trigger variable is either a change in pressure, flow, or time; the target variable is volume or flow; and the cycle variable is volume or time. The inspiratory flow shape is usually a square wave, although some ventilators may utilize other flow waveforms.

Ref: Tobin MJ. *Principles and Practice of Mechanical Ventilation*, 3rd ed. New York, NY: McGraw Hill; 2013.

34.   Which ventilator mode allows the patient to breathe spontaneously, without support, between machine-cycled breaths, which are delivered regardless of respiratory timing?

(F)   intermittent mandatory ventilation (IMV)

Intermittent mandatory ventilation (IMV) provides a preset number of mandatory breaths and allows the patient to breath spontaneously between the mandatory breaths. When IMV breaths are synchronized with the patient's inspiratory effort, the mode of ventilation is called synchronized intermittent mandatory ventilation (SIMV).

IMV breaths are generally either volume controlled (flow-targeted and volume-cycled) or pressure controlled (pressure-targeted and time-cycled).

Ref: Tobin MJ. *Principles and Practice of Mechanical Ventilation*, 3rd ed. New York, NY: McGraw Hill; 2013.

35.   Which ventilator mode provides partial ventilator support to patients with preserved respiratory drive by increasing the pressure at the airway above the expiratory pressure in response to an inspiratory effort?

(H)   pressure support

Pressure support ventilation provides a preset level of pressure support during patient-initiated inspiration. Pressure support ventilation is initiated by the patient (either pressure- or flow-triggered), pressure-targeted, and flow-cycled

Ref: Tobin MJ. *Principles and Practice of Mechanical Ventilation*, 3rd ed. New York: NY: McGraw Hill; 2013.

36.   Which ventilator mode is a form of airway pressure release ventilation (APRV)?

(I)   biphasic positive airway pressure (BIPAP)

Biphasic positive airway pressure (BIPAP) and bilevel airway pressure (Bilevel) are synonyms for airway pressure release ventilation (APRV). Note, for trademark reasons, different ventilator brands may use different names for this mode of ventilation. APRV is a form of ventilation meant to help patients with acute lung injury. APRV is time-cycled between two pressure levels and allows spontaneous breathing in any phase of the cycle. Important to note, the majority of time is spent at the higher set pressure with a brief time at the lower set pressure. In this way, the lungs are recruited and oxygenation improves. If there is no spontaneous ventilation, APRV is really a form of inverse-ratio, pressure-controlled ventilation (pressure-targeted, time-cycled). (Inverse-ratio indicates more time is spent in inhalation rather than exhalation.)

Ref: Tobin MJ. *Principles and Practice of Mechanical Ventilation*, 3rd ed. New York, NY, McGraw Hill; 2013.

37. Which ventilator mode is flow-controlled and time-cycled?

(C) **volume-control**

Volume control is flow-controlled, and either time-cycled or volume-cycled; pressure control is pressure-controlled, pressure-targeted, time-cycled ventilation; pressure support is pressure-targeted, flow-cycled ventilation. Note, because volume and flow are inverse functions of each other, volume-control ventilation controls both volume and flow.

Ref: Tobin MJ. *Principles and Practice of Mechanical Ventilation*, 3rd ed. New York, NY: McGraw Hill; 2013.

38. With respect to ventilator phase variables, the inspiratory phase ends when either a preset pressure, volume, flow, or time is reached. This preset variable that ends inspiration is referred to as the:

(A) trigger variable
(B) target variable
(C) **cycle variable**
(D) baseline variable
(E) limit variable

Phases of the respiratory cycle may be regulated by a ventilator via a variety of different variables (known as "phase variables"):

- the trigger variable equals the initiation, or "trigger," of inspiration. A preset change in pressure, volume, flow, or time may be the trigger variable (e.g., a drop in pressure triggers ventilation in a pressure triggered ventilator).
- the target variable equals the preset upper bounds, or "target," of flow, volume, or pressure to reach and maintain during inspiration. Note, time cannot be a target variable (cannot be "maintained").
- the cycle variable equals the preset pressure, volume, flow, or time that ends inspiration (e.g., a volume-

cycled ventilator will deliver flow until the preset volume is achieved).
- the baseline variable is controlled during expiration. All modern ventilators use pressure as the baseline variable.

Note, a limit variable is commonly confused with a target variable. Nomenclature standards define a limit variable only in reference to ventilator alarm limits.

Ref: Tobin MJ. *Principles and Practice of Mechanical Ventilation*, 3rd ed. New York, NY: McGraw Hill; 2013.

39. Which of the following will cause an increase in peak inspiratory pressure (PIP) without a change in plateau pressure?

(A) increased tidal volume
(B) pulmonary edema
(C) ascites
(D) endobronchial intubation
(E) **bronchospasm**

An increase in peak inspiratory pressure (PIP) and unchanged plateau pressure occurs with an increase in inspiratory gas flow rate or an increase in airway resistance (bronchospasm, secretions, foreign body aspiration, airway compression).

An increase in both PIP and plateau pressure occurs when either tidal volume is increased or pulmonary compliance decreases (pulmonary edema, ascites, endobronchial intubation).

Ref: Butterworth JF IV, Mackey DC, Wasnick JD. *Morgan & Mikhail's Clinical Anesthesiology*, 5th ed. New York, NY: McGraw Hill; 2013:77–79.

40. Which of the following conditions will alter a static pressure-volume (PV) curve?

(A) pulmonary embolus
(B) mucous plugging
(C) bronchospasm
(D) endotracheal cuff herniation
(E) **tension pneumothorax**

A tension pneumothorax (or atelectasis, pneumonia, or pulmonary edema) will reduce lung compliance ($\Delta V/\Delta P$) and alter both static and dynamic pressure-volume (PV) curves. Dynamic refers to measurements during gas flow as opposed to a static curve which is measured during the absence of flow.

Mucous plugging, bronchospasm, and endotracheal cuff herniation are examples of conditions that increase airway resistance—this will affect a dynamic PV curve but not a static PV curve.

Refs: Butterworth JF IV, Mackey DC, Wasnick JD. *Morgan & Mikhail's Clinical Anesthesiology*, 5th ed. New York, NY: McGraw Hill; 2013.
Miller RD. *Miller's Anesthesia*, 8th ed. Philadelphia, PA: Elsevier; 2015.

41. The diagram in Figure 21-12 shows an inspiratory and expiratory pressure-volume (PV) curve for an intubated and ventilated patient with an acute lung injury (ALI). In order to maintain alveolar recruitment and minimize the risk of alveolar overdistention, at what point should positive end-expiratory pressure (PEEP) be set?

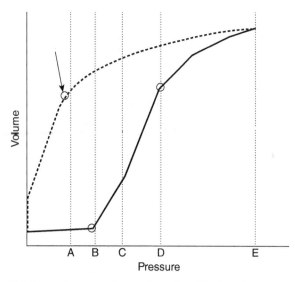

FIG. 21-12. Pressure volume relationship of the lung showing inflation (solid line) and deflation (dashed line) limbs.

(A) A
(B) B
(C) C
(D) D
(E) E

Point A is slightly above the deflection point. The deflection point represents the "critical closing pressure" at which recruited alveoli begin to close during expiration. Point B, the lower inflection point, is due to the recruitment of alveoli during inspiration; the corresponding pressure is termed the "opening pressure." Point D, the upper inflection point, is the point where alveoli start to become overdistended during inspiration. The inspiratory and expiratory limbs of the PV curve display hysteresis because the compliance of the lung changes during inspiration, and higher volumes are observed at lower pressure during deflation. Evidence suggests that optimal PEEP should be set slightly above Point A, the deflection point.

Ref: Miller RD. *Miller's Anesthesia*, 8th ed. Philadelphia, PA: Elsevier; 2015.

42. Which of the following methods is the best to detect postoperative apnea in a nonintubated patient?

(A) **pulse oximeter**
(B) nasal-oral airflow system
(C) electrocardiographic transthoracic impedance system
(D) respiratory inductive plethysmography
(E) photoplethysmography

A pulse oximeter (and end-tidal CO_2 monitor) rapidly detects changes in gas exchange. Pulse oximetry is reported as superior to methods such as airflow monitors or respiratory movement monitors. Respiratory movement can be detected with changes in transthoracic impedance as measured by electrocardiographic systems or respiratory inductive plethysmography. Photoplethysmography measures changes in venous blood flow that occur during respiration. Any of the respiratory movement monitoring systems for apnea detection is limited due to the fact that a patient may have airway obstruction but intact respiratory effort.

Ref: Miller RD. *Miller's Anesthesia*, 8th ed. Philadelphia, PA: Elsevier; 2015.

CHAPTER 22

Monitoring Methods, Instrumentation, and Alarms

1. A surgical procedure requires the strict avoidance of any sudden patient movement. Anesthetic includes large doses of a nondepolarizing neuromuscular blocking drug. Which method of electrical nerve stimulation is the best to monitor this degree of neuromuscular blockade?

   (A) double burst stimulation
   (B) train-of-four stimulation
   (C) single-twitch stimulation
   (D) tetanic stimulation
   (E) post-tetanic count stimulation

2. The evoked response of peripheral nerve stimulation can be recorded by a variety of methods. Which method records compound action potentials produced by stimulation of a peripheral nerve?

   (A) mechanomyography (MMG)
   (B) electromyography (EMG)
   (C) acceleromyography (AMG)
   (D) piezoelectric neuromuscular monitor (P_zEMG)
   (E) phonomyography (PMG)

3. Adequate neuromuscular recovery, as assessed by EMG or MMG TOF (train-of-four), requires a TOF ratio of at least:

   (A) 0.5
   (B) 0.6
   (C) 0.7
   (D) 0.8
   (E) 0.9

4. A patient in the ICU is intubated and requiring a ventilator for respiratory support. Which of the following factors is predictive of successful weaning and extubation?

   (A) frequency-to-tidal volume ratio (f/V_T) of 120
   (B) PaO_2 of 50
   (C) minute ventilation of 14 L/min
   (D) maximum inspiratory pressure (MIP) of -30 cm H_2O
   (E) vital capacity (VC) of 5 mL/kg

5. A respirometer (or spirometer) measures the exhaled tidal volume in the anesthetic breathing circuit. A Wright respirometer incorporates the following design:

   (A) a rotating vane of low mass in the expiratory limb
   (B) a platinum wire that is electrically heated at a constant temperature
   (C) a change in internal diameter to generate a drop in pressure
   (D) a Pitot tube at the Y-connection
   (E) piezoelectric crystals that generate ultrasonic beams

6. Which spirometry measurement most reflects the caliber of the large airways?

   (A) forced vital capacity (FVC)
   (B) forced expiratory volume in 1 second (FEV_1)
   (C) peak expiratory flow (PEF)
   (D) forced expiratory flow 25%–75% ($FEF_{25\%-75\%}$)
   (E) DLCO

7. Figure 22-1 shows a capnogram. Which labeled point is the best reflection of alveolar CO_2 partial pressure?

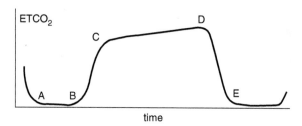

FIG. 22-1. Capnogram.

(A) A
(B) B
(C) C
(D) D
(E) E

8. Which method of measuring inspired oxygen concentration utilizes oxygen's structure of having unpaired electrons in outer shell orbits?

(A) paramagnetic oxygen analysis
(B) galvanic cell analysis
(C) polarographic oxygen analysis
(D) infrared absorption spectrophotometry
(E) mass spectrometry

9. A rise in exhaled nitrogen (N_2) can be associated with:

(A) circuit disconnection
(B) vaporizer malfunction
(C) hypoventilation
(D) endotracheal cuff leak
(E) airway obstruction

10. For most surgical patients, the most likely cause of perioperative heat loss is due to:

(A) radiation
(B) conduction
(C) convection
(D) evaporation

11. Core temperature is best measured at which of the following sites?

(A) oral
(B) axillary
(C) rectal
(D) tympanic
(E) bladder

12. In order to measure a temperature increase accurately, which of the following devices relies on using a semiconductor to measure a decrease in resistance?

(A) resistance thermometer
(B) thermistor
(C) thermocouple
(D) infrared tympanic thermometer
(E) mercury-in-glass thermometer

13. Which noninvasive method of determining oxygen saturation (SO_2) can accurately measure methemoglobin (MetHb) concentrations?

(A) co-oximetry
(B) pulse co-oximetry
(C) pulse oximetry
(D) transcutaneous oximetry
(E) reflectance pulse oximetry

14. What is the effect of significant carboxyhemoglobin (COHb) concentrations on measured pulse oximetry (SpO_2) values?

(A) SpO_2 is not significantly effected.
(B) SpO_2 remains at 85% over a wide range of COHb concentrations.
(C) SpO_2 is transiently reduced.
(D) SpO_2 is significantly reduced.
(E) SpO_2 is falsely elevated.

15. Noninvasive blood pressure monitoring equipment typically used in the operating room uses which of the following measures to calculate systolic blood pressure?

(A) presence of 1st Korotkoff sound
(B) determination of dicrotic notch
(C) maximal rate of decrease of oscillation
(D) maximal rate of increase of oscillation
(E) Doppler measurement of sound waves

16. In preoperative anesthesia clinic, a medical student performs cardiac auscultation on a patient and reports the following findings: expiration—normal S_1, narrowly split A_2P_2; inspiration—normal S_1, increase in A_2P_2 interval. This is indicative of which of the following conditions?

    (A) normal finding
    (B) atrial septal defect
    (C) right bundle branch block
    (D) aortic stenosis
    (E) pulmonary hypertension

17. An arterial blood sample is taken from a patient who is 35°C and sent for blood gas analysis. As the sample is heated and analyzed at 37°C, which of the following changes will occur?

    (A) pH will increase
    (B) gas solubility will increase
    (C) hemoglobin affinity for O_2 will increase
    (D) hemoglobin affinity for CO_2 will increase
    (E) measured PO_2 will be higher than at 35°C

18. A blood gas analyzer uses a Stow-Severinghaus electrode to measure:

    (A) pH
    (B) PO_2
    (C) PCO_2
    (D) sodium (Na^+)
    (E) potassium (K^+)

19. An arterial blood gas sample is left on the anesthesia workstation for 30 minutes before being sent for analysis. Artifactual changes in the arterial blood gas values may include:

    (A) increased PCO_2
    (B) no change in PCO_2
    (C) increased PO_2
    (D) decreased PO_2 if there is an air bubble in the sample
    (E) increased pH

20. In the operating room, the most common method to monitor carbon dioxide (CO_2), nitrous oxide (N_2O), and volatile anesthetic gas concentrations is with:

    (A) Raman scatter analysis
    (B) mass spectrometry
    (C) infrared absorption spectrophotometry
    (D) paramagnetic analysis
    (E) polarographic electrodes

21. In order to measure the concentrations of exhaled volatile anesthetics, mass spectrometry relies on the concentration of gas being related to the:

    (A) intensity of transmitted light
    (B) amount of current generated
    (C) change in resonant frequency
    (D) movement of an ionized sample
    (E) amount of emitted photons

22. For an invasive measurement of arterial blood pressure (arterial line), the natural frequency (F_n) of the system should be optimized by:

    (A) adding lengths of pressure tubing as required
    (B) limiting the number of stopcocks
    (C) adding an air bubble as required
    (D) decreasing the stiffness of the pressure tubing as required
    (E) "zeroing" at the level of the right atrium

23. How can an elevated damping coefficient (ζ) for an arterial blood pressure waveform alter blood pressure measurements?

    (A) Diastolic blood pressure is falsely decreased.
    (B) Systolic blood pressure is falsely decreased.
    (C) Systolic blood pressure if falsely increased.
    (D) Mean arterial pressure is falsely decreased.
    (E) Mean arterial pressure is falsely increased.

24. Auscultation of Korotkoff sounds allows for indirect measurement of arterial blood pressure. Which phase corresponds to systolic blood pressure?

    (A) phase I
    (B) phase II
    (C) phase III
    (D) phase IV
    (E) phase V

25. Most automatic noninvasive blood pressure (NIBP) monitors use which of the following methods to determine blood pressure?

    (A) Doppler
    (B) motion of the arterial wall
    (C) photo-oscillometry
    (D) oscillometry
    (E) Riva-Rocci method

26. In a cell salvage machine for autotransfusion, which of the following methods is used to separate red blood cells from waste?

    (A) large bore, dual lumen, low pressure suction
    (B) citrate-based anticoagulant
    (C) 40–150 μm filters
    (D) centrifuge
    (E) photo-optical density filter

27. Which of the following methods for blood warming is useful for large-volume transfusion of red blood cells (>100 mL/min)?

    (A) countercurrent metal warming
    (B) convection air warming
    (C) magnetic induction
    (D) prewarming in a convection cabinet
    (E) dry heat warming plates

28. Which of the following strategies to maintain normothermia in an operating room surgical patient would be most successful?

    (A) increase room temperature to 21°C
    (B) warm cotton blanket
    (C) space blanket
    (D) circulating-water mattress
    (E) forced-air blanket

29. In the United States, what color is an E-cylinder of oxygen?

    (A) yellow
    (B) blue
    (C) green
    (D) black
    (E) black and white

30. Which method is used to connect the pipeline medical gas supply to an anesthesia machine?

    (A) quick-couplers
    (B) pin index safety system
    (C) diameter index safety system
    (D) yoke inlet assembly
    (E) pipeline check valve

31. During surgery, the line isolation monitor (LIM) begins to alarm, indicating that leakage current exceeds 5 mA. A piece of equipment identified as faulty is considered life supporting. What should happen next?

    (A) continue surgery; connect the faulty equipment to a ground-fault circuit interrupter (GFCI)
    (B) continue surgery; do not connect any additional electronic equipment
    (C) continue surgery; do not use the electrosurgical unit (ESU)
    (D) stop surgery; patient is at imminent risk of macroshock
    (E) stop surgery; patient is at imminent risk of microshock

32. Of all the methods employed to prevent the delivery of a hypoxic mixture, which safety feature of the anesthesia workstation is the most fail-safe?

    (A) low oxygen pressure alarm
    (B) vaporizer interlock device
    (C) oxygen flush mechanism
    (D) oxygen concentration monitor
    (E) oxygen/nitrous oxide ratio controller

33. What is the NIOSH-recommended limit for operating room waste gas concentrations when both nitrous oxide and a halogenated agent are used?

    (A) time-weighted average of 25 ppm for nitrous oxide; 0.5 ppm for halogenated agent
    (B) time-weighted average of 25 ppm for nitrous oxide; 2 ppm for halogenated agent
    (C) time-weighted average of 50 ppm for nitrous oxide; 0.5 ppm for halogenated agent
    (D) time-weighted average of 50 ppm for nitrous oxide; 2 ppm for halogenated agent
    (E) time-weighted average of 2 ppm for nitrous oxide; 0.5 ppm for halogenated agent

Answers and Explanations: Monitoring Methods, Instrumentation, and Alarms

1. A surgical procedure requires the strict avoidance of any sudden patient movement. Anesthetic includes large doses of a nondepolarizing neuromuscular blocking drug. Which method of electrical nerve stimulation is the best to monitor this degree of neuromuscular blockade?

   (A) double burst stimulation
   (B) train-of-four stimulation
   (C) single-twitch stimulation
   (D) tetanic stimulation
   (E) post-tetanic count stimulation

   Post-tetanic count (PTC) can be used to assess neuromuscular blockade when large doses of nondepolarizing neuromuscular blocking drugs have been used and there is no reaction to single-twitch or train-of-four stimulation (TOF). PTC applies tetanic stimulation (50-Hz for 5 seconds) then 3 seconds later single-twitch stimulation at 1 Hz.

   Double burst stimulation is two short bursts of 50-Hz stimulation 750 msec apart. It correlates to TOF stimulation.

   TOF stimulation applies four supramaxial stimuli every 0.5 second (2 Hz). Each stimulus in the train causes "fade." Dividing the fourth response by the first response allows for calculation of TOF ratio.

   Single-twitch stimulation applies a single supramaximal stimulus over a set frequency. This is sometimes used during induction.

   Tetanic stimulation is a rapid delivery of stimuli (50-Hz for 5 seconds) that causes a sustained muscle contraction.

   Ref: Miller RD. *Miller's Anesthesia*, 8th ed. Philadelphia, PA: Elsevier; 2015.

2. The evoked response of peripheral nerve stimulation can be recorded by a variety of methods. Which method records compound action potentials produced by stimulation of a peripheral nerve?

   (A) mechanomyography (MMG)
   (B) electromyography (EMG)
   (C) acceleromyography (AMG)
   (D) piezoelectric neuromuscular monitor (P_zEMG)
   (E) phonomyography (PMG)

   Electromyography (EMG) records compound action potentials produced by stimulation of a peripheral nerve.

   Mechanomyography (MMG) records the force of muscle contraction with a force-displacement transducer. It typically requires careful positioning of the studied muscle.

   Acceleromyography (AMG) measures the acceleration of the thumb after ulnar nerve stimulation.

   Piezoelectric neuromuscular monitors (P_zEMG) record the voltage generated in a piezoelectric film attached to the thumb after ulnar nerve stimulation.

   Phonomyography (PMG) records low-frequency sounds generated by skeletal muscles during contraction.

   Ref: Miller RD. *Miller's Anesthesia*, 8th ed. Philadelphia, PA: Elsevier; 2015.

3. Adequate neuromuscular recovery, as assessed by EMG or MMG TOF (train of four), requires a TOF ratio of at least:

   (A) 0.5
   (B) 0.6
   (C) 0.7
   (D) 0.8
   (E) 0.9

Adequate recovery of neuromuscular function, as assessed by EMG or MMG, requires a TOF ratio of 0.9 or greater. When the TOF is 0.4 or less, patients usually cannot lift their arms or head. When TOF is 0.6, vital capacity is reduced, but most patients can lift their heads for 3 seconds. When the TOF is 0.8, vital capacity is normal, but patients may still have diplopia.

Ref: Miller RD. *Miller's Anesthesia*, 8th ed. Philadelphia, PA: Elsevier; 2015.

4. A patient in the ICU is intubated and requiring a ventilator for respiratory support. Which of the following factors is predictive of successful weaning and extubation?

   (A) frequency-to-tidal volume ratio (f/V_T) of 120

   (B) PaO_2 of 50

   (C) minute ventilation of 14 L/min

   (D) **maximum inspiratory pressure (MIP) of –30 cm H_2O**

   (E) vital capacity (VC) of 5 mL/kg

A maximum inspiratory pressure (MIP) of more than –30 cm H_2O is predictive of successful weaning.

Rapid, shallow breathing is not predictive of successful extubation. A frequency-to-tidal volume ratio (f/V_T) < 100 is considered the threshold for successful weaning.

Weaning attempts are not recommended for hypoxic patients (PaO_2 < 55–60).

A vital capacity (VC) of greater than 10–15 mL/kg is suggested to predict successful weaning.

Ref: Tobin MJ. *Principles and practice of mechanical ventilation*, 3rd ed. New York, NY: McGraw Hill; 2013.

5. A respirometer (or spirometer) measures the exhaled tidal volume in the anesthetic breathing circuit. A Wright respirometer incorporates the following design:

   (A) **a rotating vane of low mass in the expiratory limb**

   (B) a platinum wire that is electrically heated at a constant temperature

   (C) a change in internal diameter to generate a drop in pressure

   (D) a Pitot tube at the Y-connection

   (E) piezoelectric crystals that generate ultrasonic beams

A Wright respirometer uses a rotating vane of low mass in the expiratory limb.

A hot-wire anemometer uses a platinum wire that is heated to a constant temperature.

Variable-orifice flowmeters use a change in internal diameter to generate a drop in pressure.

A type of fixed-orifice flowmeter uses a Pitot tube at the Y-connection.

Ultrasonic flow sensors use piezoelectric crystals that generate ultrasonic beams.

Ref: Butterworth JF IV, Mackey DC, Wasnick JD. *Morgan & Mikhail's Clinical Anesthesiology*, 5th ed. New York, NY: McGraw Hill; 2013.

6. Which spirometry measurement most reflects the caliber of the large airways?

   (A) forced vital capacity (FVC)

   (B) forced expiratory volume in 1 second (FEV_1)

   (C) **peak expiratory flow (PEF)**

   (D) forced expiratory flow 25%–75% ($FEF_{25\%–75\%}$)

   (E) DLCO

PEF is the maximum flow achieved during forced exhalation, and it reflects the caliber of the large airways.

FVC is the maximal volume of air forcefully exhaled after a maximal inspiration.

FEV_1 is the amount of air exhaled during the first second of the FVC.

$FEF_{25\%–75\%}$ is the mean forced expiratory flow between 25% and 75% of the FVC. A reduction in $FEF_{25\%–75\%}$ is suggestive of small airway disease.

D_{LCO} is the diffusing capacity for carbon monoxide and is a measure of gas transfer in the lungs.

Ref: Levitzky MG. *Pulmonary Physiology*, 8th ed. New York, NY: McGraw Hill; 2013.

7. Figure 22-1 shows a capnogram. Which labeled point is the best reflection of alveolar CO_2 partial pressure?

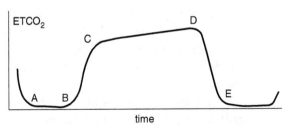

FIG. 22-1. Capnogram.

(A) A

(B) B

(C) C

(D) D

(E) E

Point D is the end-tidal CO_2 ($ETCO_2$), which best reflects $PaCO_2$.

A-B is phase I of expiration and reflects anatomic dead space.

B-C is phase II of expiration and reflects a mixture of both dead space and alveolar gas.

C-D is phase III of expiration (alveolar gas plateau) and reflects alveolar gas.

D-E is due to inspiration.

Ref: Butterworth JF IV, Mackey DC, Wasnick JD. *Morgan & Mikhail's Clinical Anesthesiology*, 5th ed. New York, NY: McGraw Hill; 2013.

8. Which method of measuring inspired oxygen concentration utilizes oxygen's structure of having unpaired electrons in outer shell orbits?

(A) paramagnetic oxygen analysis

(B) galvanic cell analysis

(C) polarographic oxygen analysis

(D) infrared absorption spectrophotometry

(E) mass spectrometry

Oxygen is paramagnetic, meaning it has unpaired electrons in outer shell orbits. Paramagnetic oxygen analysis utilizes this to correlate oxygen's behavior in a magnetic field to oxygen concentration.

Galvanic cell analysis measures current as oxygen diffuses through a membrane and is reduced at the anode.

Polarographic oxygen analysis measures current between an anode and cathode of a polarographic electrode. A polarographic electrode requires a small voltage to be applied to the two electrodes.

Infrared absorption spectrophotometry is used for analyzing anesthetic gases and relies on absorption of infrared light passing through gas. Oxygen does not absorb infrared light and requires other monitoring methods.

Mass spectrometry creates ion fragments that are magnetically separated based on mass and charge.

Ref: Butterworth JF IV, Mackey DC, Wasnick JD. *Morgan & Mikhail's Clinical Anesthesiology*, 5th ed. New York, NY: McGraw Hill; 2013.

9. A rise in exhaled nitrogen (N_2) can be associated with:

(A) circuit disconnection

(B) vaporizer malfunction

(C) hypoventilation

(D) endotracheal cuff leak

(E) airway obstruction

Gas analysis can detect many critical events:

- Endotracheal cuff leak is detected by a rise in N_2 (or decrease in CO_2).
- Circuit disconnection is detected by a sudden drop in CO_2, O_2, or anesthetic agent.
- Vaporizer malfunction is detected by a change in anesthetic agent.
- Hypoventilation is detected by a change in CO_2.
- Airway obstruction is detected by a change in CO_2.

Ref: Barash PG. *Clinical Anesthesia*, 7th ed. Philadelphia, PA: Lippincott Williams & Wilkins; 2013.

10. For most surgical patients, the most likely cause of perioperative heat loss is due to:

(A) radiation

(B) conduction

(C) convection

(D) evaporation

Radiant heat transfer means that objects of higher temperature will radiate heat and objects of lower temperature will absorb heat. Radiation is the most significant cause of heat loss in most surgical patients.

Conductive heat transfer occurs when two surfaces with a temperature difference are in close contact. This usually accounts for minimal heat loss in the operating room.

Convective heat transfer occurs when air currents act to transfer heat from the patient to the environment. This is usually the second-most significant cause of heat loss in most surgical patients.

Evaporative heat transfer from sweating (or surgical wounds) is significant for premature infants but usually not for adults.

Ref: Miller RD. *Miller's Anesthesia*, 8th ed. Philadelphia, PA: Elsevier; 2015.

11. Core temperature is best measured at which of the following sites?

   (A) oral

   (B) axillary

   (C) rectal

   (D) **tympanic**

   (E) bladder

Core temperature can be measured with tympanic membrane, pulmonary artery, distal esophageal, or nasopharyngeal temperatures.

Core temperature can be *estimated* with oral, axillary, rectal, or bladder temperatures (note that bladder temperature is sensitive to urine flow).

Ref: Miller RD. *Miller's Anesthesia*, 8th ed. Philadelphia, PA: Elsevier; 2015.

12. In order to measure a temperature increase accurately, which of the following devices relies on using a semiconductor to measure a decrease in resistance?

   (A) resistance thermometer

   (B) **thermistor**

   (C) thermocouple

   (D) infrared tympanic thermometer

   (E) mercury-in-glass thermometer

Resistance thermometers, thermistors, and thermocouples are examples of electrical techniques for measuring temperature. A thermistor is a semiconductor and its resistance decreases when it is heated. They can be made very small and are commonly used in anesthesia (pulmonary artery catheters and esophageal temperature probes).

A resistance thermometer is based on the principle that a metal's resistance increases with temperature.

A thermocouple is a device made of two different metals. A change in temperature results in a change in voltage or current.

An infrared tympanic thermometer measures radiant infrared emissions from the tympanic membrane via a thermopile (collection of thermocouples).

Mercury thermometers are based on the expansion of mercury as its temperature increases.

Refs: Miller RD. *Miller's Anesthesia*, 8th ed. Philadelphia, PA: Elsevier; 2015.

Sullivan G, Campbell E. Heat and temperature: continuing education in anaesthesia. *Crit Care Pain* 2008;8(3):104–107.

13. Which noninvasive method of determining oxygen saturation (SO_2) can accurately measure methemoglobin (MetHb) concentrations?

   (A) co-oximetry

   (B) **pulse co-oximetry**

   (C) pulse oximetry

   (D) transcutaneous oximetry

   (E) reflectance pulse oximetry

Pulse co-oximetry is a noninvasive method that uses multiple wavelengths of light to detect oxygen saturation and other hemoglobin species including MetHb and carboxyhemoglobin.

A co-oximeter can accurately measure MetHb concentrations but it is invasive as it requires a blood sample.

Pulse oximetry is noninvasive and analyzes pulsatile blood flow to measure arterial saturation (SpO_2). Two light-emitting diodes are used to discriminate between oxygenated and deoxygenated blood. A pulse co-oximeter cannot accurately measure methemoglobin (MetHb). SpO_2 approaches 85% at high levels of MetHb.

Transcutaneous oximetry uses the same principles as pulse oximetry but does not discriminate between arterial and venous blood. It cannot measure MetHb.

Reflectance pulse oximetry typically uses probes on the forehead to measure reflected light and measure SpO_2. It does not measure MetHb.

Ref: Barash PG. *Clinical Anesthesia*, 7th ed. Philadelphia, PA: Lippincott Williams & Wilkins; 2013.

14. What is the effect of significant carboxyhemoglobin (COHb) concentrations on measured pulse oximetry (SpO_2) values?

   (A) SpO_2 is not significantly effected.

   (B) SpO_2 remains at 85% over a wide range of COHb concentrations.

   (C) SpO_2 is transiently reduced.

   (D) SpO_2 is significantly reduced.

   (E) **SpO_2 is falsely elevated.**

A traditional two-wavelength pulse oximeter cannot distinguish COHb from oxyhemoglobin. Therefore, SpO_2 will be falsely elevated.

SpO_2 remains at 85% over a wide range of *methemoglobin* concentrations.

SpO_2 is transiently reduced when dyes such as indigo carmine are used.

Ref: Butterworth JF IV, Mackey DC, Wasnick JD. *Morgan & Mikhail's Clinical Anesthesiology*, 5th ed. New York, NY: McGraw Hill; 2013.

15. Noninvasive blood pressure monitoring equipment typically used in the operating room uses which of the following measures to calculate systolic blood pressure?

    (A) presence of 1st Korotkoff sound
    (B) determination of dicrotic notch
    (C) maximal rate of decrease of oscillation
    (D) maximal rate of increase of oscillation
    (E) Doppler measurement of sound waves

Blood pressure may be assessed via a variety of different noninvasive blood pressure (NIBP) measurement techniques:

- palpation: cuff is inflated above systolic blood pressure then deflated, systolic blood pressure is estimated when palpated pulse appears (this often underestimates systolic blood pressure).
- Doppler: cuff is inflated above systolic blood pressure then deflated, systolic blood pressure is estimated with detection of pulse by Doppler flow probe.
- auscultation: cuff is inflated above systolic blood pressure then deflated, systolic blood pressure is estimate with detection of the first Korotkoff sound (disappearance of Korotkoff sounds correlates with diastolic blood pressure).
- oscillometry: cuff is inflated above systolic blood pressure then deflated in a step-wise or continuous fashion. Systolic blood pressure correlates with the point of maximal rate of *increase* of oscillation (diastolic blood pressure correlates with the point of maximal rate of *decrease* of oscillation).

Typically, in the operating room, NIBP measurement relies on the oscillometric method (indeed, use of the term "NIBP" is often assumed to be referencing an oscillometric method).

The dicrotic notch may be noted on invasive blood pressure monitoring. It corresponds to the closure of the aortic valve, which causes a transient upstroke (dicrotic notch) in the descending portion of the arterial waveform.

Ref: Ward M, Langton JA. Blood pressure measurement: continuing education in anaesthesia. *Criti Care Pain* 2007;7(4):122–126.

16. In preoperative anesthesia clinic, a medical student performs cardiac auscultation on a patient and reports the following findings: expiration—normal S_1, narrowly split A_2P_2; inspiration—normal S_1, increase in A_2P_2 interval. This is indicative of which of the following conditions?

    (A) normal finding
    (B) atrial septal defect
    (C) right bundle branch block
    (D) aortic stenosis
    (E) pulmonary hypertension

S_1, the first heart sound, indicates closure of the mitral and tricuspid valves. S_2, the second heart sound, indicates closure of the aortic (A_2) and pulmonic (P_2) valves. Physiologic splitting of the A_2P_2 interval may occur in normal patients. Physiologic splitting is demonstrated when the A_2P_2 interval *increases with inspiration* and *decreases with expiration*.

Right bundle branch block causes a widely split A_2P_2 interval as pulmonic valve closure is delayed (this also occurs in severe mitral regurgitation as the aortic valve closes early). Pulmonary hypertension results in a narrowly split and fixed A_2P_2 interval, while an atrial septal defect results in a widely split and fixed A_2P_2 interval (fixed = no change during the respiratory cycle). Aortic stenosis (or other conditions that delay closure of the aortic valve such as left bundle branch block, hypertrophic obstructive cardiomyopathy, and myocardial ischemia) results in reversed (paradoxical) splitting. Reversed splitting means P_2 is the initial sound followed by A_2, and the interval widens on *expiration*.

Ref: Kasper D, Fauci A, Hauser S, et al. *Harrison's Principles of Internal Medicine*, 19th ed. New York, NY: McGraw Hill; 2015.

17. An arterial blood sample is taken from a patient who is 35°C and sent for blood gas analysis. As the sample is heated and analyzed at 37°C, which of the following changes will occur?

    (A) pH will increase
    (B) gas solubility will increase
    (C) hemoglobin affinity for O_2 will increase
    (D) hemoglobin affinity for CO_2 will increase
    (E) measured PO_2 will be higher than at 35°C

At 37°C, measured PO_2 (and PCO_2) are higher than at 35°C. Heating a blood sample causes a decrease in pH, gas solubility, and hemoglobin affinity for O_2 and CO_2. Modern blood gas analyzers correct pH, PO_2, and PCO_2 for temperature.

Ref: Miller RD. *Miller's Anesthesia*, 8th ed. Philadelphia, PA: Elsevier; 2015.

18. A blood gas analyzer uses a Stow-Severinghaus electrode to measure:

(A) pH

(B) PO_2

(C) PCO_2

(D) sodium (Na^+)

(E) potassium (K^+)

The Stow-Severinghaus electrode measures PCO_2. A Clark electrode measures PO_2. A pH-sensitive glass electrode measures pH. Other specific electrodes can measure electrolytes such as sodium and potassium.

Refs: Miller RD. *Miller's Anesthesia*, 8th ed. Philadelphia, PA: Elsevier; 2015.

Langton JA, Hutton A. Respiratory gas analysis: continuing education in anaesthesia. *Crit Care Pain* 2009;9(1): 19–23.

19. An arterial blood gas sample is left on the anesthesia workstation for 30 minutes before being sent for analysis. Artifactual changes in the arterial blood gas values may include:

(A) increased PCO_2

(B) no change in PCO_2

(C) increased PO_2

(D) decreased PO_2 if there is an air bubble in the sample

(E) increased pH

Storage longer than 20 minutes can cause increases in PCO_2 and decreases in PO_2 and pH due to cellular metabolism. An air bubble can erroneously elevate PO_2 with little effect on PCO_2 and pH.

Ref: Miller RD. *Miller's Anesthesia*, 8th ed. Philadelphia, PA: Elsevier; 2015.

20. In the operating room, the most common method to monitor carbon dioxide (CO_2), nitrous oxide (N_2O), and volatile anesthetic gas concentrations is with:

(A) Raman scatter analysis

(B) mass spectrometry

(C) infrared absorption spectrophotometry

(D) paramagnetic analysis

(E) polarographic electrodes

Infrared absorption spectrophotometry (IRAS) is the most common type of expired gas analyzer in anesthesia. It relies on differences in absorption of infrared light and can measure CO_2, N_2O, and volatile anesthetic gas concentrations.

Raman scatter analysis and mass spectrometry are not commonly used in the operating room. Both Raman scatter analysis and mass spectrometry can measure CO_2, N_2O, and volatile anesthetic gas concentrations. However, cost considerations have lead to IRAS supplanting both Raman scatter analysis and mass spectrometry in the operating room. Mass spectrometry creates ion fragments that are magnetically separated based on mass and charge. Raman scatter analysis uses a laser beam and detection of emitted photons that are proportional to the gas concentration.

Paramagnetic analyzers correlate oxygen's behavior in a magnetic field to measure *oxygen* concentration.

Polarographic analyzers measure the current between an anode and cathode of a polarographic electrode. They are used to measure *oxygen* concentration.

Refs: Butterworth JF IV, Mackey DC, Wasnick JD. *Morgan & Mikhail's Clinical Anesthesiology*, 5th ed. New York, NY: McGraw Hill; 2013.

Langton JA, Hutton A. Respiratory gas analysis: continuing education in anaesthesia. *Crit Care Pain* 2009; 9(1): 19–23.

21. In order to measure the concentrations of exhaled volatile anesthetics, mass spectrometry relies on the concentration of gas being related to the:

(A) intensity of transmitted light

(B) amount of current generated

(C) change in resonant frequency

(D) movement of an ionized sample

(E) amount of emitted photons

Mass spectrometry moves a gas sample through a near-vacuum. The sample then moves to a second chamber where it is ionized. The ions are accelerated through a magnetic field and separated according to their mass-charge ratio.

Infrared absorption spectrophotometry analyzes a gas sample based on the intensity of transmitted light.

Polarographic (Clark) electrodes use the amount of current generated to determine oxygen concentration.

Piezoelectric absorption uses two quartz crystals mounted between electrodes. As volatile anesthetics are absorbed, a change in resonant frequency occurs.

Raman scatter analysis uses a laser beam and detection of emitted photons that are proportional to the gas concentration.

Refs: Miller RD. *Miller's Anesthesia*, 8th ed. Philadelphia, PA: Elsevier; 2015.

Langton JA, Hutton A. Respiratory gas analysis: continuing education in anaesthesia. *Crit Care Pain* 2009; 9(1):19–23.

22. For an invasive measurement of arterial blood pressure (arterial line), the natural frequency (F_n) of the system should be optimized by:

(A) adding lengths of pressure tubing as required
(B) **limiting the number of stopcocks**
(C) adding an air bubble as required
(D) decreasing the stiffness of the pressure tubing as required
(E) "zeroing" at the level of the right atrium

Natural frequency (F_n) describes the likelihood of the measuring system to resonate. An optimal or high-fidelity arterial blood pressure monitoring system should have:

• limited number of stopcocks
• short length of stiff pressure tubing
• no air bubbles (air bubbles decrease the F_n of the system)

In the supine patient, arterial lines are usually zeroed at the level of the right atrium. This does not affect F_n.

Ref: Miller RD. *Miller's Anesthesia*, 8th ed. Philadelphia, PA: Elsevier; 2015.

23. How can an elevated damping coefficient (ζ) for an arterial blood pressure waveform alter blood pressure measurements?

(A) Diastolic blood pressure is falsely decreased.
(B) **Systolic blood pressure is falsely decreased.**
(C) Systolic blood pressure if falsely increased.
(D) Mean arterial pressure is falsely decreased.
(E) Mean arterial pressure is falsely increased.

The damping coefficient (ζ) describes the tendency of fluid in the measuring system to damp motion. An increased damping coefficient causes underestimation of systolic blood pressure (falsely decreased).

Overdamping also causes falsely narrowed pulse pressure and elevated diastolic blood pressure (mean pressure is relatively unchanged).

Ref: Longnecker DE, Brown DL, Newman MF, et al. *Anesthesiology*, 2nd ed. New York, NY: McGraw Hill; 2012.

24. Auscultation of Korotkoff sounds allows for indirect measurement of arterial blood pressure. Which phase corresponds to systolic blood pressure?

(A) **phase I**
(B) phase II
(C) phase III
(D) phase IV
(E) phase V

Phase I, when the first Korotkoff sound is audible, is accepted as the systolic blood pressure.

During phases II and III, the character of the sound changes. In phase IV, the sound becomes muffled. In phase V, the sound is absent.

Ref: Longnecker DE, Brown DL, Newman MF, et al. *Anesthesiology*, 2nd ed. New York, NY: McGraw Hill; 2012.

25. Most automatic noninvasive blood pressure (NIBP) monitors use which of the following methods to determine blood pressure?

(A) Doppler
(B) motion of the arterial wall

(C)   photo-oscillometry

(D)   **oscillometry**

(E)   Riva-Rocci method

Most NIPB monitors use oscillometry to determine blood pressure. Mean blood pressure corresponds to the point of peak oscillations. Systolic and diastolic blood pressure is then calculated.

Other methods of NIPB measurement include Doppler, motion of the arterial wall, and photo-oscillometric techniques.

The Riva-Rocci method estimates systolic blood pressure as the pressure when palpated radial pulse disappears with cuff inflation.

Ref: Longnecker DE, Brown DL, Newman MF, et al. *Anesthesiology*, 2nd ed. New York, NY: McGraw Hill; 2012.

26.   In a cell salvage machine for autotransfusion, which of the following methods is used to separate red blood cells from waste?

(A)   large bore, dual lumen, low pressure suction

(B)   citrate-based anticoagulant

(C)   40–150 μm filters

(D)   **centrifuge**

(E)   photo-optical density filter

Cell salvage machines use a centrifuge to separate red blood cells (RBCs) from plasma. The RBCs are more dense and separate against the outer wall of the centrifuge while plasma stays in the center where it moves to a waste bag.

Large bore, dual lumen, low pressure suction is used to collect blood from the operative field. Either heparin or citrate can be used as an anticoagulant; this does not aid in separation. Filters (40–150 μm) are used to separate debris and large clots. When the collected RBCs reach a certain density, as determined by photo-optics, washing is initiated.

Ref: Kuppurao L, Wee M. Perioperative cell salvage: continuing education in anaesthesia. *Crit Care Pain* 2010;10(4): 104–108.

27.   Which of the following methods for blood warming is useful for large-volume transfusion of red blood cells (>100 mL/min)?

(A)   countercurrent metal warming

(B)   convection air warming

(C)   **magnetic induction**

(D)   prewarming in a convection cabinet

(E)   dry heat warming plates

Two methods of blood warming that are compatible with high-flow (>100 mL/min) blood transfusion include countercurrent *water* baths (Level 1 H-1200) and magnetic induction (FMS 2000, Belmont). Both also have safety features to prevent air emboli. Countercurrent metal warming, convection air warming, and dry heat warming plates are used in a variety of warming devices that are compatible with moderate transfusion requirements (<100 mL/min). Prewarming in a convection cabinet is useful for warming crystalloids. This device should not be used for blood products.

Ref: Smith CE, Wagner K. Principles of fluid and blood warming in trauma. *Int Trauma Care* 2008;18(1): 71–79.

28.   Which of the following strategies to maintain normothermia in an operating room surgical patient would be most successful?

(A)   increase room temperature to 21°C

(B)   warm cotton blanket

(C)   space blanket

(D)   circulating-water mattress

(E)   **forced-air blanket**

Warm- forced-air blankets maintain normothermia, as they reduce heat loss from the skin. Room temperature is an important factor for heat loss. However, room temperature usually must be >23°C to maintain normothermia. This is usually too warm for OR staff! Cotton blankets (warm or room temperature) or space blankets work by adding passive insulation to the skin. Passive insulation alone is usually insufficient to maintain normothermia. Warm circulating-water mattresses are not effective, as insignificant amounts of heat are lost from the back. Warm circulating-water garments placed *over* the patient are effective.

Ref: Miller RD. *Miller's Anesthesia*, 8th ed. Philadelphia, PA: Elsevier; 2015.

29. In the United States, what color is an E-cylinder of oxygen?

    (A) yellow
    (B) blue
    (C) **green**
    (D) black
    (E) black and white

    Medical gas cylinders are color-coded. In the United States:

    - oxygen = green
    - air = yellow
    - nitrous oxide = blue
    - nitrogen = black

      Internationally, color codes for medical gas cylinders differ from those in the United States:

    - oxygen = white
    - air = black and white
    - nitrous oxide = blue
    - nitrogen = black

    Ref: Butterworth JF IV, Mackey DC, Wasnick JD. *Morgan & Mikhail's Clinical Anesthesiology*, 5th ed. New York, NY: McGraw Hill; 2013.

30. Which method is used to connect the pipeline medical gas supply to an anesthesia machine?

    (A) quick-couplers
    (B) pin index safety system
    (C) **diameter index safety system**
    (D) yoke inlet assembly
    (E) pipeline check valve

    The diameter index safety system (DISS) ensures the central (pipeline) supply of medical gas for oxygen, air, and nitrous oxide is correctly attached to the anesthesia machine. The pin index safety system (PISS) ensures the gas cylinder (usually oxygen) is correctly attached to the anesthesia machine. Holes in the cylinder valve correspond to pins in the yoke of the anesthesia machine.

    Ref: Butterworth JF IV, Mackey DC, Wasnick JD. *Morgan & Mikhail's Clinical Anesthesiology*, 5th ed. New York, NY: McGraw Hill; 2013.

31. During surgery, the line isolation monitor (LIM) begins to alarm, indicating that leakage current exceeds 5 mA. A piece of equipment identified as faulty is considered life supporting. What should happen next?

    (A) continue surgery; connect the faulty equipment to a ground-fault circuit interrupter (GFCI)
    (B) **continue surgery; do not connect any additional electronic equipment**
    (C) continue surgery; do not use the electrosurgical unit (ESU)
    (D) stop surgery; patient is at imminent risk of macroshock
    (E) stop surgery; patient is at imminent risk of microshock

    A line isolation monitor (LIM) indicates when the power system is no longer isolated from ground. A second fault in the system is required for an electrical shock. If the LIM alarms, it could mean that a faulty piece of equipment is plugged into the isolated power system. The equipment should be identified and removed if possible. If the piece of equipment is deemed to be life supporting, surgery can continue but no other pieces of electronic equipment should be connected, as the power system is no longer isolated from ground.

    A ground-fault circuit interrupter (GFCI) prevents electrical shocks, but it would interrupt power delivery to the life-supporting piece of equipment, rendering it nonfunctional.

    Ref: Barash PG. *Clinical Anesthesia*, 7th ed. Philadelphia, PA: Lippincott Williams & Wilkins; 2013.

32. Of all the methods employed to prevent the delivery of a hypoxic mixture, which safety feature of the anesthesia workstation is the most fail-safe?

    (A) low oxygen pressure alarm
    (B) vaporizer interlock device
    (C) oxygen flush mechanism
    (D) **oxygen concentration monitor**
    (E) oxygen/nitrous oxide ratio controller

    The oxygen concentration monitor is in the inspiratory or expiratory limb of the breathing circuit. This will alarm if oxygen concentration falls below a critical level. It will detect a leak in the low-pressure circuit of the anesthesia machine. It directly measures oxygen concentration and does not rely on measuring gas pressure.

The low oxygen pressure alarm is activated if inlet gas pressure drops below a certain threshold. The oxygen/nitrous oxide ratio controller device is a proportioning system that reduces nitrous oxide gas flow as oxygen pressure decreases. Both of these can be defeated if the gas line is misconnected and the pressurizing gas contains inadequate oxygen.

The oxygen flush mechanism delivers oxygen to the common gas outlet and bypasses the flowmeters and vaporizers.

The vaporizer interlock device prevents the administration of more than one volatile anesthetic at a time.

Ref: Butterworth JF IV, Mackey DC, Wasnick JD. *Morgan & Mikhail's Clinical Anesthesiology*, 5th ed. New York, NY: McGraw Hill; 2013.

33. What is the NIOSH-recommended limit for operating room waste gas concentrations when both nitrous oxide and a halogenated agent are used?

(A) time-weighted average of 25 ppm for nitrous oxide; 0.5 ppm for halogenated agent

(B) time-weighted average of 25 ppm for nitrous oxide; 2 ppm for halogenated agent

(C) time-weighted average of 50 ppm for nitrous oxide; 0.5 ppm for halogenated agent

(D) time-weighted average of 50 ppm for nitrous oxide; 2 ppm for halogenated agent

(E) time-weighted average of 2 ppm for nitrous oxide; 0.5 ppm for halogenated agent

NIOSH-recommended limits for time-weighted average exposure to both nitrous oxide and halogenated agent are 25 ppm and 0.5 ppm, respectively. If halogenated agent is used alone, the recommended limit is 2 ppm. If nitrous oxide is used alone, the recommended limit is 25 ppm.

Ref: Miller RD. *Miller's Anesthesia*, 8th ed. Philadelphia, PA: Elsevier; 2015.

CHAPTER 23

Electrical Safety and Defibrillation

1. Preoperatively, a patient is wearing a metal umbilical (belly button) ring. The planned surgical procedure is on the left arm and it requires the use of an electrosurgical unit (ESU). The patient is informed of potential risks but refuses to remove the item. Of the following options, what is the most appropriate course of action?

   (A) no alteration is required as the line isolation monitor (LIM) will detect potential microshock

   (B) lift and tape the umbilical ring so the smallest possible area is in contact with the skin

   (C) tape the umbilical ring flat to the abdomen

   (D) place the dispersive electrode (grounding pad) on the opposite side of the surgical site

   (E) have the surgeon use a unipolar ESU rather than a bipolar ESU

2. An operating room is equipped with a line isolation monitor (LIM). What does activation of the LIM alarm mean?

   (A) The ground fault circuit interrupter (GFCI) is now active.

   (B) The patient is grounded.

   (C) The power supply is grounded.

   (D) A piece of electrical equipment is grounded.

   (E) There is significant static buildup on the operating room floor.

3. A patient is undergoing surgery with a general anesthetic, standard monitors, a central venous catheter, and the use of a unipolar electrosurgery unit (ESU). In order to minimize a patient's risk of microshock, which factor is the LEAST important?

   (A) ensure all electrical equipment has intact ground wires

   (B) wear gloves before handling the central venous catheter

   (C) avoid touching electrical devices and the central venous catheter at the same time

   (D) do not let nerve stimulator wires come in contact with central venous catheter

   (E) use a line isolation monitor (LIM) to ensure an ungrounded power source

4. Microshock, or direct current to the heart, can cause ventricular fibrillation at relatively low currents. What is the maximum recommended leakage current for catheters or electrodes contacting the heart?

   (A) 1 μA

   (B) 10 μA

   (C) 100 μA

   (D) 10 mA

   (E) 100 mA

5. A patient is having a superficial surgical procedure on the posterior aspect of the neck. Anesthetic technique includes local anesthesia with intravenous sedation. Oxygen is supplied to the patient via face mask at 5 L/min. Chlorhexidine digluconate is used to prepare the skin. After use of an electrosurgery unit (ESU), a fire starts in the drape material. The FIRST course of action should be to:

(A) remove the drapes and burning material
(B) extinguish the fire with saline
(C) extinguish the fire with a CO_2 fire extinguisher
(D) turn off the oxygen supply
(E) activate the fire alarm

6. A patient is in cardiac arrest with a rhythm of pulseless ventricular fibrillation (VF). A monophasic defibrillator is rapidly prepared for a one-shock protocol. According to the 2015 American Heart Association (AHA) guidelines for cardiopulmonary resuscitation (CPR), what is the correct energy to select?

(A) 100 J
(B) 150 J
(C) 200 J
(D) 300 J
(E) 360 J

7. Synchronized cardioversion is most effective treating which of the following cardiac rhythms?

(A) junctional tachycardia
(B) multifocal atrial tachycardia
(C) atrial flutter
(D) polymorphic ventricular tachycardia
(E) ventricular fibrillation

8. Depending on the type of device, external defibrillators may deliver energy via a variety of different waveforms. A general classification includes monophasic and biphasic waveforms. In comparison to monophasic waveform defibrillators, in which of the following ways are biphasic waveform defibrillators superior?

(A) Biphasic waveforms have a higher defibrillation threshold.
(B) Biphasic waveforms require more energy for successful defibrillation.
(C) Biphasic waveforms permit reduction in the size of the defibrillator.
(D) Biphasic waveforms are associated with a higher rate of return to spontaneous circulation.
(E) Biphasic waveforms increase the survival rate of cardiac arrest patients.

9. Only a fraction of the energy of a defibrillator reaches the heart due to transthoracic impedance. To increase the current that reaches the heart, which of the following techniques should be employed?

(A) use smaller electrode pads or paddles
(B) place electrode pads or paddles in the anterior-posterior position
(C) use pressure on the electrode pads or paddles
(D) avoid use of conductive material at skin-electrode interface
(E) deliver shock in the inspiratory phase of ventilation

10. Automated external defibrillators (AEDs) may perform which of the following functions?

(A) synchronized cardioversion for atrial fibrillation
(B) shock ventricular tachycardia with a pulse
(C) warn if AED poses a shock hazard to rescuer
(D) identify if patient has signs of circulation
(E) identify if transthoracic impedance is too low

Answers and Explanations:
Electrical Safety and Defibrillation

1. Preoperatively, a patient is wearing a metal umbilical (belly button) ring. The planned surgical procedure is on the left arm and it requires the use of an electrosurgical unit (ESU). The patient is informed of potential risks but refuses to remove the item. Of the following options, what is the most appropriate course of action?

   (A) no alteration is required as the line isolation monitor (LIM) will detect potential microshock
   (B) lift and tape the umbilical ring so the smallest possible area is in contact with the skin
   (C) tape the umbilical ring flat to the abdomen
   (D) place the dispersive electrode (grounding pad) on the opposite side of the surgical site
   (E) have the surgeon use a unipolar ESU rather than a bipolar ESU

An electrosurgical unit (ESU) operates at high frequencies and applies high current via a small surface area electrode. Unipolar electrosurgery applies electric current through one electrode that is collected by a dispersive electrode (grounding pad) placed remote from the surgical site. Bipolar electrosurgery applies and collects electric current through a set of forceps; there is no need for a dispersive electrode (grounding pad).

Metal jewelry can potentially cause a burn when an ESU is used, as the metal jewelry can reconcentrate some of the electric current passing nearby. Remove all metal jewelry to eliminate this risk. If this is not possible, tape metal jewelry against the skin with as large a contact area as possible—in this case, tape the umbilical ring flat to the abdomen. Also, for unipolar electrosurgery, place the dispersive electrode (grounding pad)

so that jewelry is not in the path of the current traveling to the grounding pad; in this case it should be placed on the same side as the surgical site. A line isolation monitor will not protect a patient wearing metal jewelry from potential burn risks.

Ref: Miller RD. *Miller's Anesthesia*, 8th ed. Philadelphia, PA: Elsevier; 2015.

2. An operating room is equipped with a line isolation monitor (LIM). What does activation of the LIM alarm mean?

   (A) The ground fault circuit interrupter (GFCI) is now active.
   (B) The patient is grounded.
   (C) The power supply is grounded.
   (D) A piece of electrical equipment is grounded.
   (E) There is significant static buildup on the operating room floor.

Power supplied to most operating rooms is ungrounded. A line isolation monitor (LIM) alerts personnel if the power system becomes grounded.

A GFCI interrupts power to prevent electrical shock. It will turn off if it detects a power line connected to ground.

Historically, operating rooms were constructed with conductive flooring to reduce risk of fire due to buildup of static charge igniting flammable anesthetics.

Neither a GFCI nor static buildup is monitored by a LIM.

Ref: Miller RD. *Miller's Anesthesia*, 8th ed. Philadelphia, PA: Elsevier; 2015.

3. A patient is undergoing surgery with a general anesthetic, standard monitors, a central venous catheter, and the use of a unipolar electrosurgery unit (ESU). In order to minimize a patient's risk of microshock, which factor is the LEAST important?

(A) ensure all electrical equipment has intact ground wires

(B) wear gloves before handling the central venous catheter

(C) avoid touching electrical devices and the central venous catheter at the same time

(D) do not let nerve stimulator wires come in contact with central venous catheter

(E) **use a line isolation monitor (LIM) to ensure an ungrounded power source**

A line isolation monitor (LIM) does not protect from microshock. To minimize the risk of microshock, ensure all electrical equipment has intact ground wires, wear gloves before handling a central venous catheter, avoid touching electrical devices and a central venous catheter at the same time, and do not let nerve stimulator wires come in contact with the central venous catheter.

Ref: Barash PG. *Clinical Anesthesia*, 7th ed. Philadelphia, PA: Lippincott Williams & Wilkins; 2013.

4. Microshock, or direct current to the heart, can cause ventricular fibrillation at relatively low currents. What is the maximum recommended leakage current for catheters or electrodes contacting the heart?

(A) 1 μA

(B) **10 μA**

(C) 100 μA

(D) 10 mA

(E) 100 mA

10 μA is the maximum allowable leakage current for electrodes or catheters contacting the heart.

A microshock of 100 μA can cause ventricular fibrillation.

For macroshock current through the body:

• 1 mA is the threshold of perception

• 10–20 mA is the maximum "let-go" current before a person is unable to release contact

• 100–300 mA can cause ventricular fibrillation.

(A LIM will alarm at 5 mA.)

Ref: Miller RD. *Miller's Anesthesia*, 8th ed. Philadelphia, PA: Elsevier; 2015.

5. A patient is having a superficial surgical procedure on the posterior aspect of the neck. Anesthetic technique includes local anesthesia with intravenous sedation. Oxygen is supplied to the patient via face mask at 5 L/min. Chlorhexidine digluconate is used to prepare the skin. After use of an electrosurgery unit (ESU), a fire starts in the drape material. The FIRST course of action should be to:

(A) remove the drapes and burning material

(B) extinguish the fire with saline

(C) extinguish the fire with a CO_2 fire extinguisher

(D) **turn off the oxygen supply**

(E) activate the fire alarm

According to the "ASA Practice Advisory for the Prevention and Management of Operating Room Fires" (2008), for a fire on a patient:

• turn off gases;

• remove drapes and burning materials;

• extinguish flames with water, saline, or fire extinguisher;

• assess patient's status, devise care plan, assess for smoke inhalation.

Ref: Barash PG. *Clinical Anesthesia*, 7th ed. Philadelphia, PA: Lippincott Williams & Wilkins; 2013.

6. A patient is in cardiac arrest with a rhythm of pulseless ventricular fibrillation (VF). A monophasic defibrillator is rapidly prepared for a one-shock protocol. According to the 2015 American Heart Association (AHA) guidelines for cardiopulmonary resuscitation (CPR), what is the correct energy to select?

(A) 100 J

(B) 150 J

(C) 200 J

(D) 300 J

(E) **360 J**

Optimal energy level for defibrillation is unknown. Recommendations attempt to balance the risks of myocardial damage with the benefits of rapid termination of VF. The 2015 AHA guidelines for CPR recommend 360 J for the first shock (and subsequent shocks) with a monophasic defibrillator. Energy level for a biphasic defibrillator should follow the manufacturer's recommendation (120–200 J); if the recommended dose is unknown, the maximal dose may be considered. Currently all manufactured defibrillators use biphasic waveforms.

Ref: Link MS, Berkow LC, Kudenchuk PJ, et al. Part 7: Adult advanced cardiovascular life support: 2015 American Heart Association Guidelines Update for Cardiopulmonary Resuscitation and Emergency Cardiovascular Care. *Circulation* 2015;132:S444–S464

7. Synchronized cardioversion is most effective treating which of the following cardiac rhythms?

   (A) junctional tachycardia
   (B) multifocal atrial tachycardia
   (C) atrial flutter
   (D) polymorphic ventricular tachycardia
   (E) ventricular fibrillation

   Synchronized cardioversion is recommended to treat atrial flutter and other arrhythmias due to re-entry such as atrial fibrillation, atrioventricular nodal re-entrant tachycardia (AVNRT), and monomorphic ventricular tachycardia (VT) with a pulse. Cardioversion is ineffective for treatment of multifocal atrial tachycardia and junctional tachycardia. Polymorphic VT or pulseless monomorphic VT requires high-energy unsynchronized shocks. If synchronized cardioversion is attempted for ventricular fibrillation, a shock may not be delivered due to failure to detect a QRS wave.

   Ref: White RD, Cudnik MT, Berg MD, et al. Part 6: Electrical therapies: automated external defibrillators, defibrillation, cardioversion, and pacing: 2010 American Heart Association guidelines for cardiopulmonary resuscitation and emergency cardiovascular care. *Circulation* 2010;122: S706–S719.

8. Depending on the type of device, external defibrillators may deliver energy via a variety of different waveforms. A general classification includes monophasic and biphasic waveforms. In comparison to monophasic waveform defibrillators, in which of the following ways are biphasic waveform defibrillators superior?

   (A) Biphasic waveforms have a higher defibrillation threshold.
   (B) Biphasic waveforms require more energy for successful defibrillation.
   (C) Biphasic waveforms permit reduction in the size of the defibrillator.
   (D) Biphasic waveforms are associated with a higher rate of return to spontaneous circulation.
   (E) Biphasic waveforms increase the survival rate of cardiac arrest patients.

Biphasic waveform defibrillators are smaller in size and weigh less than monophasic waveform defibrillators. This has enabled the development of automated external defibrillators (AEDs) for placement in the community as part of lay rescuer AED programs. A monophasic waveform defibrillator delivers current in only one direction while a biphasic waveform defibrillator delivers current in one direction followed by a reversal of flow in the opposite direction. Biphasic waveform defibrillators require less energy for successful defibrillation, as the defibrillation threshold is lower as compared to that of monophasic waveform defibrillators. Biphasic defibrillators are superior to monophasic defibrillators as they are more likely to terminate either atrial or ventricular arrhythmias. However, there is no evidence from human studies to show that biphasic waveforms increase survival after cardiac arrest or are associated with a higher rate of return to spontaneous circulation.

Refs: White RD, Cudnik MT, Berg MD, et al. Part 6: Electrical therapies: automated external defibrillators, defibrillation, cardioversion, and pacing: 2010 American Heart Association guidelines for cardiopulmonary resuscitation and emergency cardiovascular care. *Circulation* 2010;122: S706–S719.

Link MS, Berkow LC, Kudenchuk PJ, et al. Part 7: Adult advanced cardiovascular life support: 2015 American Heart Association Guidelines Update for Cardiopulmonary Resuscitation and Emergency Cardiovascular Care. *Circulation* 2015;132:S444–S464

9. Only a fraction of the energy of a defibrillator reaches the heart due to transthoracic impedance. To increase the current that reaches the heart, which of the following techniques should be employed?

   (A) use smaller electrode pads or paddles
   (B) place electrode pads or paddles in the anterior-posterior position
   (C) use pressure on the electrode pads or paddles
   (D) avoid use of conductive material at skin-electrode interface
   (E) deliver shock in the inspiratory phase of ventilation

   The use of pressure on the electrode pads or paddles can reduce transthoracic impedance and increase the current delivered to the heart. Other methods of reducing transthoracic impedance include:

   • use of larger electrode pads or paddles
   • use of conductive gel pads or electrode paste
   • delivery of shock in the expiratory phase of ventilation

Transthoracic impedance is not significantly altered by position of the electrode pads or paddles (anterior-apex, apex-posterior, or anterior-posterior).

Ref: Delgado H, Toquero J, Mitroi C, Castro V, and Fernández Lozano I, Principles of external defibrillators, cardiac defibrillation, Dr. Damir Erkapic (Ed.), *InTech*, doi: 10.5772/52512. Available from: http://www.intechopen.com/books/cardiac-defibrillation/principles-of-external-defibrillators

10. Automated external defibrillators (AEDs) may perform which of the following functions?

(A) synchronized cardioversion for atrial fibrillation

(B) shock ventricular tachycardia with a pulse

(C) warn if AED poses a shock hazard to rescuer

(D) identify if patient has signs of circulation

(E) identify if transthoracic impedance is too low

Automated external defibrillators (AEDs) may shock ventricular tachycardia with a pulse. AEDs analyze the ECG signal and are designed to identify and shock ventricular fibrillation (VF). AEDs cannot identify if a patient has signs of circulation and may recommend to shock monomorphic or polymorphic ventricular tachycardia if the rate exceeds preset values. This reinforces that AEDs should only be used for unresponsive patients who are not breathing and without signs of circulation. AEDs cannot deliver synchronized shocks. AEDs cannot warn if the rescuer is at risk of shock, such as when the patient is in freestanding water. The rescuer must identify this situation and move the patient to a safe location. AEDs will warn if transthoracic impedance is too high with a "check electrodes" message. If necessary, remove hair or dry the chest to improve electrode pad contact.

Ref: The American Heart Association in collaboration with the International Liaison Committee on Resuscitation. Guidelines for cardiopulmonary resuscitation and emergency cardiovascular care. Part 4: the automated external defibrillator: key link in the chain of survival. *Circulation* 2000;102:I60–I76.

CHAPTER 24

Mathematics

1. Which of the following is an example of a logarithmic scale?

   (A) Likert scale
   (B) pH scale
   (C) visual analog scale
   (D) verbal rating scale
   (E) centigrade temperature scale

2. A resident puts a sandwich contaminated with *S. aureus* in her bag at 9 a.m. in the morning and keeps it at room temperature until noon. Assuming there were 200 colony-forming units (CFU)/mL at 9 a.m. and the bacteria divide every 20 minutes at room temperature, what will the population density of bacteria be when she takes a big juicy bite of it at noon?

   (A) 2^9 CFU/mL
   (B) 51,200 CFU/mL
   (C) 102,400 CFU/mL
   (D) 200^9 CFU/mL
   (E) too gross to bother answering

3. The following figure (Figure 24-1) plots cumulative incidence of recurrence versus time in groups that were at high or normal risk for the recurrent event. Which of the following can be correctly stated regarding this curve?

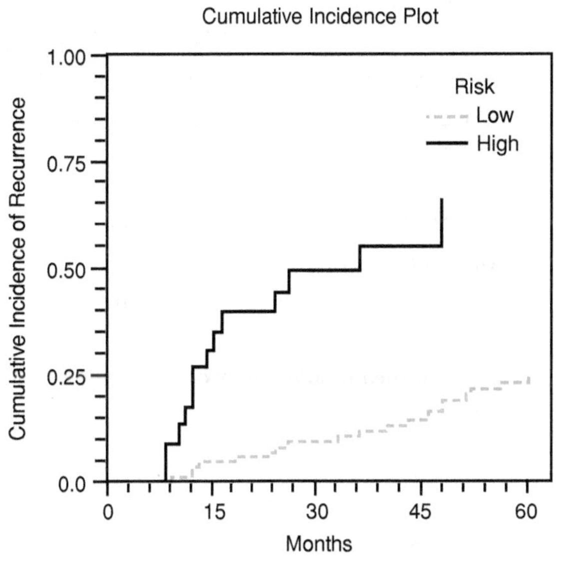

FIG. 24-1. Kaplan–Meier survival curve for recurrence of stones in patients at high versus normal risk. (Drawn from data in Borghi L, Schianchi T, Meschi T, et al. Comparison of two diets for the prevention of recurrent stones in idiopathic hypercalciuria. *N Engl J Med* 2002;346:77–88.)

   (A) Significance between the two groups can be calculated using McNemar's test.
   (B) The risk classification system is valid.
   (C) The risk classification should have been initiated 9 months earlier.
   (D) At 30 months the high-risk patients had 300% more recurrence than did low-risk patients.
   (E) The high-risk curve is invalid because of the multiple prolonged flat segments.

4. Which of the following statements is TRUE regarding the Forest plot shown in Figure 24-2?

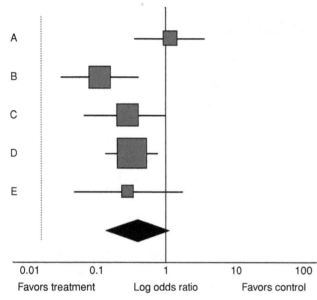

FIG. 24-2. A Forest plot summarizing the odds ratio for five studies (labeled A–E).

(A) Study B has the narrowest confidence interval.
(B) Study C is statistically significant.
(C) Study E is statistically significant.
(D) Their is a significant difference between the summed total of the two groups.
(E) Study D has the largest weight.

5. You have plotted a set of data regarding hospital length of stay for hip fracture patients. The distribution curve looks like this:

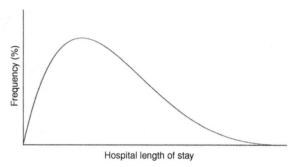

FIG. 24-3. A distribution curve for hospital length of stay.

Which of the following calculated values would you expect to be LOWEST?

(A) mean
(B) median
(C) mode
(D) midpoint
(E) range

6. A set of data is normally distributed. What proportion of that data will be within 2 standard deviations of the mean?

(A) 68.2%
(B) 72.5%
(C) 87.5%
(D) 95.4%
(E) 99.7%

7. Which of the following statements regarding confidence intervals (CI) is NOT TRUE?

(A) CI are derived from the standard error of the mean.
(B) CI can be used to assess the precision of population parameter estimates.
(C) The width of the CI depends on the degree of confidence required.
(D) The width of the CI depends on the sample size.
(E) The width of the CI depends on the mean value of the sample.

8. An analysis of variance (ANOVA) compares:

   (A) standard deviations
   (B) means
   (C) standard errors of the mean
   (D) proportions
   (E) variances

9. A resident is conducting a research project on the efficacy of a new noninvasive cardiac output apparatus. If the resident rejects a true null hypothesis, this is known as which type of error?

   (A) Type I
   (B) Type A
   (C) Type II
   (D) Type B
   (E) A waste of his research elective

10. You present a meta-analysis at your department's journal club. The conclusions of a meta-analysis can be rendered invalid by which of the following?

    (A) clinical heterogeneity
    (B) statistical heterogeneity
    (C) database bias
    (D) symmetrical funnel plot
    (E) English-language bias

11. The chi-square test for independence assesses which of the following?

    (A) whether the minimum number of cases exceed recommended boundaries
    (B) whether there is a relationship between the population and the sample
    (C) whether there is a relationship between two categorical variables
    (D) whether there is a significant difference between values taken at time 1 and values taken at time 2
    (E) none of the above

12. One hundred patients with a headache receive a new non-steroidal anti-inflammatory drug (NSAID) for treatment of their pain. If 25 patients, who would still have had a headache had they received placebo, experienced relief, then the number needed to treat (NNT) for this NSAID to relieve headache pain is:

    (A) 1.3
    (B) 4
    (C) 12.5
    (D) 25
    (E) 100

13. Microsoft Windows and Mac OS X are examples of:

    (A) graphic programs
    (B) operating systems
    (C) file management suites
    (D) database programs
    (E) email and communication software

14. The defining characteristic of a computer virus is:

    (A) it replicates itself when executed without the user's consent
    (B) it damages the host computer/device in some manner
    (C) it renders the computer/device open to other viruses
    (D) it only attacks Windows-based computers
    (E) it only stops when it has succeeded in corrupting a certain number of files

15. Which of the following is LEAST likely to cause hard disk drive failure?

    (A) head crash
    (B) extreme heat
    (C) excessive magnetic fields
    (D) normal wear and tear
    (E) a virus intended to divert fractions of a cent with every transaction

16. As it applies to anesthesiology, the term "Big Data" refers to:

   (A) data from studies recruiting >500 subjects
   (B) large-scale, compiled patient data from electronic health records
   (C) data analyzed and presented by only large, reputable journals
   (D) data from only prospectively collected databases
   (E) data from one of 12 approved studies from the ASA

Answers and Explanations: Mathematics

1. Which of the following is an example of a logarithmic scale?

   (A) Likert scale
   (B) **pH scale**
   (C) visual analog scale
   (D) verbal rating scale
   (E) centigrade temperature scale

   The logarithm of a given number is the exponent to which a fixed base number must be raised to produce that number. As an example, the logarithm of 10,000 to base 10 is 4, since 10^4 is 10,000. Logarithmic scales are common in physiology and medicine. Half-lives of drugs or radioactivity are measured using logarithmic scales, as are decibels and pH. They are a useful way of presenting information graphically on a single page that would otherwise be difficult due to the large range of values.

   pH is a measure of the concentration of hydrogen ions in aqueous solution. It is defined as the negative logarithm of that concentration and mathematically can be written as:

   $$pH = -\log_{10}[H+]$$

   Since the scale is logarithmic, every unit change increases or decreases the concentration by a factor of 10. The number of hydrogen ions in solution at a pH of 6 is 10 times that in a solution with a pH of 7.

   The visual analog, verbal rating, Likert, and centigrade scales are all linear scales, where any integer increase in value is equal in intensity or degree of change to any other similar integer increase.

   Ref: Barrett KE, Boitano S, Barman SM, et al. *Ganong's Review of Medical Physiology*, 24th ed. New York, NY: McGraw Hill; 2012.

2. A resident puts a sandwich contaminated with *S. aureus* in her bag at 9 a.m. in the morning and keeps it at room temperature until noon. Assuming there were 200 colony-forming units (CFU)/mL at 9 a.m. and the bacteria divide every 20 minutes at room temperature, what will the population density of bacteria be when she takes a big juicy bite of it at noon?

   (A) 2^9 CFU/mL
   (B) 51,200 CFU/mL
   (C) **102,400 CFU/mL**
   (D) 200^9 CFU/mL
   (E) too gross to bother answering

   This problem involves exponential growth (in this case, of bacteria). In general, we describe exponential growth in biological systems in terms of doubling times, or the time it takes for the population to increase by 100%. Using this methodology, the total population can be solved by:

   Total amount (accumulated) = (initial amount)
   $$[1 + (\text{rate of growth per period})]^N$$

   Where N = number of periods
   Solving here, we get:

   Total amount (accumulated) = $(200)[1 + 1.0]^9$

   Total amount (accumulated) = 200×5120
   $$= 102,400$$

   Ref: Brooks GF, Carroll KC, Butel JS, Morse SA, Mietzner TA. *Jawetz, Melnick, & Adelberg's Medical Microbiology*, 26th ed. New York, NY: McGraw Hill; 2013.

3. The following figure (Figure 24-1) plots cumulative incidence of recurrence versus time in groups that were at high or normal risk for the recurrent event. Which of the following can be correctly stated regarding this curve?

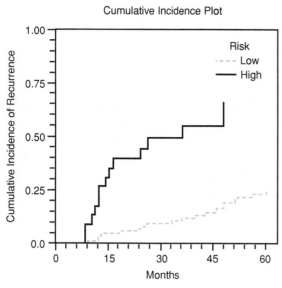

Cumulative Incidence Plot

FIG. 24-1. Kaplan–Meier survival curve for recurrence of stones in patients at high versus normal risk. (Drawn from data in Borghi L, Schianchi T, Meschi T, et al. Comparison of two diets for the prevention of recurrent stones in idiopathic hypercalciuria. *N Engl J Med* 2002;346:77–88.)

(A) Significance between the two groups can be calculated using McNemar's test.

(B) The risk classification system is valid.

(C) The risk classification should have been initiated 9 months earlier.

(D) At 30 months the high-risk patients had 300% more recurrence than did low-risk patients.

(E) The high-risk curve is invalid because of the multiple prolonged flat segments.

Kaplan-Meier (KM) curves are a very useful way of displaying differing survival or recurrence times in a study that change over time. The stepwise decline or incline in value shows the change over time. One particular advantage is that KM curves can demonstrate subject loss or withdrawal from the study before the outcome of interest is observed. This is typically shown by small vertical tick marks.

A time point can be chosen and the position of the two curves compared. In our example, examination of the 30-month time point shows that recurrence for the low-risk group was approximately 10%, whereas extending that vertical line up to meet the high-risk

curve brings us to about 50%. In order to calculate significance between the two curves, the log rank test must be applied.

The flat segments in the high-risk group only indicate that no recurrences were observed for multiple data collection intervals, so that the slope was zero for a period of time.

Ref: Dawson B, Trapp RG. *Basic & Clinical Biostatistics*, 4th ed. New York, NY: McGraw Hill; 2004.

4. Which of the following statements is TRUE regarding the Forest plot shown in Figure 24-2?

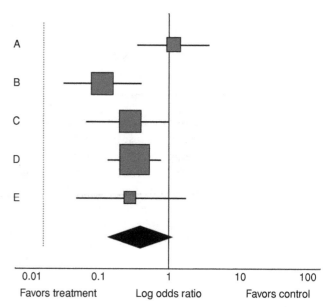

FIG. 24-2. A Forest plot summarizing the odds ratio for five studies (labeled A–E).

(A) Study B has the narrowest confidence interval.

(B) Study C is statistically significant.

(C) Study E is statistically significant.

(D) Their is a significant difference between the summed total of the two groups.

(E) Study D has the largest weight.

A Forest plot (so called because it looks like a tree with branches) is a useful way to graphically represent the effect of multiple studies on an overall outcome in a meta-analysis or systematic review. The relative risk ratio, hazard ratio, or odds ratio for each of the constituent studies are represented on the y-axis by a horizontal line and a square. The width of the line relates to the size of the 95% confidence interval for that study. In our example, study D has a fairly narrow confidence interval, while study E has a wide confidence interval (i.e., not as precise as study D). If the line crosses the vertical line in the center (i.e., if the confidence interval of the odds ratio), then the study is not statistically significant. The 95% CI lines for studies A and E both cross the line, and C touches it, indicating that those studies lack statistical significance, since their 95% CI contains the number 1.0.

The size of the square is related to the weight of the study, which is based on the number of participants and the spread of results. Bigger sample sizes and narrower 95% CIs lead to bigger weights and larger boxes. The overall result is represented by the diamond. Like the individual studies, the width of the diamond is proportional to the overall 95% CI. Since the diamond crosses the vertical line, we can conclude that overall there is no significant difference between the two groups when these five studies are compared as a whole.

Ref: McKean SC, Ross JJ, Dressler DD, et al. *Principles and Practice of Hospital Medicine*, 1st ed. New York, NY: McGraw Hill; 2012.

5. You have plotted a set of data regarding hospital length of stay for hip fracture patients. The distribution curve looks like this:

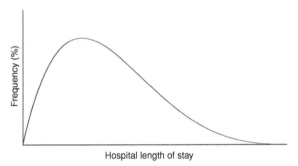

FIG. 24-3. A distribution curve for hospital length of stay.

Which of the following calculated values would you expect to be LOWEST?

(A) mean
(B) median
(C) mode
(D) midpoint
(E) range

Mean, median, and mode are all measures of central tendency for a data set. The mean is a simple average, calculated by adding up the values and dividing by the number of values in the set. The median is the middle value. If all the values are arranged from smallest to largest, the one in the center is the median. The mode is the value that is most common (this is frankly the least valuable of the three measures; no one really uses mode in clinical research).

If all three values are equal, bingo! You've got a perfectly normal distribution, with a beautiful bell-shaped curve. However, things rarely work out like that in real life, and it's more likely that your curve will be "skewed." The curve in our example is positively skewed, meaning that there are values that stretch further away from the mean on the right side. A negatively skewed curve would be a horizontal mirror image of that.

In our example, the mode is the most common value and is the highest point on the peak. Median is skewed to the right, since there are more overall values on the right side of the mode than on the left. The mean is even more right-shifted in a positively skewed curve because of the small number of outliers far to the right. You can see how this can be misleading. While mean hospital length of stay is "x" number of days, most patients actually have a lower length of stay (Figure 24-4).

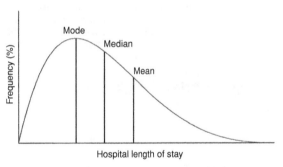

FIG. 24-4. A distribution curve for hospital length of stay, labeled with mean, median, and mode.

Ref: Dawson B, Trapp RG. *Basic & Clinical Biostatistics*, 4th ed. New York, NY: McGraw Hill; 2004.

6. A set of data is normally distributed. What proportion of that data will be within 2 standard deviations of the mean?

(A) 68.2%
(B) 72.5%
(C) 87.5%
(D) 95.4%
(E) 99.7%

The standard deviation (SD) is used for normally distributed data to describe how much the data vary around the mean (i.e., the spread of the curve). A range of 1 SD above and below the mean (±1 SD) will include 68.2% of values. Likewise, extending that out to ±2 SD will include 95.4% of the values, and ±3 SD will include 99.7%.

The reason that SD is so important is that simply stating the mean tells us very little about the shape of the bell curve. Looking at Figure 24-5, we see two curves that have the same mean. However, the tall, narrow curve has smaller standard deviations compared to the broad, shallower curve. In general, the smaller the SD, the closer the values are to the mean, and the more useful your mean value becomes.

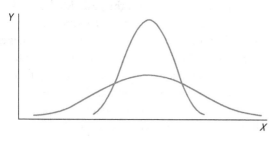

FIG. 24-5. Two normal distributions with identical means but different standard deviations. (From: LaDou J, Harrison RJ: *CURRENT diagnosis & treatment: occupational & environmental medicine*, 5th Ed. New York, NY: McGraw Hill; 2014.)

Ref: Dawson B, Trapp RG. *Basic & Clinical Biostatistics*, 4th ed. New York, NY: McGraw Hill; 2004.

7. Which of the following statements regarding confidence intervals (CI) is NOT TRUE?

(A) CI are derived from the standard error of the mean.

(B) CI can be used to assess the precision of population parameter estimates.

(C) The width of the CI depends on the degree of confidence required.

(D) The width of the CI depends on the sample size.

(E) **The width of the CI depends on the mean value of the sample.**

The confidence interval (CI) is used to define a range around the mean that is likely to contain the true population value (i.e., the mean of the entire population as a whole, not just the sample). For example, if you studied the mean age of patients presenting for their first total knee arthroplasty, you might get a value of 65 years. This would only be for the sample you stud-

ied, however. If you studied a sample in the next state, it might be different, for a number of reasons. The CI gives the range in which the true value (the age if we studied an infinite number of patients) is likely to be.

CI is usually set at a percent level of 95%. This means that the process you used will capture the true parameter 95% of the time in the long run. If you wanted to capture 99%, your CI would be larger and less precise. The size of a CI is inversely related to sample size, which makes intuitive sense: the larger your sample, the more confident you are that the true mean is close to your observed mean. A narrow CI implies high precision.

The CI is calculated using the standard error of the mean (SEM):

$$95\% \text{ CI} = \text{mean} \pm 1.96 \text{ SEM}$$

The SEM is a marker of the precision of the mean, like the standard deviation, but also takes into account the sample size:

$$\text{SEM} = \text{SD}/\sqrt{n}$$

The CI does not depend on the value of the mean itself.

Ref: Dawson B, Trapp RG. *Basic & Clinical Biostatistics*, 4th ed. New York, NY: McGraw Hill; 2004.

8. An analysis of variance (ANOVA) compares:

(A) standard deviations

(B) **means**

(C) standard errors of the mean

(D) proportions

(E) variances

Analysis of variance (ANOVA) is a group of statistical techniques used to compare the *means* of two or more samples. It is a way of generalizing the t-test (used to compare two means) to three or more groups, since applying the t-test to more than two groups would increase the likelihood of a type I error.

ANOVA tests are categorized as to the number of independent variables they are comparing. A one-way ANOVA has one independent variable (also known as a "factor") with three or more conditions (e.g., for studying the Mallampati score factor, possible conditions are MPI, MPII, MPIII, and MPIV). A two-way ANOVA has two independent variables (two factors), each with multiple conditions. This is where ANOVA really gets cool (I know, something you never thought you'd see written). An example here could be studying class of obesity versus Mallampati scores:

- Factor A: Obesity (class I, class II, class III)
- Factor B: Mallampati score (I, II, III, IV)

Ref: Dawson B, Trapp RG. *Basic & Clinical Biostatistics*, 4th ed. New York, NY: McGraw Hill; 2004.

9. A resident is conducting a research project on the efficacy of a new noninvasive cardiac output apparatus. If the resident rejects a true null hypothesis, this is known as which type of error?

(A) **Type I**
(B) Type A
(C) Type II
(D) Type B
(E) A waste of his research elective

In statistics, a type I error is the erroneous rejection of a true null hypothesis. Let's assume that the resident here has hypothesized that the cardiac output monitor will allow for significantly less crystalloid to be administered during abdominal cases than without its use. The null hypothesis is that it *doesn't* result in a significant difference. At the conclusion of the experiment, if the device did not in fact lead to a significant difference (true null hypothesis), but the resident believed that there was a difference (rejection of the null hypothesis), this would be a type I error. Bad science.

A type II error is the failure to reject a false null hypothesis. So, in our example, if the resident believed that there was no difference, when in fact there was (hooray!), that would be a type II error.

A statistical test's probability of making a type I error is denoted as $\propto$; the probability of making a type II error is denoted as β. The error rates are typically reciprocal—an effort made to reduce the likelihood of a type I error will usually result in an increase in the likelihood of a type II error. We usually set the confidence level, or 1-$\propto$, at 0.05 (*95 times out of 100, when there is no effect, we'll say there is none*). Similarly, power (1-β) is usually set at 0.8, but sometimes is set higher.

The only way the resident could say his research elective was a waste was if he didn't learn something. Most experiments have negative results. Don't get discouraged.

Ref: Dawson B, Trapp RG. *Basic & Clinical Biostatistics*, 4th ed. New York, NY: McGraw Hill; 2004.

10. You present a meta-analysis at your department's journal club. The conclusions of a meta-analysis can be rendered invalid by which of the following?

(A) clinical heterogeneity
(B) statistical heterogeneity
(C) database bias
(D) **symmetrical funnel plot**
(E) English-language bias

Meta-analyses combine results from a number of independent studies to give one overall estimate of effect. The main advantage to the meta-analysis is that by combining multiple studies, one is able to overcome small sample sizes of individual studies and analyze end points that require larger sample sizes. They are also useful in generating new hypotheses for future studies. A meta-analysis can be a very powerful way to show an effect, if conducted correctly.

There are several pitfalls that can plague a meta-analysis. First and foremost, the conclusions may be called into question if the results in the primary trials are statistically incompatible with one another (statistical heterogeneity) or if the research subjects differ significantly from one another (clinical heterogeneity). If either of these conditions occurs, the results in the primary trials cannot be validly combined together mathematically.

Bias may also occur in a number of ways. Publication bias occurs because studies with positive results are more likely to get published than are studies with negative results. Meta-analyses can also suffer from search bias, if studies were missed in the search phase. Most meta-analyses conducted these days must include a list of search terms. Selection bias occurs when clear criteria are not used to filter the initial set of studies and good studies are excluded, and/or irrelevant or poor studies included. The principal criteria are that studies be similar in terms of design, patient population, and outcomes. Occasionally, studies are excluded because they are not published in English (English-language bias).

The funnel plot is used to assess the presence of publication bias. The sample size of each primary study is plotted against its effect size. An asymmetrical funnel plot suggests that publication bias is present (Figure 24-6).

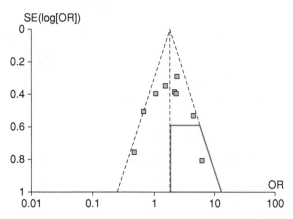

FIG. 24-6. A funnel plot; individual studies are represented by the small squares; if there is publication bias, the studies will not be equally distributed within the inverted V. The usual sign of publication bias is the absence of studies in the red box that represents where small negative studies lie. (Reproduced with permission from McKean SC, Ross JJ, Dressler DD, Brotman DJ, Ginsberg JS. *Principles and practice of hospital medicine*, 1st ed. New York, NY: McGraw Hill; 2012.)

Ref: Dawson B, Trapp RG. *Basic & Clinical Biostatistics*, 4th ed. New York, NY: McGraw Hill; 2004.

11. The chi-square test for independence assesses which of the following:

(A) whether the minimum number of cases exceed recommended boundaries

(B) whether there is a relationship between the population and the sample

(C) **whether there is a relationship between two categorical variables**

(D) whether there is a significant difference between values taken at time 1 and values taken at time 2

(E) none of the above

First things first. The "chi" is pronounced like "sky" without the s. Not like your spicy tea latte drink that gets you feeling centered in the morning.

The chi-square (or chi-squared, or χ^2) test for independence is used to determine if there is a relationship between two sets of categorical (i.e., nominal or ordinal) data from a single population. For example, you would use this test when studying the relationship between gender (variable 1) and adherence to preoperative instructions (variable 2). In contrast, the χ^2 test of homogeneity is applied to a single categorical variable from two different populations (e.g., you could ask what residents versus attendings prefer as their favorite laryngoscope blade). Note that the data must be able to be parceled into categories; the test cannot be used with continuous data such as height in inches or blood pressure in mm Hg.

Let's work through an example of patients who took a new antihypertensive medication on the morning of their operation and the effect on significant hypotension. Data analyzed with the χ^2 test for independence are commonly presented in a contingency table like this one:

TABLE 24-1. Contingency table.

	Hypotension	No hypotension	Total
Took medication	25	6	31
Didn't take medication	8	15	23
Total	33	21	54

Our job is to disprove the null hypothesis (taking medication does NOT result in hypotension). Looking at this table, we see that more patients who took the medication became hypotensive than those who didn't, so it's tempting to see an association.

We all know, however, that the bottom line to this whole shebang is the ol' p-value. Nothing is anything without a p-value—and that is the whole point of the χ^2 test. Getting a p-value. How does it do that? There's no point in going into how the χ^2 value is calculated, as it's fairly complicated. All you need to know is that a χ^2 value is derived from the contingency table, which can then be used to calculate the p-value.

In our example, the value is 11.686. Not a terrifically meaningful number to the average anesthesiologist. However, the p-value is 0.0006, which means that there is a very significant relationship between taking the medication and developing hypotension.

Ref: Dawson B, Trapp RG. *Basic & Clinical Biostatistics*, 4th ed. New York, NY: McGraw Hill; 2004.

12. One hundred patients with a headache receive a new non-steroidal anti-inflammatory drug (NSAID) for treatment of their pain. If 25 patients, who would still have had a headache had they received placebo, experienced relief, then the number needed to treat (NNT) for this NSAID to relieve headache pain is:

(A) 1.3

(B) 4

(C) 12.5

(D) 25

(E) 100

The number needed to treat (NNT) is an epidemiological concept used to assess an intervention's utility.

The NNT is the number of patients that need to receive the intervention in order for 1 patient to gain benefit from that intervention. Clearly, the lower the NNT, the better the intervention. A similar concept is the number needed to harm (NNH). The NNT should always be considered in the context of the NNH. A perfect drug would have a NNT of 1 and a NNH of infinity. The NNT is also useful in pharmacoeconomics, where the cost-effectiveness of various treatments is being weighed.

The NNT is calculated first by determining the absolute risk reduction (ARR):

$$ARR = \text{event rate in control group} - \text{event rate in treatment group}$$
$$ARR = 1 - 0.75$$
$$ARR = 0.25$$

The NNT is the reciprocal of the ARR:

$$NNT = 1/ARR$$
$$NNT = 1/0.25$$
$$NNT = 4$$

Ref: Dawson B, Trapp RG. *Basic & Clinical Biostatistics*, 4th ed. New York, NY: McGraw Hill; 2004.

13. Microsoft Windows and Mac OS X are examples of:

(A) graphic programs
(B) **operating systems**
(C) file management suites
(D) database programs
(E) email and communication software

All microcomputers require an operating system, which is a set of preprogrammed software that manages the multiple simultaneous behind-the-scenes tasks that make a computer function, as well as serve as the interface between the computer hardware and software applications. Operating systems manage memory access, organize data for long-term storage, execute programs, provide user interfaces, and manage security, I/O, device driver, and networking functions. Examples of common operating systems include Microsoft Windows, Mac OS X, and Linux. Mobile devices also use operating systems such as Android or iOS, the mobile equivalents to Windows and Mac OS X.

Programs, or applications, are sets of software instructions that tell a computer what to do. Examples of programs include word processing programs, database programs, video and image viewers, communication software (e.g., Skype, Facetime), etc. Computerized health record systems are also computer programs.

Ref: https://en.wikipedia.org/wiki/Operating_system. Accessed July 10, 2016.

14. The defining characteristic of a computer virus is:

(A) **it replicates itself when executed without the user's consent**
(B) it damages the host computer/device in some manner
(C) it renders the computer/device open to other viruses
(D) it only attacks Windows-based computers
(E) it only stops when it has succeeded in corrupting a certain number of files

A computer virus is a software program that is inadvertently executed by a host computer. When initiated, it begins to replicate itself in one or more areas, including files on the hard drive, the boot disk, or other applications. This is its defining characteristic. Viruses may wreak complete havoc on a computer, wiping out data and making the operating system unusable, or they may hide quietly in the background, collecting personal information about the user or logging keystrokes in order to send confidential information to a third party. While the vast majority of viruses are developed to infect computers that run a Windows platform, there are some that attack other types of computers as well. Billions of dollars are spent every year on antivirus software as well as in time/resources spent recovering and treating infected computers.

Ref: https://en.wikipedia.org/wiki/Computer_virus. Accessed July 10, 2016.

15. Which of the following is LEAST likely to cause hard disk drive failure?

(A) head crash
(B) extreme heat
(C) excessive magnetic fields
(D) normal wear and tear
(E) **a virus intended to divert fractions of a cent with every transaction**

Hard disk drive (HDD) failure is potentially catastrophic since, that is the location for all data file storage. When a hard disk fails, occasionally some or all of the data can be recovered, but this depends on the cause of the failure and the state of the drive. It is important to known that because they have moving parts, HDDs will eventually wear out on their own over time. Heat commonly causes HDD failure due to improper ventilation or a faulty CPU fan. Storage of a computer in a very hot location for extended periods of time can damage the HDD, but temperatures usually have to exceed 70°C. A severe jolt to the computer while the HDD is running may cause the read/write head to impact the platter where the electromagnetic information is stored. This is called a head crash and can cause physical and irreparable damage to the platter (indicated by the dreaded "click of death"). Sometimes the HDD may simply fail to spin due to failure of the circuit or the motor that spins the platter.

Since computer files are written using electromagnetism, exposure to strong electromagnetic fields may damage files and cause HDD failure. Viruses are an uncommon means by which HDD failure occurs, although it has been reported. Many of these reports are unconfirmed, and users often assume that the failure was because of an infection, when it may just have been normal wear-and-tear or nonviral corruption of a sector.

Ref: https://en.wikipedia.org/wiki/Hard_disk_drive_failure. Accessed July 10, 2016.

16. As it applies to anesthesiology, the term "Big Data" refers to:

(A) data from studies recruiting >500 subjects

(B) large-scale, compiled patient data from electronic health records

(C) data analyzed and presented by only large, reputable journals

(D) data from only prospectively collected databases

(E) data from one of 12 approved studies from the ASA

The concept of Big Data refers to the ability to rapidly collect, manage, and analyze enormous amounts of data that are otherwise too large, complex, and dynamic for conventional data tools to capture, store, and analyze properly. With the advent of the electronic health record (EHR), Big Data has made headway in health care, since the amount of information about patients, health, interventions, and outcomes is increasing exponentially as computerized record keeping becomes the standard. Effective use of Big Data allows analysts to identify trends and respond to them with measures and innovations much faster than they can when using conventional methods. With the use of very large databases, patterns emerge that are not obvious when looking at several hundred or even several thousand patients. This is particularly important in anesthesiology, since many of our big-ticket adverse outcomes (mortality, brain death, MH, nerve injury, etc.) are very rare, requiring big numbers to study properly.

Sources of data in health care include the EHR as well as billing and closed-claims databases. Anesthesiology has a unique opportunity in that Anesthesia Information Management Systems (intraoperative computerized record keeping) are collecting enormous amounts of physiologic, demographic, pharmacologic, and other data every day; with about 50 million operative cases per year, a lot of data is being collected going forward. There are many unanswered questions about how this information will best be collected and used, especially since there is very little in the way of standardization of software and applications, even within the specialty.

Ref: Simpao AF, Ahumada LM, Rehman MA. Big data and visual analytics in anaesthesia and health care. *Br J Anaesth* 2015;115(3): 350–356.

PART 4

Clinical Anesthesia Topics

CHAPTER 25

Evaluation of the Patient and Preoperative Preparation

1. Airway evaluation is recommended in all patients to detect characteristics suggestive of difficult intubation. For a male patient, which of the following findings on airway evaluation may suggest difficult intubation?

   (A) presence of a beard
   (B) neck thickness of 16 inches
   (C) narrow palate
   (D) uvula visible when tongue protruded
   (E) thyromental distance greater than 3 finger breadths

2. According to the Mallampati classification of the airway, direct visualization of a Class III airway would reveal:

   (A) hard palate only
   (B) soft palate, fauces, uvula
   (C) soft palate, tip of epiglottis
   (D) soft palate, fauces, uvula, pillars
   (E) soft palate, base of uvula

3. A 44-year-old ASA I patient scheduled for a mandibular osteotomy requires which of the following routine preoperative tests?

   (A) PTT/PT
   (B) electrolytes
   (C) ECG
   (D) CXR
   (E) no tests

4. In which of the following scenarios is a preoperative resting 12-lead electrocardiogram (ECG) considered a reasonable test as part of the preoperative evaluation?

   (A) cataract surgery; 85-year-old patient
   (B) open inguinal hernia repair; asymptomatic patient
   (C) robotic prostatectomy; patient with history of congestive heart failure
   (D) femoral-popliteal bypass; patient with no risk factors for coronary heart disease
   (E) laparoscopic hemicolectomy; patient with history of diet-controlled diabetes mellitus

5. A patient scheduled for an elective inguinal hernia repair has a myocardial infarction (MI). Subsequent testing after the MI reveals no evidence of further myocardium at risk. The patient has no other cardiac risk factors. According to ACC/ AHA recommendations, for this elective procedure what is the best course of action?

   (A) proceed with surgery
   (B) delay surgery for 4 weeks
   (C) delay surgery for 8 weeks
   (D) delay surgery for 3 months
   (E) delay surgery for 6 months

6. Which of the following patient factors increases the risk of perioperative cardiac events?

   (A) smoking
   (B) hypertension
   (C) hypercholesterolemia
   (D) family history of coronary artery disease
   (E) creatinine >2 mg/dL

7. A patient is scheduled for total knee arthroplasty. He has a history of a past MI, but has had stable symptoms for the past year. He is on insulin for diabetes, and is unable to climb stairs (due to knee pain), but can push his power mower around his backyard without any difficulty. Which of the following tests is indicated prior to his procedure?

   (A) treadmill EKG
   (B) dobutamine stress echocardiogram
   (C) radionuclide perfusion imaging
   (D) cardiopulmonary exercise testing
   (E) nothing

8. What is the ASA physical status (ASA-PS) for a patient who is moribund and not expected to survive without the operation?

   (A) 2
   (B) 3
   (C) 4
   (D) 5
   (E) 6

9. A patient's ASA physical status (ASA-PS) classification correlates with:

   (A) risk of cancellation of surgery
   (B) cost of surgery
   (C) unplanned admission after surgery
   (D) adverse cardiopulmonary complications
   (E) surgical procedure risk

10. A patient is given clonidine preoperatively in an effort to improve postoperative pain management. What is a likely side effect of administering clonidine as a preoperative medication?

    (A) tachycardia
    (B) amnesia
    (C) respiratory depression
    (D) increased gastric fluid volume
    (E) hypotension

11. A patient scheduled for surgery is thought to be at risk for aspiration pneumonitis. A premedication is given in an attempt to reduce this risk. A short time after administration the patient exhibits manifestations of acute dystonia including torticollis. Which premedication was most likely administered?

    (A) metoclopramide
    (B) sodium citrate
    (C) ranitidine
    (D) glycopyrrolate
    (E) dimenhydrinate

12. A 78-year-old patient is administered an antisialagogue, atropine, before a planned awake fiberoptic intubation. Aside from the intended xerostomia (dry mouth), what is a possible side effect of atropine administration?

    (A) confusion
    (B) miosis
    (C) bronchoconstriction
    (D) hypothermia
    (E) bradycardia

13. STOP-BANG is a popular screening questionnaire for obstructive sleep apnea (OSA). Which of the following criteria is **NOT** part of the STOP-BANG questionnaire?

    (A) Snoring
    (B) BMI >30
    (C) Hypertension
    (D) Neck size >16 inches
    (E) Age >50

14. A patient with a past medical history significant for Graves' disease is evaluated in the preoperative clinic. Which of the following clinical features is suggestive of hyperthyroidism?

    (A) weight gain
    (B) constipation
    (C) cold intolerance
    (D) bradycardia
    (E) warm skin

15. A patient requires emergency surgery. Preoperative examination indicates the patient is clinically hyperthyroid. Management of the patient with thyrotoxicosis may include all of the following **EXCEPT**:

(A) propranolol
(B) insulin
(C) iodide solutions
(D) propylthiouracil
(E) hydrocortisone

16. General recommendations regarding severe hypertension and elective surgery suggest that procedures should be delayed until blood pressure is less than:

(A) 180/110 mm Hg
(B) 140/90 mm Hg
(C) 130/80 mm Hg
(D) 160/100 mm Hg
(E) 120/80 mm Hg

17. A patient with a cecal carcinoma is scheduled for open hemicolectomy. Preoperative assessment identifies a past medical history of COPD. Which of the following is an additional risk factor for postoperative pulmonary complications?

(A) age >60
(B) asthma
(C) exercise tolerance <2 blocks
(D) abnormal pulmonary functions tests (PFTs)
(E) abnormal arterial blood gas (ABG)

18. A morbidly obese patients presents for preoperative evaluation. Which of the following comorbid conditions is **NOT** associated with increased body mass index (BMI)?

(A) metabolic syndrome
(B) type 2 diabetes
(C) mitral valve regurgitation
(D) cancer
(E) obstructive sleep apnea

19. A patient with chronic kidney disease (CKD) requiring hemodialysis is evaluated preoperatively. Which of the following abnormalities is common for a patient with CKD?

(A) hypercalcemia
(B) polycythemia
(C) secondary hypoparathyroidism
(D) hypovolemia
(E) hypertension

20. A patient with a history of medically managed glaucoma presents for preoperative anesthetic assessment. Which glaucoma treatment may increase the duration of action of succinylcholine?

(A) acetazolamide
(B) brimonidine
(C) cyclopentolate
(D) echothiophate
(E) bimatoprost

21. A patient with a history of drug abuse presents for preoperative assessment. History is notable for previous seizures. Physical exam is notable for cognitive dysfunction, tremors, and hypertension. Laboratory results are significant for macrocytic anemia. Which of the following is most likely the substance of abuse?

(A) cocaine
(B) ethanol
(C) marijuana
(D) 3, 4-methylenedioxy-methamphetamine (MDMA, "ecstasy")
(E) heroin

22. A patient with an intracranial mass is scheduled for urgent craniotomy. Presenting symptoms included headache, nausea, and a seizure. Methods to reduce intracranial pressure (ICP) include all of the following **EXCEPT**:

(A) dexamethasone
(B) fosphenytoin
(C) moderate hyperventilation (PaCO$_2$ 30–33 mm Hg)
(D) hypertonic saline
(E) mannitol

23. Preoperative assessment identifies a patient who chronically takes prednisone 25 mg PO once a day for asthma. The patient is scheduled for a major abdominal operation. What is a recommended course of action for perioperative corticosteroid management?

    (A) usual morning steroid dose, no supplementation required

    (B) usual morning steroid dose, single dose of hydrocortisone 25 mg

    (C) usual morning steroid dose, single dose of hydrocortisone 50 mg

    (D) usual morning steroid dose, hydrocortisone 50–100 mg q8h for 24 hours

    (E) usual morning steroid dose, hydrocortisone 200 mg/70 kg body weight q8h for 24 hours

24. A 4-year-old pediatric patient is assessed preoperatively before surgery. The child is very anxious with significant separation anxiety and is noncooperative. In order to administer a sedative premedication for this child, what is the most reliable route of administration?

    (A) rectal

    (B) intramuscular

    (C) sublingual

    (D) intranasal

    (E) oral

25. A geriatric patient is scheduled for surgery. Which of the following intravenous premedications is **least** likely to require a dosage adjustment?

    (A) midazolam

    (B) fentanyl

    (C) dexmedetomidine

    (D) ranitidine

    (E) metoclopramide

26. During preoperative evaluation, a patient states that they are allergic to local anesthetics. Further history elucidates that the patient developed a cardiac arrhythmia after receiving an injection of 2% lidocaine with 1:200,000 epinephrine at a dentist's office. What is the most likely explanation for this reaction?

    (A) anaphylactoid reaction to lidocaine

    (B) allergic reaction to lidocaine

    (C) allergy to para-aminobenzoic acid (PABA) preservative in local anesthetic solution

    (D) adverse side effect due to epinephrine

    (E) allergic reaction to epinephrine

27. An otherwise healthy 1-year-old infant is scheduled for elective surgery. For the child, whose diet is infant formula, what is the recommended preoperative fasting (NPO) period?

    (A) 2 hours

    (B) 4 hours

    (C) 6 hours

    (D) 8 hours

    (E) 10 hours

28. Which of the following factors **DOES NOT** increase the risk of pulmonary aspiration?

    (A) pregnancy

    (B) hiatal hernia

    (C) obesity without comorbidity

    (D) patients receiving acute opioid therapy

    (E) GERD

29. A patient with normal airway anatomy is not NPO and is considered a "full stomach." A rapid sequence induction (RSI) is indicated. What are the classic components of an RSI in the order they are performed?

    (A) preoxygenation; cricoid pressure; propofol induction; rocuronium; endotracheal intubation

    (B) preoxygenation; awake fiberoptic laryngoscopy; endotracheal intubation

    (C) preoxygenation; cricoid pressure; propofol induction; mask ventilation; succinylcholine; endotracheal intubation

    (D) preoxygenation; propofol induction; succinylcholine; endotracheal intubation

    (E) preoxygenation; inhalation induction with sevoflurane; succinylcholine; endotracheal intubation

30. Preoperatively, a patient is evaluated and felt to be at increased risk of pulmonary aspiration. Best evidence suggests which of the following preoperative pharmacologic agents is most effective at reducing gastric acidity?

    (A) metoclopramide
    (B) ranitidine
    (C) lansoprazole
    (D) ondansetron
    (E) glycopyrrolate

31. Preoperatively, a patient is evaluated and felt to be at increased risk of pulmonary aspiration. Best evidence suggests which of the following preoperative pharmacologic agents is most effective at increasing lower esophageal sphincter (LES) tone?

    (A) metoclopramide
    (B) ranitidine
    (C) lansoprazole
    (D) ondansetron
    (E) glycopyrrolate

32. A patient is scheduled for elective knee arthroscopy. Three months ago, the patient had a myocardial infarction. Management at that time included percutaneous transluminal coronary angioplasty (PTCA) with placement of a single drug eluting stent (DES). The patient is currently on clopidogrel (Plavix). According to the American College of Cardiology and American Heart Association (ACC/AHA) guidelines, what is appropriate management for this elective surgery?

    (A) proceed with surgery and hold clopidogrel for 7 days preoperatively

    (B) proceed with surgery and hold clopidogrel for 10 days preoperatively

    (C) proceed with surgery and continue clopidogrel perioperatively

    (D) cancel surgery until patient completes at least 6 months of clopidogrel therapy

    (E) cancel surgery until patient completes at least 12 months of clopidogrel therapy

33. A patient's medical therapy for type 2 diabetes mellitus includes oral hypoglycemic agents. Which of the following medications should be discontinued at least 24 hours before surgery to reduce the risk of drug-induced lactic acidosis?

    (A) glyburide
    (B) glipizide
    (C) gliclazide
    (D) metformin
    (E) repaglinide

34. A patient with medically managed hypertension is scheduled for ambulatory surgery. Antihypertensive medications, including an angiotensin II antagonist, are administered the morning of surgery. After anesthetic induction, refractory hypotension is noted. What is the best treatment?

    (A) vasopressin
    (B) ephedrine
    (C) phenylephrine
    (D) epinephrine
    (E) norepinephrine

35. A patient is chronically on medical therapy for treatment of depression. The patient is scheduled for surgery and a preoperative anesthetic consultation is performed. Which antidepressant can cause rare, but serious, side effects associated with the use of opioids?

    (A) amitriptyline
    (B) fluoxetine
    (C) trazodone
    (D) bupropion
    (E) phenelzine

36. A female patient with a complex medical history is taking multiple medications. Preoperative assessment should include instructions to discontinue which of the following medications before the day of surgery?

    (A) oxycodone
    (B) conjugated estrogens
    (C) atorvastatin
    (D) isosorbide dinitrate
    (E) fluoxetine

37. Perioperative beta-blocker therapy is recommended for a number of different clinical situations. According to the American College of Cardiology and American Heart Association (ACC/AHA) guidelines on perioperative cardiovascular evaluation and care for noncardiac surgery, the strongest recommendation for perioperative beta-blockade is for which of the following scenarios?

    (A) vascular surgery; patient without evidence of myocardial ischemia
    (B) intermediate-risk surgery; patient with one or more clinical risk factors for coronary heart disease
    (C) vascular surgery; patient with one or more clinical risk factors for coronary heart disease
    (D) intermediate-risk surgery; patient with known coronary heart disease
    (E) low-risk surgery; patient currently taking a beta-blocker

38. A patient with no known cardiac risk factors is scheduled for major vascular surgery. Which of the following techniques or medications should be used in order to reduce cardiac risk?

    (A) induced hypothermia
    (B) atorvastatin
    (C) clonidine
    (D) verapamil
    (E) dilutional anemia

39. An adult patient, with no known drug allergies, is scheduled for a total knee arthroplasty. The institutional incidence of surgical site infections (SSIs) caused by MRSA is less than 5%. In order to reduce the risk of SSI for this clean surgery, which of the following regimens for antibiotic prophylaxis is indicated?

    (A) no antibiotics indicated
    (B) cefazolin 1 g IV q3–4h
    (C) cefazolin 2 g IV q3–4h
    (D) vancomycin 1 g IV
    (E) metronidazole 500 mg IV

40. In an effort to reduce surgical site infections (SSIs), antibiotic prophylaxis is often administered preoperatively. What is the optimal time for administration of the preoperative dose?

    (A) within 30 minutes of surgical incision for cefazolin
    (B) within 2 hours of surgical incision for cefazolin
    (C) within 4 hours of surgical incision for cefazolin
    (D) within 1 hour of surgical incision for vancomycin
    (E) within 2 hours of surgical incision for ciprofloxacin

41. Which patient requires antibiotic prophylaxis for prevention of infective endocarditis?

    (A) patient with severe mitral valve prolapse (MVP) scheduled for routine dental cleaning

    (B) patient with a previous history of endocarditis scheduled for routine transesophageal echocardiography

    (C) patient with a prosthetic aortic valve scheduled for routine tonsillectomy

    (D) cardiac transplant recipient scheduled for routine bronchoscopy

    (E) patient with completely repaired congenital heart defect (15 years prior) scheduled for routine vaginal delivery

Answers and Explanations: Evaluation of the Patient and Preoperative Preparation

1. Airway evaluation is recommended in all patients to detect characteristics suggestive of difficult intubation. For a male patient, which of the following findings on airway evaluation may suggest difficult intubation?

   (A) presence of a beard
   (B) neck thickness of 16 inches
   (C) **narrow palate**
   (D) uvula visible when tongue protruded
   (E) thyromental distance greater than 3 finger breadths

   Narrow palate is considered a nonreassuring airway exam finding suggestive of difficult intubation. Other nonreassuring airway exam findings include:

   - relatively long incisors
   - prominent "overbite"
   - inability to bring mandibular incisors in front of maxillary incisors
   - interincisor distance <3 cm
   - Mallampati class >2 (uvula not visible when tongue is protruded)
   - highly arched palate
   - thyromental distance <3 finger breadths
   - short, thick neck (>17 inches in men, >16 inches in women)
   - inability to touch tip of chin to chest

   Refs: Miller RD. *Miller's Anesthesia*, 8th ed. Philadelphia, PA: Elsevier; 2015.
   American Society of Anesthesiologists, Practice guidelines for management of the difficult airway: an updated report. *Anesthesiology* 2013;118:1269–1277.

2. According to the Mallampati classification of the airway, direct visualization of a Class III airway would reveal:

   (A) hard palate only
   (B) soft palate, fauces, uvula
   (C) soft palate, tip of epiglottis
   (D) soft palate, fauces, uvula, pillars
   (E) **soft palate, base of uvula**

   For the Mallampati classification of the airway, the following anatomic landmarks are visible during direct visualization with the patient seated:

   - I—soft palate, fauces, uvula, pillars
   - II—soft palate, fauces, uvula
   - III—soft palate, base of uvula
   - IV—hard palate only

   The epiglottis is typically viewed with direct laryngoscopy. Cormack and Lehane's classification is used to describe laryngoscopic views.

   Ref: Miller RD. *Miller's Anesthesia*, 8th ed. Philadelphia, PA: Elsevier; 2015.

3. A 44-year-old ASA I patient scheduled for a mandibular osteotomy requires which of the following routine preoperative tests?

   (A) PTT/PT
   (B) electrolytes
   (C) ECG
   (D) CXR
   (E) **no tests**

   Determining appropriate preoperative laboratory studies is a controversial topic.

Studies should only be ordered if an abnormality is suspected *and* if this result impacts perioperative management. Under these circumstances, a healthy 44-year-old scheduled for mandibular surgery does not require any routine preoperative tests. If significant blood loss were anticipated, a CBC to establish baseline hemoglobin would be reasonable to order.

Ref: Miller RD. *Miller's Anesthesia*, 8th ed. Philadelphia, PA: Elsevier; 2015.

4. In which of the following scenarios is a preoperative resting 12-lead electrocardiogram (ECG) considered a reasonable test as part of the preoperative evaluation?

   (A) cataract surgery; 85-year-old patient
   (B) open inguinal hernia repair; asymptomatic patient
   (C) **robotic prostatectomy; patient with history of congestive heart failure**
   (D) femoral-popliteal bypass; patient with no risk factors for coronary heart disease
   (E) laparoscopic hemicolectomy; patient with history of diet-controlled diabetes mellitus

According to the ACC/AHA 2014 guidelines on perioperative cardiovascular evaluation, a resting 12-lead ECG is *reasonable (Class IIa recommendation)* for patients with known coronary heart disease, significant arrhythmia, peripheral arterial disease, cerebrovascular disease, or other significant structural heart disease, *except* for those undergoing low-risk surgery. The guidelines considers low-risk surgery to be that for which the patient and surgical risk factors confer a <1% risk of a major adverse cardiac event (MACE). This calculation is usually performed using the Revised Cardiac Risk Index, whereby each one of six factors (history of ischemic heart disease, history of congestive heart failure, history of cerebrovascular disease, diabetes mellitus requiring insulin, creatinine >2 mg/dL, and intrathoracic/intra-abdominal/suprainguinal vascular surgery) is given a 1-point value. The risk of a MACE is related to the number of points: 0 = 0.4%, 1 = 0.9%, 2 = 6.6%, and 3 or more = 11%. From this we can see that unless the patient has two or more risk factors as described by this index, they are considered low risk.

A resting EKG may be considered for asymptomatic patients without known coronary heart disease *except* those undergoing low-risk surgery (Class IIb). In other words, there is some thought that a preoperative ECG may have benefit as a baseline standard against

which to measure any postoperative change and provide some prognostic information. In the case of the asymptomatic patient undergoing a femoral-popliteal bypass, an ECG may indeed be considered but the strength of evidence is stronger to order an ECG for the patient with CHF undergoing a robotic prostatectomy. There is no benefit (Class III) in asymptomatic patients undergoing low-risk surgical procedures.

Note that there is no age cutoff for which an EKG becomes an indicated preoperative test, as there is an increased incidence of abnormal findings of unclear significance with increasing age. The utility of the EKG does increase with the risk of the surgical procedure.

Ref: Fleisher LA, Fleischmann KE, Auerbach AD, et al. 2014 ACC/AHA guidelines on perioperative cardiovascular evaluation and management of patients undergoing noncardiac surgery: a report of the American College of Cardiology/American Heart Association Task Force on practice guidelines. *J Am Coll Cardiol* 2014;64:e77–137.

5. A patient scheduled for an elective inguinal hernia repair has a myocardial infarction (MI). Subsequent testing after the MI reveals no evidence of further myocardium at risk. The patient has no other cardiac risk factors. According to ACC/AHA recommendations, for this elective procedure what is the best course of action?

   (A) proceed with surgery
   (B) delay surgery for 4 weeks
   (C) delay surgery for 8 weeks
   (D) delay surgery for 3 months
   (E) **delay surgery for 6 months**

Previous iterations of guidelines used myocardium at risk to delineate the likelihood of an ischemic event during non-cardiac surgery. Recent data has shown that at least 60 days should elapse after a myocardial infarction before noncardiac surgery in the absence of some type of revascularization in order to achieve the greatest reduction in risk. Note, coronary artery bypass grafting improves outcomes more than coronary stenting for patients with a recent MI who require surgery within 30 days. Current guidelines DO NOT recommend coronary revascularization before surgery solely to reduce perioperative cardiac events.

However, an MI occurring within 6 months of noncardiac surgery has been shown to be an independent risk factor for perioperative stroke, which itself is associated with an 8-fold increase in the risk of death. For these reasons, truly elective surgery should be delayed for at least 6 months after an MI.

Ref: Fleisher LA, Fleischmann KE, Auerbach AD, et al. 2014 ACC/AHA guidelines on perioperative cardiovascular evaluation and management of patients undergoing noncardiac surgery: a report of the American College of Cardiology/American Heart Association Task Force on practice guidelines. *J Am Coll Cardiol* 2014;64:e77–137.

6. Which of the following patient factors increases the risk of perioperative cardiac events?

   (A) smoking
   (B) hypertension
   (C) hypercholesterolemia
   (D) family history of coronary artery disease
   (E) **creatinine >2 mg/dL**

Lee's revised cardiac risk index (RCRI) includes the following risk factors:

- high-risk surgery (intraperitoneal, intrathoracic, suprainguinal vascular)
- ischemic heart disease
- congestive heart failure
- cerebrovascular disease
- diabetes mellitus
- creatinine >2 mg/dL

These factors identify increased incidence of perioperative cardiac events.

Other factors such as smoking, hypertension, age, male gender, hypercholesterolemia, and family history are not part of the RCRI.

Ref: Fleisher LA, Fleischmann KE, Auerbach AD, et al. 2014 ACC/AHA guidelines on perioperative cardiovascular evaluation and management of patients undergoing noncardiac surgery: a report of the American College of Cardiology/American Heart Association Task Force on practice guidelines. *J Am Coll Cardiol* 2014;64:e77–137.

7. A patient is scheduled for total knee arthroplasty. He has a history of a past MI, but has had stable symptoms for the past year. He is on insulin for diabetes, and is unable to climb stairs (due to knee pain), but can push his power mower around his backyard without any difficulty. Which of the following tests is indicated prior to his procedure?

   (A) treadmill EKG
   (B) dobutamine stress echocardiogram

   (C) radionuclide perfusion imaging
   (D) cardiopulmonary exercise testing
   (E) **nothing**

One of the biggest changes to the way that we approach patient evaluation in the last several years is the emphasis on functional capacity. Functional status can be measured in the lab with formal exercise testing, but is more commonly estimated by activities of daily living, where it is expressed in terms of metabolic equivalents (or METS). One MET is the resting basal oxygen consumption for an average 70-kg man. As oxygen demand goes up with activity, so do the METS required. For example, according to the Duke Activity Status Index (*Go Blue Devils!*) while walking around the house burns only 1–2 METS, climbing a flight of stairs or walking up a hill requires approximately 5.5 METS. Doing heavy work around the house would be between 4 and 8 METS. Strenuous sports like swimming or singles tennis are approximately 7–10 METS. Studies have shown that patients that are unable to complete 4 METS are at elevated risk for perioperative myocardial ischemia and cardiovascular events.

In the 2014 ACC/AHA guidelines for evaluation of patients undergoing noncardiac surgery, the algorithm for deciding who to test is presented as a series of decision points. After eliminating those patients who need emergency surgery and who are having acute coronary syndromes, the clinician is asked to calculate risk of a major adverse cardiac event (MACE) (see question 4). If the risk is >1%, as is the case with our example here, the patient gets 2 points (or risk of MACE of 6.6%) for coronary disease and diabetes requiring insulin—the functional capacity must be evaluated. If the patient can exert his/herself at 4 METS or more, there is no need for preoperative myocardial testing. Only if the functional capacity is low, or if it cannot be determined because of limitations from arthritis, etc., should testing be considered. Pushing a power mower around the yard is moderately intense, and is associated with >4 METS, so our patient can avoid further testing.

Ref: Fleisher LA, Fleischmann KE, Auerbach AD, et al. 2014 ACC/AHA guidelines on perioperative cardiovascular evaluation and management of patients undergoing noncardiac surgery: a report of the American College of Cardiology/American Heart Association Task Force on practice guidelines. *J Am Coll Cardiol* 2014;64:e77–137.

8. What is the ASA physical status (ASA-PS) for a patient who is moribund and not expected to survive without the operation?

(A) 2

(B) 3

(C) 4

(D) 5

(E) 6

A moribund patient who is not expected to survive without the operation is ASA-PS 5. The ASA-PS classification:

- 1—healthy without disease
- 2—mild systemic disease; no significant impact on daily activity
- 3—significant or severe disease that limits normal activity
- 4—severe disease that is a constant threat to life
- 5—moribund patient who is not expected to survive without the operation
- 6—brain-dead organ donor

Ref: Miller RD. *Miller's Anesthesia*, 8th ed. Philadelphia, PA: Elsevier; 2015; AS Awebsite: www.asahq.org.

9. A patient's ASA physical status (ASA-PS) classification correlates with:

(A) risk of cancellation of surgery

(B) cost of surgery

(C) unplanned admission after surgery

(D) adverse cardiopulmonary complications

(E) surgical procedure risk

ASA-PS is an attempt to classify risk based on a patient's preoperative medical history. It does not consider the anesthetic technique, type of surgery, or location of surgery. ASA-PS correlates with mortality and some measures of morbidity such as:

- unanticipated ICU admission
- adverse cardiopulmonary complications
- length of hospital stay for some procedures

ASA-PS does not correlate with case cancellations, cost, or unplanned admission.

Ref: Miller RD. *Miller's Anesthesia*, 8th ed. Philadelphia, PA: Elsevier; 2015.

10. A patient is given clonidine preoperatively in an effort to improve postoperative pain management. What is a likely side effect of administering clonidine as a preoperative medication?

(A) tachycardia

(B) amnesia

(C) respiratory depression

(D) increased gastric fluid volume

(E) hypotension

Alpha-2 agonists (clonidine, dexmedetomidine) can be administered as premedication to cause sedation, blunt the hemodynamic changes associated with laryngoscopy or awake fiberoptic intubation, and improve analgesia. Common side effects of alpha-2 agonists include hypotension and bradycardia. Clinically, alpha-2 agonists are not felt to have significant effect on memory, respiratory depression, or gastric fluid volume.

Ref: Barash PG. *Clinical Anesthesia*, 7th ed. Philadelphia, PA: Lippincott Williams & Wilkins; 2013.

11. A patient scheduled for surgery is thought to be at risk for aspiration pneumonitis. A premedication is given in an attempt to reduce this risk. A short time after administration the patient exhibits manifestations of acute dystonia including torticollis. Which premedication was most likely administered?

(A) metoclopramide

(B) sodium citrate

(C) ranitidine

(D) glycopyrrolate

(E) dimenhydrinate

Metoclopramide can cause acute dystonic reactions including oculogyric crisis, torticollis (head turned to side), opisthotonus (forceful extension of neck/back), spasticity, and laryngospasm. Treatment includes diphenhydramine or benztropine (anticholinergic effects). Sodium citrate, ranitidine, glycopyrrolate, and dimenhydrinate do not cause dystonic reactions.

Ref: Brunton LL, Chabner BA, Knollman BC. *Goodman & Gilman's the Pharmacological Basis of Therapeutics*, 12th ed. New York, NY: McGraw Hill; 2011.

12. A 78-year-old patient is administered an antisialagogue, atropine, before a planned awake fiberoptic intubation. Aside from the intended xerostomia (dry mouth), what is a possible side effect of atropine administration?

(A) confusion

(B) miosis

(C) bronchoconstriction

(D) hypothermia

(E) bradycardia

Anticholinergic drugs may cause confusion or delirium. Other anticholinergic side effects include: mydriasis, cycloplegia, bronchodilation, hyperthermia, and tachycardia.

Ref: Brunton LL, Chabner BA, Knollman BC. *Goodman & Gilman's the Pharmacological Basis of Therapeutics*, 12th ed. New York, NY: McGraw Hill; 2011.

13. STOP-BANG is a popular screening questionnaire for obstructive sleep apnea (OSA). Which of the following criteria is **NOT** part of the STOP-BANG questionnaire?

(A) Snoring

(B) BMI >30

(C) Hypertension

(D) Neck size >16 inches

(E) Age >50

The STOP-BANG screening questionnaire for OSA records "yes/no" responses for the following criteria:

• Snoring

• Tired (fatigue)

• Observed (observed apnea)

• Pressure (hypertension)

• BMI >35

• Age >50

• Neck size >16 inches

• Gender (male)

Answering "yes" to >5 questions equals a "high risk" of OSA.

Ref: Chung F, Yegneswaran B, Liao P, et al. STOP questionnaire: a tool to screen patients for obstructive sleep apnea. *Anesthesiology* 2008;108:812–821.

14. A patient with a past medical history significant for Graves' disease is evaluated in the preoperative clinic.

Which of the following clinical features is suggestive of hyperthyroidism?

(A) weight gain

(B) constipation

(C) cold intolerance

(D) bradycardia

(E) warm skin

Hyperthyroidism is characterized by: warm moist skin, weight loss, diarrhea, heat intolerance, tachycardia, cardiac arrhythmias, and heart failure.

Ref: Miller RD. *Miller's Anesthesia*, 8th ed. Philadelphia, PA: Elsevier; 2015.

15. A patient requires emergency surgery. Preoperative examination indicates the patient is clinically hyperthyroid. Management of the patient with thyrotoxicosis may include all of the following **EXCEPT:**

(A) propranolol

(B) insulin

(C) iodide solutions

(D) propylthiouracil

(E) hydrocortisone

Hyperthyroid patients requiring emergency surgery are managed with beta blockade for rate control, antithyroid medications (propylthiouracil and methimazole), iodide solutions to reduce hormone secretion, and hydrocortisone to prevent complications due to co-existing adrenal suppression. Insulin is not typically part of the management of hyperthyroidism.

Ref: Butterworth JF IV, Mackey DC, Wasnick JD. *Morgan & Mikhail's Clinical Anesthesiology*, 5th ed. New York, NY: McGraw Hill; 2013.

16. General recommendations regarding severe hypertension and elective surgery suggest that procedures should be delayed until blood pressure is less than:

(A) 180/110 mm Hg

(B) 140/90 mm Hg

(C) 130/80 mm Hg

(D) 160/100 mm Hg

(E) 120/80 mm Hg

Elective surgery should be delayed until severe hypertension is treated and blood pressure is less than 180/110 mm Hg. Overall, end organ damage (ischemic heart disease, heart failure, renal failure, stroke) correlate with severity and duration of hypertension. However, perioperative risk does not seem to be significantly associated with BP less than 180/110 mm Hg.

Ref: Miller RD. *Miller's Anesthesia*, 8th ed. Philadelphia, PA: Elsevier; 2015.

17. A patient with a cecal carcinoma is scheduled for open hemicolectomy. Preoperative assessment identifies a past medical history of COPD. Which of the following is an additional risk factor for postoperative pulmonary complications?

    (A) age >60
    (B) asthma
    (C) exercise tolerance <2 blocks
    (D) abnormal pulmonary functions tests (PFTs)
    (E) abnormal arterial blood gas (ABG)

Exercise tolerance of less than 2 blocks (or one flight of stairs) is a risk factor for postoperative pulmonary complications. Other risk factors for postoperative pulmonary complications include:

- COPD
- age >70 years
- cigarette use (current or >40 pack-years)
- ASA-PS >2
- surgery >2 hours
- general anesthesia with endotracheal tube
- BMI >30
- albumin <3 g/dL

Asthma is not a risk factor for postoperative pulmonary complications unless there is a history of recent exacerbation. Pulmonary function tests and arterial blood analysis are not predictive of postoperative pulmonary complications for nonthoracic surgery.

Ref: Miller RD. *Miller's Anesthesia*, 8th ed. Philadelphia, PA: Elsevier; 2015.

18. A morbidly obese patients presents for preoperative evaluation. Which of the following comorbid conditions is **NOT** associated with increased body mass index (BMI)?

    (A) metabolic syndrome
    (B) type 2 diabetes
    (C) mitral valve regurgitation
    (D) cancer
    (E) obstructive sleep apnea

Obesity is associated with metabolic syndrome (abdominal obesity, reduced high- density lipoprotein, hyper-

triglyceridemia, hypertension, and elevated fasting glucose), type 2 diabetes, cancer, and obstructive sleep apnea. Valvular heart disease is not typically considered a comorbid condition associated with increased BMI. Mitral valve regurgitation (and pulmonary hypertension) is associated with the now withdrawn weight loss regimen of fenfluramine and phentermine (fen-phen).

Ref: Butterworth JF IV, Mackey DC, Wasnick JD. *Morgan & Mikhail's Clinical Anesthesiology*, 5th ed. New York, NY: McGraw Hill; 2013.

19. A patient with chronic kidney disease (CKD) requiring hemodialysis is evaluated preoperatively. Which of the following abnormalities is common for a patient with CKD?

    (A) hypercalcemia
    (B) polycythemia
    (C) secondary hypoparathyroidism
    (D) hypovolemia
    (E) hypertension

Hypertension is a common abnormality associated with CKD. Other abnormalities include:

- hypocalcemia
- hyperphosphatemia
- Vit D deficient osteomalacia
- anemia
- secondary hyperparathyroidism
- hypervolemia
- hyperkalemia
- abnormal bleeding time, coagulopathy
- metabolic acidosis
- congestive heart failure
- pericarditis
- fatigue, lethargy, seizures

Ref: Miller RD. *Miller's Anesthesia*, 8th ed. Philadelphia, PA: Elsevier; 2015.

20. A patient with a history of medically managed glaucoma presents for preoperative anesthetic assessment. Which glaucoma treatment may increase the duration of action of succinylcholine?

    (A) acetazolamide
    (B) brimonidine
    (C) cyclopentolate
    (D) echothiophate
    (E) bimatoprost

Echothiophate is a cholinesterase inhibitor. It will prolong the duration of action of succinylcholine (for an additional 2 to 14 minutes). Acetazolamide inhibits carbonic anhydrase and reduces aqueous humor production. Brimonidine (Alphagan) is an alpha-2 receptor agonist. Cyclopentolate is a muscarinic antagonist. Bimatoprost (Lumigan) is a prostaglandin analog that increases uveoscleral outflow.

Ref: Brunton LL, Chabner BA, Knollman BC. *Goodman & Gilman's the Pharmacological Basis of Therapeutics*, 12th ed. New York, NY: McGraw Hill; 2011.

21. A patient with a history of drug abuse presents for preoperative assessment. History is notable for previous seizures. Physical exam is notable for cognitive dysfunction, tremors, and hypertension. Laboratory results are significant for macrocytic anemia. Which of the following is most likely the substance of abuse?

    (A) cocaine

    (B) ethanol

    (C) marijuana

    (D) 3,4-methylenedioxy-methamphetamine (MDMA, "ecstasy")

    (E) heroin

Ethanol abuse has multi-system effects including: withdrawal seizures, cognitive dysfunction, tremors, hypertension, and macrocytic anemia. Other effects of ethanol abuse include: cardiac arrhythmias, coronary artery disease, cardiomyopathy, stroke, skeletal muscle myopathy, esophageal reflux, chronic gastritis, acute and chronic pancreatitis, alcoholic cirrhosis, and nutritional deficiencies.

Cocaine abuse is notable for toxicity including: cardiac arrhythmias, myocardial ischemia, seizures, and stroke. Macrocytic anemia is not typically a finding of cocaine abuse.

Marijuana is notable for withdrawal symptoms including: restlessness, irritability, insomnia, and nausea.

3,4-methylenedioxy-methamphetamine (MDMA, "ecstasy") is notable for acute effects of: altered sensorium, hallucinations, tachycardia, dry mouth, and hyperthermia.

Heroin abuse is notable for withdrawal symptoms including: irritability, nausea, cramps, insomnia, pupillary dilation, sweating, hypertension, yawning, and piloerection ("gooseflesh").

Refs: Brunton LL, Chabner BA, Knollman BC. *Goodman & Gilman's the Pharmacological Basis of Therapeutics*, 12th ed. New York, NY: McGraw Hill; 2011.
Miller RD. *Miller's Anesthesia*, 8th ed. Philadelphia, PA: Elsevier; 2015.

22. A patient with an intracranial mass is scheduled for urgent craniotomy. Presenting symptoms included headache, nausea, and a seizure. Methods to reduce intracranial pressure (ICP) include all of the following **EXCEPT**:

    (A) dexamethasone

    (B) fosphenytoin

    (C) moderate hyperventilation (PaCO$_2$ 30–33 mm Hg)

    (D) hypertonic saline

    (E) mannitol

Fosphenytoin is indicated for the treatment and prevention of seizures. It does not affect intracranial pressure (ICP). For increased ICP, treatment measures include:

- Dexamethasone to reduce vasogenic edema associated with tumors

- Hypertonic saline and mannitol to reduce brain water content

- Moderated hyperventilation (PaCO$_2$ 30–33 mm Hg) to acutely reduce ICP. Note that more aggressive hyperventilation can decrease cerebral blood flow and potentially worsen ischemic injury.

Refs: Butterworth JF IV, Mackey DC, Wasnick JD. *Morgan & Mikhail's Clinical Anesthesiology*, 5th ed. New York, NY: McGraw Hill; 2013.
Mortazavi MM, Romeo AK, Deep A, et al. Hypertonic saline for treating raised intracranial pressure: literature review with meta-analysis. *J Neurosurg* 2012;116:210–221.

23. Preoperative assessment identifies a patient who chronically takes prednisone 25 mg PO once a day for asthma. The patient is scheduled for a major abdominal operation. What is a recommended course of action for perioperative corticosteroid management?

    (A) usual morning steroid dose, no supplementation required

    (B) usual morning steroid dose, single dose of hydrocortisone 25 mg

    (C) usual morning steroid dose, single dose of hydrocortisone 50 mg

    (D) usual morning steroid dose, hydrocortisone 50–100 mg q8h for 24 hours

    (E) usual morning steroid dose, hydrocortisone 200 mg/70 kg body weight q8h for 24 hours

A patient chronically taking corticosteroids undergoing a major "stress" operation should take their usual morning steroid dose and hydrocortisone 50–100 mg q8h for 24 hours.

Patients who chronically take steroids may be at risk of inadequate "stress response" perioperatively and potentially suffer significant hypotension or shock. Stress dose steroid coverage is a controversial topic and recommendations vary greatly as there is limited research evidence available. Most anesthesiology textbooks agree that hydrocortisone supplementation perioperatively should vary according to the invasiveness of the proposed surgical procedure:

- Minimal "stress" surgery = usual maintenance steroid dose + low dose hydrocortisone supplementation or no supplementation necessary.

- Intermediate "stress" surgery = usual maintenance steroid dose + hydrocortisone 25–50 mg q8h for 24 hours with either a short taper or resumption of usual dose.

- Major "stress" surgery = usual maintenance steroid dose + hydrocortisone 50–100 mg q8h for 24 hours with either a short taper or resumption of usual dose.

Refs: Garcia JE, Hill GE, Joshi GP. Perioperative stress dose steroids: is it really necessary? *ASA Newsletter* 2013;77(11): 32–35.
Miller RD. *Miller's Anesthesia*, 8th ed. Philadelphia, PA: Elsevier; 2015.

24. A 4-year-old pediatric patient is assessed preoperatively before surgery. The child is very anxious with significant separation anxiety and is noncooperative. In order to administer a sedative premedication for this child, what is the most reliable route of administration?

(A) rectal
(B) intramuscular
(C) sublingual
(D) intranasal
(E) oral

Intramuscular premedication is reliable and does not require cooperation; it is painful. Oral, sublingual, and intranasal routes of drug administration require a degree of cooperation and can be challenging if a child refuses or spits out the medication. Rectal medications are typically reserved for children still in diapers.

Ref: Miller RD. *Miller's Anesthesia*, 8th ed. Philadelphia, PA: Elsevier; 2015.

25. A geriatric patient is scheduled for surgery. Which of the following intravenous premedications is **least** likely to require a dosage adjustment?

(A) midazolam
(B) fentanyl
(C) dexmedetomidine
(D) ranitidine
(E) metoclopramide

For a geriatric patient, ranitidine is least likely to require dosage adjustment. In general, due to pharmacokinetic or pharmacodynamic changes, elderly patients often require a decreased dose of medication compared to younger adults. Ranitidine, due to age related decreases in renal function, may require a longer interval (q12–24h) for repeated dosing but the initial dose (50 mg IV) remains the same. Mainly due to changes in brain sensitivity, both midazolam and fentanyl require significant dosage reduction for geriatric patients. Dexmedetomidine may have a higher incidence of bradycardia and hypotension in patients younger than 65 years, and a dose reduction may be required. Geriatric patients may be at increased risk of side effects of metoclopramide (sedation, confusion, parkinsonian-like symptoms, and tardive dyskinesia) and a dosage reduction may be required.

Ref: Miller RD. *Miller's Anesthesia*, 8th ed. Philadelphia, PA: Elsevier; 2015.

26. During preoperative evaluation, a patient states that they are allergic to local anesthetics. Further history elucidates that the patient developed a cardiac arrhythmia after receiving an injection of 2% lidocaine with 1:200,000 epinephrine at a dentist's office. What is the most likely explanation for this reaction?

(A) anaphylactoid reaction to lidocaine
(B) allergic reaction to lidocaine
(C) allergy to para-aminobenzoic acid (PABA) preservative in local anesthetic solution
(D) adverse side effect due to epinephrine
(E) allergic reaction to epinephrine

Epinephrine in the local anesthetic solution can cause adverse side effects including palpitations. Patients may erroneously associate this with an "allergic" reaction.

PABA can be associated with allergies, but it is used with ester local anesthetics. True allergic or anaphylactoid reactions during anesthesia are relatively rare (1:6000).

Ref: Miller RD. *Miller's Anesthesia*, 8th ed. Philadelphia, PA: Elsevier; 2015.

27. An otherwise healthy 1-year-old infant is scheduled for elective surgery. For the child, whose diet is infant formula, what is the recommended preoperative fasting (NPO) period?

    (A) 2 hours
    (B) 4 hours
    (C) 6 hours
    (D) 8 hours
    (E) 10 hours

    The ASA practice guidelines suggest a fasting period of 6 hours for infants receiving formula and solids. For all age groups, a fasting period of 2 hours is recommended for clear fluids. For infants, a fasting period of 4 hours is recommended for breast milk. For noninfants, a fasting period of 6 hours is recommended after a light meal, and 8 hours after a meal of fatty or fried food.

    Ref: American Society of Anesthesiologists. Practice guidelines for preoperative fasting and the use of pharmacologic agents to reduce the risk of pulmonary aspiration: Application to healthy patients undergoing elective procedures. An updated report by the American Society of Anesthesiologists Task Force on Preoperative Fasting. *Anesthestology* 2011;114:495–511.

28. Which of the following factors **DOES NOT** increase the risk of pulmonary aspiration?

    (A) pregnancy
    (B) hiatal hernia
    (C) obesity without comorbidity
    (D) patients receiving acute opioid therapy
    (E) GERD

    Obesity and the risk of pulmonary aspiration is a controversial subject. Unfortunately major anesthesiology textbooks often disagree. Obese patients are at higher risk of hiatal hernia, GERD, and comorbidities including DM2. Research on obese patients and gastric emptying is not straightforward. Both delayed gastric emptying and faster gastric emptying have both been reported in obese patients. Most texts agree that obese patients without comorbidity associated with delayed emptying or esophageal sphincter incompetence are not at increased risk of pulmonary aspiration.

The patient with a "full stomach" or esophageal sphincter incompetence is considered at risk of pulmonary aspiration. This includes:

- pregnancy
- diabetes
- acute opioid therapy
- GERD
- hiatal hernia
- not NPO as per guidelines
- currently nauseous/vomiting

Ref: Butterworth JF IV, Mackey DC, Wasnick JD. *Morgan & Mikhail's Clinical Anesthesiology*, 5th ed. New York, NY: McGraw Hill; 2013.

29. A patient with normal airway anatomy is not NPO and is considered a "full stomach." A rapid sequence induction (RSI) is indicated. What are the classic components of an RSI in the order they are performed?

    (A) preoxygenation; cricoid pressure; propofol induction; rocuronium; endotracheal intubation
    (B) preoxygenation; awake fiberoptic laryngoscopy; endotracheal intubation
    (C) preoxygenation; cricoid pressure; propofol induction; mask ventilation; succinylcholine; endotracheal intubation
    (D) preoxygenation; propofol induction; succinylcholine; endotracheal intubation
    (E) preoxygenation; inhalation induction with sevoflurane; succinylcholine; endotracheal intubation

The classic components of a rapid sequence induction (RSI) are: preoxygenation, intravenous anesthesia, rapid-onset neuromuscular blockade, cricoid pressure, and endotracheal intubation. Both succinylcholine and rocuronium are considered rapid-onset neuromuscular blockers. Cricoid pressure, although controversial in its efficacy, is considered a classic component of an RSI.

Ref: Miller RD. *Miller's Anesthesia*, 8th ed. Philadelphia, PA: Elsevier; 2015.

30. Preoperatively, a patient is evaluated and felt to be at increased risk of pulmonary aspiration. Best evidence suggests which of the following preoperative pharmacologic agents is most effective at reducing gastric acidity?

    (A) metoclopramide

    (B) **ranitidine**

    (C) lansoprazole

    (D) ondansetron

    (E) glycopyrrolate

H$_2$ receptor antagonists (ranitidine, cimetidine) reduce gastric acidity and volume (Category A1 evidence). Proton pump inhibitors (lansoprazole, omeprazole) also reduce gastric acidity and volume (Category A2 evidence). There is equivocal evidence that anticholinergics (glycopyrrolate, atropine) reduce gastric acidity and volume (Category C2 evidence). Metoclopramide reduces gastric volume but there is equivocal evidence that is reduces gastric acidity (Category C1 evidence). Ondansetron reduces nausea and vomiting but does not alter gastric pH or motility.

   Evidence:

   • Category A1—multiple randomized controlled trials (RCTs), supported by meta-analysis.

   • Category A2—multiple RCTs, no meta-analysis.

   • Category B—suggestive literature

   • Category C1—meta-analysis did not find significant differences

   • Category C2—RCTs report inconsistent results or no differences, no meta-analysis.

   Ref: American Society of Anesthesiologists. Practice guidelines for preoperative fasting and the use of pharmacologic agents to reduce the risk of pulmonary aspiration: Application to healthy patients undergoing elective procedures. An updated report by the American Society of Anesthesiologists Task Force on Preoperative Fasting. *Anesthesiology* 2011;114:495–511.

31. Preoperatively, a patient is evaluated and felt to be at increased risk of pulmonary aspiration. Best evidence suggests which of the following preoperative pharmacologic agents is most effective at increasing lower esophageal sphincter (LES) tone?

    (A) **metoclopramide**

    (B) ranitidine

    (C) lansoprazole

    (D) ondansetron

    (E) glycopyrrolate

Metoclopramide increases LES tone and stimulates stomach and small intestine contractions. Ranitidine, lansoprazole, ondansetron, and sodium citrate have no effect on LES tone. A variety of factors will decrease LES tone including: cricoid pressure, hiatal hernia, and medications such as anticholinergics (atropine or glycopyrrolate), opioids, propofol, and inhaled anesthetics.

   Ref: Butterworth JF IV, Mackey DC, Wasnick JD. *Morgan & Mikhail's Clinical Anesthesiology*, 5th ed. New York, NY: McGraw Hill; 2013.

32. A patient is scheduled for elective knee arthroscopy. Three months ago, the patient had a myocardial infarction. Management at that time included percutaneous transluminal coronary angioplasty (PTCA) with placement of a single drug eluting stent (DES). The patient is currently on clopidogrel (Plavix). According to the American College of Cardiology and American Heart Association (ACC/AHA) guidelines, what is appropriate management for this elective surgery?

    (A) proceed with surgery and hold clopidogrel for 7 days preoperatively

    (B) proceed with surgery and hold clopidogrel for 10 days preoperatively

    (C) proceed with surgery and continue clopidogrel perioperatively

    (D) cancel surgery until patient completes at least 6 months of clopidogrel therapy

    (E) **cancel surgery until patient completes at least 12 months of clopidogrel therapy**

According to the 2014 ACC/AHA guidelines, elective noncardiac surgery is not recommended when clopidogrel therapy needs to be continued. The minimum prescribed time for clopidogrel therapy is 12 months for DES, and elective noncardiac surgery should optimally be delayed until after this time. For bare metal stents, the minimum prescribed time for clopidogrel therapy is 1 month. Elective noncardiac surgery should be delayed for 14 days following balloon angioplasty.

   Ref: Fleisher LA, Fleischmann KE, Auerbach AD, et al. 2014 ACC/AHA guidelines on perioperative cardiovascular evaluation and management of patients undergoing noncardiac surgery: a report of the American College of Cardiology/American Heart Association Task Force on practice guidelines. *J Am Coll Cardiol* 2014; 64:e77–137.

33. A patient's medical therapy for type 2 diabetes mellitus includes oral hypoglycemic agents. Which of the following medications should be discontinued at least 24 hours before surgery to reduce the risk of drug-induced lactic acidosis?

(A) glyburide

(B) glipizide

(C) gliclazide

(D) **metformin**

(E) repaglinide

Metformin (a biguanide) should be held for at least 24 hours preoperatively to reduce the risk of drug-induced lactic acidosis. The sulfonylurea class of medications includes glyburide, glipizide, and gliclazide; while repaglinide is a noninsulin secretagogue—none of which are associated with lactic acidosis.

Ref: Miller RD. *Miller's Anesthesia*, 8th ed. Philadelphia, PA: Elsevier; 2015.

34. A patient with medically managed hypertension is scheduled for ambulatory surgery. Antihypertensive medications, including an angiotensin II antagonist, are administered the morning of surgery. After anesthetic induction, refractory hypotension is noted. What is the best treatment?

(A) **vasopressin**

(B) ephedrine

(C) phenylephrine

(D) epinephrine

(E) norepinephrine

Vasopressin is the treatment of choice for refractory hypotension associated with the use of ACE inhibitors or angiotensin II antagonists. Antihypertensive medications are generally continued throughout the perioperative period, but conflicting opinion exists regarding the continuation or discontinuation of ACE inhibitors and angiotensin II antagonists because of increased risk of significant hypotension.

Ref: Miller RD. *Miller's Anesthesia*, 8th ed. Philadelphia, PA: Elsevier; 2015.

35. A patient is chronically on medical therapy for treatment of depression. The patient is scheduled for surgery and a preoperative anesthetic consultation is performed. Which antidepressant can cause rare, but serious, side effects associated with the use of opioids?

(A) amitriptyline

(B) fluoxetine

(C) trazodone

(D) bupropion

(E) **phenelzine**

Phenelzine is an irreversible inhibitor of the enzyme monoamine oxidase (MAO). Perioperatively, MAOIs can have serious interactions with indirect acting sympathomimetics (ephedrine, tyramine) and opioids. The reaction with opioids can present with hyperthermia, seizures, and coma. Typical recommendations are to discontinue irreversible MAOIs such as phenelzine for 2 to 3 weeks before surgery. Although other classes of antidepressants can have side effects related to their blockade of neurotransmitter reuptake, they should be continued throughout the perioperative period to avoid withdrawal symptoms or recurrence of psychiatric illness.

Refs: Miller RD. *Miller's Anesthesia*, 8th ed. Philadelphia, PA: Elsevier; 2015.

Butterworth JF IV, Mackey DC, Wasnick JD. *Morgan & Mikhail's Clinical Anesthesiology*, 5th ed. New York, NY: McGraw Hill; 2013.

36. A female patient with a complex medical history is taking multiple medications. Preoperative assessment should include instructions to discontinue which of the following medications before the day of surgery?

(A) oxycodone

(B) **conjugated estrogens**

(C) atorvastatin

(D) isosorbide dinitrate

(E) fluoxetine

Conjugated estrogens (Premarin) should be discontinued prior to surgery to reduce the potential risk related to development of perioperative DVT/PE. Most medications should be continued throughout the perioperative period. Exceptions are for: anticoagulants (warfarin, clopidogrel ± aspirin, NSAIDs, or COX-2 inhibitors depending on the type of surgery), oral hypoglycemics, insulin preparations, supplements (vitamins, herbals), phosphodiesterase 5 inhibitors (Viagra), topical medications (as absorption can vary during surgery and anesthesia), and MAOIs.

Ref: Miller RD. *Miller's Anesthesia*, 8th ed. Philadelphia, PA: Elsevier; 2015.

37. Perioperative beta-blocker therapy is recommended for a number of different clinical situations. According to the American College of Cardiology and American Heart Association (ACC/AHA) guidelines on perioperative cardiovascular evaluation and care for noncardiac surgery, the strongest recommendation for perioperative beta-blockade is for which of the following scenarios?

    (A) vascular surgery; patient without evidence of myocardial ischemia

    (B) intermediate-risk surgery; patient with one or more clinical risk factors for coronary heart disease

    (C) vascular surgery; patient with one or more clinical risk factors for coronary heart disease

    (D) intermediate-risk surgery; patient with known coronary heart disease

    (E) low-risk surgery; patient currently taking a beta-blocker

    Patients currently taking β-blocker therapy should continue therapy throughout the perioperative period (even for low-risk surgery). This is a Class I recommendation (*should* be performed). The guidelines emphasize that the management of beta-blockers after surgery should be dictated by clinical circumstances, regardless of when the drug was started (Class IIa recommendations). For example, hypotension, bleeding or bradycardia are all good reasons to hold/stop beta-blockers, and the potential harm of continuing these drugs in such settings likely outweighs any potential benefits. In patients with 3 or more Revised Cardiac Risk Index factors, it may be reasonable (Class IIb) to start beta blockers before surgery. However, if this is done, it should be done well enough in advance to be able to assess efficacy and tolerability. It is NOT recommended to start beta-blockers on the day of surgery (Class III, harm).

    Note, some sources may be out of date with respect to current perioperative beta-blockade guidelines. Early studies of perioperative beta blockade which demonstrated benefits including reduced mortality rates have NOT been borne out by more recent studies. The POISE study found perioperative beta blockade increased the risk of stroke and death from noncardiac complications. Further complicating the data, a number of studies by the Dutch researcher Poldermans were put into question with allegations of academic misconduct. Current ACC/AHA guidelines from 2014 have EXCLUDED ALL of the Poldermans studies (known as the Dutch Echocardiography Cardiac Risk Evaluation Applying Stress Echocardiography, or DECREASE, trials).

Note: Perioperative beta-blockade guidelines have been tainted by apparent fraudulent data. New research questions the validity of perioperative beta-blockade. Most anesthesiology texts are out of date with respect to these findings. Revisions to major guidelines are pending. Despite this, it is still recommended that a patient taking beta-blocker therapy continue with the medication throughout the perioperative period.

Ref: Fleisher LA, Fleischmann KE, Auerbach AD, et al. 2014 ACC/AHA guidelines on perioperative cardiovascular evaluation and management of patients undergoing noncardiac surgery: a report of the American College of Cardiology/American Heart Association Task Force on practice guidelines. *J Am Coll Cardiol* 2014;64:e77–137.

38. A patient with no known cardiac risk factors is scheduled for major vascular surgery. Which of the following techniques or medications should be used in order to reduce cardiac risk?

    (A) induced hypothermia

    (B) atorvastatin

    (C) clonidine

    (D) verapamil

    (E) dilutional anemia

    According to the American College of Cardiology and American Heart Association (ACC/AHA) guidelines on perioperative cardiovascular evaluation and care for noncardiac surgery, initiating statin therapy in patients not already on the drugs who are undergoing vascular surgery is a reasonable practice (Class IIa). Evidence suggests that statins stabilize atherosclerotic plaque and reduce mortality after vascular surgery. Other risk reduction strategies include alpha-2 agonists, and calcium channel blockers. However, the evidence is not as robust and alpha-2 agonists are recommended for perioperative control of hypertension in patients with known CAD or at least 1 clinical risk factor. The best evidence for calcium channel blockers is for diltiazem; with evidence of reduced ischemia and trends towards reduced mortality. Large scale trials for verapamil are needed. Other factors that are associated with **increased** perioperative risk and should be avoided include: hypothermia, anemia/polycythemia, unnecessary use of vasopressors, and prolonged operations.

Ref: Fleisher LA, Fleischmann KE, Auerbach AD, et al. 2014 ACC/AHA guidelines on perioperative cardiovascular evaluation and management of patients undergoing noncardiac surgery: a report of the American College of Cardiology/American Heart Association Task Force on practice guidelines. *J Am Coll Cardiol* 2014;64:e77–137.

39. An adult patient, with no known drug allergies, is scheduled for a total knee arthroplasty. The institutional incidence of surgical site infections (SSIs) caused by MRSA is less than 5%. In order to reduce the risk of SSI for this clean surgery, which of the following regimens for antibiotic prophylaxis is indicated?

    (A) no antibiotics indicated
    (B) cefazolin 1 g IV q3–4h
    (C) cefazolin 2 g IV q3–4h
    (D) vancomycin 1 g IV
    (E) metronidazole 500 mg IV

Cefazolin 2 g IV q3–4h is indicated to reduce the risk of SSI for a total joint arthroplasty in a patient without allergies. Most SSIs are due to gram-positive cocci (staphylococci) so first-generation cephalosporins are indicated. If the institution has a high rate of MRSA SSIs (>20% of all SSIs caused by MRSA) vancomycin is indicated. If the patient has a significant penicillin allergy, then either vancomycin or clindamycin is indicated. If anaerobic or gram-negative antibiotic coverage is desired, then a second-generation cephalosporin (e.g., cefoxitin) or cefazolin and metronidazole is indicated.

> **Ref:** Bratzler DW, Dellinger EP, Olsen KM, et al. Clinical practice guidelines for antimicrobial prophylaxis in surgery. *Am J Health Syst Pharm* 2013;70(3):195–283.

40. In an effort to reduce surgical site infections (SSIs), antibiotic prophylaxis is often administered preoperatively. What is the optimal time for administration of the preoperative dose?

    (A) within 30 minutes of surgical incision for cefazolin
    (B) within 2 hours of surgical incision for cefazolin
    (C) within 4 hours of surgical incision for cefazolin
    (D) within 1 hour of surgical incision for vancomycin
    (E) within 2 hours of surgical incision for ciprofloxacin

According to clinical practice guidelines for antimicrobial prophylaxis in surgery, the optimal time for administration of the preoperative dose is within 2 hours of surgical incision for ciprofloxacin or vancomycin. Cefazolin should be given within 60 minutes of surgical incision.

> **Ref:** Bratzler DW, Dellinger EP, Olsen KM, et al. Clinical practice guidelines for antimicrobial prophylaxis in surgery. *Am J Health Syst Pharm* 2013;70(3):195–283.

41. Which patient requires antibiotic prophylaxis for prevention of infective endocarditis?

    (A) patient with severe mitral valve prolapse (MVP) scheduled for routine dental cleaning
    (B) patient with a previous history of endocarditis scheduled for routine transesophageal echocardiography
    (C) patient with a prosthetic aortic valve scheduled for routine tonsillectomy
    (D) cardiac transplant recipient scheduled for routine bronchoscopy
    (E) patient with completely repaired congenital heart defect (15 years prior) scheduled for routine vaginal delivery

A patient with a prosthetic aortic valve scheduled for routine tonsillectomy requires antibiotic prophylaxis for prevention of infective endocarditis.

Cardiac conditions for which infective endocarditis prophylaxis may be reasonable include:

- Prosthetic cardiac valve
- Previous history of infective endocarditis
- Congenital heart disease (CHD):
  - unrepaired cyanotic CHD, including shunts
  - completely repaired CHD with prosthetic material (during first 6 months after procedure)
  - repaired CHD with residual defects near prosthetic material
- Cardiac transplant patients with valvular disease

Only patients with the aforementioned cardiac conditions require antibiotic prophylaxis if they undergo the following procedures:

- Dental procedures that involves manipulation of gingival tissue, periapical region of teeth, or disruption of oral mucosa.
- Respiratory tract mucosal incision or biopsy including tonsillectomy or adenoidectomy; or respiratory tract procedure to treat infection.
- GI or GU tract procedure with established GI or GU tract infection.
- Procedure involving infected skin or musculoskeletal tissue.

> **Ref:** Miller RD. *Miller's Anesthesia*, 8th ed. Philadelphia, PA: Elsevier; 2015.

General Anesthesia, Monitored Anesthetic Care, and Sedation

1. Guedel classically described four stages of anesthesia for inhalation anesthetics. Which of the following findings occurs only in the stage of "surgical anesthesia"?

    (A) unconsciousness and amnesia

    (B) apnea

    (C) no movement except respiration

    (D) increased muscular movement

    (E) hypertension and tachycardia

2. During a preoperative consultation, a patient expresses concern about anesthetic awareness for their upcoming surgery. A discussion of risk factors for anesthetic awareness ensues. Which of the following situations has the lowest likelihood of anesthetic awareness?

    (A) trauma surgery

    (B) caesarean section

    (C) maintenance of anesthesia with a BIS number of 60

    (D) maintenance of anesthesia with end-tidal anesthetic gas concentration >0.5 MAC

    (E) maintenance of anesthesia with nitrous oxide (N_2O)

3. Sevoflurane is used to perform an inhalation induction on a pediatric patient. Which of the following side effects is most likely?

    (A) laryngospasm

    (B) breath-holding

    (C) coughing

    (D) excitement

    (E) bronchospasm

4. For maintenance of anesthesia, a combined technique of isoflurane and fentanyl is selected. If fentanyl concentrations are maintained in the analgesic range, how is the MAC of isoflurane altered?

    (A) increased by 50%

    (B) increased by 25%

    (C) unchanged

    (D) decreased by 25%

    (E) decreased by 50%

5. As a sole intravenous anesthetic, propofol is selected for procedural sedation. What is typically suggested as the starting dose of propofol for sedation?

    (A) loading dose of 0.25–1 mg/kg

    (B) maintenance infusion of 50–150 mcg/kg/min

    (C) loading dose of 1–3 mcg/kg

    (D) maintenance infusion of 10–20 mcg/kg/min

    (E) loading dose of 0.5–1 mcg/kg

6. A patient requires an awake nasal fiberoptic intubation. Anesthesia of the nasal mucosa requires blockade of which sensory nerve?

    (A) glossopharyngeal nerve

    (B) vagus nerve

    (C) hypoglossal nerve

    (D) facial nerve

    (E) trigeminal nerve

7. A Cormack and Lehane grade 2 view is best described by which of the following?

    (A) full view of vocal cords

    (B) view of epiglottis only

    (C) view of soft palate only

    (D) view of arytenoid cartilages only

    (E) no view of vocal cords

8. The Mallampati classification is a preoperative airway screening test that attempts to identify patients "at risk" of difficult tracheal intubation. If a patient is identified as a Mallampati class 3 or 4 airway, what is the sensitivity of this test to actually predict difficult tracheal intubation?

   (A) 10%
   (B) 25%
   (C) 50%
   (D) 75%
   (E) 95%

9. Which of the following characteristics is NOT an independent predictor of difficult mask ventilation?

   (A) obstructive sleep apnea
   (B) age >40
   (C) BMI >30 kg/m²
   (D) limited mandibular protrusion
   (E) snoring

10. An otherwise normal patient is assessed preoperatively, and no concerns regarding difficult tracheal intubation are identified. However, the first attempt at tracheal intubation fails. According to the ASA practice guidelines for management of the difficult airway, from this point onward what is the initial consideration?

   (A) call for help
   (B) return patient to spontaneous ventilation
   (C) awaken the patient
   (D) place a laryngeal mask
   (E) initiate a surgical airway

11. Preoperative assessment identifies an otherwise well but uncooperative patient as potentially difficult to intubate. Of the following options, which is the preferred method to secure the airway?

   (A) propofol; rocuronium; direct laryngoscopy
   (B) propofol; succinylcholine; direct laryngoscopy
   (C) awake surgical airway
   (D) awake fiber-optic-guided intubation
   (E) inhalation induction; direct laryngoscopy

12. To facilitate tracheal intubation, a variety of medications may be used. Instead of an induction agent and a neuromuscular blocking drug, the use of an induction agent with remifentanil will result in:

   (A) better conditions for direct laryngoscopy
   (B) lower frequency of failed intubation
   (C) lower frequency of airway trauma
   (D) less hypotension
   (E) more difficult mask ventilation

13. A retrograde intubation technique traditionally includes which of the following steps?

   (A) patient placed supine with neck in flexion
   (B) insert the introducer needle at the level of the cricotracheal membrane
   (C) insert the introducer needle in a cephalad direction
   (D) confirm placement of the introducer needle position with aspiration of air
   (E) after passage of retrograde guide wire; retrograde passage of stiffer plastic sheath

14. Preoperatively, a patient is identified as difficult to intubate, and an awake intubation technique is attempted. However, the awake intubation technique is unsuccessful. Surgery cannot be canceled. After this failure of the awake intubation technique, which of the following is an option for noninvasive airway management?

   (A) surgical airway
   (B) face mask
   (C) percutaneous airway
   (D) jet ventilation
   (E) retrograde intubation

15. Which of the following videolaryngoscopes has a built-in channel for passage of the tracheal tube?

   (A) McGrath
   (B) GlideScope
   (C) Airtraq
   (D) C-Mac
   (E) DCI (direct coupler interface)

16. For tracheal intubation a paraglossal technique of laryngoscopy with a Miller laryngoscope is employed. Where is the optimal position for the tip of the Miller laryngoscope?

    (A) in the vallecula
    (B) in the piriform fossa
    (C) the posterior surface of epiglottis
    (D) in the esophagus
    (E) near the posterior pharyngeal wall

17. Flexible fiber-optic intubation is often performed for patients with difficult airways. However, there are certain clinical situations that increase the technical difficulty of flexible fiber-optic intubation. Which of the following situations makes flexible fiber-optic intubation LEAST likely to succeed?

    (A) small mouth opening
    (B) airway hemorrhage
    (C) upper airway tumor
    (D) facial deformity
    (E) unstable cervical spine

18. Which laryngoscope blade has a flexible tip that is operated by a lever on the handle?

    (A) McCoy
    (B) Macintosh
    (C) Miller
    (D) Magill
    (E) Wisconsin

19. Transillumination with a lighted stylet is a useful method to aid in tracheal intubation. For which one of the following situations is transillumination with a lighted stylet indicated?

    (A) patient with an unstable cervical spine
    (B) patient with an airway infection
    (C) patient with airway trauma
    (D) patient with an airway foreign body
    (E) patient with an airway tumor

20. A patient is induced with propofol and rocuronium. Tracheal intubation is attempted with direct laryngoscopy using a Macintosh blade. The epiglottis obscures the view of the vocal cords. A second attempt at tracheal intubation is performed. For the second attempt at tracheal intubation, which of the following techniques should be **avoided**?

    (A) blind nasotracheal intubation
    (B) direct laryngoscopy with Macintosh blade and gum elastic bougie
    (C) flexible fiber-optic intubation
    (D) intubating laryngeal mask airway
    (E) direct laryngoscopy with Miller blade

21. A laryngeal mask airway (LMA) is placed and the cuff is inflated to form an adequate seal for gas exchange. What is the maximum recommended cuff pressure for an LMA?

    (A) 20 cm H_2O
    (B) 30 cm H_2O
    (C) 40 cm H_2O
    (D) 50 cm H_2O
    (E) 60 cm H_2O

22. The original technique for laryngeal mask airway (LMA) placement includes which of the following steps?

    (A) patient is supine with neck extended
    (B) before insertion, the LMA cuff is inflated and lubricated
    (C) index finger presses tip of LMA cuff upward against the soft palate
    (D) LMA is advanced until cuff is no longer visible
    (E) LMA cuff is inflated and outward movement of the tube is observed

23. A supraglottic airway with drain tube access to the stomach (e.g., ProSeal laryngeal mask airway) is placed and positive-pressure ventilation is planned. Before the initiation of positive-pressure ventilation, which of the following methods is most helpful to confirm correct airway placement?

    (A) a self-inflating bulb is deflated and will not fill when placed at the drain tube
    (B) the presence of end-tidal CO_2
    (C) chest movement with manual ventilation
    (D) soapy film or gel placed at drain tube moves with positive-pressure ventilation
    (E) airway cuff leak at a minimum of 10 cm H_2O

24. A pre-hospital emergency medical services team uses a Combitube to manage a patient's airway. Which of the following is the best classification of a Combitube?

    (A) cuffed pharyngeal sealer without esophageal sealing
    (B) cuffed pharyngeal sealer with esophageal sealing
    (C) cuffed perilaryngeal sealer with nondirectional sealing
    (D) cuffed perilaryngeal sealer with directional sealing
    (E) uncuffed anatomically shaped sealer

25. A patient in a "cannot intubate, cannot ventilate" situation requires an emergency airway. For experienced and well-trained staff, which of the following techniques is generally the fastest way to insert a cuffed tube into the trachea?

    (A) surgical cricothyrotomy
    (B) surgical tracheotomy
    (C) needle cricothyrotomy
    (D) percutaneous dilational cricothyrotomy
    (E) percutaneous dilational tracheotomy

26. In a "cannot intubate, cannot ventilate" situation, a patient develops increasing hypoxemia. An emergency percutaneous airway is made with a needle (cannula) cricothyrotomy. Effective ventilation with this type of airway requires which of the following?

    (A) high-frequency jet ventilation
    (B) a flexible cannula
    (C) confirmation of exhalation through the upper airway
    (D) confirmation of tracheal position via aspiration of saline
    (E) an initial inflation pressure of at least 55 psi (4 kPa)

27. Of the various options for one-lung ventilation, which of the following methods allows for bronchoscopy to the isolated lung?

    (A) double-lumen tube
    (B) bronchial blocker
    (C) Univent tube
    (D) endobronchial tube
    (E) endotracheal tube advanced into bronchus

28. A left-sided double-lumen tube (DLT) needs to fit correctly within a patient's left bronchus. The patient is a male who is 180 cm (71 inches) tall. Based on sex and height, what is the correct size of DLT for this patient?

    (A) 32 Fr
    (B) 35 Fr
    (C) 37 Fr
    (D) 39 Fr
    (E) 41 Fr

29. Direct laryngoscopy is used to place a left-sided double-lumen tube (DLT). The DLT is turned 90 degrees counterclockwise after the endobronchial cuff passes the vocal cords. Which of the following methods is useful to confirm proper DLT placement in the left bronchus?

   (A) auscultation alone
   (B) bronchoscopy; tracheal view shows blue endobronchial cuff 5 mm above carina
   (C) bronchoscopy; right upper lobe view shows two orifices
   (D) bronchoscopy; left endobronchial view shows two orifices
   (E) bronchoscopy; endobronchial blocker in the right mainstem bronchus

30. In preparation for a thoracotomy and one-lung ventilation, a left-sided double-lumen tube (DLT) is placed without difficulty, and the patient is moved to the lateral position. During positioning, the endobronchial cuff migrates to a more proximal position. Which of the following complications is most likely?

   (A) protrusion of the endobronchial cuff into the surgical field
   (B) failure of the lung to collapse
   (C) subcutaneous emphysema
   (D) massive airway bleeding
   (E) unexpected air leak

31. Options for lung isolation and one-lung ventilation (OLV) include double-lumen tubes (DLTs) and bronchial blockers. Compared to a DLT, which of the following is an advantage of a bronchial blocker for OLV?

   (A) less time for airway positioning
   (B) bronchoscopy not necessary
   (C) easier for postoperative two-lung ventilation
   (D) easier to apply suction to the isolated lung
   (E) easier to alternate OLV to either lung

32. After completion of a thoracic surgery procedure, a patient requires postoperative ventilation. A left-sided double-lumen tube (DLT) was placed for the surgery. Rather than exchanging the DLT for a single lumen endotracheal tube, which of the following is a **benefit** of a DLT for postoperative ventilation?

   (A) less airflow resistance
   (B) decreased risk of lost airway
   (C) easier suctioning
   (D) less risk of airway edema
   (E) decreased risk of mucous plugging

33. A patient who requires a thoracotomy is difficult to intubate. A single lumen tube (SLT) is successfully placed. However, one-lung ventilation with a DLT is desired. An exchange catheter is used to switch the SLT to a DLT. Which of the following correctly describes how to use an exchange catheter?

   (A) place the patient supine with neck extended
   (B) select an exchange catheter that is flexible with no outer markings
   (C) select an exchange catheter at least 100 cm long
   (D) advance exchange catheter through the tracheal lumen of the DLT
   (E) insert exchange catheter no more than 24 cm at the lips

34. A bougie, or endotracheal tube introducer, is used to aid direct laryngoscopy and placement of an endotracheal tube. What is a relative contraindication for use of a bougie?

   (A) Grade III Cormack-Lehane view
   (B) suspected cervical spine injury
   (C) laryngeal disruption
   (D) pediatric patient
   (E) use of a videolaryngoscope

35. Which of the following tracheal tube introducers (or "intubating stylets") has the ability to jet ventilate a patient?

   (A) Eschmann tracheal tube introducer
   (B) Frova tracheal tube introducer
   (C) gum elastic bougie
   (D) SunMed tracheal tube introducer
   (E) Flex-Guide tracheal tube introducer

36. A tracheal tube introducer, or bougie, is selected to facilitate placement of a standard endotracheal tube (ETT). The tracheal tube introducer is successfully placed, but the ETT does not pass into the trachea. To facilitate passage of the ETT over the tracheal tube introducer, which of the following maneuvers should be attempted?

    (A) rotate the ETT 180 degrees clockwise
    (B) switch to a smaller diameter bougie
    (C) switch to a flexible ETT
    (D) remove the laryngoscope blade
    (E) switch to a larger diameter ETT

37. Direct laryngoscopy is performed on an adult patient. The larynx is not visualized and a blind technique with a tracheal tube introducer, or bougie, is attempted. Which of the following is most suggestive of successful placement of the bougie in the trachea?

    (A) no resistance to passage of entire bougie
    (B) tactile clicks during passage of bougie
    (C) proximal holdup at 10 cm
    (D) distal holdup at 50 cm
    (E) visualization of the bougie passing ventral to the epiglottis

38. An uncuffed endotracheal tube (ETT) is placed for a pediatric anesthetic. At peak inflation, what is an appropriate cuff leak pressure?

    (A) 15 cm H_2O
    (B) 25 cm H_2O
    (C) 35 cm H_2O
    (D) 45 cm H_2O
    (E) 55 cm H_2O

39. Compared to an uncuffed endotracheal tube (ETT) of the same size, what is an advantage of a *cuffed* ETT in young children?

    (A) less expensive
    (B) larger internal diameter
    (C) lower ETT exchange rate
    (D) lower risk of mucosal injury
    (E) less work of breathing for patient

40. An endotracheal tube (ETT) is placed using a flexible fiberoptic technique for a neurosurgical procedure. Which of the following ETTs may be prone to irreversible compression?

    (A) standard PVC ETT
    (B) microlaryngeal ETT
    (C) wire-reinforced ETT
    (D) Lanz valve ETT
    (E) nasal RAE ETT

41. An ENT surgeon plans to excise an adult patient's vocal cord lesion without using a laser. General anesthesia with airway protection and positive pressure ventilation is desired. For endotracheal tubes (ETTs) of comparable size, which type of ETT is the best choice?

    (A) standard PVC ETT
    (B) microlaryngeal ETT
    (C) wire-reinforced ETT
    (D) Lanz valve ETT
    (E) pediatric ETT

42. In the ICU, a critically ill patient requires intubation and positive pressure ventilation. In order to reduce the risk of microaspiration and ventilator-associated pneumonia (VAP), a number of ETT design modifications have been proposed. Which of the following ETT designs or features may reduce the risk of microaspiration or VAP?

    (A) use of high volume–low pressure (HVLP) cuff rather than a high pressure-low volume (HPLV) cuff
    (B) use of a polyurethane cuff rather than a polyvinyl chloride cuff
    (C) use of barrel-shaped cuff rather than a tapered cuff
    (D) maintenance of HVLP cuff pressure at 15 cm H_2O with a pneumatic valve
    (E) intermittent aspiration of tracheal secretions rather than continuous aspiration of subglottic secretions

43. Endotracheal tubes (ETTs) can be made with a variety of materials including latex, silicone, polyvinyl chloride (PVC), or polyurethane (PU). In order to reduce the risk of airway mucosal injury, most ETT cuff designs are *high volume–low pressure (HVLP)*. However, there are ETT cuffs that are *high pressure–low volume (HPLV)*. Which of the following ETTs has a *HPLV* cuff?

    (A) standard PVC ETT
    (B) silicone ETT for intubating LMA
    (C) PVC ETT with Lanz valve
    (D) PVC ETT with tapered cuff
    (E) PU ETT with tapered cuff and drain for subglottic secretions

44. Laser surgery of the airway requires the selection of a laser-safe endotracheal tube (ETT). Which of the following ETTs is NOT approved by the Food and Drug Administration (FDA) as laser resistant?

    (A) flexible stainless steel with plastic surface
    (B) red rubber with copper foil wrap
    (C) silicone with aluminum wrap and Teflon coating
    (D) silicone with layer of aluminum powder in silicone
    (E) PVC wrapped in aluminum foil tape

45. There are a variety of ways to assess endotracheal tube cuff pressures. How does an endotracheal tube with the Lanz system ensure adequate cuff pressure?

    (A) uses a pressure limiting valve
    (B) requires a manometer
    (C) measures minimal occlusive volume
    (D) performs a minimal leak test
    (E) requires palpation of the pilot balloon

46. A patient is scheduled for a laparoscopic hemicolectomy. For general anesthesia, which of the following is NOT an ASA standard monitor?

    (A) low oxygen concentration alarm
    (B) Foley catheter
    (C) continuous electrocardiogram
    (D) temperature probe
    (E) measurement of volume of expired gas

47. According to the ASA practice guidelines for sedation and analgesia by nonanesthesiologists, the definition of moderate or "conscious" sedation includes which of the following features?

    (A) purposeful response to verbal stimuli
    (B) cardiovascular function may be impaired
    (C) airway intervention may be required
    (D) spontaneous ventilation may be inadequate
    (E) unarousable to painful stimuli

48. Which of the following is the LEAST acceptable technique for providing sedation during a minor surgical procedure?

    (A) intermittent boluses of propofol
    (B) continuous infusion of propofol
    (C) target controlled infusion of propofol
    (D) continuous infusion of dexmedetomidine
    (E) intermittent boluses of fentanyl and droperidol

49. According to closed-claims data, which of the following mechanisms is the most likely to cause injury leading to litigation following monitored anesthetic care (MAC)?

    (A) respiratory event
    (B) inadequate oxygenation or ventilation
    (C) cardiovascular event
    (D) equipment failure of malfunction
    (E) cautery fires

50. According to the American Society of Anesthesiologists Practice Guidelines for Sedation and Analgesia by Non-Anesthesiologists, which of the following is TRUE regarding moderate sedation?

    (A) The fasting time for a meal of tea and toast is 4 hours.
    (B) A designated individual may engage both in monitoring of the patient and assisting the practitioner performing the procedure.
    (C) Propofol is associated with an increased incidence of adverse outcomes compared to midazolam.
    (D) Patients receiving moderate sedation for brief procedures may bypass the recovery room and proceed straight to discharge.
    (E) Fixed combinations of sedatives and analgesics provide good patient satisfaction while reducing risks for adverse events.

Answers and Explanations: General Anesthesia, Monitored Anesthetic Care, and Sedation

1. Guedel classically described four stages of anesthesia for inhalation anesthetics. Which of the following findings occurs only in the stage of "surgical anesthesia"?

   (A) unconsciousness and amnesia
   (B) apnea
   (C) **no movement except respiration**
   (D) increased muscular movement
   (E) hypertension and tachycardia

   Although Guedel's four stages and signs of anesthesia are mostly of historic interest, it is still frequently referenced:

   - Stage 1: awake to unconscious, analgesia increases
   - Stage 2: "excitement" stage to onset of automatic breathing, sympathetic activity (hypertension, tachycardia), purposeless movements, irregular respiration
   - Stage 3: "surgical anesthesia," regular breathing, stable heart rate and blood pressure, no movement except respiration
   - Stage 4: anesthetic overdose, from cessation of respiration and collapse of circulation to death

   Refs: Hewer CL. The stages and signs of general anaesthesia. *Br Med J*.1937;2(3996):274–276.
   Urban BW, Bleckwenn M. Concepts and correlations relevant to general anaesthesia. *Br J Anaesth*. 2002;89(1):3–16.

2. During a preoperative consultation, a patient expresses concern about anesthetic awareness for their upcoming surgery. A discussion of risk factors for anesthetic awareness ensues. Which of the following situations has the lowest likelihood of anesthetic awareness?

   (A) trauma surgery
   (B) caesarean section

   (C) **maintenance of anesthesia with a BIS number of 60**
   (D) maintenance of anesthesia with end-tidal anesthetic gas concentration >0.5 MAC
   (E) maintenance of anesthesia with nitrous oxide (N₂O)

   Evidence suggests a maintenance anesthetic using a BIS-guided technique with the BIS titrated to 40 to 60 is effective at preventing awareness (as is an end-tidal anesthetic gas concentration >0.7 MAC). Anesthetic awareness can occur with:

   - low anesthetic delivery: error or interruption of delivery; use of only N₂O for maintenance anesthesia
   - patients with low cardiovascular reserve: pregnancy, hypovolemia, or cardiac failure (caesarean section, cardiac surgery, emergency surgery, trauma surgery)
   - patients with high anesthetic requirement: tolerance to sedative medications (chronic alcohol, benzodiazepine, or opioid use)

   Ref: Miller RD. *Miller's Anesthesia*, 8th ed. Philadelphia, PA: Elsevier; 2015.

3. Sevoflurane is used to perform an inhalation induction on a pediatric patient. Which of the following side effects is most likely?

   (A) laryngospasm
   (B) breath-holding
   (C) coughing
   (D) **excitement**
   (E) bronchospasm

   Of the listed complications, excitement during induction is the most common side effect of a sevoflurane induction (14%). Inhalation induction with sevoflurane is a common technique for pediatric patients. Other complications with this technique include:

- laryngospasm (3%)
- breath-holding (5%)
- coughing (6%)
- bronchospasm (0.3%)

Ref: Miller RD. *Miller's Anesthesia*, 8th ed. Philadelphia, PA: Elsevier; 2015.

4. For maintenance of anesthesia, a combined technique of isoflurane and fentanyl is selected. If fentanyl concentrations are maintained in the analgesic range, how is the MAC of isoflurane altered?

(A) increased by 50%
(B) increased by 25%
(C) unchanged
(D) decreased by 25%
(E) decreased by 50%

If fentanyl is maintained in the analgesic range, the MAC of isoflurane is reduced by 50%. MAC is a measure of anesthetic gas that prevents movement after surgical incision in 50% of patients. Balanced anesthesia with an opioid and a volatile anesthetic results in a decrease in the MAC of the volatile anesthetic.

Ref: Miller RD. *Miller's Anesthesia*, 8th ed. Philadelphia, PA: Elsevier; 2015.

5. As a sole intravenous anesthetic, propofol is selected for procedural sedation. What is typically suggested as the starting dose of propofol for sedation?

(A) loading dose of 0.25–1 mg/kg
(B) maintenance infusion of 50–150 mcg/kg/min
(C) loading dose of 1–3 mcg/kg
(D) maintenance infusion of 10–20 mcg/kg/min
(E) loading dose of 0.5–1 mcg/kg

The dose of propofol for sedation is typically suggested as a loading dose of 0.25–1 mg/kg and a maintenance infusion of 10–50 mcg/kg/min. For anesthesia, the dose of propofol is suggested as a loading dose 1–2 mg/kg and a maintenance infusion of 50–150 mcg/kg/min. For sedation, a suggested loading dose of fentanyl is 1–3 mcg/kg. For sedation, a suggested maintenance dose of ketamine is 10–20 mcg/kg/min. For sedation, a

suggested loading dose of dexmedetomidine is 0.5–1 mcg/kg (over 10 minutes).

Ref: Miller RD. *Miller's Anesthesia*, 8th ed. Philadelphia, PA: Elsevier; 2015.

6. A patient requires an awake nasal fiberoptic intubation. Anesthesia of the nasal mucosa requires blockade of which sensory nerve?

(A) glossopharyngeal nerve
(B) vagus nerve
(C) hypoglossal nerve
(D) facial nerve
(E) trigeminal nerve

Anesthesia of the nasal mucosa requires blockade of the trigeminal nerve (the ophthalmic branch, V1, innervates the anterior portion of the nasal mucosa and the maxillary branch, V2, innervates the posterior portion of the nasal mucosa). The glossopharyngeal nerve innervates the oral mucosa and the posterior 1/3 of the tongue. The vagus nerve provides sensory innervation to the trachea below the epiglottis. The hypoglossal nerve provides the motor supply of the tongue. A branch of the facial nerve (chorda tympani) supplies taste to the anterior 2/3 of the tongue.

Ref: Butterworth JF IV, Mackey DC, Wasnick JD. *Morgan & Mikhail's Clinical Anesthesiology*, 5th ed. New York, NY: McGraw Hill; 2013.

7. A Cormack and Lehane grade 2 view is best described by which of the following?

(A) full view of vocal cords
(B) view of epiglottis only
(C) view of soft palate only
(D) view of arytenoid cartilages only
(E) no view of vocal cords

A Cormack and Lehane grade 2 view includes a partial view of the vocal cords and a full view of the arytenoid cartilage. The modified Cormack/Lehane grading system is shown in Figure 26-1.

- Grade 1: Full view of vocal cords
- Grade 2a: Partial view of vocal cords
- Grade 2b: View of arytenoid cartilages only
- Grade 3a: View of epiglottis only, no vocal cords (epiglottis able to be lifted off posterior hypopharynx)

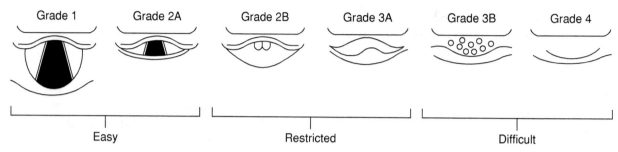

FIG. 26-1. Modified Cormack/Lehane grading system of laryngoscopic view. (Reproduced with permission from Hung O, Murphy MF. *Management of the difficult and failed airway*, 2nd ed. New York, NY: McGraw Hill; 2012.)

- Grade 3b: View of epiglottis only, no vocal cords (epiglottis cannot be lifted off posterior hypopharynx)
- Grade 4: View of soft palate only, no epiglottis

Ref: Hung O, Murphy MF. *Management of the Difficult and Failed Airway*, 2nd ed. New York, NY: McGraw Hill; 2012.

8. The Mallampati classification is a preoperative airway screening test that attempts to identify patients "at risk" of difficult tracheal intubation. If a patient is identified as a Mallampati class 3 or 4 airway, what is the sensitivity of this test to actually predict difficult tracheal intubation?

    (A) 10%
    (B) 25%
    (C) 50%
    (D) 75%
    (E) 95%

If a patient is identified as a Mallampati class 3 or 4 airway, there is an ~50% likelihood that the patient will actually be difficult to intubate (sensitivity = ~50%). There are a variety of bedside screening tests that attempt to identify those patients "at risk" of difficult tracheal intubation. Unfortunately, there is no ideal bedside screening test, as sensitivity (true positives) and specificity (true negatives) tend to be unsatisfactory.

Refs: Hung O, Murphy MF. *Management of the Difficult and Failed Airway*, 2nd ed. New York, NY: McGraw Hill; 2012.

Shiga T, Wajima Z, Inoue T, et al. Predicting difficult intubation in apparently normal patients: a meta-analysis of bedside screening test performance. *Anesthesiology* 2005; 103(2):429–437.

9. Which of the following characteristics is NOT an independent predictor of difficult mask ventilation?

    (A) obstructive sleep apnea
    (B) age >40
    (C) BMI >30 kg/m²
    (D) limited mandibular protrusion
    (E) snoring

Age >57 is an independent predictor of difficult mask ventilation. Other independent predictors of difficult mask ventilation include:

- BMI >30 kg/m²
- presence of a beard
- history of snoring
- history of obstructive sleep apnea
- limited mandibular protrusion
- thick/obese neck anatomy

Refs: Miller RD. *Miller's Anesthesia*, 8th ed. Philadelphia, PA: Elsevier; 2015.

Kheterpal S, Han R, Tremper KK, et al. Incidence and predictors of difficult and impossible mask ventilation. *Anesthesiology* 2006;105:885–891.

10. An otherwise normal patient is assessed preoperatively, and no concerns regarding difficult tracheal intubation are identified. However, the first attempt at tracheal intubation fails. According to the ASA practice guidelines for management of the difficult airway, from this point onward what is the initial consideration?

    (A) call for help
    (B) return patient to spontaneous ventilation
    (C) awaken the patient
    (D) place a laryngeal mask
    (E) initiate a surgical airway

According to the ASA practice guidelines for management of the difficult airway, after the initial intubation attempt fails, the first consideration is to call for help. The ASA difficult airway algorithm has a pathway for the unanticipated difficult airway. After the initial intubation attempt is unsuccessful, the practitioner is supposed to consider:

- calling for help
- returning patient to spontaneous ventilation
- awakening the patient

The next step is to determine if face mask ventilation is adequate with or without a supraglottic airway. Depending on the adequacy of ventilation, the patient will enter either the "nonemergency" pathway or the "emergency" pathway.

Ref: Apfelbaum JL, Hagberg CA, Caplan RA, et al. Practice guidelines for management of the difficult airway—an updated report by the American Society of Anesthesiologists task force on management of the difficult airway. *Anesthesiology* 2013;118(2):251–270.

11. Preoperative assessment identifies an otherwise well but uncooperative patient as potentially difficult to intubate. Of the following options, which is the preferred method to secure the airway?

(A) propofol; rocuronium; direct laryngoscopy

(B) propofol; succinylcholine; direct laryngoscopy

(C) awake surgical airway

(D) awake fiber-optic-guided intubation

(E) **inhalation induction; direct laryngoscopy**

If a patient is uncooperative yet potentially difficult to intubate, an inhalation induction that preserves spontaneous ventilation followed by direct laryngoscopy (or other airway management technique) is the preferred method of securing the airway. According to the ASA practice guidelines for management of the difficult airway, an uncooperative patient may limit the options for airway management, particularly awake techniques. Techniques that abolish spontaneous ventilation should also be avoided in situations where difficult intubation is anticipated.

Refs: Apfelbaum JL, Hagberg CA, Caplan RA, et al. Practice guidelines for management of the difficult airway—an updated report by the American Society of Anesthesiologists task force on management of the difficult airway. *Anesthesiology* 2013;118(2):251–270.

Miller RD. *Miller's Anesthesia*, 8th ed. Philadelphia, PA: Elsevier; 2015.

12. To facilitate tracheal intubation, a variety of medications may be used. Instead of an induction agent and a neuromuscular blocking drug, the use of an induction agent with remifentanil will result in:

(A) better conditions for direct laryngoscopy

(B) lower frequency of failed intubation

(C) lower frequency of airway trauma

(D) less hypotension

(E) **more difficult mask ventilation**

The use of an induction agent with remifentanil will result in more difficult mask ventilation, due to either vocal cord closure or chest wall rigidity, compared to a technique with an induction agent and a neuromuscular blocking drug. Other disadvantages of an induction agent and remifentanil technique to facilitate tracheal intubation include:

- poorer conditions for tracheal intubation
- higher frequency of failed intubation
- higher frequency of airway trauma
- hypotension is more likely

Ref: Miller RD. *Miller's Anesthesia*, 8th ed. Philadelphia, PA: Elsevier; 2015.

13. A retrograde intubation technique traditionally includes which of the following steps?

(A) patient placed supine with neck in flexion

(B) insert the introducer needle at the level of the cricotracheal membrane

(C) insert the introducer needle in a cephalad direction

(D) **confirm placement of the introducer needle position with aspiration of air**

(E) after passage of retrograde guide wire; retrograde passage of stiffer plastic sheath

Although there are many variations, retrograde intubation technique typically involves the following steps:

- patient positioned supine with neck in extension
- the introducer needle insertion site is at the level of the *cricothyroid* membrane
- the introducer needle is inserted directly *posteriorly* with the bevel in a cephalad direction to minimize risk of vocal cord injury

- confirm placement of the introducer needle in the trachea with aspiration of air
- after passage of the retrograde guide wire, some retrograde intubation sets include a stiffer plastic catheter that is introduced via the nose or mouth over the retrograde guide wire.

Ref: Miller RD. *Miller's Anesthesia*, 8th ed. Philadelphia, PA: Elsevier; 2015.

14. Preoperatively, a patient is identified as difficult to intubate, and an awake intubation technique is attempted. However, the awake intubation technique is unsuccessful. Surgery cannot be canceled. After this failure of the awake intubation technique, which of the following is an option for noninvasive airway management?

    (A) surgical airway

    (B) face mask

    (C) percutaneous airway

    (D) jet ventilation

    (E) retrograde intubation

    If an awake intubation strategy fails and surgery cannot be canceled, face mask anesthesia is an option for noninvasive airway management. According to the ASA practice guidelines for management of the difficult airway, if the primary strategy of awake intubation fails, there are three options:

    - cancel the case
    - invasive airway access—surgical or percutaneous airway, jet ventilation, or retrograde intubation
    - other options—face mask, supraglottic airway, local anesthesia, or regional nerve block.

    Ref: Apfelbaum JL, Hagberg CA, Caplan RA, et al. Practice guidelines for management of the difficult airway—an updated report by the American Society of Anesthesiologists task force on management of the difficult airway. *Anesthesiology* 2013;118(2):251–270.

15. Which of the following videolaryngoscopes has a built-in channel for passage of the tracheal tube?

    (A) McGrath

    (B) GlideScope

    (C) Airtraq

    (D) C-Mac

    (E) DCI (direct coupler interface)

    The Airtraq video laryngoscope has a built-in channel for passage of the tracheal tube. Other examples of vid-

eolaryngoscopes with built-in channels for the tracheal tube include the Bullard laryngoscope and the AirWay laryngoscope. The McGrath, GlideScope, C-Mac, and DCI video laryngoscopes do not have built-in channels for passage of the tracheal tube and typically they require a rigid stylet to aid tracheal tube placement.

Ref: Butterworth JF IV, Mackey DC, Wasnick JD. *Morgan & Mikhail's Clinical Anesthesiology*, 5th ed. New York, NY: McGraw Hill; 2013.

16. For tracheal intubation a paraglossal technique of laryngoscopy with a Miller laryngoscope is employed. Where is the optimal position for the tip of the Miller laryngoscope?

    (A) in the vallecula

    (B) in the piriform fossa

    (C) the posterior surface of epiglottis

    (D) in the esophagus

    (E) near the posterior pharyngeal wall

    The optimal position for the tip of the Miller laryngoscope is the posterior surface of the epiglottis. If a paraglossal technique of laryngoscopy with a Miller laryngoscope is employed and the larynx is not visible, the tip of the laryngoscope is likely in the:

    - vallecula
    - piriform fossa
    - esophagus
    - posterior pharyngeal wall.

    The optimal position for the tip of a Macintosh laryngoscope is in the vallecula.

    Ref: Miller RD. *Miller's Anesthesia*, 8th ed. Philadelphia, PA: Elsevier; 2015.

17. Flexible fiber-optic intubation is often performed for patients with difficult airways. However, there are certain clinical situations that increase the technical difficulty of flexible fiber-optic intubation. Which of the following situations makes flexible fiber-optic intubation LEAST likely to succeed?

    (A) small mouth opening

    (B) airway hemorrhage

    (C) upper airway tumor

    (D) facial deformity

    (E) unstable cervical spine

    Flexible fiber-optic intubation is least likely to succeed in the presence of airway hemorrhage, as bleeding can obscure the field of view, leading to "red-out" and inability to identify anatomic landmarks. Flexible fiber-optic intubation is useful in a variety of potentially difficult airway scenarios including:

- small mouth opening
- upper airway obstruction (tumor or angioedema)
- facial deformities or trauma
- minimizing cervical spine movement

Ref: Miller RD. *Miller's Anesthesia*, 8th ed. Philadelphia, PA: Elsevier; 2015.

18. Which laryngoscope blade has a flexible tip that is operated by a lever on the handle?

(A) **McCoy**
(B) Macintosh
(C) Miller
(D) Magill
(E) Wisconsin

The McCoy laryngoscope blade is curved and has a flexible tip that is operated by a lever on the handle. The Macintosh blade is a curved laryngoscope blade while the Miller, Magill, and Wisconsin blades are examples of straight laryngoscope blades.

Refs: Butterworth JF IV, Mackey DC, Wasnick JD. *Morgan & Mikhail's Clinical Anesthesiology*, 5th ed. New York, NY: McGraw Hill; 2013.

Gabbott DA. Laryngoscopy using the McCoy laryngoscope after application of a cervical collar. *Anaesthesia* 1996; 51(9):812–814.

19. Transillumination with a lighted stylet is a useful method to aid in tracheal intubation. For which one of the following situations is transillumination with a lighted stylet indicated?

(A) **patient with an unstable cervical spine**
(B) patient with an airway infection
(C) patient with airway trauma
(D) patient with an airway foreign body
(E) patient with an airway tumor

A lighted stylet is a blind technique that has been used successfully in patients with cervical spine disorders. Contraindications to this technique include airway tumors, infection, trauma, and foreign bodies.

Ref: Miller RD. *Miller's Anesthesia*, 8th ed. Philadelphia, PA: Elsevier; 2015.

20. A patient is induced with propofol and rocuronium. Tracheal intubation is attempted with direct laryngoscopy using a Macintosh blade. The epiglottis obscures the view of the vocal cords. A second attempt at tracheal intubation is performed. For the second attempt at tracheal intubation, which of the following techniques should be **avoided**?

(A) **blind nasotracheal intubation**
(B) direct laryngoscopy with Macintosh blade and gum elastic bougie
(C) flexible fiber-optic intubation
(D) intubating laryngeal mask airway
(E) direct laryngoscopy with Miller blade

A secondary plan for tracheal intubation should always be ready if the initial plan for tracheal intubation fails. A secondary plan of blind nasotracheal intubation should be avoided in a patient who is not breathing spontaneously. Blind nasotracheal intubation is performed on patients breathing spontaneously (either under anesthesia or awake). Tracheal tube placement is guided by noting changes in breath sounds. Blind nasotracheal intubation performed on an apneic patient increases the likelihood of failure and trauma. Other options for tracheal intubation after failure of direct laryngoscopy include:

- same laryngoscope with use of tracheal tube introducer (bougie or stylet)
- different laryngoscope blade (Miller)
- flexible fiber-optic laryngoscope
- intubating supraglottic airway device (intubating laryngeal mask airway)

Ref: Miller RD. *Miller's Anesthesia*, 8th ed. Philadelphia, PA: Elsevier; 2015.

21. A laryngeal mask airway (LMA) is placed and the cuff is inflated to form an adequate seal for gas exchange. What is the maximum recommended cuff pressure for an LMA?

(A) 20 cm H_2O
(B) 30 cm H_2O
(C) 40 cm H_2O
(D) 50 cm H_2O
(E) **60 cm H_2O**

The maximum recommended cuff pressure for an LMA is 60 cm H_2O. Higher pressures can decrease pharyngeal mucosal perfusion and cause nerve injury. A manometer is used to measure cuff pressure. A cuff *leak* pressure of at least 20 cm H_2O is a useful test to assess the position and function of a laryngeal mask airway.

Ref: Miller RD. *Miller's Anesthesia*, 8th ed. Philadelphia, PA: Elsevier; 2015.

22. The original technique for laryngeal mask airway (LMA) placement includes which of the following steps?

    (A)   patient is supine with neck extended
    (B)   before insertion, the LMA cuff is inflated and lubricated
    (C)   index finger presses tip of LMA cuff upward against the soft palate
    (D)   LMA is advanced until cuff is no longer visible
    (E)   **LMA cuff is inflated and outward movement of the tube is observed**

    The original technique for LMA placement includes LMA cuff inflation and outward movement of the tube. The original technique for LMA placement is as follows:

    • patient is placed in a "sniffing" position (neck flexed and head extended)
    • before insertion, the LMA cuff is *deflated* and lubricated
    • index finger presses the tip of LMA cuff upward against the *hard* palate
    • LMA is advanced until definite resistance is felt
    • LMA cuff is inflated and outward movement of the tube is observed

    Ref: Miller RD. *Miller's Anesthesia*, 8th ed. Philadelphia, PA: Elsevier; 2015.

23. A supraglottic airway with drain tube access to the stomach (e.g., ProSeal laryngeal mask airway) is placed and positive-pressure ventilation is planned. Before the initiation of positive-pressure ventilation, which of the following methods is most helpful to confirm correct airway placement?

    (A)   **a self-inflating bulb is deflated and will not fill when placed at the drain tube**
    (B)   the presence of end-tidal CO_2
    (C)   chest movement with manual ventilation
    (D)   soapy film or gel placed at drain tube moves with positive-pressure ventilation
    (E)   airway cuff leak at a minimum of 10 cm H_2O

    A supraglottic airway with drain tube access to the esophagus and stomach (e.g., ProSeal LMA) is correctly positioned when the drain tube is at the upper esophageal sphincter. The upper esophageal sphincter is a potential space and is generally collapsed. Thus, the airway position is confirmed when a self-inflating bulb is deflated and will not fill when placed at the drain tube. (If the airway is malpositioned in the hypopharynx or glottic opening, the deflated bulb will refill.) This is particularly important for positive-pressure ventilation, as a malpositioned airway can lead to gastric distension and aspiration. There are a variety of other tests to check the placement of a supraglottic airway device with drain tube access to the esophagus and stomach. These include:

    • observation of chest movement with manual ventilation
    • capnography
    • cuff leak pressure >20 cm H_2O
    • soapy film or gel placed at drain tube does not move with positive pressure ventilation (or airway pressures of at least 20 cm H_2O)
    • examination with a flexible fiber-optic laryngoscope

    Note that observation of chest movement with manual ventilation, capnography, and cuff leak pressure >20 cm H_2O help confirm the airway's ability to ventilate the patient but do not confirm that the tip of the airway is placed in the upper esophageal sphincter.

    Ref: Miller RD. *Miller's Anesthesia*, 8th ed. Philadelphia, PA: Elsevier; 2015.

24. A pre-hospital emergency medical services team uses a Combitube to manage a patient's airway. Which of the following is the best classification of a Combitube?

    (A)   cuffed pharyngeal sealer without esophageal sealing
    (B)   **cuffed pharyngeal sealer with esophageal sealing**
    (C)   cuffed perilaryngeal sealer with nondirectional sealing
    (D)   cuffed perilaryngeal sealer with directional sealing
    (E)   uncuffed anatomically shaped sealer

    A Combitube is a cuffed pharyngeal sealer with esophageal sealing. Another example of this type of airway device includes the laryngeal tube. There are many classifications for supraglottic airways. A basic classification includes:

    • Perilaryngeal sealers:
      • nondirectional sealing (e.g., LMA)

- directional sealing (e.g., ProSeal LMA)
- Pharyngeal sealers:
  - without esophageal sealing (e.g., Cobra or COPA)
  - with esophageal sealing (Combitube)
- Uncuffed preshaped sealers (e.g., SLIPA or I-gel)

Refs: Miller RD. *Miller's Anesthesia*, 8th ed. Philadelphia, PA: Elsevier; 2015.

Jolliffe L, Jackson I. Airway management in the outpatient setting: new devices and techniques. *Curr Opin Anaesthesiol* 2008;21:719–722.

25. A patient in a "cannot intubate, cannot ventilate" situation requires an emergency airway. For experienced and well-trained staff, which of the following techniques is generally the fastest way to insert a cuffed tube into the trachea?

(A) surgical cricothyrotomy

(B) surgical tracheotomy

(C) needle cricothyrotomy

(D) percutaneous dilational cricothyrotomy

(E) percutaneous dilational tracheotomy

For experienced and well-trained staff, a surgical cricothyrotomy is the fastest way to insert a cuffed tube into the trachea (within 30 seconds). The technique requires a No. 20 scalpel to make a horizontal incision, insertion of a tracheal hook, caudal and outward traction on the cricoid cartilage with the tracheal hook, and insertion of the cuffed tube. Anesthesiologists may not be as familiar with the surgical cricothyrotomy and prefer the percutaneous dilational cricothyrotomy (Seldinger cricothyrotomy). This procedure is fast, safe, and easily learned, especially by physicians who are familiar with Seldinger techniques for vascular access. The cricothyroid membrane is punctured using a needle attached to a syringe filled with fluid so that the presence of air bubbles alerts the operator to correct needle placement within the trachea. A wire is inserted through the needle into the trachea and advanced caudally. A curved plastic 5 mm internal diameter airway catheter with internal dilator is advanced over the wire into the trachea and then the dilator removed. This can then be connected via a standard 15 mm connector to a bag-valve-mask or ventilator.

Surgical *tracheotomy* with skin incision, separation of strap muscles, +/− division of the isthmus of the thyroid gland, incision of the anterior wall of the trachea, and placement of a cuffed tube takes a few minutes even for the most skilled surgeon. The percutaneous dilational tracheotomy is an elective procedure performed under bronchoscopic guidance with a guidewire and progressive dilation. Needle (cannula) cricothyrotomy, where a large-gauge IV catheter is inserted through the cricothyroid membrane and attached to a jet ventilator, is fast but does not result in placement of a cuffed tube into the trachea. Note: tracheotomy refers to a surgical procedure; tracheostomy refers to the resulting stoma or hole. The terms are often used interchangeably.

Ref: Miller RD. *Miller's Anesthesia*, 8th ed. Philadelphia, PA: Elsevier; 2015.

26. In a "cannot intubate, cannot ventilate" situation, a patient develops increasing hypoxemia. An emergency percutaneous airway is made with a needle (cannula) cricothyrotomy. Effective ventilation with this type of airway requires which of the following?

(A) high-frequency jet ventilation

(B) a flexible cannula

(C) confirmation of exhalation through the upper airway

(D) confirmation of tracheal position via aspiration of saline

(E) an initial inflation pressure of at least 55 psi (4 kPa)

Effective ventilation with a needle (cannula) cricothyrotomy requires confirmation of exhalation through the upper airway. A needle (cannula) cricothyrotomy also requires the following:

- confirmation of tracheal position via aspiration of air with a syringe
- a rigid cannula
- an initial inflation pressure of *less* than 55 psi (4 kPa)
- low-frequency jet ventilation

If proper technique is not followed, barotrauma may result if the lungs fail to deflate, or subcutaneous emphysema may result if the cannula becomes dislodged.

Ref: Miller RD. *Miller's Anesthesia*, 8th ed. Philadelphia, PA: Elsevier; 2015.

27. Of the various options for one-lung ventilation, which of the following methods allows for bronchoscopy to the isolated lung?

(A) **double-lumen tube**

(B) bronchial blocker

(C) Univent tube

(D) endobronchial tube

(E) endotracheal tube advanced into bronchus

Of the various options for one-lung ventilation, a double-lumen tube allows for bronchoscopy to the isolated lung. The other methods of lung isolation do not allow for access to the isolated lung for bronchoscopy.

Ref: Butterworth JF IV, Mackey DC, Wasnick JD. *Morgan & Mikhail's Clinical Anesthesiology,* 5th ed. New York, NY: McGraw Hill; 2013.

28. A left-sided double-lumen tube (DLT) needs to fit correctly within a patient's left bronchus. The patient is a male who is 180 cm (71 inches) tall. Based on sex and height, what is the correct size of DLT for this patient?

(A) 32 Fr

(B) 35 Fr

(C) 37 Fr

(D) 39 Fr

(E) **41 Fr**

A male who is >170 cm (67 inches) tall typically requires a 41 Fr DLT. Shorter males typically require a 39 Fr DLT. A woman who is >170 cm (67 inches) tall typically requires a 37 Fr DLT. Shorter females typically require a 35 Fr DLT.

Ref: Miller RD. *Miller's Anesthesia,* 8th ed. Philadelphia, PA: Elsevier; 2015.

29. Direct laryngoscopy is used to place a left-sided double-lumen tube (DLT). The DLT is turned 90 degrees counterclockwise after the endobronchial cuff passes the vocal cords. Which of the following methods is useful to confirm proper DLT placement in the left bronchus?

(A) auscultation alone

(B) bronchoscopy; tracheal view shows blue endobronchial cuff 5 mm above carina

(C) bronchoscopy; right upper lobe view shows two orifices

(D) **bronchoscopy; left endobronchial view shows two orifices**

(E) bronchoscopy; endobronchial blocker in the right mainstem bronchus

To confirm proper left-sided DLT placement, a left endobronchial view should show two orifices (left upper and left lower bronchi). Auscultation alone is not a reliable method to confirm proper DLT placement. Bronchoscopy should be performed with the following views:

• tracheal view shows blue endobronchial cuff 5 mm *below* carina

• right upper lobe shows *three* orifices (apical, anterior, and posterior) (Note: this is the only portion of the tracheobronchial tree with three orifices. A DLT does not involve the use of an endobronchial blocker.)

Ref: Miller RD. *Miller's Anesthesia,* 8th ed. Philadelphia, PA: Elsevier; 2015.

30. In preparation for a thoracotomy and one-lung ventilation, a left-sided double-lumen tube (DLT) is placed without difficulty, and the patient is moved to the lateral position. During positioning, the endobronchial cuff migrates to a more proximal position. Which of the following complications is most likely?

(A) protrusion of the endobronchial cuff into the surgical field

(B) **failure of the lung to collapse**

(C) subcutaneous emphysema

(D) massive airway bleeding

(E) unexpected air leak

A malpositioned DLT, where the endobronchial cuff migrates to a more proximal position, can lead to failure of the lung to collapse. Both malposition and airway trauma are relatively common problems due to DLTs. Airway trauma can occur if the DLT is inappropriately undersized or oversized (the undersized DLT can migrate distally and damage both the bronchus and/or distal trachea). Airway trauma may present as the following:

• protrusion of the endobronchial cuff into the surgical field

• subcutaneous emphysema

• massive airway bleeding

• unexpected air leak

Inability to ventilate can occur when bronchial blockers are used for one-lung ventilation, if the bronchial blocker is incorrectly inflated in the trachea or if it migrates above the carina.

Ref: Miller RD. *Miller's Anesthesia*, 8th ed. Philadelphia, PA: Elsevier; 2015.

31. Options for lung isolation and one-lung ventilation (OLV) include double-lumen tubes (DLTs) and bronchial blockers. Compared to a DLT, which of the following is an advantage of a bronchial blocker for OLV?

    (A) less time for airway positioning
    (B) bronchoscopy not necessary
    (C) easier for postoperative two-lung ventilation
    (D) easier to apply suction to the isolated lung
    (E) easier to alternate OLV to either lung

    Compared to a DLT, an advantage of a bronchial blocker for OLV is that it is easier for postoperative two-lung ventilation. Instead of removing a DLT and placing an endotracheal tube, the bronchial blocker is simply withdrawn and two-lung ventilation can begin. Bronchial blockers (either via a standard endotracheal tube or a Univent tube) are placed in the desired mainstem bronchus and allow for collapse of the lung for same-sided surgery. Disadvantages of a bronchial blocker include:

    • more time for positioning
    • a bronchoscope is essential
    • minimal suction to the isolated lung
    • difficult to alternate OLV to either lung

    Ref: Miller RD. *Miller's Anesthesia*, 8th ed. Philadelphia, PA: Elsevier; 2015.

32. After completion of a thoracic surgery procedure, a patient requires postoperative ventilation. A left-sided double-lumen tube (DLT) was placed for the surgery. Rather than exchanging the DLT for a single lumen endotracheal tube, which of the following is a **benefit** of a DLT for postoperative ventilation?

    (A) less airflow resistance
    (B) decreased risk of lost airway
    (C) easier suctioning
    (D) less risk of airway edema
    (E) decreased risk of mucous plugging

A benefit of a DLT for postoperative ventilation is a decreased risk of lost airway (as the need for tube exchange is avoided). Risks of leaving a DLT for postoperative ventilation include:

• increased airflow resistance (and difficulty weaning from ventilator)
• malposition (and hypoxia)
• mucous plugging
• difficulty suctioning
• airway edema and trauma
• vocal cord injury

Ref: Hung O, Murphy MF. *Management of the Difficult and Failed Airway*, 2nd ed. New York, NY: McGraw Hill; 2012.

33. A patient who requires a thoracotomy is difficult to intubate. A single lumen tube (SLT) is successfully placed. However, one-lung ventilation with a DLT is desired. An exchange catheter is used to switch the SLT to a DLT. Which of the following correctly describes how to use an exchange catheter?

    (A) place the patient supine with neck extended
    (B) select an exchange catheter that is flexible with no outer markings
    (C) select an exchange catheter at least 100 cm long
    (D) advance exchange catheter through the tracheal lumen of the DLT
    (E) insert exchange catheter no more than 24 cm at the lips

    When an exchange catheter is used to switch a SLT to a DLT, it should be inserted no more than 24 cm at the lips (to avoid airway injury). Other aspects of a successful tube exchange include:

    • place the patient supine in the "sniffing" position (neck flexion and head extension)
    • select an exchange catheter that is flexible with outer markings (to control depth of insertion)
    • select an exchange catheter that is at least 83 cm long (for DLT exchange)
    • advance the exchange catheter through the endobronchial lumen of the DLT

    Ref: Miller RD. *Miller's Anesthesia*, 8th ed. Philadelphia, PA: Elsevier; 2015.

34. A bougie, or endotracheal tube introducer, is used to aid direct laryngoscopy and placement of an endotracheal tube. What is a relative contraindication for use of a bougie?

    (A) Grade III Cormack-Lehane view
    (B) suspected cervical spine injury
    (C) laryngeal disruption
    (D) pediatric patient
    (E) use of a videolaryngoscope

    Laryngeal disruption is a relative contraindication for the use of a bougie. If the airway is disrupted, the bougie may migrate outside the airway. A bougie is often a useful adjunct to direct laryngoscopy for patients with a grade III Cormack-Lehane view (a bougie tends *not* to be useful for a grade IV Cormack-Lehane view). Other uses for a bougie as an airway adjunct include for pediatric patients, those with possible cervical spine injury, and in conjunction with videolaryngoscopy.

    Ref: Miller RD. *Miller's Anesthesia*, 8th ed. Philadelphia, PA: Elsevier; 2015.

35. Which of the following tracheal tube introducers (or "intubating stylets") has the ability to jet ventilate a patient?

    (A) Eschmann tracheal tube introducer
    (B) Frova tracheal tube introducer
    (C) gum elastic bougie
    (D) SunMed tracheal tube introducer
    (E) Flex-Guide tracheal tube introducer

    The Frova tracheal tube introducer (Cook, Inc.) is a hollow tube with a curved tip that can both aid in intubation and jet ventilate a patient. Other tracheal tube introducers that can jet ventilate a patient include the Cook Airway Exchange Cather and the Sheridan Tube Exchanger (Sheridan Catheter Corp.). The Eschmann tracheal tube introducer (Portex Limited), often referred to as a gum elastic bougie, is a straight stylet with a curved tip. It does not have a hollow core to allow for jet ventilation. Other variations of this solid design include single-use devices such as the SunMed tracheal tube introducer and the Flex-Guide tracheal tube introducer, both of which are flexible with curved distal tips.

    Ref: Hung O, Murphy MF. *Management of the Difficult and Failed Airway*, 2nd ed. New York, NY: McGraw Hill; 2012.

36. A tracheal tube introducer, or bougie, is selected to facilitate placement of a standard endotracheal tube (ETT). The tracheal tube introducer is successfully placed, but the ETT does not pass into the trachea. To facilitate passage of the ETT over the tracheal tube introducer, which of the following maneuvers should be attempted?

    (A) rotate the ETT 180 degrees clockwise
    (B) switch to a smaller diameter bougie
    (C) switch to a flexible ETT
    (D) remove the laryngoscope blade
    (E) switch to a larger diameter ETT

    To facilitate passage of an ETT over a tracheal tube introducer, or bougie, switch to a flexible ETT. Passage of an ETT over a tracheal tube introducer (or flexible fiberoptic bronchoscope) may be difficult if the tip of the ETT becomes obstructed against the right arytenoid cartilage. A number of different measures are proven to facilitate passage:

    - use a flexible ETT. Depending on the manufacturer, either the inherent flexibility of the ETT or a posterior location of the bevel (rather than a left-sided bevel as for a standard ETT) translates to an increased rate of success.
    - rotate the ETT 90 degrees anticlockwise. For a standard ETT the bevel is on the left side, which means the tip of the ETT is prone to impingement on the right arytenoid cartilage. A 90-degree anticlockwise rotation moves the bevel in a posterior direction and increases the likelihood of successful passage into the trachea. A 180-degree rotation will increase the likelihood of tip impingement against the left arytenoid cartilage.
    - keep the laryngoscope blade in place. This improves successful passage by keeping oropharyngeal tissues from obstructing passage.
    - minimize the gap between the tracheal tube introducer and the ETT, either by using a smaller ETT or a larger diameter tracheal tube introducer (or flexible fiberoptic bronchoscope).

    Refs: Miller RD. *Miller's Anesthesia*, 8th ed. Philadelphia, PA: Elsevier; 2015.

    Asai T, Shingu K. Difficulty in advancing a tracheal tube over a fibreoptic bronchoscope: incidence, causes, and solutions. *Br J Anaesth* 2004;92(6):870–881.

37. Direct laryngoscopy is performed on an adult patient. The larynx is not visualized and a blind technique with a tracheal tube introducer, or bougie, is attempted. Which of the following is most suggestive of successful placement of the bougie in the trachea?

(A) no resistance to passage of entire bougie
(B) **tactile clicks during passage of bougie**
(C) proximal holdup at 10 cm
(D) distal holdup at 50 cm
(E) visualization of the bougie passing ventral to the epiglottis

A reliable sign of successful placement of a bougie in the trachea is the presence of clicks and distal holdup of the bougie between 24 cm and 40 cm. This is indicative of the bougie moving across the tracheal cartilages and then obstructing in the distal airway. No resistance to passage of the entire bougie is indicative of placement in the esophagus. When the larynx is obstructed by a down-folded epiglottis (Grade III view), the bougie is passed under the dorsal (posterior) surface of the epiglottis and a blind attempt is made at placement in the trachea.

Refs: Miller RD. *Miller's Anesthesia*, 8th ed. Philadelphia, PA: Elsevier; 2015.
Kidd JF, Dyson A, Latto IP. Successful difficult intubation: use of the gum elastic bougie. *Anaesthesia* 1998;43(6): 437–438.

38. An uncuffed endotracheal tube (ETT) is placed for a pediatric anesthetic. At peak inflation, what is an appropriate cuff leak pressure?

(A) 15 cm H₂O
(B) **25 cm H₂O**
(C) 35 cm H₂O
(D) 45 cm H₂O
(E) 55 cm H₂O

For pediatric patients, an appropriately sized uncuffed ETT should have a cuff leak pressure between 20 cm and 30 cm H_2O at peak inflation pressure. Higher pressure may result in tracheal mucosal injury and airway morbidity, while lower pressure may be inadequate for effective ventilation and airway protection.

Ref: Miller RD. *Miller's Anesthesia*, 8th ed. Philadelphia, PA: Elsevier; 2015.

39. Compared to an uncuffed endotracheal tube (ETT) of the same size, what is an advantage of a *cuffed* ETT in young children?

(A) less expensive
(B) larger internal diameter
(C) **lower ETT exchange rate**
(D) lower risk of mucosal injury
(E) less work of breathing for patient

For pediatric patients, a cuffed ETT decreases the need for ETT exchange. An ETT exchange is required if an uncuffed ETT is placed and the leak pressure is not between 20 cm and 30 cm H_2O. Higher pressure may result in tracheal mucosal injury and airway morbidity, while lower pressure may be inadequate for effective ventilation and airway protection. Depending on the pediatric population studied, the risk of ETT exchange can be up to 30% when an uncuffed ETT is used. Cuffed ETTs are more expensive than uncuffed ETTs. Compared to a similarly sized uncuffed ETT, cuffed ETTs have a larger *external* diameter. Due to this increase in external diameter, a smaller cuffed ETT is required to replace an uncuffed ETT. This theoretically results in increased work of breathing when using a cuffed ETT. The overall risk of mucosal injury is the same between cuffed and uncuffed ETTs.

Refs: Miller RD. *Miller's Anesthesia*, 8th ed. Philadelphia, PA: Elsevier; 2015.
Khine HH, Corddry DH, Kettrick RG, et al. Comparison of cuffed and uncuffed endotracheal tubes in young children during general anesthesia. *Anesthesiology* 1997;86:627–631.

40. An endotracheal tube (ETT) is placed using a flexible fiberoptic technique for a neurosurgical procedure. Which of the following ETTs may be prone to irreversible compression?

(A) standard PVC ETT
(B) microlaryngeal ETT
(C) **wire-reinforced ETT**
(D) Lanz valve ETT
(E) nasal RAE ETT

Although wire-reinforced ETTs are indicated in situations to reduce the risk of ETT kinking, a wire-reinforced ETT may be prone to irreversible compression. Situations of near-complete airway obstruction have been described when a patient bites down on a wire-reinforced tube. All of the other ETTs listed are typically made of polyvinyl chloride (PVC) or other flexible materials. This avoids the risk of irreversible compression but does make the ETTs prone to kinking, particularly when the patient's neck (and airway) is flexed or extended as for certain neurosurgical or ENT procedures.

Ref: Miller RD. *Miller's Anesthesia*, 8th ed. Philadelphia, PA: Elsevier; 2015.

41. An ENT surgeon plans to excise an adult patient's vocal cord lesion without using a laser. General anesthesia with airway protection and positive pressure ventilation is desired. For endotracheal tubes (ETTs) of comparable size, which type of ETT is the best choice?

   (A)   standard PVC ETT
   (B)   **microlaryngeal ETT**
   (C)   wire-reinforced ETT
   (D)   Lanz valve ETT
   (E)   pediatric ETT

For an adult airway procedure requiring an ETT, a microlaryngeal ETT is the best choice. A microlaryngeal ETT is specifically designed for airway surgery; it has a small diameter to avoid obstructing the view of the surgical field while it is long enough and has a large enough cuff for use in adults. If laser is indicated for the procedure, then a laser-resistant ETT is indicated. A pediatric ETT has a small enough diameter for airway surgery but it is not long enough, and the cuff tends to be too small to use in an adult. The external diameter of the other ETTs (standard PVC, wire-reinforced, and Lanz valve ETT) may obstruct the surgical field for airway surgery.

Ref: Dorsch JA, Dorsch SE. *Understanding Anesthesia Equipment,* 5th ed. Philadelphia, PA: Lippincott Williams & Wilkins; 2008.

42. In the ICU, a critically ill patient requires intubation and positive pressure ventilation. In order to reduce the risk of microaspiration and ventilator-associated pneumonia (VAP), a number of ETT design modifications have been proposed. Which of the following ETT designs or features may reduce the risk of microaspiration or VAP?

   (A)   use of high volume–low pressure (HVLP) cuff rather than a high pressure-low volume (HPLV) cuff
   (B)   **use of a polyurethane cuff rather than a polyvinyl chloride cuff**
   (C)   use of barrel-shaped cuff rather than a tapered cuff
   (D)   maintenance of HVLP cuff pressure at 15 cm H_2O with a pneumatic valve
   (E)   intermittent aspiration of tracheal secretions rather than continuous aspiration of subglottic secretions

The use of a polyurethane (PU) cuff rather than a polyvinyl chloride (PVC) cuff may reduce the risk of microaspiration and VAP. PU cuffs are thinner than PVC cuffs and can create a stronger seal (at a safe pressure). HPLV cuffs may offer superior protection against aspiration compared to HVLP cuffs. However, HPLV cuffs are not typically used for long-term ventilation given the risk of ischemic damage to the tracheal mucosa. Typically HPLV cuffs are used only for short procedures.

A tapered cuff design also has superior sealing properties than a barrel-shaped cuff, which may reduce the risk of microaspiration and VAP. Maintenance of adequate cuff pressure is an important factor to reduce microaspiration and VAP. Intermittent manometry or specialized ETTs (Lanz valve or electronically monitored) can be used to maintain intracuff pressure at typically 25 cm H_2O, while 20 cm H_2O is usually considered the safe lower limit for HVLP cuffs.

Continuous aspiration of subglottic secretions (CASS) may reduce the risk of microaspiration while intermittent tracheal suctioning may actually increase the risk of microaspiration by creating negative pressure below the ETT cuff.

Refs: Dorsch JA, Dorsch SE. *Understanding Anesthesia Equipment,* 5th ed. Philadelphia, PA: Lippincott Williams & Wilkins; 2008.
Jaillette E, Martin-Loeches I, Artigas A, et al. Optimal care and design of the tracheal cuff in the critically ill patient. *Ann Intensive Care* 2014;4:7.

43. Endotracheal tubes (ETTs) can be made with a variety of materials including latex, silicone, polyvinyl chloride (PVC), or polyurethane (PU). In order to reduce the risk of airway mucosal injury, most ETT cuff designs are *high volume–low pressure (HVLP)*. However, there are ETT cuffs that are *high pressure–low volume (HPLV)*. Which of the following ETTs has a *HPLV* cuff?

   (A)   standard PVC ETT
   (B)   **silicone ETT for intubating LMA**
   (C)   PVC ETT with Lanz valve
   (D)   PVC ETT with tapered cuff
   (E)   PU ETT with tapered cuff and drain for subglottic secretions

A silicone ETT for an intubating LMA has a high pressure–low volume (HPLV) cuff. This is an exception to the more standard high volume–low pressure (HVLP) cuff, which reduces the risk of mucosal injury. A HPLV cuff does offer some advantages as the cuff seals closely against the ETT:

• improves visibility of ETT during intubation

• eases passage of ETT for nasal intubation or for passage through intubating LMA

Ref: Dorsch JA, Dorsch SE. *Understanding Anesthesia Equipment,* 5th ed. Philadelphia, PA: Lippincott Williams & Wilkins; 2008.

44. Laser surgery of the airway requires the selection of a laser-safe endotracheal tube (ETT). Which of the following ETTs is NOT approved by the Food and Drug Administration (FDA) as laser resistant?

(A) flexible stainless steel with plastic surface

(B) red rubber with copper foil wrap

(C) silicone with aluminum wrap and Teflon coating

(D) silicone with layer of aluminum powder in silicone

(E) **PVC wrapped in aluminum foil tape**

A standard PVC ETT wrapped in aluminum foil tape (or other noncombustible tape) is *not* approved by the FDA as a laser-resistant method. If an anesthesiologist creates their own laser-resistant ETT by wrapping a PVC ETT with noncombustible tape, they assume product liability if injury occurs. Laser-resistant ETTs approved by the FDA include:

• flexible stainless steel with plastic surface (Laser-Flex)

• red rubber with copper foil wrap (Sheridan Laser-Trach tube)

• silicone with aluminum wrap and Teflon coating (Laser Shield II)

• silicone with layer of aluminum powder in silicone (Laser Shield)

Ref: Miller RD. *Miller's Anesthesia,* 8th ed. Philadelphia, PA: Elsevier; 2015.

45. There are a variety of ways to assess endotracheal tube cuff pressures. How does an endotracheal tube with the Lanz system ensure adequate cuff pressure?

(A) **uses a pressure limiting valve**

(B) requires a manometer

(C) measures minimal occlusive volume

(D) performs a minimal leak test

(E) requires palpation of the pilot balloon

A Lanz cuff system is a pressure-limiting valve with a reservoir that acts to maintain cuff pressure within a preset range of approximately 25 to 30 cm H_2O. Electronic devices are also available that automatically maintain cuff pressure within set limits. A manometer directly measures cuff pressure, yet they are infrequently used in the operating room. Downsides of manometers include expense and the need for calibration. Although the technique is inaccurate, palpation of the pilot balloon is a commonly employed method in the operating room to assess cuff pressure. Minimal occlusive volume (MOV) requires a stethoscope to auscultate the cessation of air leak at peak inspiratory pressure; minimal leak technique (MLT) also requires a stethoscope to auscultate the cessation of air leak at peak inspiratory pressure; then a small amount of air is removed to create a leak.

Ref: Dorsch JA, Dorsch SE. *Understanding Anesthesia Equipment,* 5th ed. Philadelphia, PA: Lippincott Williams & Wilkins; 2008.

46. A patient is scheduled for a laparoscopic hemicolectomy. For general anesthesia, which of the following is NOT an ASA standard monitor?

(A) low oxygen concentration alarm

(B) **Foley catheter**

(C) continuous electrocardiogram

(D) temperature probe

(E) measurement of volume of expired gas

ASA monitoring standards for general anesthesia includes evaluation of oxygenation, ventilation, circulation, and temperature. A Foley catheter is not a standard monitor for general anesthesia. Measures of oxygenation include breathing system oxygen concentration, low oxygen concentration alarm, and pulse oximetry. Measures of ventilation include end-tidal carbon dioxide analysis, end-tidal carbon dioxide alarm, and volume of expired gas. Measures of circulation include continuous electrocardiogram, blood pressure and heart evaluated at least every 5 minutes, and continual peripheral pulse monitoring (pulse plethysmography or oximetry). Measures of temperature are required when "clinically significant changes" in body temperature are expected.

Ref: ASA Standards for Basic Anesthetic Monitoring (Effective July 1, 2011). Available at: http://www.asahq.org/For-Members/Clinical-Information/Standards-Guidelines-and- Statements.aspxf

47. According to the ASA practice guidelines for sedation and analgesia by nonanesthesiologists, the definition of moderate or "conscious" sedation includes which of the following features?

    (A) **purposeful response to verbal stimuli**
    (B) cardiovascular function may be impaired
    (C) airway intervention may be required
    (D) spontaneous ventilation may be inadequate
    (E) unarousable to painful stimuli

The ASA practice guidelines for sedation and analgesia by non-anesthesiologists defines moderate or "conscious" sedation as the following:

- responsiveness: purposeful response to verbal or tactile stimuli
- airway: no intervention required
- spontaneous intervention: adequate
- cardiovascular function: usually maintained

Airway intervention may be required and spontaneous ventilation may be inadequate during deep sedation. A patient may be unarousable to painful stimuli and cardiovascular function may be impaired during general anesthesia.

Ref: Gross JB, Bailey PL, Connis RT, et al. Practice guidelines for sedation and analgesia by non-anesthesiologists. *Anesthesiology* 2002; 96(4):1004–1017.

48. Which of the following is the LEAST acceptable technique for providing sedation during a minor surgical procedure?

    (A) intermittent boluses of propofol
    (B) continuous infusion of propofol
    (C) target controlled infusion of propofol
    (D) continuous infusion of dexmedetomidine
    (E) **intermittent boluses of fentanyl and droperidol**

There are multiple ways to administer sedation for minor surgical and interventional procedures safely and efficiently. In addition to propofol, other agents and common adjuncts include midazolam, opioids (especially short-acting agents such as fentanyl, alfentanil, and remifentanil), dexmedetomidine, and sub-hypnotic doses of ketamine. Multimodal analgesia (e.g., NSAIDs and/or acetaminophen) and antiemetic prophylaxis are also important ingredients for successful monitored anesthetic care. Both intermittent bolus and continuous infusions of propofol are very common. The latter tends to provide more predictable plasma concentrations, improved cardiopulmonary stability, and faster recovery times. Target controlled infusions utilize a computerized algorithm to calculate the infusion rate required to maintain a specific plasma level of a drug based on parameters such as height, weight, and sex; they appear to provide equivalent, but not superior, outcomes compared to manually controlled infusions with propofol.

Fentanyl and droperidol administered together were used for some time as the basis for "neuroleptanalgesia," a technique used for sedation that rendered patients in a detached, pain-free state of immobilization and insensitivity to pain. Downsides to this technique included prolonged sedation, dysphoria, and dyskinesia, and this has largely been abandoned since the advent of newer agents with fewer side effects.

Ref: Longnecker DE, Brown DL, Newman MF, Zapol WM. *Anesthesiology*, 2nd ed. New York, NY: McGraw Hill; 2012.

49. According to closed-claims data, which of the following mechanisms is the most likely to cause injury leading to litigation following monitored anesthetic care (MAC)?

    (A) **respiratory event**
    (B) inadequate oxygenation or ventilation
    (C) cardiovascular event
    (D) equipment failure of malfunction
    (E) cautery fires

Monitored anesthetic care (MAC) is not necessarily simple and safe, as may be believed by some. In analyzing the ASA closed-claims database, patients receiving MAC tended to be older and more ill than those receiving general anesthesia. While regional anesthetic cases were obviously different mechanistically, MAC and GA shared many commonalities (Table 26-1): the proportion of claims related to respiratory (24% vs. 22%) and cardiovascular (14% vs. 17%) events were similar. However, there was a far higher proportion of cases caused by inadequate oxygenation or ventilation (18% vs. 2%). This probably reflects the lack of airway control and the high proportion (50%) of head and neck cases where the anesthesiologist had restricted access to the airway.

TABLE 26-1. Mechanisms of injury in the American society of anesthesiologist closed claims study in different anesthetic techniques.

	MAC (n = 121), n (%)	GA (n = 1519), n (%)	RA (n = 312), n (%)
Respiratory event	29 (24%)	337 (22%)	11 (4%)
Inadequate oxygenation or ventilation	22 (18%)	33 (2%)	5 (2%)
Cardiovascular event	17 (14%)	253 (17%)	23 (7%)
Equipment failure or malfunction	25 (21%)	199 (13%)	8 (3%)
Cautery fires	20 (17%)	10 (1%)	1 (0%)
Related to regional block	2 (2%)	7 (0%)	168 (54%)
Inadequate anesthesia/ patient movement	13 (11%)	42 (3%)	7 (2%)
Medication related	11 (9%)	95 (6%)	11 (4%)
Other events	24 (20%)	586 (39%)	84 (27%)

GA, general anesthesia; MAC, monitored anesthesia care; RA, regional anesthesia. (Reprinted from Longnecker DE, Brown DL, Newman MF, Zapol WM: *Anesthesiology*, 2nd Ed. New York, NY: McGraw Hill; 2012. After Bhananker SM, Posner KL, Cheney FW, et al. Injury and liability associated with monitored anesthesia care: a closed claims analysis. *Anesthesiology*. 2006;104:228–234.)

Ref: Longnecker DE, Brown DL, Newman MF, Zapol WM. *Anesthesiology*, 2nd ed. New York, NY: McGraw Hill; 2012.

50. According to the American Society of Anesthesiologists Practice Guidelines for Sedation and Analgesia by Non-Anesthesiologists, which of the following is TRUE regarding moderate sedation?

(A) The fasting time for a meal of tea and toast is 4 hours.

(B) A designated individual may engage both in monitoring of the patient and assisting the practitioner performing the procedure.

(C) Propofol is associated with an increased incidence of adverse outcomes compared to midazolam.

(D) Patients receiving moderate sedation for brief procedures may bypass the recovery room and proceed straight to discharge.

(E) Fixed combinations of sedatives and analgesics provide good patient satisfaction while reducing risks for adverse events.

The 2002 ASA practice guidelines for sedation and analgesia by non-anesthesiologists were designed to assist in decision making of non-anesthesiologist practitioners engaged in sedation for a diagnostic/therapeutic procedures. These include procedures performed in freestanding clinics, physician offices, dental offices, and so on, as well as in a hospital environment.

The fasting guidelines for moderate or deep sedation are exactly the same as for other anesthetic types. Therefore, a light meal would require a 6-hour fast.

During deep sedation, the guidelines recommend that the individual monitoring the patient should have no other responsibilities. For moderate sedation, the guidelines allow that the individual monitoring the patient may assist the practitioner with brief ancillary tasks, providing these tasks are interruptible. The practitioner should not monitor the patient by his/herself without assistance.

While the consultants involved in creating the guidelines agree that both propofol and methohexital can result in rapid, profound decreases in levels of consciousness and apnea, there are no data supporting a superior safety profile of midazolam over propofol in this setting.

All patients receiving moderate or deep sedation should be observed in an appropriately staffed and equipped area until they are near their baseline level of consciousness and are stable from a cardiorespiratory perspective.

Safe sedation practice is based on titration of sedative and/or analgesic medications to each individual's needs, rather than administration of predetermined fixed combinations of drugs (e.g., fentanyl and midazolam mixed in the same syringe).

Ref: Gross JB, Bailey PL, Connis RT, et al. Practice guidelines for sedation and analgesia by non-anesthesiologists. *Anesthesiology* 2002;96:1004–1017.

Regional Anesthesia

1. Midazolam is a useful premedication for regional anesthetic procedures because it:

    (A) decreases the incidence of hallucinations
    (B) elevates the seizure threshold
    (C) produces a retrograde amnestic effect
    (D) does not interact with anticholinergics
    (E) is synergistic with opioids for respiratory depression

2. Which of the following pairs of spinal levels best identifies where the spinal cord terminates in adults and infants, respectively?

    (A) L1 in adults, S1 in infants
    (B) L1 in adults, S3 in infants
    (C) L1 in adults L3 in infants
    (D) L3 in adults, S1 in infants
    (E) L3 in adults, S3 in infants

3. An epidural is being placed for labor analgesia. Which of the following monitors should be used during the administration of the epidural?

    (A) fetal heart rate monitor
    (B) tocograph
    (C) temperature
    (D) electrocardiogram
    (E) impedance pneumography for respiratory rate

4. Which of the following is the BEST indication for thoracic epidural analgesia?

    (A) hemorrhoidectomy
    (B) total knee arthroplasty
    (C) midline laparotomy
    (D) axillary node dissection
    (E) hip arthroscopy

5. Which of the following is an absolute contraindication to spinal anesthesia?

    (A) severe kyphoscoliosis
    (B) chronic backache
    (C) aortic stenosis
    (D) INR of 1.4
    (E) increased intracranial pressure

6. A 3-month-old, 6-kg infant is undergoing a caudal block for analgesia following inguinal hernia surgery. The MOST appropriate medication to administer in the caudal space is:

    (A) 1 mL 0.25% ropivacaine with epinephrine
    (B) 3 mL 0.25% ropivacaine with epinephrine
    (C) 3 mL 0.5% ropivacaine with epinephrine
    (D) 6 mL 0.25% ropivacaine with epinephrine
    (E) 6 mL 0.5% ropivacaine with epinephrine

7. Which of the following statements regarding spinal anesthesia is TRUE?

    (A) The largest nerve roots in the cauda equina are blocked more profoundly than smaller nerve roots.
    (B) When performing lumbar spinal anesthesia, local anesthetics are not taken up by the spinal cord.
    (C) B-fibers are blocked first and remain blocked the longest.
    (D) 5% to 10% of elimination of local anesthetics occurs via intrathecal metabolism.
    (E) Absorption of local anesthetic occurs primarily by vessels in the dura layer.

8. Local anesthetic placed in the epidural space must cross the dura in order to reach the nerve fibers. This is achieved by:

   (A) venous transfer across the dura
   (B) diffusion across the dura at the nerve root
   (C) transfer across arachnoid granulations
   (D) bulk transfer through intervertebral foraminae
   (E) dissociation into the free base

9. In performing a combined spinal-epidural via the midline approach, the correct order of structures that one or more needles passes through is:

   (A) supraspinous ligament, ligamentum flavum, dura mater, arachnoid mater
   (B) interspinous ligament, anterior longitudinal ligament, ligamentum flavum, dura mater
   (C) interspinous ligament, supraspinous ligament, ligamentum flavum, arachnoid mater
   (D) supraspinous ligament, ligamentum flavum, posterior longitudinal ligament, pia mater
   (E) interspinous ligament, ligamentum flavum, dura mater, pia mater

10. Which of the following factors is MOST likely to influence intrathecal spread of local anesthetics and block height?

    (A) baricity of the local anesthetic
    (B) patient height
    (C) age
    (D) gender
    (E) obesity

11. A patient is to undergo a procedure on the perineum. Which combination of position for the spinal anesthetic and local anesthetic baricity would best achieve an adequate spinal block for the proposed procedure?

    (A) hypobaric bupivacaine in the sitting position
    (B) hypobaric bupivacaine in the lateral position
    (C) isobaric bupivacaine in the lateral position
    (D) hyperbaric bupivacaine in the jackknife position
    (E) hyperbaric bupivacaine in the sitting position

12. Which of the following is the most common sign/symptom of local anesthetic systemic toxicity (LAST)?

    (A) agitation
    (B) perioral numbness
    (C) dizziness
    (D) loss of consciousness
    (E) seizure

13. You are placing an epidural in a 70-kg woman for saphenous vein stripping. Loss of resistance to saline is achieved at the L4-5 interspace and a catheter is passed easily; 15 mL of 0.5% bupivacaine is administered through the catheter. Approximately 90 seconds later, the patient complains of dizziness. Her blood pressure, which was 130/80 mm Hg at baseline, is now 85/45 mm Hg and the heart rate has dropped to 52 beats/min. Several moments later, she begins to seize. The BEST medication to administer first is:

    (A) phenytoin 100 mg IV
    (B) epinephrine 100 mcg IV
    (C) vasopressin 40 U IV
    (D) lipid emulsion 20% 100 mL IV
    (E) propofol 20 mL IV

14. An epidural catheter is placed in a healthy young man for knee arthroscopy, and a 3-mL test dose of 1.5% lidocaine with 15 mcg of epinephrine is administered. Which of the following is NOT a criterion for a positive test dose?

    (A) an increase in heart rate of 20 beats/min or greater
    (B) an increase in systolic blood pressure of 15 mm Hg or greater
    (C) a decrease in T-wave amplitude of 25% or greater
    (D) an inability to dorsiflex the ankle
    (E) more than three premature ventricular contractions in 1 minute

15. A patient reports having back pain after an uneventful spinal anesthetic. Which of the following features is MOST consistent with a diagnosis of transient neurologic symptoms (TNS)?

(A) paresthesia or numbness in a lumbar radicular distribution

(B) surgery in the prone position

(C) obesity

(D) ropivacaine 0.75% as the spinal drug

(E) pain immediately after resolution of the spinal block

16. Administering epidural morphine during cesarean delivery has been shown to increase the risk of:

(A) herpes simplex virus type 1 reactivation

(B) herpes simplex virus type 2 reactivation

(C) hepatitis B virus reactivation

(D) hepatitis C virus reactivation

(E) group B streptococcal infection

17. Which of the following is a risk factor for the development of a spinal hematoma following neuraxial anesthesia?

(A) male sex

(B) younger age

(C) spinal (compared with epidural) technique

(D) spinal stenosis

(E) diabetes mellitus

18. According to the American Society of Regional Anesthesia and Pain Medicine (ASRA) Evidence-Based Guidelines on regional anesthesia in patients receiving antithrombotic/thrombolytic therapy, which of the following situations represents a contraindication to neuraxial anesthesia?

(A) placing an epidural for a vascular surgical procedure 90 minutes prior to anticipated intravenous administration of 5,000 units of heparin

(B) conducting a spinal anesthetic 11 hours after the last dose of enoxaparin used for thromboprophylaxis

(C) performing a combined spinal-epidural on a patient taking warfarin with an INR of 1.4

(D) placing an epidural catheter in a patient receiving 5,000 units of heparin subcutaneously twice daily

(E) administering a single-shot spinal in a patient who stopped their clopidogrel 5 days ago

Answers and Explanations: Regional Anesthesia

1. Midazolam is a useful premedication for regional anesthetic procedures because it:

   (A) decreases the incidence of hallucinations
   (B) **elevates the seizure threshold**
   (C) produces a retrograde amnestic effect
   (D) does not interact with anticholinergics
   (E) is synergistic with opioids for respiratory depression

The benzodiazepine midazolam is a very common anxiolytic administered prior to regional anesthetic procedures. In addition to being short-acting (half-life of 2 hours) and providing a titratable level of sedation, midazolam produces a dose-dependent *antero*grade amnesia that can be helpful in eliminating recall during the procedure. However, one of the principal advantages of midazolam is that it is a potent anticonvulsant, raising the seizure threshold and increasing the plasma concentration of local anesthetic required to cause seizures. This is likely to be most valuable in preventing signs and symptoms of mild CNS toxicity. Some have suggested that its use can in fact mask the early premonitory signs of severe toxicity. This has not been evaluated rigorously, and most regional anesthesiologists use midazolam for all of the reasons cited above, including alteration of seizure thresholds.

Ref: Hadzic A. *Hadzic's Peripheral Nerve Blocks and Anatomy for Ultrasound Guided Regional Anesthesia*, 2nd ed. New York, NY: McGraw Hill; 2012.

2. Which of the following pairs of spinal levels best identifies where the spinal cord terminates in adults and infants, respectively?

   (A) L1 in adults, S1 in infants
   (B) L1 in adults, S3 in infants
   (C) **L1 in adults L3 in infants**
   (D) L3 in adults, S1 in infants
   (E) L3 in adults, S3 in infants

The spinal cord normally extends from the foramen magnum to the level of L1 in adults and L3 in infants and children (Figure 27-1). The dural sac continues for several more levels so that it ends at S1 in adults and S3 in children (these are convenient numbers to remember: L1, L3; S1, S3). Based on this anatomical knowledge, it would be reasonable to suggest that a spinal needle could be safely placed below the L1 level without fear of contacting the conus medullaris of the spinal cord.

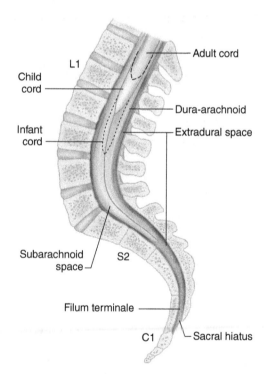

FIG. 27-1. Sagittal view through the lumbar vertebrae and sacrum. Note the end of the spinal cord rises with development from approximately L3 to L1. The dural sac normally ends at S2. (Reproduced with permission from Butterworth JF IV, Mackey DC, Wasnick JD. *Morgan & Mikhail's Clinical Anesthesiology,* 5th ed. New York, NY: McGraw Hill; 2013.)

There are two problems with this simplistic thinking. First, there is some natural variation among individuals in where the cord ends, and it is possible that the conus extends to the L2 level. More importantly, anesthesiologists are notoriously poor at determining which level is the correct level using palpation. The traditional teaching is that a line connecting the iliac crests (Tuffier's line) crosses the midline at L4, or according to some sources, the L3/4 interspace. Studies have shown that palpation is more likely than not to result in misidentification of the spinal level, sometimes by as many as two levels. In misjudging the level, there is a tendency to believe the space identified is lower than it really is. In addition, Tuffier's line does intersect L4 radiologically, but of course patients have soft tissue that overlies the iliac crests. By using surface landmarks, Tuffier's line crosses the L2/3 interspace in 30% to 50% of cases, which explains why we are typically off by one to two spaces.

There continue to be reports of cord damage with spinal needles, which is a preventable complication. Knowing the limitations of the physical exam and deliberately choosing as low a space as possible are good first steps to improving patient safety with spinal anesthesia. The use of ultrasound to identify the spinal level precisely has been shown to be simple, easy to teach, and reliable.

Ref: Butterworth JF IV, Mackey DC, Wasnick JD. *Morgan & Mikhail's Clinical Anesthesiology*, 5th ed. New York, NY: McGraw Hill; 2013.

3. An epidural is being placed for labor analgesia. Which of the following monitors should be used during the administration of the epidural?

   (A) fetal heart rate monitor
   (B) tocograph
   (C) temperature
   (D) electrocardiogram
   (E) impedance pneumography for respiratory rate

The range of monitors that should be used during the conduction of regional anesthesia includes many of the same monitors used for general anesthesia. Oxygenation should be quantified using pulse oximetry. The circulation should be monitored by measuring blood pressure (either noninvasively or via an arterial line) and an electrocardiogram (EKG). These three monitors are essential for identifying complications from

regional anesthesia as early as possible, especially high or total spinal, and local anesthetic systemic toxicity. The delivery of a significant amount (>2–3 mL) of local anesthetics should never take place without these three monitors being in place.

The ASA guideline on monitoring references monitoring of ventilation, which should also be done, if only in a qualitative manner by observing the patient's respiration, speaking with the patient throughout the procedure, and watching for condensation on the inside of the oxygen face mask. Capnography is a nice monitor to have, and is easily done when regional anesthesia is performed in the operating room, but is not mandatory. Impedance pneumography, in which respiratory rate is inferred from the changes in impedance via the EKG leads, is also not compulsory. Temperature should be monitored whenever clinically significant changes in temperature are anticipated or suspected; this is typically not the case for the duration of time it takes to place an epidural, but may be indicated during the subsequent surgical procedure.

Fetal heart rate monitoring and tocography (monitoring of uterine tone) are not required monitors during the performance of epidural labor analgesia, but can be helpful if it can be done from a practical point of view.

Ref: Butterworth JF IV, Mackey DC, Wasnick JD. *Morgan & Mikhail's Clinical Anesthesiology*, 5th ed. New York, NY: McGraw Hill; 2013.

4. Which of the following is the BEST indication for thoracic epidural analgesia?

   (A) hemorrhoidectomy
   (B) total knee arthroplasty
   (C) midline laparotomy
   (D) axillary node dissection
   (E) hip arthroscopy

In order for epidural analgesia to be maximally effective, the blocked area must match the spinal level corresponding to the surgical or painful stimulus. For example, a midline laparotomy is likely to extend from T7 to T12 (Figure 27-2). The safest and most efficient approach (from the point of view of volume of local anesthetic used) is to insert the needle somewhere within that T7-T12 range. Local anesthetic can be expected to spread cranially and caudally from the catheter tip, with 1 to 2 mL of injectate covering approximately one spinal

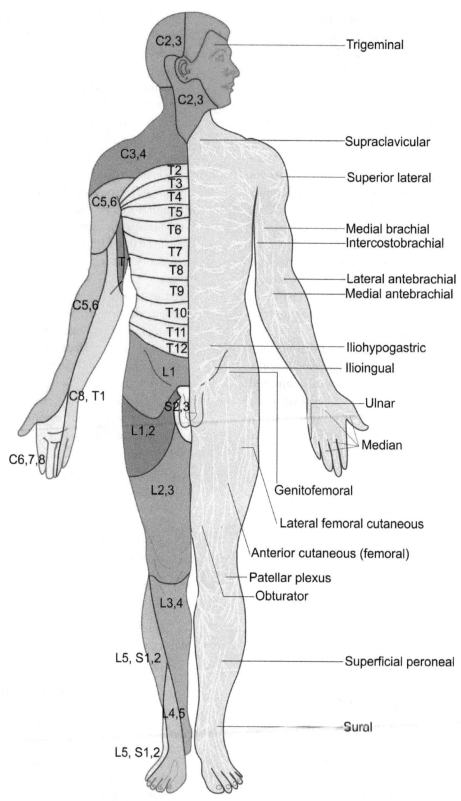

FIG. 27-2. Dermatomes and corresponding peripheral nerves: front. (Reproduced with permission from Hadzic A. *Hadzic's Peripheral Nerve Blocks and Anatomy for Ultrasound Guided Regional Anesthesia*, 2nd ed. New York, NY: McGraw Hill; 2012.)

level. Spread within the thoracic epidural space tends to travel preferentially toward the mid-thoracic region; a bolus via a high thoracic (C7-T2) epidural catheter will tend to spread more caudally than cranially, whereas a bolus via a low thoracic (T7-L1) epidural catheter will tend to spread more cranially than caudally. Injection in the mid-thoracic region will spread equally in both directions. In our example, we wish to cover T7-T12, so a low thoracic epidural catheter is indicated. Since we can expect a greater degree of cranial than caudal spread in this region, an insertion point in the *lower* end of that range (T10-T11) would best cover all the dermatomes.

Some anesthesiologists advocate placing a lumbar catheter for abdominal indications and administering a large (>20 mL) bolus in order to cover the low thoracic dermatomes. This may be done due to familiarity with lumbar epidural techniques, or as a result of perceived risk of spinal cord injury with thoracic epidural analgesia. The problem with this approach is that the initial bolus may well work (although it often takes a large volume of local anesthetic), but when the continuous infusion is initiated and the extensive block wears off, the background rate is usually insufficient to reach the abdominal (T6-L1) dermatomes. The result is the worst of both worlds: the patient has an excellent blockade of their lower limbs, is confined to bed, has an indwelling urinary catheter due to blockade of the sacral autonomic fibers, and has little coverage of their incision. A thoracic epidural that is thoughtfully placed allows for leg movement and in many cases ambulation (because the lumbar roots are not extensively blocked), avoids the need for a urinary catheter, and provides high-quality analgesia with few side effects.

Axillary node dissection is a procedure that requires low cervical and very high thoracic blockade (C5-8 and T1-2). This can be accomplished through a combination of brachial plexus block and thoracic paravertebral block at the T2 level.

Ref: Longnecker DE, Brown DL, Newman MF, Zapol WM. *Anesthesiology*, 2nd ed. New York, NY: McGraw Hill; 2012.

5. Which of the following is an absolute contraindication to spinal anesthesia?

(A) severe kyphoscoliosis

(B) chronic backache

(C) aortic stenosis

(D) INR of 1.4

(E) **increased intracranial pressure**

There are relatively few absolute contraindications to neuraxial anesthesia. These include patient refusal and an inability to remain still during the spinal or epidural procedure. Raised intracranial pressure is considered by many experts to be an absolute contraindication, since creating a hole in the dura and arachnoid membrane (either deliberately or accidentally) may result in brainstem herniation if a sufficient volume of cerebrospinal fluid leaks out of the intrathecal space.

Relative contraindications to spinal or epidural anesthesia must be weighed against the potential benefits of the neuraxial technique (or, in some cases, the benefits of avoiding general anesthesia and the attendant risks of airway manipulation, etc.). Severe hypotension and/or hypovolemia may be difficult to treat if the patient is not adequately resuscitated with fluids and/or pressor agents before or during the block; local infection overlying the puncture site or sepsis may increase the risk of meningitis with neuraxial instrumentation; altered hemostasis, either intrinsic or through the use of anticoagulant or antiplatelet medications, is another relative contraindication. The American Society of Regional Anesthesia and Pain Medicine (ASRA) has published a consensus guideline aimed at providing decision support to clinicians who are considering neuraxial anesthesia in patients with altered hemostasis. For example, in patients who are taking Coumadin, the guideline states that an INR <1.5 should be a safe threshold for placing a spinal or epidural, or for removing an epidural catheter. It is important to recognize that these are expert opinion guidelines, and their use is designed to be an aid to clinical judgment. Many anesthesiologists routinely administer spinal anesthesia in patients who have an INR >1.4 if, after performing a risk-benefit analysis, it is thought that the reason to place a spinal or epidural is strong enough. For example, in the patient with a fractured hip who has an INR of 1.6 and severe cardiopulmonary disease, the risk of spinal hematoma may be estimated to be far less than an adverse event related to general anesthesia with tracheal intubation.

Aortic stenosis is a consideration with neuraxial anesthesia, as a rapid reduction in afterload and preload (and the reflexive tachycardia) can precipitate life-threatening hypotension due to a fixed stroke volume. This can be overcome by using gradually titrated techniques such as epidural anesthesia or continuous spinal anesthesia. These patients also benefit from establishing invasive monitoring of arterial pressure beforehand and judicious use of fluid and pressor therapy during and after the block.

Ref: Miller RD. *Miller's Anesthesia*, 8th ed. Philadelphia, PA: Elsevier; 2015.

6. A 3-month-old, 6-kg infant is undergoing a caudal block for analgesia following inguinal hernia surgery. The MOST appropriate medication to administer in the caudal space is:

(A) 1 mL 0.25% ropivacaine with epinephrine
(B) 3 mL 0.25% ropivacaine with epinephrine
(C) 3 mL 0.5% ropivacaine with epinephrine
(D) **6 mL 0.25% ropivacaine with epinephrine**
(E) 6 mL 0.5% ropivacaine with epinephrine

Caudal analgesia is frequently used for children in combination with general anesthesia. The single-shot technique involves passing an intravenous catheter over-needle through the sacrococcygeal ligament, which is a "roof" over the sacral hiatus that is created by the unfused S4 and S5 laminae. Once the needle is passed through, the cannula is slipped off and advanced into the caudal space, which is the caudad terminus of the epidural space. The dural sac ends at S3 in children, so there is usually little danger of puncturing the dura and accessing the subarachnoid space, but this can happen, and care must be taken not to advance the sharp needle too far in the space.

Once the cannula is in place and negative aspiration rules out intravascular placement, an injection of local anesthetic takes place. A reliable and well-validated recipe for volume in children is that high sacral blockade can be achieved with 0.5 mL/kg of local anesthetic, and high lumbar with 1.0 mL/kg. Higher volumes may be administered to achieve thoracic analgesia, but this increases the risk of toxicity, and consideration to choosing an alternate technique such as a high lumbar or low thoracic epidural is warranted.

Since the goal with pediatric caudal techniques is almost always analgesia and not surgical anesthesia, a low concentration of local anesthetic is indicated, such as 0.25% ropivacaine. Epinephrine is a useful safety adjuvant, since the caudal space is quite vascular, and epinephrine will truncate the peak plasma levels of local anesthetic.

Ref: Butterworth JF IV, Mackey DC, Wasnick JD. *Morgan & Mikhail's Clinical Anesthesiology*, 5th ed. New York, NY: McGraw Hill; 2013.

7. Which of the following statements regarding spinal anesthesia is TRUE?

(A) The largest nerve roots in the cauda equina are blocked more profoundly than smaller nerve roots.
(B) When performing lumbar spinal anesthesia, local anesthetics are not taken up by the spinal cord.
(C) **B-fibers are blocked first and remain blocked the longest.**
(D) 5% to 10% of elimination of local anesthetics occurs via intrathecal metabolism.
(E) Absorption of local anesthetic occurs primarily by vessels in the dura layer.

Spinal nerve roots in the cauda equina lack the protective covering of dura and arachnoid, and are therefore very susceptible to the effects of local anesthetics. Uptake of local anesthetic is dependent on the surface area. The smallest nerve roots have the largest relative surface area and are more extensively and rapidly penetrated by the drug. The spinal cord also absorbs some local anesthetic, especially since these lipid soluble drugs are taken up easily by highly myelinated nerves. However, only the most superficial portions of the cord are affected, and the clinical significance is likely minimal.

Different fiber types have different susceptibilities to local anesthetics. Preganglionic sympathetic B-fibers are most sensitive, followed by C-fibers (sensation to cold, post-ganglionic sympathetic), A-delta fibers (pin-prick), A-beta fibers (touch), and lastly A-alpha (motor) fibers. Since deposition of local anesthetic in the lumbar intrathecal space creates a concentration gradient from high to low as we proceed cranially, it is easy to imagine that a point will be reached where the motor fibers return. Several spinal levels above that, sensation to touch returns. Finally, there is a zone of one to three spinal levels where only the sympathetic fibers are blocked, which is indicated by vasodilation and color change from the normal area above it. This is termed "differential nerve blockade" (Figure 27-3). It is challenging to detect the break point where the motor fibers return to function, since it is usually on the abdomen and not a limb. The easiest break point to detect is between the zone where both sensory and sympathetic fibers are blocked (no sensation to pin prick) and the zone where only sympathetic fibers are blocked (sensation to pin prick but not cold).

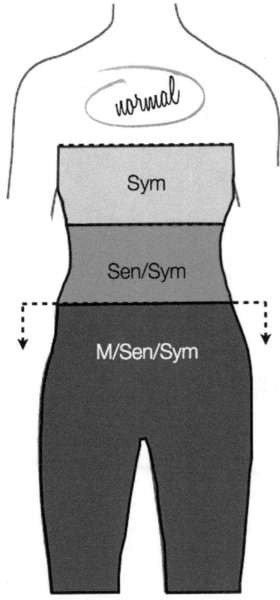

FIG. 27-3. Differential nerve blockade during spinal anesthesia. Note that since the concentration of local anesthetic is most dense at the site of insertion (lumbar spine), the patient will exhibit a motor (M), sensory (Sen), and sympathetic (Sym) in the lower limbs, pelvis, and lower abdomen. At a certain level, the function of the resistant motor fibers will return, leaving a zone of sensory and sympathetic block. Above this will be a zone of just sympathetic block, where the patient will report feeling pinprick or soft touch sensation, but will not react to cold. Normal neural function returns several dermatomal levels cranial to this.

Elimination of local anesthetics during spinal block occurs entirely by vascular absorption. No local metabolism occurs in the subarachnoid space. All of the local anesthetic is taken up by blood vessels, primarily those lying in the pia layer of the meninges. Some local anesthetic also diffuses across the dura to the epidural space, where it is rapidly taken up by large epidural vessels.

Ref: Cousins MJ, Carr DB, Horlocker TT, Bridenbaugh PO. *Cousins & Bridenbaugh's Neural Blockade in Clinical Anesthesia and Pain Medicine*, 4th ed. Philadelphia, PA: Lippincott Williams & Wilkins; 2009.

8. Local anesthetic placed in the epidural space must cross the dura in order to reach the nerve fibers. This is achieved by:

   (A) venous transfer across the dura

   (B) diffusion across the dura at the nerve root

   (C) transfer across arachnoid granulations

   (D) bulk transfer through intervertebral foraminae

   (E) dissociation into the free base

The dura is a tough, acellular connective tissue sack that extends from the skull to the spinal canal in the sacrum. Dura is made up of both collagen and elastin, separated by clefts of ground substance that improve its permeability. The dura is variably thick among individuals and between spinal levels in the same individual, but is typically thickest in the midline.

Local anesthetic is thought to leave the epidural space and cross the dura laterally at the nerve root rather than at the midline. Two factors are likely responsible for this location being the site of action. First, the dura is thinnest at the nerve root before the nerve exits the intervertebral foramen, and resistance to passive diffusion is less than in other locations. More importantly, the roots are close to the dura, and the volume of CSF surrounding them is minimal, resulting in less dilution of the local anesthetic as it passes across the dural layer.

The fact that epidural local anesthetics exert their action at the nerve roots confers one of its prime advantages: a segmental block can be achieved by blocking selective spinal levels, while allowing for intact function of the spinal cord. For example, the entire abdomen or thoracic wall can be profoundly blocked with a thoracic epidural while leaving the lower limbs spared in order to ambulate.

Ref: Cousins MJ, Carr DB, Horlocker TT, Bridenbaugh PO. *Cousins & Bridenbaugh's Neural Blockade in Clinical Anesthesia and Pain Medicine*, 4th ed. Philadelphia, PA: Lippincott Williams & Wilkins; 2009.

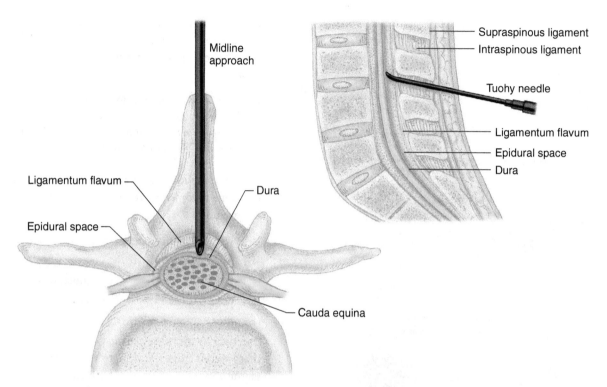

FIG. 27-4. Lumbar epidural anesthesia; midline approach. (Reproduced with permission from Butterworth JF IV, Mackey DC, Wasnick JD. *Morgan and Mikhail's Clinical Anesthesiology*, 5th ed. New York, NY: McGraw Hill; 2013.)

9. In performing a combined spinal-epidural via the midline approach, the correct order of structures that one or more needles passes through is:

(A) **supraspinous ligament, ligamentum flavum, dura mater, arachnoid mater**

(B) interspinous ligament, anterior longitudinal ligament, ligamentum flavum, dura mater

(C) interspinous ligament, supraspinous ligament, ligamentum flavum, arachnoid mater

(D) supraspinous ligament, ligamentum flavum, posterior longitudinal ligament, pia mater

(E) interspinous ligament, ligamentum flavum, dura mater, pia mater

The correct order of structures passed through from skin to subarachnoid space is (Figure 27-4):

• skin

• subcutaneous fat

• supraspinous ligament

• interspinous ligament

• ligamentum flavum

• epidural space

• dura mater

• arachnoid mater (usually not appreciable as a separate layer from dura)

The anterior and posterior longitudinal ligaments run along the anterior and posterior aspects of the vertebral body and are thus substantially deeper than a needle should travel. The pia mater surrounds the spinal cord and each individual nerve root in the cauda equina. Traversing the pia mater is not a goal, and elevates the risk of neural injury.

During the paramedian approach, the paraspinal muscles are substituted for the supraspinous and interspinous ligaments. The first ligament encountered in this approach is the ligamentum flavum.

Refs: Butterworth JF IV, Mackey DC, Wasnick JD. *Morgan & Mikhail's Clinical Anesthesiology*, 5th ed. New York, NY: McGraw Hill; 2013.

10. Which of the following factors is MOST likely to influence intrathecal spread of local anesthetics and block height?

(A) **baricity of the local anesthetic**

(B) patient height

(C) age

(D) gender

(E) obesity

The two principal factors that influence the cranial spread of local anesthetic in the intrathecal space are

(1) dose and (2) baricity and position. Importantly, dose should be thought of as the mass in mg, not in volume or concentration. It is possible to vary both volume and concentration to arrive at the same milligram dose and obtain the same effect. Therefore, it makes much more sense to speak about spinal dosing in the following way: "I usually use 12.5 mg of bupivacaine for my total knee patients," or "the ED95 for bupivacaine in cesarean delivery is 13 mg," etc. Don't fall into a trap of talking in terms of milliliters.

Baricity and position are the other big factor. For example, a hyperbaric solution, or one that has a higher specific gravity than CSF, will tend to sink to the floor. If a patient is positioned in Trendelenburg (head down), the block height will be higher than if they were slightly head up. A hypobaric solution would produce the opposite results. Isobaric solutions tend to stay in the same place no matter what you do with the position.

Other factors that increase the height of the block are a reduced volume of CSF and "aiming" the local anesthetic cranially using a directional needle such as a Whitacre or Sprotte. Factors shown to have an effect in some but not all studies include age, weight, extremes of height, and temperature of the solution: solutions straight out of a refrigerator will tend to act as hyperbaric ones; body temperature solutions tend to be slightly hypobaric.

Other proposed factors have been shown to have no effect. These include barbotage (the act of repeatedly withdrawing CSF into the syringe during injection to admix with the local anesthetic and increase the volume), gender, and, as mentioned above, the volume or concentration of the local anesthetic (providing dose in milligrams remains the same).

Ref: Cousins MJ, Carr DB, Horlocker TT, Bridenbaugh PO. *Cousins & Bridenbaugh's Neural Blockade in Clinical Anesthesia and Pain Medicine*, 4th ed. Philadelphia, PA: Lippincott Williams & Wilkins; 2009.

11. A patient is to undergo a procedure on the perineum. Which combination of position for the spinal anesthetic and local anesthetic baricity would best achieve an adequate spinal block for the proposed procedure?

    (A) hypobaric bupivacaine in the sitting position

    (B) hypobaric bupivacaine in the lateral position

    (C) isobaric bupivacaine in the lateral position

    (D) hyperbaric bupivacaine in the jackknife position

    (E) **hyperbaric bupivacaine in the sitting position**

The baricity of a local anesthetic solution refers to its specific gravity in relation to CSF. Most local anesthetics reconstituted in normal saline are isobaric, and do not appreciably sink or float when administered into the subarachnoid space. The addition of a small amount of dextrose will render these solutions hyperbaric, so that they sink to the most dependent areas after injection. In contrast, adding sterile water to an isobaric solution will create a hypobaric solution that rises to nondependent areas of the thecal sac.

Clearly, any discussion of baricity should also involve patient position. The manipulation of the baricity of solutions and the deliberate positioning of patients during and immediately after the spinal anesthetic can be very useful in achieving specific clinical effects. For example, ambulatory hemorrhoidal surgery involves only the sacral nerve roots. Rather than administer a large dose of isobaric solution, which would provide a mid- to high lumbar block that far outlasts the duration of the procedure, a relatively small (e.g., 5 mg) dose of hyperbaric bupivacaine can be administered at the lumbar level and the patient instructed to sit for 10 minutes or so. This allows the solution to "sink" down to the sacral roots, preserving the lower limb function and establishing what is called a "saddle block." Local anesthetics do persist for some time in the CSF and therefore can move after this time, but not to a clinically significant degree. After the 10-minute "soak time," much of the block has been established by absorption into the nerve roots and will not change even with repositioning.

A related example is the use of hypobaric solutions in the jackknife position for anorectal surgery. When placed in the lumbar spinal space, these local anesthetics will "float" up and create a similar effect at the sacral roots. Care must be taken in the head-down jackknife position to not mistakenly use hyperbaric solutions—this could cause progressive cranial spread and a high or total spinal. Unilateral spinal anesthesia is advocated by some by using either hyper- or hypobaric solutions with the patient on their side, such as in operative fixation of a fractured hip. The purpose of doing this is to reduce the effect of a bilateral sympathectomy and minimize hypotension in what are often hemodynamically challenged patients.

The downside to attempting to achieve very precise results with hyper- or hypobaric solutions is twofold. First, clinicians often (relatively) overdose the spinal, using similar doses to what would be expected if one were using isobaric for standard lumbar spinal anesthesia. This obviates any specific anatomic or duration-related advantage. Second, frequently not enough time is spent in the sitting or lateral position, and moving the patient to supine or prone results in unwanted spread of local anesthetic that is still unbound in the CSF.

Ref: Butterworth JF IV, Mackey DC, Wasnick JD. *Morgan & Mikhail's Clinical Anesthesiology,* 5th ed. New York, NY: McGraw Hill; 2013.

12. Which of the following is the most common sign/symptom of local anesthetic systemic toxicity (LAST)?

    (A) agitation
    (B) perioral numbness
    (C) dizziness
    (D) loss of consciousness
    (E) seizure

Local anesthetic systemic toxicity (LAST) is a serious and potentially fatal complication of the regional anesthesia. While the presentation of LAST is varied, the classic teaching has for decades been that rising plasma levels of local anesthetic produce a sequential series of signs and symptoms starting with a prodrome (dizziness, drowsiness, tinnitus, perioral numbness, confusion, dysphoria, dysarthria), followed by frank signs of central nervous system excitatory activity (seizures), followed by loss of consciousness. If plasma levels are sufficiently high, cardiovascular toxicity follows, with either bradycardia or tachycardia, hypotension, QRS widening, ventricular ectopy, ST segment changes, and lethal arrhythmias such as ventricular tachycardia or fibrillation and asystole.

In reality, the presentation is much less straightforward and sequential. While about 45% of patient present with CNS signs/symptoms alone, another 45% first present with both CNS and CVS symptoms and signs. The remainder (about 10%) present with CVS toxicity alone. Among the reported signs and symptoms of CNS toxicity, 18% had prodromal signs, while over two-thirds of patients present with seizures. Among CVS signs, bradycardia (27%) and hypotension (18%) are the most common.

Ref: Di Gregorio G, Neal JM, Rosenquist RW, Weinberg GL. Clinical presentation of local anesthetic systemic toxicity: a review of published cases, 1979 to 2009. *Reg Anesth Pain Med* 2010; 35:181–187.

13. You are placing an epidural in a 70-kg woman for saphenous vein stripping. Loss of resistance to saline is achieved at the L4-5 interspace and a catheter is passed easily; 15 mL of 0.5% bupivacaine is administered through the catheter. Approximately 90 seconds later, the patient complains of dizziness. Her blood pressure, which was 130/80 mm Hg at baseline, is now 85/45 mm Hg and the heart rate has dropped to 52 beats/min. Several moments later, she begins to seize. The BEST medication to administer first is:

    (A) phenytoin 100 mg IV
    (B) epinephrine 100 mcg IV
    (C) vasopressin 40 U IV
    (D) lipid emulsion 20% 100 mL IV
    (E) propofol 20 mL IV

The differential diagnosis of dizziness and hypotension after a neuraxial block should include high or total spinal (and for completeness, anaphylaxis and drug error), but a seizure pushes the diagnosis toward local anesthetic systemic toxicity (LAST). Until proven otherwise, this episode should be treated as such.

As with all crises in acute care medicine, the initial treatment algorithm should focus on the ABCs. Ventilate the patient with 100% oxygen and provide circulatory support as per BLS and ACLS. Seizure suppression is important in order to reduce the hypermetabolism and production of carbon dioxide; hypercarbia will increase cerebral blood flow and exacerbate the delivery of toxic local anesthetic to the brain. Benzodiazepines are the drug of choice, and as anesthesiologists, we typically have midazolam somewhere handy. *Small* doses of propofol have been used as well for seizure suppression, but care must be taken in the setting of hypotension; 20 mL of propofol is not a small dose in this context.

While the initial steps of the resuscitation are taking place, a team member should be preparing lipid emulsion. 20% lipid emulsion solution is superior to epinephrine and vasopressin in achieving return of spontaneous circulation and improving rate-pressure product in animal models of bupivacaine-induced cardiac arrest. While the mechanism is not yet entirely clear, various theories of how this simple drug works as an antidote to LAST include its acting as a lipid phase in the plasma to "soak up" the lipid soluble local anesthetic; acting at the mitochondrial level to provide substrate for respiration; and most recently, acting as a shuttle to drive local anesthetic into skeletal muscle cells and away from neurons and cardiac myocytes. Whatever the mechanism of action, it is clear that lipid emulsion works, and it should be stocked wherever local anesthetics are used in the hospital. For more information about lipid emulsion and LAST, see www.lipidrescue.org.

The recommended initial dose is 1.5 mL/kg of lean body mass: for most average-sized people, just give 100 mL as a bolus. This is not a situation where you need to be doing math in your head, so memorize 100 mL as your starting number. An infusion can then be started at 0.25 mL/kg/min (or about 18 mL/min).

Ref: http://www.lipidrescue.org. Accessed July 10, 2016

14. An epidural catheter is placed in a healthy young man for knee arthroscopy, and a 3-mL test dose of 1.5% lidocaine with 15 mcg of epinephrine is administered. Which of the following is NOT a criterion for a positive test dose?

(A) an increase in heart rate of 20 beats/min or greater

(B) an increase in systolic blood pressure of 15 mm Hg or greater

(C) a decrease in T-wave amplitude of 25% or greater

(D) an inability to dorsiflex the ankle

(E) **more than three premature ventricular contractions in 1 minute**

It is well known that aspirating an epidural catheter may yield some false negative results—in other words, the initial aspiration may reveal no blood or CSF, but subsequent aspiration after time has passed shows that the catheter is located in the intravascular or intrathecal space. The purpose and method of the test dose during epidural anesthesia is twofold. First, a local anesthetic (usually 3 mL of 1.5% lidocaine) is administered to rule out inadvertent intrathecal placement. The total of 45 mg of lidocaine is sufficient to cause a clinically appreciable (but not dangerously high) spinal block.

The addition of 15 mcg of epinephrine is sufficient to reliably warn of an intravascular catheter placement through an increase in heart rate of 20 beats/min or greater, an increase in systolic blood pressure of 15 mm Hg or greater, and a decrease in T-wave amplitude of 25% or greater. This last criterion, while sensitive, is challenging from a practical point of view to detect, especially on a wall-mounted monitor in a preoperative block area, or in a labor suite. Premature ventricular contractions, while associated with epinephrine-induced irritability of the myocardium, are not a strict criterion.

Note that the sensitivity of the hemodynamic responses to epinephrine is confounded by contrac-

tions during labor, as well as in the elderly who have a blunted response to catecholamines.

Ref: Hadzic A. *NYSORA Textbook of Regional Anesthesia and Acute Pain Medicine*, 1st ed. New York, NY: McGraw Hill; 2007.

15. A patient reports having back pain after an uneventful spinal anesthetic. Which of the following features is MOST consistent with a diagnosis of transient neurologic symptoms (TNS)?

(A) paresthesia or numbness in a lumbar radicular distribution

(B) surgery in the prone position

(C) **obesity**

(D) ropivacaine 0.75% as the spinal drug

(E) pain immediately after resolution of the spinal block

Transient neurologic symptoms (TNS) is the name of a specific pain syndrome described in patients that have received a spinal anesthetic. It is characterized by transient, self-limiting lower back and lower limb pain that varies in intensity from barely noticeable to moderately or severely intense. Its etiology is not entirely clear; predominant theories include muscular or ligamentous stretching following positioning in a patient with a motor blockade of the lumbar musculature, and direct stretching of the sciatic nerve. These two "stretching" theories are supported by the fact that patients undergoing lidocaine spinal anesthesia in the lithotomy position have an incidence of TNS of 30% to 35%, compared to 4% to 8% in the supine position. Lidocaine is far and away the agent most likely to cause TNS, although it has been described rarely with other local anesthetics such as mepivacaine and prilocaine. Other risk factors include knee arthroscopy and obesity. Outpatient surgical status has been implicated in some studies, but not others. Pregnant patients do not appear to be at greater risk than nonpregnant patients.

One thing is clear regarding TNS: it is NOT due to direct neurotoxicity of the local anesthetic. This is supported by the following:

- Symptoms are limited to pain; abnormal sensory or motor findings should prompt the evaluation for other causes of back pain such as spinal hematoma or nerve root compression.

- Pain does not start immediately after resolution of the block (as would be expected if neuropathy was involved). Instead, it typically starts 24 to 48 hours after the spinal anesthetic, further supporting the muscular/ligamentous stretch theory—kind of like how your muscles are sore the day *after* you work out, not while you're leaving the gym.

- Changes in concentration of the local anesthetic (using 0.5% lidocaine in place of 5%) or addition of vasoconstrictors does not affect the incidence of TNS.

- Electrophysiologic testing during episodes of TNS are normal in volunteer studies.

TNS can be prevented almost entirely by avoiding spinal lidocaine. However, in those cases where it does occur, treatment centers around reassurance (it only lasts 7 to 10 days at most), NSAIDs, and warm heat applied to the lower back. If spasm is present, muscle relaxant drugs can be useful.

Ref: Pollock J. Transient neurologic symptoms: etiology, risk factors. *Reg Anesth Pain Med* 2002; 27:581–586.

16. Administering epidural morphine during cesarean delivery has been shown to increase the risk of:

(A) **herpes simplex virus type 1 reactivation**

(B) herpes simplex virus type 2 reactivation

(C) hepatitis B virus reactivation

(D) hepatitis C virus reactivation

(E) group B streptococcal infection

Herpes labialis (e.g., oral herpes or "cold sores") is typically caused by herpes simplex virus (HSV) type 1. In contrast, genital herpes is typically caused by HSV-2. While HSV-1 and HSV-2 usually cause infection "above the belt" and "below the belt," respectively, each virus can infect either area, although it is unusual. The prevalence of HSV-1 within women of childbearing age is estimated to be approximately 50% to 70%.

Why is herpes infection during pregnancy and childbirth of interest? Firstly, *primary* herpes infection (women who acquire the virus for the first time) during pregnancy presents a profound threat to the fetus; congenital herpes is associated with severe fetal anomalies and fetal loss. Herpes can also be passed to the newborn either by passage through the genital tract during active HSV-2 infection or (much less commonly) by transmission from contact with other individuals who have active oral HSV-1 lesions. Neonatal herpes can cause skin, eye, and mouth disease, encephalitis, or disseminated infection; mortality with widespread infection reaches 30% even with prompt antiviral treatment. Mothers, family members, and caregivers

should be actively treated if they have oral lesions, and contact with the neonate should be limited.

So, why is this relevant to anesthesia? Administration of epidural or spinal morphine has been shown to lead to reactivation of HSV-1 lesions in women undergoing cesarean delivery. This may occur in as many as 40% of women with latent HSV-1 infection. Intravenous or oral opioids do not appear to increase the risk, which raises questions about the mechanism. Currently, it is unclear exactly why this occurs, but some have proposed that opioid-induced suppression of host immunity is the underlying mechanism. This may lead to replication of the virus in the dorsal root ganglion where it normally remains dormant.

Despite the fact that spinal and epidural morphine increases the risk of HSV-1 reactivation, there is little data to support the idea that these recrudescences are associated with neonatal infection, and the analgesic benefit outweighs this theoretical risk in most cases. Note that neuraxial morphine does *not* increase the rate of genital herpes reactivation.

Ref: Chestnut DH. *Chestnut's Obstetric Anesthesiology: Principles and Practice,* 5th ed. Philadelphia, PA: Elsevier; 2014.

17. Which of the following is a risk factor for the development of a spinal hematoma following neuraxial anesthesia?

(A) male sex

(B) younger age

(C) spinal (compared with epidural) technique

(D) **spinal stenosis**

(E) diabetes mellitus

Several patient, anesthetic, and pharmacologic factors have been associated with increased risk of a spinal hematoma following neuraxial anesthesia. These include:

- Female sex
- Increased age
- Spinal stenosis or ankylosing spondylitis (due to decreased space for hematoma to collect and increased pressure on neurologic structures)
- Renal insufficiency (due to decreased clearance of low molecular weight heparin)
- Traumatic needle/catheter placement
- Epidural technique (compared with spinal technique, it involves a larger needle and usually an indwelling catheter)
- Preexisting coagulopathy (e.g., HELLP syndrome)

- Perioperative low-molecular-weight heparin (LMWH) administration
- Combined antiplatelet or anticoagulant medication with LMWH
- Twice-daily LMWH (vs. once daily)

Ref: Horlocker et al. *Regional Anesthesia in the Patient Receiving Antithrombotic or Thrombolytic Therapy: American Society of Regional Anesthesia and Pain Medicine Evidence-based Guidelines,* 3rd ed. *Reg Anesth Pain Med* 2010;35:64–101.

18. According to the American Society of Regional Anesthesia and Pain Medicine (ASRA) Evidence-Based Guidelines on regional anesthesia in patients receiving antithrombotic/thrombolytic therapy, which of the following situations represents a contraindication to neuraxial anesthesia?

   (A) placing an epidural for a vascular surgical procedure 90 minutes prior to anticipated intravenous administration of 5,000 units of heparin

   (B) conducting a spinal anesthetic 11 hours after the last dose of enoxaparin used for thromboprophylaxis

   (C) performing a combined spinal-epidural on a patient taking warfarin with an INR of 1.4

   (D) placing an epidural catheter in a patient receiving 5,000 units of heparin subcutaneously twice daily

   (E) administering a single-shot spinal in a patient who stopped their clopidogrel 5 days ago

The ASRA Evidence-Based Guidelines on regional anesthesia in patients receiving antithrombotic/thrombolytic therapy are a consensus statement put together by key opinion leaders, which aids in clinical decision making. One of the caveats to these guidelines is that these are for individual agents only. The authors stress that if patients are on multiple agents, hemostasis may be effectively impaired despite each individual agent meeting the threshold for neuraxial puncture. For example, it is not known to what degree the risk of a spinal hematoma is increased in the patient taking aspirin, unfractionated heparin, *and* garlic supplements, even though all three are not problematic by themselves. As always, clinical judgment and careful weighing of risks and benefits should not be supplanted by a generalized guideline.

Intravenous unfractionated heparin may be given 1 hour after neuraxial anesthesia, provided that the spi-

nal or epidural placement was uncomplicated. A traumatic (bloody) tap can present a dilemma; if the dose of heparin is 5,000 to 10,000 units, as might be used for vascular surgery, a discussion with the surgeon and weighing of the risks/benefits is recommended, although there is little data to guide clinicians either way. In the case of a bloody tap prior to full heparinization for cardiopulmonary bypass, it is recommended that surgery be delayed for 24 hours. Epidural catheters should be removed only after a normal aPTT is obtained, usually 2 to 4 hours after the bolus or infusion has ceased. Heparin can be restarted 1 hour after removal.

Subcutaneous unfractionated heparin (e.g., 5,000 units twice daily) is not a contraindication to neuraxial procedures; however, the risk of bleeding is theoretically highest in the 2 hours following administration, so consideration of timing may increase the margin of safety.

Neuraxial procedures are thought to be safe with once-daily dosing of low-molecular-weight heparin (LMWH), providing the timing is carefully managed. Instrumentation of the neuraxis should be delayed for 10 to 12 hours after the last dose of LMWH; the subsequent dose should not be administered any sooner than 2 hours after the spinal/epidural procedure. Epidural catheters can be safely maintained with this regimen. Twice-daily dosing or treatment doses of LMWH are not compatible with indwelling epidural catheters. Placement should be delayed for 24 hours after the last dose. After removal, 2 hours should elapse before the subsequent dose is administered.

Patients taking warfarin should not be instrumented with an INR of 1.5 or greater, per the guidelines. An INR of 1.5 represents mean activity levels of all four vitamin K-dependent factors (II, VII, IX, X) at near or over 50%; since it is generally felt that 40% activity level is enough for adequate hemostasis, this guideline seems appropriate.

The suggested time interval between discontinuation of clopidogrel and neuraxial blockade is 7 days. If spinal or epidural anesthesia is indicated in the meantime, platelet function assays may be helpful to establish exact degree of platelet inhibition.

Ref: Horlocker et al. *Regional Anesthesia in the Patient Receiving Antithrombotic or Thrombolytic Therapy: American Society of Regional Anesthesia and Pain Medicine Evidence-based Guidelines,* 3rd ed. *Reg Anesth Pain Med* 2010; 35:64–101.

CHAPTER 28

Complications in Anesthesia

1. Which of the following is the most common complication of nasotracheal intubation?

   (A) arytenoid dislocation
   (B) submucosal tear of the posterior pharyngeal wall
   (C) avulsion of the turbinate bone
   (D) epistaxis
   (E) esophageal perforation

2. Which of the following statements regarding sore throat following general anesthesia are TRUE?

   (A) The rates of sore throat for endotracheal tube (ETT) and laryngeal mask airway (LMA) are similar.
   (B) The most common injury attributed to the LMA is nerve palsy.
   (C) The incidence of sore throat is directly proportional to the size of the ETT.
   (D) High-volume, low-pressure cuffs are associated with a reduced incidence of sore throat.
   (E) Cuffed tubes lead to a greater incidence of sore throat than do uncuffed tubes.

3. Which of the following is TRUE regarding dental damage during general anesthesia?

   (A) The reported incidence is approximately 1 in 50.
   (B) Roughly 50% of all anesthesia-related dental injuries occur during laryngoscopy.
   (C) Upper and lower incisors are damaged with equal frequency.
   (D) In the setting of poor dentition, mouth guards can reduce the risk of damage.
   (E) The use of an oropharyngeal airway during the case can reduce the risk of damage.

4. Which of the following is the most commonly injured structure during airway management?

   (A) teeth
   (B) tongue
   (C) pharynx
   (D) larynx
   (E) esophagus

5. Which of the following techniques is MOST likely to prevent corneal abrasions?

   (A) petroleum ointment
   (B) paraffin-based ointment
   (C) methylcellulose ointment
   (D) vertical taping of the eyelids
   (E) horizontal taping of the eyelids

6. Which of the following is NOT a risk factor for postoperative visual loss after spine surgery?

   (A) female sex
   (B) use of the Wilson bed frame
   (C) long duration of anesthesia
   (D) obesity
   (E) the use of large amounts of crystalloid solutions for fluid replacement

7. Which of the following drugs is associated with superficial thrombophlebitis following intravenous injection?

   (A) thiopental
   (B) dexmedetomidine
   (C) propofol
   (D) ketamine
   (E) etomidate

8. Which of the following drugs is MOST likely to cause tissue necrosis upon inadvertent intra-arterial injection?

   (A) thiopental
   (B) dexmedetomidine
   (C) propofol
   (D) ketamine
   (E) etomidate

9. A patient undergoing an elective coronary artery bypass graft is induced uneventfully. The resident places a right internal jugular 8.5 Fr introducer, and while passing the introducer through the skin of the neck is somewhat difficult, it eventually gives, and is advanced completely. No catheter is placed through the lumen of the introducer. Several minutes later, the attending performing the transesophageal echocardiogram notices a moderate pericardial effusion that was not present on the preoperative echo. Which of the following best explains the pericardial effusion?

   (A) perforation of the right ventricle by the guidewire
   (B) perforation of the right atrium by the guidewire
   (C) perforation of the coronary sinus by the guidewire
   (D) perforation of the right ventricle by the tissue dilator
   (E) perforation of the right atrium by the tissue dilator

10. Which of the following is the MOST useful is preventing inadvertent injury to the carotid artery during central venous cannulation of the internal jugular vein?

   (A) blood gas analysis of the aspirate
   (B) transduction of the cannula to determine the vascular waveform and pressure
   (C) ultrasound guidance
   (D) color of the blood emerging from the needle hub
   (E) pulsatile flow of blood from the needle hub

11. Which of the following statements about venous air embolism (VAE) is TRUE?

   (A) The incidence of VAE is similar between prone and sitting neurosurgical cases.
   (B) The cerebral sinuses are a common source of air emboli.
   (C) The generation of VAE requires the surgical site to be at or slightly below the level of the heart.
   (D) A drop in the end-tidal carbon dioxide level is the most sensitive sign of VAE.
   (E) Once diagnosed, PEEP should be added to prevent further air emboli.

12. Which of the following is NOT a risk factor for pulmonary artery rupture associated with the use of pulmonary artery (Swan-Ganz) catheters?

   (A) pulmonary hypertension
   (B) fever
   (C) anticoagulant use
   (D) mitral valve stenosis
   (E) advanced age

13. Which of the following practices is LEAST likely to aid in preventing an intraneural injection during peripheral nerve block?

   (A) use of a small (vs. large) gauge needle
   (B) use of a beveled (vs. pencil point) needle
   (C) use of electrical nerve stimulation
   (D) use of ultrasonographic guidance
   (E) monitoring injection pressure during injection

14. Which of the following arm positions is MOST likely to result in changes in upper limb somatosensory evoked potentials during spinal surgery in the prone position?

   (A) arms tucked in at the side, forearms supinated
   (B) arms tucked in at the side, forearms pronated
   (C) arms extended above the head ("Superman-style")
   (D) arms abducted laterally 90°, elbows extended
   (E) arms abducted laterally 90°, elbows flexed 90°

15. Which of the following statements regarding the use of pneumatic limb tourniquets for surgery is TRUE?

(A) Tourniquet cuff width is directly proportional to the inflation pressure required to occlude blood flow.

(B) The use of a straight tourniquet cuff occludes blood flow with the same inflation pressure as a contoured cuff.

(C) Tourniquet downtime, where the pressure is released for a short period of time before being reinflated, has been shown to reduce risk of injury.

(D) The pathophysiology of nerve injury related to tourniquet use is primarily ischemic damage to the nerve fibers.

(E) When setting inflation pressure, limb occlusion pressure should be directly measured.

16. Which of the following anesthetic techniques is LEAST associated with postoperative peripheral neuropathies?

(A) epidural anesthesia

(B) lithotomy position

(C) diabetes mellitus

(D) pneumatic tourniquets

(E) renal disease

17. Safety maneuvers that may prevent the occurrence of an airway fire during upper airway laser surgery include all of the following EXCEPT:

(A) maintaining the FiO_2 <30%

(B) use of a tube with a double cuff

(C) use of a tube constructed from polyvinyl chloride (PVC)

(D) use of an operative bronchoscope

(E) the avoidance of nitrous oxide

18. A patient is being ventilated with 40% oxygen during laser coagulation of laryngeal granulomas. Suddenly the surgeon shouts that the endotracheal tube has caught on fire. The most appropriate FIRST step should be to:

(A) Turn off the flows on the oxygen flowmeter.

(B) Splash sterile saline into the field.

(C) Immediately remove the burning endotracheal tube from the patient.

(D) Turn off the volatile agent.

(E) Disconnect the tube from the circle circuit and remove the tube from the patient.

19. The effect of occupational exposure to an operating room environment is most likely to increase the risk of which one of these events for female workers?

(A) spontaneous abortion

(B) congenital cleft lip abnormalities in offspring

(C) autism in offspring

(D) breast cancer

(E) sensorineural hearing loss

20. The initial drop in core body temperature during anesthesia is due to which of the following factors?

(A) decrease in metabolic rate

(B) redistribution of blood flow

(C) radiation of heat to the atmosphere

(D) evaporation from skin and exposed tissues

(E) conduction of heat to the operating room table

21. Of the four fundamental mechanisms of heat transfer, which two are MOST responsible for the linear phase of hypothermia during general anesthesia?

(A) conduction and radiation

(B) conduction and evaporation

(C) convection and radiation

(D) convection and conduction

(E) evaporation and radiation

22. Which of the following BEST describes the difference in mechanisms of hypothermia with neuraxial vs. general anesthesia?

    (A) Redistribution only plays a minor role in hypothermia.
    (B) Patients will complain of feeling cold faster.
    (C) Active vasoconstriction during the plateau phase is impaired.
    (D) There is relatively little convection of heat.
    (E) Intraoperative shivering is decreased.

23. Which of the following BEST describes the cardiac effects of mild (~1.3°C) postoperative hypothermia compared with normothermia?

    (A) There is a cardioprotective effect.
    (B) There is an increased risk of atrial fibrillation.
    (C) There is decreased myocardial contractility.
    (D) There is an increased risk of myocardial ischemia.
    (E) There is no difference in cardiac outcomes.

24. Which of the following is NOT a known effect of perioperative hypothermia?

    (A) increased incidence of wound infection
    (B) increased risk for blood loss and transfusion requirements
    (C) decreased affinity of hemoglobin for oxygen
    (D) bronchorrhea
    (E) increased duration of neuromuscular blockade

25. Which of the following is the BEST strategy in order to minimize the initial redistribution phase of hypothermia?

    (A) preoperative administration of vasoconstrictors
    (B) preoperative forced-air warming for 1 to 2 hours
    (C) elect to use spinal anesthesia when possible
    (D) wrap the patient's head in a piece of clear plastic once under general anesthesia
    (E) use of a simple cotton blanket

26. Which of the following locations gives the most accurate result when monitoring core body temperature?

    (A) tympanic membrane
    (B) bladder
    (C) axilla
    (D) esophagus
    (E) rectum

27. Which of the following is NOT a characteristic feature of heat stroke?

    (A) advanced age
    (B) hypertension
    (C) multiorgan system failure
    (D) altered mental status
    (E) rhabdomyolysis

28. Which of the following strategies is LEAST effective in preventing intraoperative bronchospasm in an asthmatic patient scheduled for open inguinal hernia repair?

    (A) advise preoperative smoking cessation of 2 months' duration
    (B) use of a laryngeal mask airway (vs. an endotracheal tube)
    (C) use of atracurium as the neuromuscular blocking agent
    (D) prescribing oral methylprednisolone 40 mg daily for 5 days
    (E) use of ketamine as an induction agent

29. A 21-year-old patient is admitted to the ICU with status asthmaticus. Her arterial blood gas reveals a PaO_2 of 72 mm Hg and a $PaCO_2$ of 46 mm Hg on a nonrebreather oxygen mask. Her peak flow rate is 35% of baseline. Which of the following therapies is MOST likely to improve her condition?

    (A) theophylline
    (B) helium-oxygen (heliox)
    (C) broad spectrum antibiotics
    (D) intravenous magnesium
    (E) leukotriene receptor antagonist therapy

30. The prevalence of latex allergy among health care workers is approximately:

    (A) 1%
    (B) 4%
    (C) 12%
    (D) 16%
    (E) 20%

31. Which of the following is LEAST likely to be a presenting feature of anaphylaxis during general anesthesia?

    (A) rash
    (B) flushing
    (C) difficulty ventilating
    (D) pulselessness
    (E) hypotension

32. Which of the following is NOT indicated for the initial management of anaphylaxis?

    (A) albuterol
    (B) hydrocortisone
    (C) epinephrine
    (D) fluids
    (E) ranitidine

33. Which of the following is the most common class of substances to cause intraoperative anaphylactic reactions?

    (A) antibiotics
    (B) propofol
    (C) neuromuscular blockers
    (D) latex
    (E) local anesthetics

34. Which of the following diagnostic tests should be performed the same day as the anaphylactic reaction?

    (A) serum histamine
    (B) serum tryptase
    (C) mast cell count
    (D) immunoglobulin E assay
    (E) radioallergosorbent test (RAST)

Directions: Use the following scenario to answer questions 35–37.

A 25-year-old male is emerging from an uneventful general anesthetic for a laparoscopic hernia repair. He has mild asthma for which he takes albuterol inhalers as needed, but has had no recent exacerbations or respiratory tract infections. He is on no other medications, has a good exercise tolerance, and a clear chest exam. The resident extubates the patient prior to awakening with an end-tidal sevoflurane concentration of 1% in order to decrease the risk of bucking on the endotracheal tube. Shortly thereafter, the patient coughs and begins to exhibit labored breathing, with high-pitched inspiratory sounds. Despite a good face mask fit, tidal volumes are minimal.

35. Which of the following is the most likely diagnosis given the above scenario?

    (A) anaphylaxis
    (B) bronchospasm
    (C) laryngospasm
    (D) airway foreign body
    (E) pneumothorax

36. The patient begins to desaturate to an SpO_2 of 89%. Which of the following therapies is most likely to result in successful termination of this event?

    (A) nebulized albuterol
    (B) racemic epinephrine
    (C) IV steroids
    (D) needle decompression of the chest
    (E) succinylcholine

37. Ten minutes later, the resident is called to the recovery room where the patient is awake but appears panicked. He is breathing at a rate of 40/min, and is tachycardic and hypertensive. His SpO_2 is 86% on face mask oxygen, and he is coughing up copious frothy secretions. Chest exam reveals bilateral coarse crackles. Which of the following is the most likely diagnosis?

    (A) panic attack
    (B) anaphylaxis
    (C) bronchospasm
    (D) pulmonary edema
    (E) myocardial infarction

38. Which of the following is NOT a risk factor for pulmonary aspiration of gastric contents?

    (A) pregnancy
    (B) progressive systemic sclerosis (scleroderma)
    (C) post-ictal state
    (D) meperidine
    (E) metoprolol

39. What is the approximate half-emptying time of clear liquids in the healthy stomach?

    (A) 6 minutes
    (B) 12 minutes
    (C) 20 minutes
    (D) 30 minutes
    (E) 45 minutes

40. Which of the following statements regarding the gastric aspiration of pulmonary contents is TRUE?

    (A) The ASA guidelines suggest a preoperative fast of 4 hours from infant formula.
    (B) Backwards-upwards-rightwards pressure (BURP) on the cricoid cartilage prevents passive regurgitation.
    (C) Omeprazole 20 mg PO as a single preoperative dose effectively increases gastric pH.
    (D) Empiric corticosteroids have no role following aspiration of gastric contents.
    (E) The incidence of aspiration with laryngeal mask airways (LMAs) is higher than with endotracheal tubes.

41. Which of the following regarding the genetics and pathophysiology of malignant hyperthermia (MH) is CORRECT?

    (A) Malignant hyperthermia is inherited in an autosomal recessive pattern.
    (B) Most patients who have an MH event have a family history of MH.
    (C) The principal genetic mutation responsible for MH lies on chromosome 17.
    (D) The inciting event in MH is the unregulated release of ryanodine.
    (E) MH is a channelopathy leading to dysregulation of calcium homeostasis.

Answers and Explanations:
Complications in Anesthesia

1. Which of the following is the most common complication of nasotracheal intubation?

   (A) arytenoid dislocation
   (B) submucosal tear of the posterior pharyngeal wall
   (C) avulsion of the turbinate bone
   (D) epistaxis
   (E) esophageal perforation

   Abrasion of the nasal mucosa as the tube passes posteriorly can lead to epistaxis, the most common complication of nasal intubation. This usually occurs in the anterior aspect of the nasal septum, and is more likely to occur with larger tubes, use of excessive force, and/or repeated attempts. The use of vasoconstrictors has been shown in some studies to reduce the rate of epistaxis. One study estimated the rate of epistaxis to be approximately 17%, although most of these cases were not severe. Epistaxis is classified anatomically as either originating anteriorly or posteriorly. It is often difficult to determine.

   If bleeding is noted on insertion, some recommend to continue with the intubation, provided it can be completed quickly. This will serve to use the tube to tamponade the bleeding. If bleeding is brisk, the tube can be withdrawn slightly and the balloon inflated so that blood does not contaminate the oropharynx. In addition, while the balloon serves to tamponade the bleeding site, the tube lumen acts as a nasal airway. If bleeding continues, it can usually be controlled by the insertion of a bacitracin-coated absorbent tampon. Once placed, 10 mL of saline should be instilled in the nare (using a 22-guage angiocath) to speed the expansion of the tampon.

   Ref: Butterworth JF IV, Mackey DC, Wasnick JD. *Morgan & Mikhail's Clinical Anesthesiology,* 5th ed. New York, NY: McGraw Hill; 2013.

2. Which of the following statements regarding sore throat following general anesthesia are TRUE?

   (A) The rates of sore throat for endotracheal tube (ETT) and laryngeal mask airway (LMA) are similar.
   (B) The most common injury attributed to the LMA is nerve palsy.
   (C) The incidence of sore throat is directly proportional to the size of the ETT.
   (D) High-volume, low-pressure cuffs are associated with a reduced incidence of sore throat.
   (E) Cuffed tubes lead to a greater incidence of sore throat than do uncuffed tubes.

   Sore throat is a common complaint after general anesthesia, affecting up to >10% of patients at 24 hours postoperatively. Up to 50% of patients who have their tracheas intubated with ETTs report sore throats; conversely, the use of an LMA reduces that risk to between 18% and 35%.

   Mechanical trauma is the main culprit with both types of devices. Injuries seen with ETTs include de-epithelialization, hematoma, edema, submucosal tears, and granuloma formation; the main concern with LMA use is pharyngeal edema, although nerve palsies (recurrent laryngeal, hypoglossal, lingual), arytenoid dislocation, and bruising of the other laryngeal cartilages and uvula have been reported. There is a direct relationship between ETT diameter and incidence of sore throat. Interestingly, while high-volume, low-pressure cuffs have decreased the incidence of post-extubation croup (a phenomenon due to the excessive pressure leading to mucosal ischemia and subsequent reperfusion edema), the high-volume, low-pressure cuffs are more likely to cause sore throat due to a greater surface area. Uncuffed tubes are associated with an increased risk of sore throat than do cuffed tubes. This has been explained by the flow of nonhumidified gas across the unprotected airway mucosa during spontaneous ventilation.

Patient factors associated with sore throat include female sex, younger patients, and those undergoing gynecological procedures.

Ref: Butterworth JF IV, Mackey DC, Wasnick JD. *Morgan & Mikhail's Clinical Anesthesiology,* 5th ed. New York, NY: McGraw Hill; 2013.

3. Which of the following is TRUE regarding dental damage during general anesthesia?

    (A) The reported incidence is approximately 1 in 50.

    (B) Roughly 50% of all anesthesia-related dental injuries occur during laryngoscopy.

    (C) Upper and lower incisors are damaged with equal frequency.

    (D) In the setting of poor dentition, mouth guards can reduce the risk of damage.

    (E) The use of an oropharyngeal airway during the case can reduce the risk of damage.

Dental trauma occurs in one out of every 2,000 to 2,500 patients undergoing general anesthesia. Fracture of the enamel surface is the most common injury, although subluxation or avulsion of the tooth may occur, as well as damage to artificial dental work such as crowns or veneers.

Poor laryngoscopic technique is to blame in roughly 50%, especially if the operator is using the upper incisors as a fulcrum. For this reason, the upper incisors are the most frequently injured teeth. Another common cause is biting, particularly when oropharyngeal airways are used inappropriately as bite blocks. Specifically designed bite blocks or a roll of gauze tend to reduce the risk of damage. Several patient factors increase the risk of damage, including previous trauma, poor dentition, protruding upper incisors, gum disease, and artificial dental work.

If a tooth is damaged, all of the fragments must be accounted for; a chest X-ray is sometimes required if the tooth is unaccounted for in the mouth of pharynx. All dental injuries should be explained to the patient and referred on for dental care.

Ref: Butterworth JF IV, Mackey DC, Wasnick JD. *Morgan & Mikhail's Clinical Anesthesiology,* 5th ed. New York, NY: McGraw Hill; 2013.

4. Which of the following is the most commonly injured structure during airway management?

    (A) teeth

    (B) tongue

    (C) pharynx

    (D) larynx

    (E) esophagus

The ASA closed-claims database registry revealed that airway trauma accounted for 6% of all respiratory claims. The claimants were typically young, healthy females undergoing routine (i.e., nondifficult) airway management. When classified by structure injured, the larynx was most common (33%), followed by pharynx (19%), esophagus (18%), trachea (15%), and temporomandibular joint (10%). Laryngeal injuries include ulceration or granuloma formation on the vocal cord, arytenoid dislocation, laceration/bleeding of the vocal cord, damage to intrinsic muscles, and infection of the soft tissue. The overwhelming majority of pharyngeal, esophageal, and tracheal injuries were perforations and tears. Several authors have implicated the use of rigid stylets within endotracheal tubes as causative factors, and advocate against their routine use. The advent of videolaryngoscopy has not reduced the incidence of airway trauma; in fact, multiple cases of soft tissue tears, perforations, and even submucosal tube advancement have been reported. The use of a rigid stylet to guide the tube with the operator's attention focused on the video image of the glottis has led to most of these complications.

Mortality from tracheal and esophageal perforation is approximately 15% to 20%, and is often due to complications related to subsequent mediastinitis and/or pneumothoraces.

Ref: Butterworth JF IV, Mackey DC, Wasnick JD. *Morgan & Mikhail's Clinical Anesthesiology,* 5th ed. New York, NY: McGraw Hill; 2013.

5. Which of the following techniques is MOST likely to prevent corneal abrasions?

    (A) petroleum ointment

    (B) paraffin-based ointment

    (C) methylcellulose ointment

    (D) vertical taping of the eyelids

    (E) horizontal taping of the eyelids

Corneal abrasions can occur as a result of direct trauma to the eye from items such as the laryngoscope, face mask, surgical drapes, or personal items such as name badges, stethoscopes, watches, etc. Postoperatively, patients can inadvertently damage their own corneas while rubbing their eyes, or by bed linens if positioned in the lateral position. However, direct trauma and chemical injury account for only 20% of corneal abrasions; the vast majority are due to failure of the eyelid to close properly (lagophthalmos), which leads to corneal drying. During normal sleep conditions, less than 5% of individuals exhibit lagophthalmos, but this jumps to up to 60% of patients while under anesthesia. In addition, general anesthesia significantly reduces tear production and stability, leading to a more rapid time to breaking of the tear film covering the cornea.

The prone position carries an increased risk for corneal abrasions, even with the head turned to the side. In these cases, the dependent eye is much more at risk than the non-dependent eye. Head and neck surgery is also a higher risk class of procedures, likely from direct trauma or pressure on the globe.

Taping of the eyelids is a popular method for preventing lagophthalmos and exposure keratopathy during general anesthesia, and is the most effective. Horizontal taping allows for full apposition of both lids; vertical taping is not recommended, as the lids may open under the tape. Taping should be done immediately after induction and before intubation, except in cases of rapid-sequence intubation where securing the airway is the first priority. Taping is not without hazards: if improperly applied, the cornea can rub on the tape. Allergic reactions have also been reported, and eyelash trauma is not infrequent. The use of bio-occlusive dressings such as Tegaderm or OpSite carries the advantage of complete coverage of both eyelids, thereby preventing evaporation of the tear film. There is some evidence showing superiority to taping in prevention of corneal abrasions.

Ointments have been used, with or without eye taping. The overall evidence from the literature, however, shows no difference in corneal abrasion rates when compared with taping alone. Moreover, the use of petroleum-based ointments disrupts the stability of the precorneal tear film, which may result in accelerated dryness. Paraffin-based ointments have been associated with blurred vision, allergic reactions, and a foreign-body sensation. Water-based methylcellulose solutions (i.e., artificial tears) appear to have a low complication rate.

Goggles may provide protection against trauma but do not protect against desiccation. Protective contact lenses appear to be effective but are relatively impractical and may cause abrasions upon insertion.

Ref: Butterworth JF IV, Mackey DC, Wasnick JD. *Morgan & Mikhail's Clinical Anesthesiology,* 5th ed. New York, NY: McGraw Hill; 2013.

6. Which of the following is NOT a risk factor for postoperative visual loss after spine surgery?

(A) female sex
(B) use of the Wilson bed frame
(C) long duration of anesthesia
(D) obesity
(E) the use of large amounts of crystalloid solutions for fluid replacement

Perioperative visual loss (POVL) is a devastating injury, and can be attributed to one of three mechanisms: ischemic optic neuropathy (ION), central retinal artery occlusion (CRAO), or cortical blindness. CRAO is typically caused by atheroemboli from an ipsilateral carotid artery. Cortical blindness is usually due either to trauma or ischemia from hypotension/arrest.

ION can occur either in the anterior portion of the optic nerve where the nerve enters the globe (AION), or the posterior aspect of the nerve where it lies in the bony orbit. Like other parts of the brain, the optic nerve enjoys autoregulatory control over a range of ocular perfusion pressures, although that range is not very large. If the MAP drops below the lower limit of autoregulation, flow is simply related directly to pressure. While the exact mechanism of ION is not completely understood, most experts believe that it is primarily elevated venous pressure in the head that leads to interstitial edema that is the initial inciting factor. This then injures the optic nerve through direct mechanical compression, venous infarction, or compression of very small pial vessels that supply the optic nerve. Although rare, this seems to be confined to certain types of procedures, such as spine surgery, cardiac surgery, and more recently robotic surgery of long duration in the head-down position.

Risk factors for ION have been derived from an analysis of a multicenter case-control study and include: obesity, male sex, use of the Wilson frame, longer duration of anesthesia, greater estimated blood loss, and a lower relative volume of colloid administered as the non-blood volume replacement. Obesity increases intra-abdominal pressure and predisposes to central venous congestion. The Wilson frame places the patient's head below the level of the heart when in the level orientation, leading to increased venous pressure in the head. Bleeding leads to inflammation, capillary leak, and replacement with non-blood fluids, which, especially when using crystalloid, leads to edema. Edema in the eye socket can increase intraocular pressure and increase venous pressure, potentially leading to a compartment syndrome of the eye. Anemia is also a risk factor for ION, partly because a steal phenomenon occurs from the ophthalmic artery to ensure oxygen delivery to the brain at the expense of the eyes.

The ASA practice advisory for perioperative visual loss associated with spine surgery outlines several strategies to prevent ION, including elevating the head of the bed to keep the head neutral with the heart or above it, keeping the head in a neutral position, using colloids along with crystalloids for volume replacement, and considering staging procedures for high-risk patients. It is also worthwhile identifying patients at high risk for POVL based on expected duration and/or blood loss. These patients should be informed about their risk profile and counseled appropriately (i.e., that there is a low but unpredictable risk of POVL). Intraoperatively, the anesthesiologist should continually monitor systemic blood pressure, periodically check hemoglobin values, and avoid direct pressure on the globe. The patient's vision should be assessed postoperatively as soon as the patient is alert if there is concern for POVL. If POVL is suspected, an urgent ophthalmologic consultation should be obtained; additional management may include optimizing hemoglobin values, hemodynamic status, and oxygenation.

Ref: Butterworth JF IV, Mackey DC, Wasnick JD. *Morgan & Mikhail's Clinical Anesthesiology*, 5th ed. New York, NY: McGraw Hill; 2013.

7. Which of the following drugs is associated with superficial thrombophlebitis following intravenous injection?

(A) thiopental
(B) dexmedetomidine
(C) propofol
(D) ketamine
(E) etomidate

Most anesthetic drugs do not cause inflammatory reactions of the venous system upon injection. However, some drugs are solubilized in agents such as propylene glycol or polyethylene glycol, both of which have been demonstrated to cause superficial thrombophlebitis.

Etomidate is one such drug, and the thrombophlebitis typically occurs 48–72 hours after injection. It is self-limiting in most cases, but subsequent clot formation in the damaged vessel has been reported. This effect is probably lessened by using a fast-flowing intravenous line. Both diazepam and lorazepam can cause thrombophlebitis from propylene glycol and polyethylene glycol, respectively. When diazepam is formulated in a lipid emulsion (Diazemuls), the incidence of thrombophlebitis is no different than that of midazolam. It has been suggested that rocuronium causes thrombophlebitis after injection; while it certainly causes pain on injection in awake subjects, the evidence supporting it being a thrombophlebitic drug is weak. Similarly, propofol is well known to cause burning pain on injection but does not cause thrombophlebitis.

Ref: Barash PG. *Clinical Anesthesia*, 7th ed. Philadelphia, PA: Lippincott Williams & Wilkins; 2013.

8. Which of the following drugs is MOST likely to cause tissue necrosis upon inadvertent intra-arterial injection?

(A) thiopental
(B) dexmedetomidine
(C) propofol
(D) ketamine
(E) etomidate

Accidental intra-arterial injection of drugs is rare, and is estimated to occur between 1 in 3,500 and 1 in 50,000 cases involving parenteral administration of drugs. At the hand or wrist level, where many intravenous cannulae are situated, arteries are small and superficial, and can be mistaken for veins, especially in vasculopathic individuals or those with low systemic blood pressure. Signs suggestive of intra-arterial cannula placement include bright red blood in the IV cannula on placement, pulsatile flow in the distal IV tubing, distal signs of ischemia (blanching, mottled appearance), and a more intense than expected degree of pain at the catheter location. Transduction of the cannula will usually confirm the diagnosis.

Intra-arterial thiopental results in a well-defined syndrome that can have disastrous outcomes. Typically, severe pain manifests immediately after injection along the distribution of the vessel (i.e., into the hand). However, this may not always be present because anesthesia is being induced. Skin pallor, redness, and cyanosis can occur. If the patient is awakened early, hypesthesia, weakness, paralysis, and anesthesia may be present, all from ischemia to the distal structures. In severe cases, significant edema, thrombosis, and ultimately gangrene may develop. The pathophysiology of thiopental-induced arterial injury relates to arterial spasm, direct tissue destruction by the drug, a chemical arteritis, and release of thromboxane that leads to vasoconstriction and thrombosis.

Once recognized, the injection should be immediately halted. If the procedure is elective, the patient should be awakened; if emergent, alternative means of continuing the induction should be undertaken (i.e., establishment of alternative venous access and induction/maintenance with other agents). Treatment centers around three strategies: first, heparin should be administered to prevent thrombosis; second, sympathetic block of the limb should be considered (i.e., stellate ganglion block/brachial plexus block) in order to cause sympathetic vasodilation; finally, vasodilators (e.g., reserpine, tolazoline), thromboxane inhibitors (aspirin, corticosteroids), and high-molecular-weight dextrans have been advocated.

While it causes pain on venous injection, propofol does not appear to cause any sequelae following intra-arterial injection.

Ref: Barash PG. *Clinical Anesthesia*, 7th ed. Philadelphia, PA: Lippincott Williams & Wilkins; 2013.

9. A patient undergoing an elective coronary artery bypass graft is induced uneventfully. The resident places a right internal jugular 8.5 Fr introducer, and while passing the introducer through the skin of the neck is somewhat difficult, it eventually gives, and is advanced completely. No catheter is placed through the lumen of the introducer. Several minutes later, the attending performing the transesophageal echocardiogram notices a moderate pericardial effusion that was not present on the preoperative echo. Which of the following best explains the pericardial effusion?

(A) perforation of the right ventricle by the guidewire
(B) perforation of the right atrium by the guidewire
(C) perforation of the coronary sinus by the guidewire

(D) perforation of the right ventricle by the tissue dilator

(E) **perforation of the right atrium by the tissue dilator**

Effusion and/or tamponade secondary to perforation of the cardiac chambers during central venous access are a relatively rare but potentially fatal complication. Depending on the severity of the perforation, the clinical presentation may occur immediately, or may be delayed by a day or weeks. One principal risk factor is a catheter tip position that is below the reflection of the pericardium on the superior vena cava. It has been recommended that a chest X-ray is performed on all central venous lines (and peripherally inserted central lines) to evaluate tip location. Proximal SVC and ipsilateral brachiocephalic veins are probably the best location. Other risk factors include the infusion of hyperosmolar solutions (which can cause erosion through vessel walls) and a catheter tip that lies at a more perpendicular orientation to the vessel/chamber wall, predisposing it to perforation with movement. Peripherally inserted central catheters (PICC lines) carry additional risk in this regard, because movement of the arm tends to move the catheter within the central veins and/or heart.

Catheter design may affect risk profile, as flexible, pigtail-style catheter tips are less likely to cause perforation. Similarly, the soft J-tip of the guidewire is unlikely to pass through a vessel/chamber wall unless an extraordinary amount of force is applied. However, the very stiff tissue dilator that accompanies the introducer is unfortunately a perfect weapon for vascular perforation; for this reason great care must be taken to only push the dilator through the soft tissue of the skin. A skin cut with the scalpel that extends down to the vein facilitates this. Once the tip of the introducer is in the vessel, the introducer can be gently slid off and advanced to an appropriate depth.

If the catheter tip is felt to be inside the pericardial sac, the tip should be aspirated and pericardiocentesis and/or surgical repair undertaken immediately.

Ref: Ha Hall JB, Schmidt GA, Kress JP. *Principles of Critical Care*, 4th ed. New York, NY: McGraw Hill; 2015.

10. Which of the following is the MOST useful is preventing inadvertent injury to the carotid artery during central venous cannulation of the internal jugular vein?

(A) blood gas analysis of the aspirate
(B) transduction of the cannula to determine the vascular waveform and pressure

(C) **ultrasound guidance**

(D) color of the blood emerging from the needle hub

(E) pulsatile flow of blood from the needle hub

Ultrasound guidance during central venous cannulation confers several advantages over the landmark-based technique. A review of 26 randomized controlled trials comparing the two methods revealed the following benefits:

- 82% relative risk reduction in failed catheter placement (CI 68%–90%)

- 75% relative risk reduction in arterial puncture (CI 58%–85%)

- 79% relative risk reduction for pneumothorax (CI 27%–94%, $p = 0.009$)

The theoretical advantage of ultrasound guidance over blood gas analysis, waveform transduction, and examination of the blood is that by the time a diagnosis has been made with these latter techniques, puncture of the artery has already occurred.

Arteriotomy is not without potentially serious complications. Localized hematoma and/or false aneurysm may expand and cause compression of other vital neck structures such as the airway. In addition, arterial dissection, thrombosis, and distal thromboembolism have all been reported. If a large-bore cannula has been inserted, prompt consultation with a vascular surgeon is indicated. There are several options for management, including percutaneous removal, surgical removal, or endovascular-assisted removal, but this complication will require a team-oriented approach.

Refs: Carmody KA, Moore CL, Feller-Kopman D. *Handbook of Critical Care and Emergency Ultrasound.* New York, NY: McGraw Hill; 2011.

Wu et al. *Real-time Two-dimensional Ultrasound Guidance for Central Venous Cannulation: A Meta-analysis. Anesthesiology* 2013;118:361–375.

11. Which of the following statements about venous air embolism (VAE) is TRUE?

(A) The incidence of VAE is similar between prone and sitting neurosurgical cases.

(B) **The cerebral sinuses are a common source of air emboli.**

(C) The generation of VAE requires the surgical site to be at or slightly below the level of the heart.

(D) A drop in the end-tidal carbon dioxide level is the most sensitive sign of VAE.

(E) Once diagnosed, PEEP should be added to prevent further air emboli.

Venous air embolism can occur whenever there is a direct connection between air and the vasculature, and a pressure gradient exists, promoting air being sucked into the vessel instead of bleeding. The most common clinical scenarios are neurosurgery procedures on the spine and head, where the operative site is located above the level of the heart. This positioning establishes the negative pressure gradient, especially when the central venous pressure is low. Adding to this is the relative abundance of venous sites that are held open by dura (e.g., venous sinuses in the head) or bone during these procedures. VAE can also occur during central venous cannulation or removal.

Air emboli obstruct the pulmonary vasculature, raising pulmonary arterial pressures and causing increased RV pressure and a decrease in CO and systemic pressure. Myocardial ischemia from hypoxia and/or RV overload can occur. In large enough volumes, air can pass through the pulmonary circulation and cause systemic emboli. A large air bubble can also become trapped in the right ventricular outflow tract, resulting in an airlock and severe hemodynamic compromise. Signs and symptoms range from nothing to cardiovascular collapse. Dyspnea, chest pain, dizziness, hypotension, and a churning "mill-wheel" murmur are typical signs.

Monitors for detection of VAE include EKG (sinus tachycardia, right heart strain, myocardial ischemia), ABG (hypoxemia, hypercarbia), a decrease in the end-tidal CO_2 due to an increase in the pulmonary dead space, precordial Doppler (mill-wheel murmur), and hemodynamic changes such as increase PA pressures and CVP with decreased CO and systemic blood pressure. Transesophageal echocardiography is significantly more sensitive than all of these, although it may not be practical or even safe, especially in long cases in the sitting position. The next best is precordial Doppler (Figure 28-1). In cases where patients are thought to be at high risk, a multi-orifice catheter can be placed with the tip 2 cm below the SVC-atrial junction, so that aspiration of air may be attempted if VAE occurs. This positioning can be accomplished by filling the CVP catheter with an electrolyte solution and attaching the left leg lead to the hub (commercial kits with the EKG adapter are available). As the catheter is advanced, a tip position in the mid-right atrium is heralded by a equi-biphasic P wave on lead II.

Treatment of VAE begins with prevention of further air entry. The surgeon should be notified and

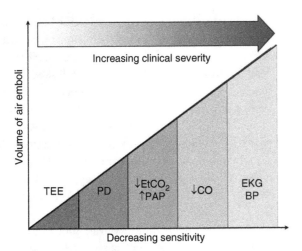

FIG. 28-1. Sensitivity of various monitors for detecting venous air embolism. BP = blood pressure, CO = cardiac output, $EtCO_2$ = end tidal carbon dioxide, PAP = pulmonary artery pressure, PD = precordial Doppler, TEE = transesophageal echocardiography.

advised to flood the field with saline or use wet gauze/bone wax on the open surfaces. Jugular compression and lowering the head level both elevate the venous back-pressure and prevent further air entry. The next step is to treat the intravascular air that is present by aspirating the right heart catheter if present, ceasing nitrous oxide administration, giving 100% oxygen, and supportive care such as pressors/inotropes and/or chest compressions. The use of PEEP to create a positive pressure gradient was once advocated but is no longer used, as it has been recognized to be ineffective and perhaps dangerous in promoting paradoxical embolism through a patent foramen ovale.

Ref: Longnecker DE, Brown DL, Newman MF, Zapol WM. *Anesthesiology*, 2nd ed. New York, NY: McGraw Hill; 2012.

12. Which of the following is NOT a risk factor for pulmonary artery rupture associated with the use of pulmonary artery (Swan-Ganz) catheters?

(A) pulmonary hypertension

(B) fever

(C) anticoagulant use

(D) mitral valve stenosis

(E) advanced age

Pulmonary artery (PA) rupture is a rare but often fatal complication of the use of PA catheters. It carries a mortality rate of approximately 30%, many of whom

die immediately from massive hemorrhage/hemoptysis. Those that do survive usually require an emergent thoracotomy for control and surgical repair. Some lesions are self-limiting and result in pseudoaneurysms; these are at risk for spontaneous hemorrhage and should be managed with endovascular coiling.

PA rupture sometimes occurs during the insertion phase, but more frequently this is the result of balloon inflation in a catheter that has inadvertently drifted into a more distal position that originally intended. Risk factors include preexisting pulmonary hypertension, advanced age, and hypothermia, all of which result in stiffer, less compliant pulmonary arterial systems. Hypothermia is an important factor to remember during cardiopulmonary bypass when the core temperature is significantly lower than normal. Other factors include anticoagulant therapy and mitral valve disease (which increases pulmonary venous and eventually arterial pressures). For high-risk patients, the pulmonary artery diastolic pressure can be used to estimate the wedge pressure (in most cases), rather than repeatedly inflating and deflating the balloon.

Ref: Longnecker DE, Brown DL, Newman MF, Zapol WM. *Anesthesiology*, 2nd ed. New York, NY: McGraw Hill; 2012.

13. Which of the following practices is LEAST likely to aid in preventing an intraneural injection during peripheral nerve block?

(A) use of a small (vs. large) gauge needle

(B) use of a beveled (vs. pencil point) needle

(C) use of electrical nerve stimulation

(D) use of ultrasonographic guidance

(E) monitoring injection pressure during injection

The goal of peripheral nerve blockade is to deposit the local very close to, but not inside, the nerve. It has been shown for decades that injection into nerve fascicles leads to neurologic injury and/or permanent disability. Peripheral nerves can be thought of as bundles of tubular fascicles that are enveloped and bound together by connective tissue, or epineurium. On the outer surface of the "bundle of fascicles" the epineurium becomes condensed to form a relatively tough membrane that provides protection and structural integrity to the nerve.

There are several measures that have been used to avoid pushing a needle through this outer epineurium.

Ultrasound guidance allows the clinician to observe the needle approach but not violate the epineurial covering of the nerve. This is a good monitor, but it relies on good needle-probe coordination and proper interpretation of the image. Similarly, it has been demonstrated that during electrical nerve stimulation, the presence of a motor response at currents less than 0.2 mA are associated with intraneural needle tip placement. In this situation it is wise to withdraw the needle and reestablish its position. It has been shown that if a needle is abutting the epineurium of the nerve, the force required to initiate flow through the needle tip is almost always high (>15 psi); monitoring the resistance to injection is an important safety tool to prevent inadvertent needle entry into the nerve. This is a nonspecific monitor—i.e., high injection pressures can be achieved with blockage of the needle lumen by tissue or clot, or needle positioning up against fascia or bone. However, if flow can be initiated with low pressures, then it is very unlikely that it is in a dangerous location with respect to nerve injury.

Low-angle (i.e., 30 degrees) beveled needles are less likely to penetrate the outer epineurium compared to sharp needles. However, if penetration does occur, sharp needles cause less fascicular damage than do beveled needles. In general, beveled needles are recommended for nerve blockade. The size of the needle is less relevant when it comes to *preventing* an intraneural injection, although nerve injury is less widespread when small needles do puncture the nerve, compared to that caused by large needles (i.e., 24 gauge vs. 19 gauge).

Ref: Hadzic A. *NYSORA Textbook of Regional Anesthesia and Acute Pain Medicine*, 1st ed. New York, NY: McGraw Hill; 2007.

14. Which of the following arm positions is MOST likely to result in changes in upper limb somatosensory evoked potentials during spinal surgery in the prone position?

(A) arms tucked in at the side, forearms supinated

(B) arms tucked in at the side, forearms pronated

(C) arms extended above the head ("Superman-style")

(D) arms abducted laterally 90°, elbows extended

(E) arms abducted laterally 90°, elbows flexed 90°

Upper extremity nerve injuries following anesthesia occur with a variety of patient positions, including supine, lateral, prone, lithotomy, and beach chair, although the pattern and distribution might differ between positions. Overall, the ulnar nerve is the most commonly injured location, followed by the brachial plexus and then the median nerve. Other isolated nerve injuries following anesthesia have been reported, including axillary nerve, radial nerve, and musculocutaneous nerve. It is generally agreed that stretch injury is the most common etiology due to non-anatomic positioning of the upper limb in relation to the shoulder/neck; compression injuries are likely also common.

Upper limb nerve injuries during prone procedures have been reported with nearly every type of arm position. SSEP changes have been observed with arms tucked by the patient's side as well as with varying degrees of abduction. However, the highest risk position appears to be with the arms extended straight above the head, due to a large degree of unnatural strain.

Ref: Butterworth JF IV, Mackey DC, Wasnick JD. *Morgan & Mikhail's Clinical Anesthesiology*, 5th ed. New York, NY: McGraw Hill; 2013.

15. Which of the following statements regarding the use of pneumatic limb tourniquets for surgery is TRUE?

(A) Tourniquet cuff width is directly proportional to the inflation pressure required to occlude blood flow.

(B) The use of a straight tourniquet cuff occludes blood flow with the same inflation pressure as a contoured cuff.

(C) Tourniquet downtime, where the pressure is released for a short period of time before being reinflated, has been shown to reduce risk of injury.

(D) The pathophysiology of nerve injury related to tourniquet use is primarily ischemic damage to the nerve fibers.

(E) When setting inflation pressure, limb occlusion pressure should be directly measured.

Tourniquet-related nerve injuries occur at a rate of approximately 1 in 6,000 for upper limb and 1 in 3,500 for lower limb. Tourniquet cuff design plays a role in the risk of injury. The wider the cuff, the less inflation pressure is required to stop blood flow. Therefore, narrow cuffs should be avoided as they require more pressure on the tissues to occlude flow, compared to wider cuffs. Similarly, a contoured cuff occludes blood flow at a lower inflation pressure than does a straight (cylindrical) cuff of equivalent width. While an attractive theory, the use of tourniquet downtime as a preventive measure for nerve or muscle injury has never been shown to be effective.

The pathology of nerve lesions related to tourniquet use is often attributed to compressive ischemia of the nerve. However, most cases of nerve damage have been shown to result from damage to the myelin sheath directly underneath the edges of the cuff, leading to a compressive neurapraxia.

Limb occlusion pressure is the minimum pressure required to halt blood flow. Studies have shown that the use of limb occlusion pressure (plus a safety margin) as opposed to an empiric value (e.g., 300 mm Hg) leads to significantly lower inflation pressures (up to 19%–42% lower). In its 2009 Recommended Practices for the Use of Pneumatic Tourniquet, the Association of peri Operative Registered Nurses (AORN) recommended that tourniquet pressure for normal adults be set at the limb occlusion pressure, plus a safety margin of 40 mm Hg for limb occlusion pressures less than 130 mm Hg, 60 mm Hg for pressures 131 to 190 mm Hg, and 80 mm Hg for those greater than190 mm Hg to account for variations in systolic pressure throughout the case. The recommendation also advocated adding 50 mm Hg in children. Limb occlusion pressure can be measured in variety of ways. The simplest is by an automated plethysmograph built into the tourniquet, which measures the occlusion pressures in the first 30 seconds of the case.

Ref: Hadzic A. *NYSORA Textbook of Regional Anesthesia and Acute Pain Medicine*, 1st ed. New York, NY: McGraw Hill; 2007.

16. Which of the following anesthetic techniques is LEAST associated with postoperative peripheral neuropathies?

   (A) epidural anesthesia
   (B) lithotomy position
   (C) diabetes mellitus
   (D) pneumatic tourniquets
   (E) renal disease

Postoperative nerve injury occurs rarely, and estimates from the largest databases quote an incidence of roughly 0.02% to 0.04%. However, nearly 20% of all claims in the closed-claims database involve injury to a specific part of the peripheral nervous system or spinal cord. Damage to three areas—the ulnar nerve, the brachial plexus, and the lumbosacral root—account for more than half of all the peripheral nerve claims. Factors implicated in postoperative nerve injury can be classified into three categories: patient-related factors, anesthetic-related factors, and surgical-related factors (Table 28-1).

TABLE 28-1. Factors associated with peripheral nerve injury.

Patient factors	Anesthetic factors	Surgical factors
Diabetes mellitus	Epidural anesthesia	Neurosurgery
Hypertension	Spinal	Orthopedics
Tobacco use	General anesthesia	Cardiac surgery
	Peripheral nerve blockade	General surgery
		Median sternotomy
		Lithotomy position >2 h
		Prone position
		Pneumatic tourniquet use

Note that the patient disease factors that are linked to postoperative injury share pathophysiologic features that lead to decreased perfusion of small vessels, a possible contributing element to nerve injury after surgery. The type of anesthetic technique may not appear to matter as much (with the exception of monitored anesthetic care, which has a lower incidence of nerve injury postoperatively), as the published rates after nerve block, neuraxial, and general all seem to be roughly similar. However, what might be different is the distribution of specific injury patterns. For example, after general anesthesia, the ulnar nerve is the most susceptible nerve; neuraxial anesthesia is obviously likely to put the lumbosacral plexus at somewhat higher risk.

Ref: Butterworth JF IV, Mackey DC, Wasnick JD. *Morgan & Mikhail's Clinical Anesthesiology*, 5th ed. New York, NY: McGraw Hill; 2013.

17. Safety maneuvers that may prevent the occurrence of an airway fire during upper airway laser surgery include all of the following EXCEPT:

(A) maintaining the FiO_2 <30%

(B) use of a tube with a double cuff

(C) use of a tube constructed from polyvinyl chloride (PVC)

(D) use of an operative bronchoscope

(E) the avoidance of nitrous oxide

Three elements are required for any fire to occur: heat (or a source of ignition), fuel, and an oxidizer. Common heat sources in the operating room include the electrocautery unit, lasers, and the fiber-optic light cord. There are plenty of fuel sources in the operating room, including drapes, gauze, hair, linens, etc. In the case of airway fires, the endotracheal tube is usually the fuel source and a laser (less commonly electrocautery) is the heat source. Oxygen itself is usually the oxidizer, but nitrous oxide also supports combustion, and during performance of airway surgery, the inspired concentrations of these two gases should be as low as possible (i.e., use air if possible).

Airway fires during laser surgery occur when the laser comes in contact with the endotracheal tube. Certain tubes are flammable and are not appropriate for airway surgery, including the usual PVC tubes that are typically used for most other cases, as well as silicone and red rubber tubes. The practice of wrapping tubes in foil tape is unsafe and should be discouraged, as the tube can kink or parts can be left unprotected where the tape fails to overlap. Specialized laser tubes that are made of metal (or rubber covered in metal) are made for this purpose. They contain two cuffs that should be inflated with saline mixed with methylene blue. In the event that the laser or a spark breaks the cuff, the surgeon will be alerted to this event by a splash of blue; the saline may also extinguish the fire. An alternative to using an endotracheal tube is to use an operative bronchoscope, either with intermittent ventilation, jet ventilation, or spontaneous ventilation. Although there is less flammable material in the airway, the downside to this is a less reliable FiO_2.

Ref: Barash PG: *Clinical Anesthesia*, 7th ed. Philadelphia, PA: Lippincott Williams & Wilkins; 2013.

18. A patient is being ventilated with 40% oxygen during laser coagulation of laryngeal granulomas. Suddenly the surgeon shouts that the endotracheal tube has caught on fire. The most appropriate FIRST step should be to:

(A) Turn off the flows on the oxygen flowmeter.

(B) Splash sterile saline into the field.

(C) Immediately remove the burning endotracheal tube from the patient.

(D) Turn off the volatile agent.

(E) Disconnect the tube from the circle circuit and remove the tube from the patient.

The first priority in managing this situation is to prevent *further* injury to the patient's airway. Disconnecting the endotracheal tube from the circuit deprives the fuel source of its oxygen, and it can then be quickly removed. In contrast, if oxygen (or nitrous oxide) continues to flow through the tube while it is removed, this creates a blowtorch effect, which will only serve to cause flame injury to previously unburned areas of the upper airway, tongue, and lips as it is withdrawn (Figure 28-2). Fiddling with flowmeter knobs will only waste precious time. The disconnection of the tube from the circuit and removal of the tube can be done in one smooth, sequential action.

Airway injury can develop very rapidly from edema caused by thermal injury. Directly affected areas will begin to swell immediately. Areas that were in direct contact with the flame may still be injured as superheated air is inspired and the soft tissues of the pharynx and larynx act as a heat sink. Tracheobronchial and pulmonary injuries associated with fires include reactive airways from aerosolized irritants (especially plastics), sloughing of mucosa, diffuse microatelectasis from loss of surfactant, and pulmonary edema from capillary leak. Once the damaged tube is removed, re-intubation should be considered immediately, as the swelling and edema can quickly progress, making laryngoscopy difficult or impossible. A large tube should be placed, as bronchoscopy will almost certainly need to be performed, and removal of charred/sloughed airway tissue may be required.

Ref: Apfelbaum JL, Caplan RA, Barker SJ, et al. *Practice Advisory for the Prevention and Management of Operating Room Fires: An Updated Report by the American Society of Anesthesiologists Task Force on Operating Room Fires. Anesthesiology* 2013:118:271–290.

Longnecker DE, Brown DL, Newman MF, Zapol WM. *Anesthesiology*, 2nd ed. New York, NY: McGraw Hill; 2012.

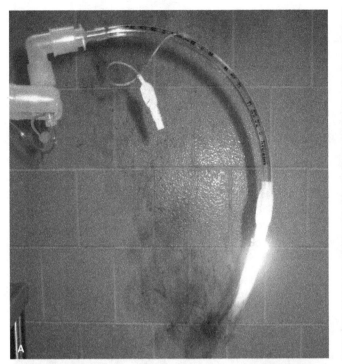

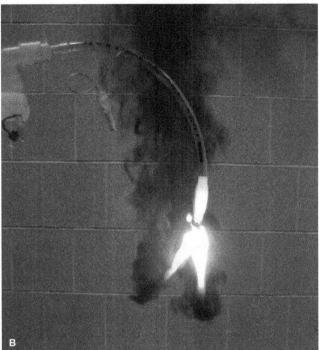

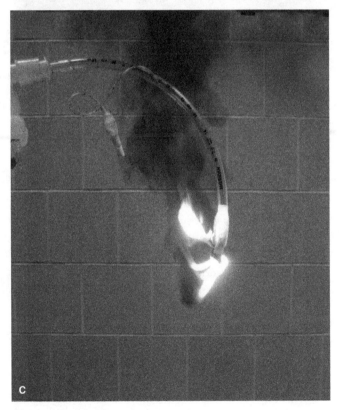

FIG. 28-2. A standard polyvinyl chloride 7.0 endotracheal tube on fire. **A.** Approximately 3 seconds after ignition while receiving 1 L of oxygen and 2 L of nitrous oxide, note the "blow torch." **B.** Approximately 10 seconds after ignition; the flame intensifies and is accompanied by a large volume of combustible products. **C.** Gas flows have been stopped, but the tube continues to burn vigorously. (Courtesy of Bil Ragan.)

19. The effect of occupational exposure to an operating room environment is most likely to increase the risk of which one of these events for female workers?

(A) spontaneous abortion

(B) congenital cleft lip abnormalities in offspring

(C) autism in offspring

(D) breast cancer

(E) sensorineural hearing loss

There have been several large-scale epidemiologic studies looking at the effect of working in the operating room on worker health. Hazards include the effect of trace gases from the anesthetic, radiation, exposure to allergens (especially latex), infections, and noise from saws and other instruments. Most of these studies are flawed in one or more ways, as multiple confounders exist and important data such as degree and duration of anesthetic exposure is missing. For example, early studies showed an association with working in the operating room and an increased risk of spontaneous abortion and congenital abnormalities in women. However, other results conflict with this and demonstrate that factors such as stress, night shifts, and standing for long periods of time are more causative.

Notwithstanding, the best evidence that we have does indeed suggest an increased relative risk of spontaneous abortion for female physicians and nurses who work in the operating room (RR = 1.3). The evidence is not as robust for congenital abnormalities. Nitrous oxide may be a causative factor: polls of female dental hygienists working in offices with unscavenged nitrous oxide revealed that these women were 2.6 times more likely to suffer spontaneous abortion that those who worked in offices where the gas was scavenged. One meta-analysis of 19 epidemiologic studies demonstrated that women with occupational exposure to anesthetic gases were at 50% higher risk of spontaneous abortion.

The data on cancer rates in operating room personnel suffers from the same weaknesses as other similar epidemiologic studies. However, women seem to have a slightly increased risk for leukemia, lymphoma, and cervical cancer.

NIOSH recommends exposure limits for waste anesthetic gases of 2 ppm (1-hour ceiling) for halogenated anesthetic agents when used alone or 0.5 ppm of a halogenated agent and 25 ppm of nitrous oxide (time-weighted average during the period of anesthetic administration). This body also recommends the following to reduce nitrous oxide exposure: (1) monitoring the air in operating rooms; (2) implementation of appropriate engineering controls, work practices, and equipment maintenance procedures; and (3) institution of a worker education program. Efforts aimed at reducing waste gases include frequent room air changes (standards for operating room construction from the American Institute of Architects require 15 to 21 air exchanges per hour), proper scavenging, attention to unnecessary circuit/mask/LMA leaks, and avoidance of open delivery systems.

There is no evidence that operating room workers suffer hearing loss at a greater rate than the general population.

Ref: Butterworth JF IV, Mackey DC, Wasnick JD. *Morgan & Mikhail's Clinical Anesthesiology,* 5th ed. New York, NY: McGraw Hill; 2013.

20. The initial drop in core body temperature during anesthesia is due to which of the following factors?

(A) decrease in metabolic rate

(B) redistribution of blood flow

(C) radiation of heat to the atmosphere

(D) evaporation from skin and exposed tissues

(E) conduction of heat to the operating room table

The core body temperature of an awake human is maintained within a very narrow range (0.1°C–0.2°C). Outside this range, thermoregulatory mechanisms are activated, namely vasoconstriction followed by shivering if the core temperature drops, or sweating if the temperature rises. Tonic vasoconstriction and arteriovenous shunting in the extremities keeps blood from losing heat to the distal extremities, which is why hands and feet are typically several degrees colder than the core.

General anesthesia defeats this shunting in two ways. First, most anesthetics are inherent vasodilators. Second, anesthetics (including volatile agents and propofol) reduce the threshold at which vasoconstriction is activated. This is a dose-dependent effect, so as concentrations of propofol or partial pressures of volatile agent increase, the patient will require a greater and greater degree of hypothermia to initiate vasoconstriction

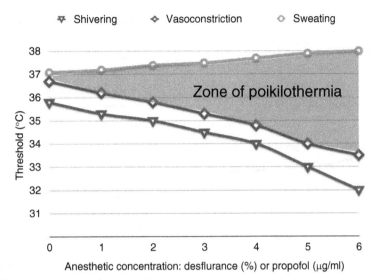

FIG. 28-3. The effect of anesthetic concentration on thermoregulatory thresholds.

(Figure 28-3). In essence, the patient becomes poikilothermic, until such time as their core body temperature falls low enough to reach the "new" threshold and stimulate vasoconstriction again.

Taken together, the loss of vasoconstriction results in a net shift of heat from the core compartment (head, thorax, abdomen, and pelvis) to the peripheral compartment (Figure 28-4). This so-called redistribution is responsible for the vast majority of core heat loss in the first 1 to 2 hours (~1.5°C). Note that the total amount of heat in the body is roughly similar during this time, but it is distributed throughout a wider volume.

Ref: Longnecker DE, Brown DL, Newman MF, Zapol WM. *Anesthesiology*, 2nd ed. New York, NY: McGraw Hill; 2012.

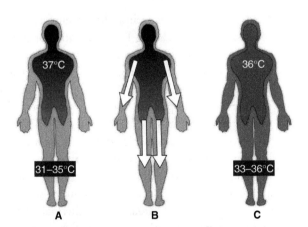

FIG. 28-4. Redistribution of heat from the core compartment to the peripheral compartment. **(A)** Normal temperature gradient between core and peripheral compartments; **(B)** with loss of arteriovenous shunting in hands/feet, blood flow to the limbs increases; **(C)** redistributed heat map, with a lowered core compartment temperature and an elevated peripheral compartment temperature.

21. Of the four fundamental mechanisms of heat transfer, which two are MOST responsible for the linear phase of hypothermia during general anesthesia?

(A) conduction and radiation

(B) conduction and evaporation

(C) convection and radiation

(D) convection and conduction

(E) evaporation and radiation

Intraoperative hypothermia follows a predictable three-phase pattern. The first phase, lasting 1 to 2 hours, is redistribution of heat from the core to periphery. Following this, the next 2 to 4 hours are characterized by a slow, linear decrease in core temperature (the linear phase), which can be quantified as the difference between heat production and heat loss. Heat production is reduced in anesthetized patients due to a decrease in the metabolic rate. The third phase is termed the plateau phase and is characterized by an attenuation of the heat loss due to reactivation of the vasoconstrictive shunts in the limbs (Figure 28-5). There are four fundamental means of heat loss:

1. Radiation: the loss of heat as infrared heat rays are emitted from an object and strike another object in their path. These emanate from all objects that exist above absolute zero, with intensity of the radiation increasing as temperature increases.

2. Convection: the loss of the thin layer of warm air on top of the skin by displacement with cold air (i.e., wind chill).

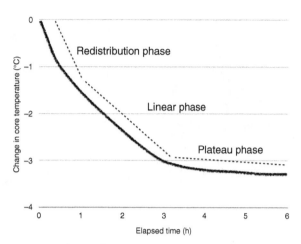

FIG. 28-5. Phases of intraoperative heat loss.

3. Conduction: the transfer of heat directly from one surface to another surface of a lower temperature (e.g., the mattress).

4. Evaporation: loss of heat required to convert water into vapor.

Since only a relatively small body surface area is in contact with the operating room mattress, there is little heat loss by conduction; in addition, foam mattresses are good insulators and do not accept heat readily. Evaporation can play a larger role in procedures with large skin incisions and exposure of internal organs to the ambient air, but this is not typically a big factor in heat loss. Most heat is lost through radiation and convection. Forced-air warmers reduce the impact of both of these processes.

Ref: Longnecker DE, Brown DL, Newman MF, Zapol WM. *Anesthesiology*, 2nd ed. New York, NY: McGraw Hill; 2012.

22. Which of the following BEST describes the difference in mechanisms of hypothermia with neuraxial vs. general anesthesia?

(A) Redistribution only plays a minor role in hypothermia.

(B) Patients will complain of feeling cold faster.

(C) Active vasoconstriction during the plateau phase is impaired.

(D) There is relatively little convection of heat.

(E) Intraoperative shivering is decreased.

Regional anesthesia results in vasodilatation of the blocked area and an increase in temperature of the skin in that part of the body (e.g., legs/pelvis with neuraxial).

This inhibits the central control of thermoregulation by "tricking" the regulatory system into accepting core temperatures that are actually lower than normal without triggering a response. Moreover, regional anesthesia directly inhibits the ability of the sympathetic system to actively respond, even once this lowered threshold has been reached. Redistribution accounts for approximately 80% of the 0.8°C reduction in core body temperature seen in the first hour. Even though regional anesthesia results in a cooling of the body, patients often feel warmer after the block, likely due to the same misinterpretation of the afferent impulses, and are less likely to complain of feeling cold. Despite this, it is not unusual for patients to begin to shiver under regional anesthesia. Unlike general anesthesia, stabilization of the temperature during the plateau phase rarely occurs because continued sympathetically mediated vasodilation permits continued heat loss.

Ref: Longnecker DE, Brown DL, Newman MF, Zapol WM. *Anesthesiology*, 2nd ed. New York, NY: McGraw Hill; 2012.

23. Which of the following BEST describes the cardiac effects of mild (~1.3°C) postoperative hypothermia compared with normothermia?

(A) There is a cardioprotective effect.

(B) There is an increased risk of atrial fibrillation.

(C) There is decreased myocardial contractility.

(D) There is an increased risk of myocardial ischemia.

(E) There is no difference in cardiac outcomes.

Mild hypothermia activates the adrenergic system, increasing the circulating levels of both norepinephrine (by 3–4 times) and epinephrine. The combined effect of this catecholamine surge serves to drive an increase in myocardial work, including heart rate, contractility, and rate-pressure product. In healthy volunteers, this is matched by a corresponding dilation of the coronary circulation. However, in those with flow-limiting atherosclerotic lesions, the increased oxygen demand associated with the cold induced catechol amine surge may predispose to myocardial ischemia.

Frank et al. compared passive thermal warming (simple drapes) to active warming (forced-air warming) in 300 high-risk patients undergoing abdominal, vascular, or thoracic surgical procedures. On arrival to the ICU, the difference in mean core temperatures was 1.3°C. After monitoring for 24 hours, patients who received active warming were 55% less likely to experience a morbid cardiac event, defined as unstable angina/ischemia, cardiac arrest, or myocardial infarction. In addition, patients in the passive warming group were three times as likely to have an episode of ventricular tachycardia.

Ref: Frank SM, Fleisher LA, Breslow MJ, et al. *Perioperative Maintenance of Normothermia Reduces the Incidence of Morbid Cardiac Events. A Randomized Clinical Trial.* *JAMA* 1997;277:1127–1134.

24. Which of the following is NOT a known effect of perioperative hypothermia?

    (A) increased incidence of wound infection
    (B) increased risk for blood loss and transfusion requirements
    (C) decreased affinity of hemoglobin for oxygen
    (D) bronchorrhea
    (E) increased duration of neuromuscular blockade

Hypothermia is known to increase the risk of wound infections (for example, by a factor of 3 in colonic resection patients) by two main mechanisms. First, hypothermia is known to directly impact both cellular and humoral immune function, including impairment of natural killer cells, macrophages, and neutrophils. In addition, lowering of the skin temperature results in thermoregulatory vasoconstriction, decreasing the oxygen tension in the area of the incision.

Bleeding and the need for transfusion are both significantly increased with even mild (~0.85°C) hypothermia. This is multifactorial, as both coagulation factor enzymatic function and qualitative platelet function are reduced.

The effects of hypothermia on the pulmonary system include tachypnea, depression of the cough reflex, and an increase in secretions (e.g., "cold bronchorrhea"). Importantly, hypothermia causes a left-shift of the oxy-hemoglobin dissociation curve, which decreases the ability of the molecule to unload oxygen at the tissue level for a given oxygen tension (i.e., there is an *increased* affinity for oxygen).

Hypothermia has pharmacologic effects. The duration of action of vecuronium is more than doubled in patients with a core temperature 2°C less than normal. In other words, the duration of action of vecuronium in these patients exceeds that of pancuronium in normothermic patients. This effect is also true of rocuronium and, to a lesser extent, atracurium. The tissue solubility

of volatile anesthetics increases with hypothermia, meaning that the anesthetic content of the body is increased when the patient is cooled. This does not affect potency (remember: potency is a factor of partial pressure, not concentration), but may prolong recovery as more anesthetic needs to be washed out. MAC decreases by about 5%/°C. Therefore, at 20°C, MAC is zero and no anesthesia is required. Hypothermia increases the steady-state concentration of both propofol and fentanyl, probably due to reduced inter-compartmental clearances between the core and peripheral compartments.

Ref: Longnecker DE, Brown DL, Newman MF, Zapol WM. *Anesthesiology,* 2nd ed. New York, NY: McGraw Hill; 2012.

25. Which of the following is the BEST strategy in order to minimize the initial redistribution phase of hypothermia?

    (A) preoperative administration of vasoconstrictors
    (B) preoperative forced-air warming for 1 to 2 hours
    (C) elect to use spinal anesthesia when possible
    (D) wrap the patient's head in a piece of clear plastic once under general anesthesia
    (E) use of a simple cotton blanket

The redistribution phase of core temperature reduction involves a loss of tonic thermoregulatory vasoconstrictor arteriovenous shunts in the hands and feet, and an increase in blood flow to the normally cooler limbs. If these shunts are defeated *before* anesthesia is induced, then there is no gradient for core heat loss, and the redistribution phase becomes negligible. This is accomplished by one of two methods. The first is cutaneous "pre-warming" with forced-air warming. In order to be effective, the temperature of the limbs must match core temperature, which is why this needs to be initiated 1 to 2 hours prior to induction. An alternative is to prescribe vasodilators (e.g., nifedipine) starting the night before surgery and continuing on the morning of surgery to pharmacologically induce a vasodilation. Both of these methods have been successful in reducing the drop in core temperature usually seen in the first 1 to 2 hours of general anesthesia.

Forced-air warming is a highly effective means of preventing heat loss and treating hypothermia. Most of the body's heat is lost through the skin by radiation and convection, and modern forced-air warming systems can transfer more than 50 W across the skin surface, counteracting both of these mechanisms. Carbon fiber electric blankets that cover the patient's skin surface appear to be as effective as forced-air warming, and are less bulky. In addition, air currents, which have been implicated by some investigators in an increase in colony-forming units on the sterile field, are not created with electric blankets.

Passive insulation with blankets, plastic, and metalloplastic covers ("space blankets") work to create and maintain a thin layer of warm air between the cover and the skin. As such, they all tend to be of equal efficacy. A single layer of passive insulation can be expected to decrease cutaneous heat loss by about 30%. Additional layers of blankets do not add much further benefit. Radiant heaters ("french fry lamps") can be effective, especially when parts of the body cannot be covered by forced-air warming covers (e.g., small children and infants).

Ref: Longnecker DE, Brown DL, Newman MF, Zapol WM. *Anesthesiology*, 2nd ed. New York, NY: McGraw Hill; 2012.

26. Which of the following locations gives the most accurate result when monitoring core body temperature?

    (A) **tympanic membrane**
    (B) bladder
    (C) axilla
    (D) esophagus
    (E) rectum

Core temperature can be monitored accurately in a number of locations. The pulmonary artery, nasopharynx, esophagus, and tympanic membrane are all located in the highly perfused core compartment and should reflect core temperature in most situations. Esophageal temperature may not reflect true core temperature in the setting of thoracic or liver surgery, or when a nasogastric tube is adjacent to the thermistor. Bladder temperature appears to reflect core temperature reliably in steady-state situations, but less so when temperatures are dynamic, such as during cardiopulmonary bypass. Similarly, rectal temperature can be reliable, and is especially useful during neuraxial anesthesia, but appears to have poor correlation with increases in temperature during malignant hyperthermia. Skin temperatures are imprecise; axillary measurements can correlate well to core temperature, but the thermistor must be positioned exactly over the axillary artery and the arm must be at 0° to the thorax.

Tympanic membrane temperature monitoring is ideal, as it is very close to the brain, and reflects core temperature even in dynamic situations such as rapid cooling or rewarming. Furthermore, evaluation of tympanic membrane temperature is easy and safe to perform, even in awake patients, especially with infrared thermometers.

Ref: Longnecker DE, Brown DL, Newman MF, Zapol WM. *Anesthesiology*, 2nd ed. New York, NY: McGraw Hill; 2012.

27. Which of the following is NOT a characteristic feature of heat stroke?

    (A) advanced age
    (B) **hypertension**
    (C) multiorgan system failure
    (D) altered mental status
    (E) rhabdomyolysis

Heat illness can be classified into heat exhaustion and heat stroke. Heat exhaustion is characterized by a temperature of up to 39°C, flu-like symptoms, myalgias, malaise, and nausea/vomiting. The primary problem is hypovolemia, and treatment centers on effective volume repletion.

Heat stroke is a life-threatening condition caused by a marked elevation in body temperature (i.e., 41°C). There are two types of heat stroke: classic heat stroke usually occurs when the environment is extremely hot (e.g., heat waves in the summer) in elderly or debilitated, those with severe heart failure, or those with a history of alcohol/drug abuse; exertional heat stroke typically occurs in young athletes and soldiers who are made to work for long periods of time with inadequate rest and hydration. Besides a hot environment, one of the risk factors is ambient humidity, as evaporation becomes ineffective above a relative humidity of 75%.

An increase in temperature results in an increase in oxygen consumption and metabolic rate, tachypnea, and tachycardia. Above 42°C, oxidative phosphorylation becomes uncoupled, and many enzymes cease to function. Blood becomes shunted away from the GI tract to the skin and muscles, leading to intestinal ischemia and increased risk for translocation of bacteria. A cytokine-related inflammatory response is mounted.

Clinical signs of heat stroke include skin flushing, neurologic dysfunction (e.g., dizziness, altered speech, agitation, delirium, convulsions, and coma), hypovolemia and hypotension, pulmonary edema, rhabdomyolysis, acute kidney injury, disseminated intravascular coagulation, hepatic injury, and hypoglycemia. Mortality is in the range of 20% to 65%, and is related to the degree of temperature elevation, the time to initiate cooling measures, and the number of systems involved.

Treatment begins with initial resuscitative measures with attention to airway, breathing, and circulation. Cooling measures are the primary means of decreasing morbidity and mortality, and include misting with cool spray, cold water immersion, and application of ice packs to the axillae, neck, and groin. More invasive measures include thoracic, peritoneal, and gastric lavage. However, peritoneal lavage is contraindicated in pregnant patients and those with prior abdominal surgery. Gastric lavage requires endotracheal intubation for airway protection and has been associated with water intoxication.

Ref: Longnecker DE, Brown DL, Newman MF, Zapol WM. *Anesthesiology*, 2nd ed. New York, NY: McGraw Hill; 2012.

28. Which of the following strategies is LEAST effective in preventing intraoperative bronchospasm in an asthmatic patient scheduled for open inguinal hernia repair?

   (A) advise preoperative smoking cessation of 2 months' duration

   (B) use of a laryngeal mask airway (vs. an endotracheal tube)

   (C) use of atracurium as the neuromuscular blocking agent

   (D) prescribing oral methylprednisolone 40 mg daily for 5 days

   (E) use of ketamine as an induction agent

Bronchoconstriction in a patient with inherently reactive airways can be provoked by a large number of stimuli (Table 28-2).

TABLE 28-2. Factors that trigger bronchospasm.

Intrinsic	Medications	Anesthetic-related
Increased secretions	Neuromuscular blockers	Latex
Increased vagal tone	Antibiotics	Endotracheal tubes
Acute respiratory infection	Beta-blockers	Nonhumidified gas
	Protamine	Airway suctioning
	Morphine	Extubation

Many of these factors are modifiable. Smokers should be advised to stop 2 months ahead of time, if possible, to allow for the greatest degree of ciliary mucus clearance recovery. If the disease is severe enough, adding corticosteroids, either inhaled or oral, has been shown to decrease post-intubation wheezing in poorly compliant patients. A dose of 40 mg PO methylprednisolone for 5 days is unlikely to cause adrenal suppression unless the patient has been on systemic steroids for more than 2 weeks in the past 6 months *and* is undergoing a major procedure with a large expected stress response. Inhaled bronchodilators should be administered up until and including the morning of surgery, either by nebulizer or MDI (either is effective if done correctly). Anticholinergic therapy such as glycopyrrolate can suppress airway vagal tone and dry secretions.

Drugs that release histamine can induce bronchospasm, such as mivacurium, atracurium, and morphine. Ketamine is probably the best choice for induction agent, provided no contraindications, as it induces bronchodilation by release of catecholamines. Co-administration of an antisialagogue is recommended because of ketamine's propensity to cause salivation. Anesthetic maintenance is often carried out with volatile anesthetics, as the potent agents are known vasodilators; desflurane, however, has been shown to provoke bronchospasm in smokers. Avoidance of endotracheal intubation and extubating patients have long been a fundamental consideration for management of the asthmatic patient. Laryngeal mask airways aid in this task by avoiding direct contact of the tracheal mucosa and preventing secretions from entering the subglottic airway.

Ref: Butterworth JF IV, Mackey DC, Wasnick JD. *Morgan & Mikhail's Clinical Anesthesiology*, 5th ed. New York, NY: McGraw Hill; 2013.

29. A 21-year-old patient is admitted to the ICU with status asthmaticus. Her arterial blood gas reveals a PaO_2 of 72 mm Hg and a $PaCO_2$ of 46 mm Hg on a nonrebreather oxygen mask. Her peak flow rate is 35% of baseline. Which of the following therapies is MOST likely to improve her condition?

   (A) theophylline

   (B) helium-oxygen (heliox)

   (C) broad-spectrum antibiotics

   (D) intravenous magnesium

   (E) leukotriene receptor antagonist therapy

This patient's blood gas demonstrates hypoxemia in the face of an augmented FiO_2, which is usually only seen in severe cases of asthma. Similarly, hypercarbia is a late sign indicating respiratory muscle fatigue and signals imminent respiratory failure. Recommended therapeutic interventions for patients with severe asthma include:

- Oxygen, titrated to keep SaO_2 >90%.
- Inhaled beta-agonists. Administered either by nebulizer or by MDI, inhaled beta-2 agonists are a mainstay of initial treatment.
- Inhaled anticholinergics. Ipratropium 500 mcg every 20 minutes × 3 doses, then prn has been shown to provide better improvement in bronchodilation when combined with albuterol than albuterol alone for severe asthma treated in the ICU.
- Systemic glucocorticoids. This is essential for refractory bronchospasm to relieve the airway inflammation and mucus plugging. These should be given in intravenous form for patients in extremis; most severe attacks will require a 10- to 14-day course.
- Magnesium sulfate. IV magnesium (2 g) is recommended for patients with life-threatening asthma or those whose condition remains severe (peak flow <40%) after 1 hour of conventional therapy. Two systematic reviews have shown it adds value to conventional treatment in severe attacks.
- Anesthetic agents. Both inhaled volatile agents and ketamine have been reported to be effective in case reports, although more robust evidence of their efficacy is lacking.

The decreased density of helium-oxygen (heliox) is the theoretical basis for improving airflow, but efficacy data is conflicting. Also, its use in severe asthma may be limited by its limited FiO_2 (e.g., 30%). Methylxanthines such as theophylline have been shown to be ineffective and predispose to side effects when combined with beta-2 agonists. Empiric antibiotics play no role in the acute management of status asthmaticus.

Ref: Hall JB, Schmidt GA, Kress JP. *Principles of Critical Care*, 4th ed. New York, NY: McGraw Hill; 2015.

30. The prevalence of latex allergy among health care workers is approximately:

(A) 1%
(B) 4%
(C) 12%
(D) 16%
(E) 20%

Latex allergy developed as a significant health concern in the 1980s with the adoption of universal precautions in response to the HIV epidemic. The estimated prevalence of latex allergy of 4% among health care workers is distinctly higher than that of the general population (0.8%).

Natural latex is the milky sap from the rubber tree *Hevea brasiliensis*. The processing of the raw product involves the addition of preservatives, accelerators, and oxidants to impart strength and stretchability to the rubber. There are no less than 14 antigenic proteins in natural latex, and these can be modified by the manufacturing process. There has been a well-documented association of latex allergy in those individuals with allergies to banana, kiwi, avocado, and chestnut. The protein portion in the product leads to a Type I hypersensitivity reaction (IgE-mediated urticaria and/or anaphylaxis); the chemicals present in the latex lead to the type IV reaction sometimes seen (contact dermatitis).

Latex exposure can occur via a number of routes, but mucosal and respiratory routes are the most important. Latex allergens are absorbed into the cornstarch powder and become aerosolized, leading to respiratory symptoms in hospital personnel. A move away from powdered gloves has been made for this reason. Many hospitals have moved to a completely nonlatex environment to prevent this occupational and patient safety hazard.

Ref: Bousquet J, Flahault A, Vandenplas O, et al. *Natural Rubber Latex Allergy Among Health Care Workers: A Systematic Review of the Evidence. J Allergy Clin Immunol* 2006;118:447–454.

31. Which of the following is LEAST likely to be a presenting feature of anaphylaxis during general anesthesia?

(A) rash
(B) flushing
(C) difficulty ventilating
(D) pulselessness
(E) hypotension

Type I, IgE-mediated hypersensitivity reactions, also known as anaphylaxis, are fatal in 3% to 10% of all cases, and prompt recognition of the syndrome and initiation of treatment is critical. This can be complicated by sedation and anesthesia while in the operating room, and the need to rely on objective signs. The most common initial presenting sign of anaphylaxis is severe hypotension and/or pulselessness (28% of patients), followed by high airway pressures/difficulty ventilating lungs (26%), and flushing (21%). Less common presenting signs include coughing (6%), rash (4%), and desaturation, cyanosis, EKG changes, wheezing, and urticaria (total 15%).

Mucocutaneous signs such as rash and urticaria are less common in moderate to severe anaphylactic reactions. This is likely because the significant hypotension caused by vasodilatation and capillary leak leads to a shunting of perfusion away from the skin and muscle tissue to critical organs such as the heart, brain, and kidneys. As such, circulating antigen may not be delivered to subcutaneous mast cells in sufficient concentration to provoke the wheal-and-flare response. Any histamine (or other mediators) that is released subcutaneously may not be enough to overcome the shunting of blood away from the skin. Once the blood pressure is stabilized, the cutaneous signs frequently appear, as perfusion returns to the skin tissues.

Ref: Longnecker DE, Brown DL, Newman MF, Zapol WM. *Anesthesiology*, 2nd ed. New York, NY: McGraw Hill; 2012.

32. Which of the following is NOT indicated for the initial management of anaphylaxis?

(A) albuterol
(B) hydrocortisone
(C) epinephrine
(D) fluids
(E) ranitidine

Anaphylaxis starts with exposure to an antigen (e.g., rocuronium, latex, peanuts). Usually the first exposure is unremarkable clinically, but this results in the generation by B cells of specific antibodies against this antigen. These are expressed on the surface of two types of cells. Mast cells are located in subcutaneous connective tissue and in the mucosa of the lung and gut; basophils are circulating granulocytes. Upon subsequent exposure to the same antigen, mast cells and basophils release the contents of their granules into the tissues (skin, lung, gut) and bloodstream. These granules contain a variety of vasoactive and inflammatory mediators such as prostaglandins, leukotrienes, proteoglycans, proteases, heparin, and platelet-activating factor; however, by far the most important mediator is histamine. Histamine is a potent vasodilator and increases capillary permeability. This largely explains the clinical picture of anaphylaxis and the four target systems:

skin (erythema, urticaria, angioedema), respiratory (edema, bronchospasm), cardiovascular (vasodilation, hypovolemia), and GI (mucosal edema, diarrhea).

Epinephrine is the drug of choice for anaphylaxis. The alpha-1 agonism reverses vasodilation, and the beta-2 agonism reverses bronchoconstriction. Epinephrine also aids in preventing the release of further mediators from mast cells and basophils. Fatalities during anaphylaxis are usually due to a delay in administration of epinephrine. In the first 10 minutes, over 50% of a patient's intravascular volume can be lost to capillary leak. Early and aggressive fluid therapy is therefore important. In mild cases where wheezing is the primary component, nebulized albuterol may be helpful, although epinephrine should be administered if cardiovascular signs begin to manifest. Early IV corticosteroids are recommended for their anti-inflammatory effects, especially if angioedema and bronchospasm are components of the reaction. These drugs take time to take effect; often 4 to 6 hours will pass before an effect is seen. Hydrocortisone is the fastest-acting steroid.

Histamine blockers make intuitive sense, since this is the ligand that is implicated in most of the disease process. However, histaminergic pharmacodynamics is complicated (Table 28-3).

TABLE 28-3. Effect of histamine 1 and 2 receptor activation on various tissues.

Effect	H₁ receptor	H₂ receptor
Positive chronotropism		✓
Positive inotropism		✓
Coronary vasodilatation	✓	✓
Decreased SVR	✓	✓
Increased vascular permeability	✓	
Bronchoconstriction	✓	
Bronchodilation		✓
Pulmonary vasoconstriction		✓
Pulmonary vasodilation	✓	

In general, histamine-1 blockers (e.g., diphenhydramine) are thought to be relatively benign in early anaphylaxis, although later use in cardiovascular collapse is controversial. Histamine-2 blockers (e.g., ranitidine, famotidine) are not recommended, as they can block the helpful effects of histamine on positive inotropy and chronotropy, as well as coronary vasodilation.

Refs: Longnecker DE, Brown DL, Newman MF, Zapol WM. *Anesthesiology*, 2nd ed. New York, NY: McGraw Hill; 2012.

Brunton LL, Chabner BA, Knollman BC. *Goodman & Gilman's the Pharmacological Basis of Therapeutics*, 12th ed. New York, NY: McGraw Hill; 2011.

33. Which of the following is the most common class of substances to cause intraoperative anaphylactic reactions?

    (A) antibiotics
    (B) propofol
    (C) neuromuscular blockers
    (D) latex
    (E) local anesthetics

Muscle relaxants account for 70% of all anaphylactic reactions under anesthesia. The benzylisoquinolines are more likely to cause a reaction than are the aminosteroids. Anaphylaxis has been reported with this class of drugs on first exposure, which suggests that there is cross-reactivity with another non-neuromuscular agent. Some studies have shown that there is indeed cross-reactivity to some cosmetic products.

Antibiotics are certainly a class that has known allergens, although the incidence of reactions to contemporary antibiotics is not nearly what it was with penicillin. In the early days of first-generation cephalosporins, there was cross-contamination of the vials with penicillin, which led to the oft-repeated 10% cross-sensitivity with this group of drugs. However, the formulations are much purer today, and if a patient gives a remote or questionable history of penicillin allergy (i.e., denies anaphylaxis), it is probably safe to administer a cephalosporin.

Latex allergy is responsible for approximately 12% to 13% of all anesthetic allergic reactions. High-risk individuals include the very atopic patient, children undergoing multiple procedures and/or bladder catheterizations, health care workers and those with other occupational latex exposure, and those with an allergy to bananas, chestnuts, kiwi, and avocado.

While thiopental has a reported incidence of 1 in 30,000 doses, there appears to be no cases of methohexital hypersensitivity. Similarly, allergic reactions to etomidate and ketamine are exceedingly rare. Propofol is formulated in a lipid vehicle containing soybean oil, egg lecithin, and glycerol. Those with a soy allergy should avoid this drug. Since there is no egg protein component to the emulsion, however, those with egg allergies are likely to be safe.

Synthetic colloids (hydroxyethyl starches, dextran, and gelatins) account for 4.5% of allergic reactions. Hyperosmolar, iodinated contrast dye can cause an anaphylactoid reaction, which is a direct (i.e., *not* IgE-mediated) degranulation of mast cells and basophils. Clinically, anaphylactoid and anaphylactic reactions are indistinguishable.

Most other classes of drugs that are used in typical anesthetic practice, including opioids and local anesthetics, are not associated with anything but a very remote risk of allergic reaction.

Ref: Longnecker DE, Brown DL, Newman MF, Zapol WM. *Anesthesiology*, 2nd ed. New York, NY: McGraw Hill; 2012.

34. Which of the following diagnostic tests should be performed the same day as the anaphylactic reaction?

    (A) serum histamine
    (B) serum tryptase
    (C) mast cell count
    (D) immunoglobulin E assay
    (E) radioallergosorbent test (RAST)

Treatment of the signs and symptoms of anaphylaxis is always the first priority, and performing diagnostic tests is of secondary importance. However, once the patient is stabilized, it is helpful to send off a serum tryptase to confirm the diagnosis of an allergic reaction. Tryptase is a preformed neutral protease that is released from mast cells. Its serum half-life is approximately 3 hours, compared with 3 minutes for histamine, making it a useful marker that can still be obtained once the crisis has been treated. It is recommended that three samples be taken to create a concentration curve over the first day: the first immediately after the reaction has been treated, the second about 1 hour later, and the third at 6 to 24 hours. Baseline tryptase levels are usually in the range of 0.8 to 1.5 ng/mL. Elevations greater than 20 ng/mL are considered diagnostic of an anaphylactic reaction.

Once confirmed, the patient should be referred to an allergist where they can undergo one or more tests. RAST involves exposing a disk coupled with a specific antigen (usually a drug in the anesthesia setting) to patient serum. However, the gold standard for determining sensitivity in IgE reactions is skin testing. The basis for this is to inject a small amount of suspected antigen into the dermis and observe the reaction. There is a small risk of anaphylaxis during skin testing. Patients with extensive skin lesions, those who are taking antihistamines, or those who have had a recent episode of anaphylaxis should avoid skin testing and undergo RAST instead.

Once a diagnosis is made, there is no benefit in pretreating allergic patients with histamine 1 or 2 blockers, or corticosteroids during subsequent anesthetics. Although they could potentially minimize the severity of anaphylaxis, these medications also blunt the early signs of an anaphylactic reaction, which can lead to a delay in diagnosis until full-blown cardiovascular collapse is the presenting sign. The best strategy is to avoid the most potent allergens.

Ref: Longnecker DE, Brown DL, Newman MF, Zapol WM. *Anesthesiology*, 2nd ed. New York, NY: McGraw Hill; 2012.

Directions: Use the following scenario to answer questions 35–37.

A 25-year-old male is emerging from an uneventful general anesthetic for a laparoscopic hernia repair. He has mild asthma for which he takes albuterol inhalers as needed, but has had no recent exacerbations or respiratory tract infections. He is on no other medications, has a good exercise tolerance, and a clear chest exam. The resident extubates the patient prior to awakening with an end-tidal sevoflurane concentration of 1% in order to decrease the risk of bucking on the endotracheal tube. Shortly thereafter, the patient coughs and begins to exhibit labored breathing, with high-pitched inspiratory sounds. Despite a good face mask fit, tidal volumes are minimal.

35. Which of the following is the most likely diagnosis given the above scenario?

(A) anaphylaxis
(B) bronchospasm
(C) **laryngospasm**
(D) airway foreign body
(E) pneumothorax

Laryngospasm is a reflexive closure of the vocal cords caused by light anesthesia and the presence of airway irritants such as saliva, blood, or foreign bodies. The protective reflex begins with stimulation of the multitude of mechanoreceptors, chemoreceptors, and thermal receptors located in the larynx. These are highly concentrated at the posterior aspect of the vocal cords. Afferent stimulation of these receptors results in a reflex tonic contraction of the intrinsic laryngeal mus-

cles, leading to adduction of the cords as well as descent of the epiglottis. Laryngospasm can be classified as either partial (with some gas exchange occurring and noisy, stridorous breathing) or complete (where the cords are firmly apposed, and no gas exchange is occurring despite the efforts of the patient). The incidence of laryngospasm has been estimated at 0.9% for patients of all ages, although that rate doubles in children under 9 years of age and triples for those under 3 months of age.

Although this patient has reactive airways disease, clues that this is more likely laryngospasm include the timing (immediately after extubation), the end-tidal volatile concentration (1% sevoflurane is approximately 0.5 MAC, which is likely too light for proper "deep" extubation), and the presence of high-pitched inspiratory sounds (i.e., stridor). Expiratory wheezes are far more likely with bronchospasm.

Ref: Longnecker DE, Brown DL, Newman MF, Zapol WM. *Anesthesiology*, 2nd ed. New York, NY: McGraw Hill; 2012.

36. The patient begins to desaturate to an SpO_2 of 89%. Which of the following therapies is most likely to result in successful termination of this event?

(A) nebulized albuterol
(B) racemic epinephrine
(C) IV steroids
(D) needle decompression of the chest
(E) **succinylcholine**

Once laryngospasm has been diagnosed, attempts to "break" it should be made immediately. Deepening the patient by the administration of IV propofol (30–50 mg) is sometimes effective, as is a jaw thrust maneuver. Frequently, all that is required to halt the reflex is the application of positive pressure with the face mask. However, complete airway obstruction due to laryngospasm cannot be treated with positive pressure and will only serve to press the arytenoepiglottic folds more closely together and force air into the stomach. If airway maneuvers do not work, succinylcholine should be administered either IV (0.1 mg/kg) or IM (3 mg/kg).

Ref: Longnecker DE, Brown DL, Newman MF, Zapol WM. *Anesthesiology*, 2nd ed. New York, NY: McGraw Hill; 2012.

37. Ten minutes later, the resident is called to the recovery room where the patient is awake but appears panicked. He is breathing at a rate of 40/min, and is tachycardic and hypertensive. His SpO_2 is 86% on face mask oxygen, and he is coughing up copious frothy secretions. Chest exam reveals bilateral coarse crackles. Which of the following is the most likely diagnosis?

    (A) panic attack
    (B) anaphylaxis
    (C) bronchospasm
    (D) pulmonary edema
    (E) myocardial infarction

This scenario is a classic case of negative-pressure pulmonary edema (NPPE). It characteristically occurs after the relief from upper airway obstruction, usually from laryngospasm, although reports have been made after bronchospasm. Other inciting events include foreign body in the airway, epiglottitis, vocal cord palsy, obstructive sleep apnea, biting of the endotracheal tube/laryngeal mask airway, and vigorous direct suctioning of the endotracheal tube adapter. The pathophysiology involves the generation of a large negative intrathoracic pressure by inspiring against an obstructed upper airway. This promotes the hydrostatic transudation of fluid from the pulmonary capillaries into the extracellular fluid and alveoli. Other factors that exacerbate the clinical picture are hypoxia, hypercarbia, and increased release of catecholamines. Hypoxia in particular increases pulmonary vascular resistance and depresses myocardial contractility, contributing to pulmonary edema formation.

The typical clinical presentation is rapid onset of respiratory distress, coughing of frothy secretions, hemoptysis, hypoxia, and widespread crackles on chest auscultation. Chest radiographs often show evidence of both interstitial edema (Kerley B lines, peribronchial cuffing, and pleural effusion) and, if intrathoracic pressures were sufficiently negative, alveolar infiltrates (consolidation). NPPE is usually self-limiting and resolution is usually within 24 hours. However, most patients that earn the diagnosis will need some form of treatment, including maintenance of a patent airway, application of oxygen, and positive airway pressure. This occasionally requires re-intubation and mechanical ventilation, but can often be accomplished with noninvasive positive-pressure ventilation such as Bi-PAP. Diuretics are frequently administered, although the evidence base for their use is very limited.

Ref: Longnecker DE, Brown DL, Newman MF, Zapol WM. *Anesthesiology*, 2nd ed. New York, NY: McGraw Hill; 2012.

38. Which of the following is NOT a risk factor for pulmonary aspiration of gastric contents?

    (A) pregnancy
    (B) progressive systemic sclerosis (scleroderma)
    (C) post-ictal state
    (D) meperidine
    (E) metoprolol

There are three principal types of risk factors for gastric aspiration: increases in gastric volume (i.e., delayed gastric emptying), impairment of the lower esophageal sphincter, and impairment of the laryngeal protective reflexes. This can be thought of as the "Swiss cheese" model—for aspiration of gastric contents to occur, all three of these conditions must be present.

Delayed gastric emptying
- Autonomic dysfunction (diabetes mellitus, chronic renal failure)
- Progressive systemic sclerosis (scleroderma)
- Neurologic disease (Parkinson's disease, multiple sclerosis, diffuse neuromuscular disease)
- Pregnancy
- Beta-2 agonism (pain, stress, trauma)
- Medications (opioids, antimuscarinics)
- Postvagotomy
- Pyloric dysfunction/altered duodenal motility
- Postviral gastroparesis

Lower esophageal incompetence/predisposition for regurgitation
- Pregnancy
- Hiatal hernia
- Obesity
- Progressive systemic sclerosis (scleroderma)
- Alcohol
- Smoking
- Achalasia
- Cricoid pressure
- Light anesthesia
- Lithotomy position
- Medications (atropine, glycopyrrolate, dopamine, sodium nitroprusside, beta-agonists, opioids, propofol, thiopental, inhaled anesthetics, glucagon)

Laryngeal incompetence

- GA/sedation
- Neurologic (bulbar disease, head injury, CVA, post-ictal, coma)
- Postintubation lasting >8 hours (mechanical effect)
- Blockade of recurrent laryngeal nerve(s)
- Opioids
- Elderly

Metoprolol is a beta-blocker, which increases LES tone and increases gastric emptying.

Ref: Longnecker DE, Brown DL, Newman MF, Zapol WM. *Anesthesiology*, 2nd ed. New York, NY: McGraw Hill; 2012.

39. What is the approximate half-emptying time of clear liquids in the healthy stomach?

(A) 6 minutes
(B) 12 minutes
(C) 20 minutes
(D) 30 minutes
(E) 45 minutes

Liquids are emptied from the stomach as a function of the pressure gradient between the stomach and duodenum. Physiologic studies have shown that in healthy humans, the time to empty half of the volume is 12 minutes. Therefore, over 90% of the volume is gone in four half-lives, or 48 minutes. Delayed gastric emptying can be caused by disease processes (e.g., diabetes mellitus, chronic renal failure), beta-2 agonism (stress, pain), medications (opioids, antimuscarinics), and the mechanical/hormonal changes associated with pregnancy.

Many systems are moving toward encouraging clear liquids up until this 2-hour mark, as it has been shown to actually reduce residual gastric volumes at induction compared to standard NPO after midnight. In addition, there is evidence that this practice enhances recovery and helps decrease length of stay after colonic surgery. Finally, allowing carbohydrate drinks up to 2 hours ahead of time may prevent dehydration, hypoglycemia, and prevent the hunger and thirst that many patients, especially children, find uncomfortable. There is no evidence that allowing clear fluids up to 2 hours prior to surgery increases morbidity or the risk of gastric aspiration.

Ref: Hauser B, Roelants M, De Schepper J, et al. Gastric emptying of liquids in children. *J Pediatr Gastroenterol Nutr* 2016;62:403–408.

40. Which of the following statements regarding the gastric aspiration of pulmonary contents is TRUE?

(A) The ASA guidelines suggest a preoperative fast of 4 hours from infant formula.
(B) Backwards-upwards-rightwards pressure (BURP) on the cricoid cartilage prevents passive regurgitation.
(C) Omeprazole 20 mg PO as a single preoperative dose effectively increases gastric pH.
(D) Empiric corticosteroids have no role following aspiration of gastric contents.
(E) The incidence of aspiration with laryngeal mask airways (LMAs) is higher than with endotracheal tubes.

The ASA fasting guidelines suggest 2 hours for clear fluids, 4 hours for breast milk, 6 hours for infant formula, nonhuman milk, and solids, and 8 hours for a large and/or fatty meal.

The BURP maneuver is advocated as a method to improve laryngoscopic view of the glottis, not a safety maneuver to prevent regurgitation of gastric contents. As initially described, and as validated in cadaver studies, the correct performance of Sellick's maneuver (or cricoid pressure) involves the application of 44 N of force directly backwards on the cricoid ring to occlude the esophagus. The efficacy of cricoid pressure is controversial, however, with MRI studies showing that the esophagus "slips out" to the anterolateral aspect of the vertebral body when pressurized from the anterior direction by the cricoid ring. Furthermore, several studies have demonstrated that cricoid pressure worsens the visualization of the larynx, as well as the ability to efficiently and correctly place endotracheal tubes and LMA devices. Finally, there is debate as to whether cricoid pressure, as it is commonly taught, is done in a proper fashion when required. For example, poorly trained assistants are likely to grasp the wrong cartilaginous structure with their fingers and/or apply an ineffective amount of pressure to that cartilage.

While a single dose of ranitidine 150 mg PO on the morning of surgery has been shown to decrease gastric volumes and increase pH, omeprazole requires two successive doses to achieve this: one the night before, and one the morning of surgery. As such, a single dose does little to change the chemistry or volume of the gastric secretions.

Once an aspiration event has occurred, therapy should be focused on preventing further pulmonary aspiration of whatever gastric contents have been regurgitated (i.e., head-down positioning), followed by immediate endotracheal intubation and suctioning of the tracheobronchial tree. The stomach should be suctioned out and, if particulate matter is suspected, bronchoscopy performed to identify the degree of soiling of the airway. Supportive care aimed at maintaining oxygenation and preventing/treating bronchospasm is initiated. Since aspiration pneumonitis is a sterile event in most cases, there is no role for empiric antibiotics. Similarly, empiric steroid therapy has shown to be ineffective and in some cases has led to worsened outcomes.

Numerous studies using a variety of methodologies including pH measurement, marker dyes, and bronchoscopic examination have shown that LMA airways are relatively resistant to the passage of regurgitated material into the tracheobronchial tree. A recent large systematic review has shown that in randomized controlled trials comparing the two devices, there is no difference in the risk of pulmonary aspiration of gastric contents for elective surgical patients.

Ref: Yu SH, Beirne OR. *Laryngeal Mask Airways have a Lower Risk of Airway Complications Compared with Endotracheal intubation: A Systematic Review. J Oral Maxillofac Surg* 2010;68:2359–2376.

41. Which of the following regarding the genetics and pathophysiology of malignant hyperthermia (MH) is CORRECT?

    (A) Malignant hyperthermia is inherited in an autosomal recessive pattern.

    (B) Most patients who have an MH event have a family history of MH.

    (C) The principal genetic mutation responsible for MH lies on chromosome 17.

    (D) The inciting event in MH is the unregulated release of ryanodine.

    (E) **MH is a channelopathy leading to dysregulation of calcium homeostasis.**

Malignant hyperthermia is a disorder of skeletal muscle that can be pharmacologically triggered to produce a combination of hypermetabolism, muscle rigidity, and rhabdomyolysis. It is of special interest to anesthesiologists, since the volatile agents and succinylcholine are both known to trigger the event.

MH is inherited in an autosomal dominant pattern, and has been seen worldwide in all races. It is estimated that its prevalence in the general population is between 1:5,000 and 1:10,000. Despite it not being a sex-linked inheritance pattern, many registries and observers have reported it being approximately three times more prevalent in males. There is some association with young age, increased muscularity, increased muscle tone (hypertonia) as well as a history of muscle cramps. Only 7% of patients in the North American MH Registry had a family history at the time of their triggering anesthetic.

The pathophysiology of MH is related to unregulated release of calcium from the sarcoplasmic reticulum in skeletal muscle. During normal depolarization of the muscle cell membrane, voltage-gated calcium channels undergo a conformational change and permit the release of calcium from the sarcoplasmic reticulum. Calcium floods the cytoplasm of the cell and binds to troponin C, initiating the mechanical contraction event. Calcium is then actively pumped back into the sarcoplasmic reticulum.

Patients susceptible to MH have a channelopathy of one or more proteins involved in this calcium release. By far the most studied is the ryanodine receptor type 1 (RYR1) protein. Activation of RYR1 by either calcium or caffeine causes the increased release of calcium into the cytosol. In contrast, dantrolene, the antidote to MH, is a potent inhibitor of RYR1. Over 60% of families that are MH susceptible are known to have mutations of the gene coding for RYR1, which is located on chromosome 19q12-13. There are currently over 30 known mutations that produce a dysfunctional RYR1 protein. These dysfunctional receptors respond to a variety of stimuli (including volatile anesthetics, large calcium and potassium fluxes, and caffeine) in two ways: (1) the receptors have a lower threshold for opening and (2) they are unable to close as quickly. This prolongs the time that calcium is able to travel down its concentration gradient and vastly increases the overall intracellular calcium concentration. This leads to unopposed contraction, rigidity, and hypermetabolism characteristic of the MH event.

Ref: Longnecker DE, Brown DL, Newman MF, Zapol WM. *Anesthesiology*, 2nd ed. New York, NY: McGraw Hill; 2012.

CHAPTER 29

Postoperative Period

1. Whenever possible, it is recommended to use multimodal analgesia for postoperative pain management. Following total knee arthroplasty, which multimodal technique for postoperative pain management is most effective?

   (A) postincisional infiltration of bupivacaine
   (B) epidural morphine
   (C) IV opioids and pregabalin
   (D) IV opioids and ketamine
   (E) IV opioids and acetaminophen

2. In an attempt to reduce the incidence of chronic postsurgical pain (CPSP), nonopioid adjuvant analgesics are often administered. Best evidence suggests which of the following adjuvants may modify the risk of CPSP?

   (A) ketamine
   (B) gabapentin
   (C) dexmedetomidine
   (D) magnesium
   (E) amitriptyline

3. Within clinically relevant dosages, which of the following nonopioid adjuvants can cause hypotension?

   (A) lidocaine infusion
   (B) ketamine
   (C) pregabalin
   (D) dexmedetomidine
   (E) dexamethasone

4. Traditional NSAIDs and COX-2 inhibitors have a variety of side effects. Compared to COX-2 inhibitors, which of the following side effects is seen MORE OFTEN in patients administered traditional NSAIDs?

   (A) GI hemorrhage
   (B) decreased renal function
   (C) myocardial infarction
   (D) asthma
   (E) headache

5. Nonopioid adjuvants for postoperative analgesia may have all of the following benefits EXCEPT:

   (A) reduced opioid induced hyperalgesia
   (B) reduced risk of chronic pain
   (C) reduced postoperative pain intensity
   (D) preventive analgesia
   (E) preemptive analgesia

6. Low-dose ketamine (0.5–1 mg/kg, with continuous infusion of 2–10 mcg/kg/min) is often used as a perioperative nonopioid adjuvant. What is considered the primary mechanism of action for low-dose ketamine's analgesic effects?

   (A) NMDA receptor antagonism
   (B) mu-opioid receptor agonism
   (C) kappa-opioid receptor agonism
   (D) muscarinic receptor agonism
   (E) Na^+ channel inhibition

7. A patient is undergoing high-risk vascular surgery. Clonidine is selected as an adjuvant for perioperative pain management. Which of the following is an additional benefit of clonidine?

    (A) earlier intake of enteral nutrition
    (B) reduced risk of respiratory depression
    (C) reduced risk of significant hypotension
    (D) reduced risk of myocardial infarction
    (E) reduced risk of death

8. For treatment of moderate to severe postoperative pain, which of the following opioids is LEAST effective?

    (A) transdermal fentanyl patch
    (B) intravenous buprenorphine
    (C) intravenous sufentanil
    (D) oral oxycodone
    (E) intramuscular meperidine

9. For an adult, which of the following single-dose analgesics provides the greatest pain relief for moderate to severe postoperative pain?

    (A) ibuprofen 400 mg PO
    (B) tramadol 50 mg PO
    (C) acetaminophen 650 mg PO
    (D) codeine 60 mg PO
    (E) aspirin 650 mg PO

10. For infiltration anesthesia in adults, what is the maximum recommended dose of bupivacaine?

    (A) 1 mg/kg
    (B) 2 mg/kg
    (C) 4.5 mg/kg
    (D) 7 mg/kg
    (E) 9 mg/kg

11. For an opioid-naive adult after surgery, what is an acceptable initial order for a fentanyl patient-controlled analgesia (PCA) regimen?

    (A) 0.5 mg IV q5min
    (B) 15 mcg IV q5min
    (C) 30 mcg IV q15min
    (D) 50 mcg IV q20min
    (E) continuous IV infusion of 0.01 mg/kg/hr

12. What is a typical dose of intrathecal opioid recommended for outpatient knee arthroscopy?

    (A) morphine 100 mcg
    (B) morphine 200 mcg
    (C) morphine 300 mcg
    (D) fentanyl 25 mcg
    (E) fentanyl 100 mcg

13. After bowel resection, a low thoracic epidural is used for postoperative analgesia. A variety of local anesthetic solutions with or without opioids are available. Rather than using 0.125% bupivacaine, what is an advantage of using a solution of 0.05% bupivacaine and fentanyl 5 mcg/mL?

    (A) less nausea and vomiting
    (B) less pruritus
    (C) less sedation
    (D) less motor block
    (E) less respiratory depression

14. An opioid-naïve adult patient requires intravenous patient-controlled analgesia (PCA) with an opioid for postoperative pain management. A continuous background infusion of opioid can be programmed in addition to the demand dose. What is an advantage of using a PCA system with a continuous infusion of opioids?

    (A) improved postoperative analgesia
    (B) improved postoperative sleep patterns
    (C) less physical requirement for patient
    (D) less overall opioid use
    (E) less respiratory depression

15. Multiple alternative and complementary therapies are available for postoperative pain management. To be effective, which of the following techniques requires patient susceptibility?

    (A) TENS
    (B) cryotherapy
    (C) acupuncture
    (D) hypnosis
    (E) ultrasound

16. Of the following alternative and complementary therapies for postoperative pain management, which is postulated to work via release of endorphins?

   (A) acupuncture
   (B) hypnosis
   (C) cryotherapy
   (D) ultrasound
   (E) therapeutic touch

17. Atelectasis is diagnosed as the cause of a patient's postoperative hypoxemia. Which of the following is the most likely mechanism for postoperative hypoxemia in a patient with atelectasis?

   (A) hypoventilation
   (B) diffusion impairment
   (C) V/Q mismatch
   (D) right-to-left shunt
   (E) hypoxic pulmonary vasoconstriction

18. Perioperatively, a number of factors may contribute to a decline in functional residual capacity (FRC). A patient is anesthetized and positioned for surgery: they are placed in the supine position, anesthesia is induced, followed by muscle paralysis, then the patient is placed in >30-degree Trendelenburg position and nonlaparoscopic upper abdominal surgery is started. Which of the following factors is LEAST LIKELY to decrease FRC?

   (A) patient in supine position
   (B) induction of general anesthesia
   (C) addition of muscle paralysis
   (D) >30-degree Trendelenburg position
   (E) nonlaparoscopic upper abdominal surgery

19. Postoperatively, a patient is noted to have significant systemic hypertension. Which of the following is the greatest risk factor for postoperative hypertension?

   (A) history of essential hypertension
   (B) increased sympathetic nervous system activity due to pain
   (C) increased sympathetic nervous system activity due to hypercapnia
   (D) shivering
   (E) hypervolemia

20. After an exploratory laparotomy for a bowel perforation, a patient is transferred to the postanesthesia care unit (PACU), and persistent hypotension is noted. Initial treatment consists of intravenous crystalloids. The hypotension is not corrected with fluid resuscitation. No ECG changes are noted; BP = 95/42; mean arterial pressure (MAP) = 60 mm Hg; HR = 96/min; CVP = 8 mm Hg, CO = 8.4 L/min. Based on this information, which of the following interventions is recommended?

   (A) continue IV fluids only
   (B) add infusion of dobutamine
   (C) add infusion of vasopressin
   (D) add infusion of norepinephrine
   (E) add infusion of epinephrine

21. Multiple patient factors independently predict the risk of postoperative nausea and vomiting (PONV) in adults. Which of the following factors is LEAST likely to predict PONV?

   (A) female sex
   (B) nonsmoking
   (C) history of motion sickness
   (D) obesity
   (E) patient <50 years old

22. The brainstem's vomiting centers may receive stimulation from all of the following EXCEPT:

   (A) the chemoreceptor trigger zone
   (B) vagal afferents of the gastrointestinal tract
   (C) the vestibular system
   (D) visceral and somatic nuclei
   (E) the cerebral cortex

23. There are many prevention strategies to reduce the baseline risk of postoperative nausea and vomiting (PONV) in adults. Which of the following strategies is most helpful?

   (A) avoid the use of neostigmine
   (B) use nitrous oxide instead of volatile anesthetic
   (C) use supplemental oxygen
   (D) routine gastric decompression
   (E) adequate hydration

24. The act of vomiting is associated with which of the following physical signs?

    (A) decreased salivation
    (B) diaphragm contraction
    (C) small intestine peristalsis
    (D) bradycardia
    (E) abdominal muscle relaxation

25. Which of the following medications is NOT indicated for prophylaxis and/or treatment of PONV?

    (A) dexamethasone
    (B) scopolamine
    (C) esomeprazole
    (D) haloperidol
    (E) perphenazine

26. Which of the following H1-receptor antagonists is indicated for treatment of postoperative nausea and vomiting (PONV) in adults?

    (A) fexofenadine
    (B) loratadine
    (C) dimenhydrinate
    (D) cetirizine
    (E) chlorpheniramine

27. Which of the following medications is the LEAST effective at reducing postoperative nausea and vomiting (PONV)?

    (A) ondansetron 4 mg IV
    (B) aprepitant 40 mg PO
    (C) dexamethasone 8 mg IV
    (D) droperidol 1.25 mg IV
    (E) metoclopramide 10 mg IV

28. In order to reduce postoperative nausea and vomiting (PONV) most effectively, when should ondansetron (5-HT3 antagonist) be administered?

    (A) induction of anesthesia
    (B) end of surgery
    (C) prior evening before surgery
    (D) 2 hours before induction of anesthesia
    (E) during maintenance phase of anesthesia

29. Despite initial prophylactic therapy with ondansetron, 4 hours after surgery a patient has significant PONV. For this patient, PONV rescue therapy may include all of the following EXCEPT:

    (A) dimenhydrinate
    (B) ondansetron
    (C) droperidol
    (D) transdermal scopolamine
    (E) dexamethasone

30. PONV management may include the use of droperidol. In 2001, the FDA published a "black box" warning regarding the use of droperidol. According to this warning, if droperidol administration is considered, which of the following measures is recommended?

    (A) avoid droperidol for patients with hyperkalemia
    (B) avoid droperidol for patients with tachycardia
    (C) droperidol only for prophylaxis of PONV
    (D) after droperidol, monitor ECG for 2 to 3 hours
    (E) after droperidol, monitor for extrapyramidal side effects

31. Multi-modal therapy is selected for a patient at high risk of PONV. Compared to monotherapy, which of the following combinations is LEAST effective at reducing PONV?

    (A) ondansetron + dexamethasone
    (B) ondansetron + droperidol
    (C) ondansetron + casopitant
    (D) dexamethasone + metoclopramide
    (E) dexamethasone + droperidol

32. Best evidence suggests which of the following non-pharmacologic modalities as most effective at reducing the incidence of postoperative nausea and vomiting (PONV)?

    (A) music therapy
    (B) ginger
    (C) hypnosis
    (D) P6 acupoint stimulation
    (E) aromatherapy with isopropyl alcohol

33. After a general anesthetic with the use of neuromuscular blocking drugs, a patient is awake and recovering in the postanesthesia care unit (PACU). The patient seems to have upper airway obstruction with a paradoxical breathing pattern. Residual neuromuscular blockade is considered in the differential diagnosis. In this situation, which of the following methods to assess for the ability to maintain and protect the airway is preferred?

   (A) train-of-four stimulation
   (B) tetanic stimulation
   (C) grip strength
   (D) sustained head lift
   (E) tongue protrusion

34. Postoperatively, which of the following complications is most common?

   (A) upper airway obstruction
   (B) hypotension
   (C) hypertension
   (D) altered mental status
   (E) nausea and vomiting

35. A physically fit, 30-year-old male patient undergoes an inpatient surgical procedure. His airway management includes the use of a defasciculating dose of rocuronium and succinylcholine. He is ambulatory shortly after the procedure but notes significant myalgias (muscle stiffness) for 3 days postoperatively. Which of the following factors IS associated with postoperative myalgias?

   (A) patient with greater muscle mass
   (B) male sex
   (C) inpatient surgery
   (D) early ambulation
   (E) use of defasciculating dose of rocuronium

36. Which of the following is a risk factor for postoperative cognitive dysfunction (POCD)?

   (A) general anesthesia
   (B) patient's age
   (C) intraoperative episodes of hypotension
   (D) intraoperative episodes of hypoxemia
   (E) ambulatory surgery

37. For an adult, which of the following is a risk factor for the development of postoperative delirium?

   (A) decreased functional status
   (B) intraoperative use of nitrous oxide
   (C) intraoperative hematocrit <35%
   (D) age >40 years
   (E) general anesthesia

38. Within 8 hours of surgery, a patient's mental function is notably altered. The patient, who previously exhibited no cognitive deficits, now exhibits altered level of attention and altered level of consciousness. The symptoms resolve after approximately 1 week. Which of the following is the best term to describe these findings?

   (A) postoperative cognitive dysfunction
   (B) postoperative delirium
   (C) emergence excitement
   (D) dementia
   (E) delayed awakening

39. A patient undergoing a laparoscopic sigmoid resection receives a general anesthetic. Sevoflurane, fentanyl, and rocuronium are selected for maintenance of anesthesia. Post-surgery, the patient fails to regain consciousness 60 minutes after the discontinuation of general anesthesia. Typically, what is the most likely explanation of this delayed emergence?

   (A) residual effects of sedative drugs
   (B) residual neuromuscular blockade
   (C) hypothermia
   (D) perioperative stroke
   (E) hypoglycemia

Answers and Explanations: Postoperative Period

1. Whenever possible, it is recommended to use multimodal analgesia for postoperative pain management. Following total knee arthroplasty, which multimodal technique for postoperative pain management is most effective?

   (A) postincisional infiltration of bupivacaine
   (B) epidural morphine
   (C) **IV opioids and pregabalin**
   (D) IV opioids and ketamine
   (E) IV opioids and acetaminophen

   Meta-analysis data shows that intravenous (IV) opioids with calcium channel blockers (gabapentin or pregabalin) are a useful multimodal technique that improves analgesia, compared to IV opioids alone.

   Multimodal pain management is defined as the administration of two or more analgesic drugs (each with a distinct mechanism of action). Therefore, although epidural morphine and postincisional infiltration of bupivacaine can both improve postoperative analgesia, in and of themselves they are not multimodal techniques.

   IV opioids with ketamine and IV opioids with acetaminophen are both multimodal techniques, but current evidence is inconsistent as to whether they are superior to IV opioids alone. However, it is currently recommended, except when contraindicated, that all surgical patients receive multimodal pain management including around-the-clock NSAIDs, COX-2 selective NSAIDs, or acetaminophen.

   Refs: American Society of Anesthesiologists Task Force on Acute Pain Management, Practice guidelines for acute pain management in the perioperative setting: an updated report by the American Society of Anesthesiologists Task Force on Acute Pain Management, *Anesthesiology* 2012; 116:248–273.
   Miller RD. *Miller's Anesthesia*, 8th ed. Philadelphia, PA: Elsevier; 2015.

2. In an attempt to reduce the incidence of chronic postsurgical pain (CPSP), nonopioid adjuvant analgesics are often administered. Best evidence suggests which of the following adjuvants may modify the risk of CPSP?

   (A) ketamine
   (B) **gabapentin**
   (C) dexmedetomidine
   (D) magnesium
   (E) amitriptyline

   Best evidence suggests that gabapentin (and pregabalin) can prevent CPSP. CPSP is defined as the presence of unexplained pain more than 2 months postoperatively. Depending on the type of surgery, the incidence of CPSP can range from ~10% to >50%. A number of different nonopioid adjuvants have been studied to reduce the incidence of CPSP. Studies of ketamine, dexmedetomidine, magnesium infusions, lidocaine infusions, and various antidepressants (TCAs—amitriptyline, SSRIs, and SNRIs) are unfortunately either limited or sometimes contradictory.

   Refs: Miller RD. *Miller's Anesthesia*, 8th ed. Philadelphia, PA: Elsevier; 2015.
   Ramaswamy S, Wilson JA, Colvin L. Non-opioid-based adjuvant analgesia in perioperative care. *Contin Educ Anaesth Crit Care* 2013;13(5):152–157.

3. Within clinically relevant dosages, which of the following nonopioid adjuvants can cause hypotension?

   (A) lidocaine infusion
   (B) ketamine
   (C) pregabalin
   (D) **dexmedetomidine**
   (E) dexamethasone

Alpha-2 agonists such as dexmedetomidine and clonidine can cause hypotension and bradycardia within clinically relevant dosages. The mechanism of action is due to the ability of alpha-2 agonists to reduce central sympathetic outflow. Other potential/theoretical side effects of nonopioid adjuvants include:

- ketamine; psychomimetic side effects such as hallucinations; tachycardia, hypertension
- pregabalin/gabapentin: dizziness, sedation, fatigue
- dexamethasone/methylprednisolone: hyperglycemia, GI bleeding, altered wound healing
- lidocaine: local anesthetic toxicity (CNS/cardiovascular)

Ref: Butterworth JF IV, Mackey DC, Wasnick JD. *Morgan & Mikhail's Clinical Anesthesiology,* 5th ed. New York, NY: McGraw Hill; 2013.

4. Traditional NSAIDs and COX-2 inhibitors have a variety of side effects. Compared to COX-2 inhibitors, which of the following side effects is seen MORE OFTEN in patients administered traditional NSAIDs?

(A) **GI hemorrhage**
(B) decreased renal function
(C) myocardial infarction
(D) asthma
(E) headache

Traditional NSAIDs cause a higher incidence of GI hemorrhage as compared to COX-2 inhibitors (celecoxib). COX-2 inhibitors are indicated for patients at risk of GI complications. Both traditional NSAIDs and COX-2 inhibitors increase the risk of:

- adverse renal events (in patients with renal disease)
- cardiovascular events (myocardial infarction, stroke)
- hypersensitivity (asthma, urticaria, angioneurotic edema)
- CNS side effects (headache, dizziness, confusion)

Ref: Brunton LL, Chabner BA, Knollman BC. *Goodman & Gilman's the Pharmacological Basis of Therapeutics,* 12th ed. New York, NY: McGraw Hill; 2011.

5. Nonopioid adjuvants for postoperative analgesia may have all of the following benefits EXCEPT:

(A) reduced opioid induced hyperalgesia
(B) reduced risk of chronic pain
(C) reduced postoperative pain intensity
(D) preventive analgesia
(E) **preemptive analgesia**

Nonopioid adjuvants for postoperative analgesia may have a number of *preventive analgesia* effects, including:

- reduced opioid-induced hyperalgesia
- reduced postoperative pain intensity
- reduced opioid consumption (and reduce opioid side effects)
- reduced risk of chronic pain

Preemptive analgesia is the term used by Patrick Wall in 1988 to describe the goal of using analgesics *before* surgical incision in order to block the induction of central sensitization and thereby improving postoperative pain control. Research to prove preemptive analgesia is not compelling; this is due to the fact that general anesthesia and systemic opioids do not completely block central sensitization (and also due to debate about the basic definition of preemptive analgesia and study design). The term *preventive analgesia* is used to describe the goal of minimizing central sensitization by using analgesics throughout the perioperative period. Central sensitization is the cascade of effects after surgical incision that leads to the amplification of postoperative pain.

Refs: Miller RD. *Miller's Anesthesia,* 8th ed. Philadelphia, PA: Elsevier; 2015.
Butterworth JF IV, Mackey DC, Wasnick JD. *Morgan & Mikhail's Clinical Anesthesiology,* 5th ed. New York, NY: McGraw Hill; 2013.
Katz J, Clarke H, Seltzer Z. Preventive analgesia: quo vadimus? *Anesth Analg* 2011;113(5):1242–1253.

6. Low-dose ketamine (0.5–1 mg/kg, with continuous infusion of 2–10 mcg/kg/min) is often used as a perioperative nonopioid adjuvant. What is considered the primary mechanism of action for low-dose ketamine's analgesic effects?

(A) **NMDA receptor antagonism**
(B) mu-opioid receptor agonism
(C) kappa-opioid receptor agonism
(D) muscarinic receptor agonism
(E) Na^+ channel inhibition

The primary mechanism of action for low-dose ketamine's analgesic effects is NMDA receptor antagonism, which activates inhibitory pain pathways. The pharmacology of ketamine is complex:

- low-dose ketamine, via its action as an NMDA antagonist, prevents opioid receptor internalization and prevents opioid-induced hyperalgesia and acute tolerance.

- higher anesthetic doses of ketamine act as mu- and kappa-opioid receptor *antagonists.*

- ketamine also acts as a monoaminergic, muscarinic, and nicotinic antagonist, and it also inhibits neuronal sodium channels (which may explain its local anesthetic properties).

Refs: Butterworth JF IV, Mackey DC, Wasnick JD. *Morgan & Mikhail's Clinical Anesthesiology,* 5th ed. New York, NY: McGraw Hill; 2013.
Pai A, Heining M. Ketamine. *Contin Educ Anaesth Crit Care Pain* 2007;7(2):59–63.
Hirota K, Lambert DG. Ketamine: new uses for an old drug? *BJA* 2011;107(2):123–126.

7. A patient is undergoing high-risk vascular surgery. Clonidine is selected as an adjuvant for perioperative pain management. Which of the following is an additional benefit of clonidine?

   (A) earlier intake of enteral nutrition
   (B) reduced risk of respiratory depression
   (C) reduced risk of significant hypotension
   (D) reduced risk of myocardial infarction
   (E) reduced risk of death

Alpha-2 agonists such as clonidine and dexmedetomidine do not increase the risk of respiratory depression.

   Alpha-2 agonists were previously thought to decrease the risk of death and myocardial infarction after vascular surgery. However, the recent POISE-2 trial found that clonidine *did not* decrease the risk of death or myocardial infarction. Clonidine increases the risk of significant hypotension.

   Intravenous lidocaine infusions may have benefits including improved bowel function after surgery.

Refs: Devereaux PJ, Sessler DI, Leslie K, et al. Clonidine in patients undergoing noncardiac surgery. *NEJM* 2014; 370(16):1504–1513.
Wijeysundera DN, Bender JS, Beattie WS. Alpha-2 adrenergic agonists for the prevention of cardiac complications among patients undergoing surgery. *Cochrane Database*

Syst Rev 2009;4(CD004126), doi: 10.1002/14651858. CD004126.pub2.
Butterworth JF IV, Mackey DC, Wasnick JD. *Morgan & Mikhail's Clinical Anesthesiology,* 5th ed. New York, NY: McGraw Hill; 2013.

8. For treatment of moderate to severe postoperative pain, which of the following opioids is LEAST effective?

   (A) transdermal fentanyl patch
   (B) intravenous buprenorphine
   (C) intravenous sufentanil
   (D) oral oxycodone
   (E) intramuscular meperidine

Transdermal fentanyl is not indicated for the routine treatment of postoperative pain, as the onset of action is too slow. It may take up to 16 hours after placement of a transdermal fentanyl patch for full analgesic effect. There are many other options for the management of moderate to severe postoperative pain, including intravenous buprenorphine (opioid agonist-antagonist), intravenous sufentanil, oral oxycodone, and intramuscular meperidine (although this route of administration may be painful).

Refs: Miller RD. *Miller's Anesthesia,* 8th ed. Philadelphia, PA: Elsevier; 2015.
Brunton LL, Chabner BA, Knollman BC. *Goodman & Gilman's the Pharmacological Basis of Therapeutics,* 12th ed. New York, NY: McGraw Hill; 2011.

9. For an adult, which of the following single-dose analgesics provides the greatest pain relief for moderate to severe postoperative pain?

   (A) ibuprofen 400 mg PO
   (B) tramadol 50 mg PO
   (C) acetaminophen 650 mg PO
   (D) codeine 60 mg PO
   (E) aspirin 650 mg PO

Of the listed analgesics, ibuprofen 400 mg PO provides the greatest pain relief for moderate to severe postoperative pain.

   Analgesics may be compared using the number needed to treat (NNT). NNT is defined as the number of patients who require treatment for one patient to receive >50% pain relief compared to placebo:

- ibuprofen 400 mg PO, NNT = 2.5
- tramadol 50 mg PO, NNT = 8.3
- acetaminophen 650 mg PO, NNT = 4.6

- codeine 60 mg PO, NNT = 16.7
- aspirin 650 mg PO, NNT = 4.4

Refs: Bandolier, available at: http://www.medicine.ox.ac.uk/ bandolier/booth/painpag/ Acutrev/Analgesics/Leagtab. html.

Miller RD. *Miller's Anesthesia*, 8th ed. Philadelphia, PA: Elsevier; 2015.

10. For infiltration anesthesia in adults, what is the maximum recommended dose of bupivacaine?

   (A) 1 mg/kg

   (B) 2 mg/kg

   (C) 4.5 mg/kg

   (D) 7 mg/kg

   (E) 9 mg/kg

For infiltration anesthesia in adults, the maximum recommended dose of bupivacaine is 2 mg/kg. Other frequently used anesthetics include lidocaine (4.5 mg/kg) and procaine (7 mg/kg). If epinephrine is added, the maximum dose can be increased by 1/3.

Ref: Brunton LL, Chabner BA, Knollman BC. *Goodman & Gilman's the Pharmacological Basis of Therapeutics*, 12th ed. New York, NY: McGraw Hill; 2011.

11. For an opioid-naive adult after surgery, what is an acceptable initial order for a fentanyl patient-controlled analgesia (PCA) regimen?

   (A) 0.5 mg IV q5min

   (B) 15 mcg IV q5min

   (C) 30 mcg IV q15min

   (D) 50 mcg IV q20min

   (E) continuous IV infusion of 0.01 mg/kg/hr

Opioid doses for an opioid-naïve adult after surgery can vary widely, but suggested starting doses for intravenous PCA regimens include:

- fentanyl 10–50 mcg IV bolus, lockout interval 4–10 minutes
- morphine 0.5–2.5 mg IV bolus, lockout interval 5–10 minutes
- hydromorphone 0.05–0.4 mg IV bolus, lockout interval 5–10 minutes

Continuous infusions are not recommended for initial regimens in opioid-naïve adult patients.

Ref: Miller RD. *Miller's Anesthesia*, 8th ed. Philadelphia, PA: Elsevier; 2015.

12. What is a typical dose of intrathecal opioid recommended for outpatient knee arthroscopy?

   (A) morphine 100 mcg

   (B) morphine 200 mcg

   (C) morphine 300 mcg

   (D) fentanyl 25 mcg

   (E) fentanyl 100 mcg

For an outpatient knee arthroscopy, typically fentanyl 10 to 25 mcg intrathecal is recommended. This dose will improve intraoperative analgesia without excessive postoperative motor blockade. Intrathecal morphine is typically not recommended for outpatient procedures, given the risk of delayed respiratory depression (>6 hours after administration).

Ref: Miller RD. *Miller's Anesthesia*, 8th ed. Philadelphia, PA: Elsevier; 2015.

13. After bowel resection, a low thoracic epidural is used for postoperative analgesia. A variety of local anesthetic solutions with or without opioids are available. Rather than using 0.125% bupivacaine, what is an advantage of using a solution of 0.05% bupivacaine and fentanyl 5 mcg/mL?

   (A) less nausea and vomiting

   (B) less pruritus

   (C) less sedation

   (D) less motor block

   (E) less respiratory depression

An epidural solution of 0.05% bupivacaine and fentanyl 5 mcg/mL has some advantages over a solution of 0.125% bupivacaine:

- less motor block
- less hypotension

Epidural solutions with opioids do have a higher risk of opioid-related complications compared to plain local anesthetic solutions (higher risk of nausea/vomiting, pruritus, sedation, and respiratory depression).

Ref: Butterworth JF IV, Mackey DC, Wasnick JD. *Morgan & Mikhail's Clinical Anesthesiology*, 5th ed. New York, NY: McGraw Hill; 2013.

14. An opioid-naïve adult patient requires intravenous patient-controlled analgesia (PCA) with an opioid for postoperative pain management. A continuous background infusion of opioid can be programmed in addition to the demand dose. What is an advantage of using a PCA system with a continuous infusion of opioids?

    (A) improved postoperative analgesia
    (B) improved postoperative sleep patterns
    (C) less physical requirement for patient
    (D) less overall opioid use
    (E) less respiratory depression

    An advantage of a PCA with a continuous background infusion of opioid is that the patient requires no cognitive or physical capabilities for its effective use. This is of particular use for pediatric patients too young to understand how to use a PCA device. A continuous infusion may also be appropriate for opioid-tolerant patients who require a basal opioid requirement.

    In adults, PCA with a continuous infusion does *not* improve postoperative analgesia or sleep patterns, uses more overall opioid, and increases the likelihood of opioid side effects including respiratory depression. There is some evidence that a continuous infusion will improve the postoperative sleep patterns of pediatric patients.

    Ref: Miller RD. *Miller's Anesthesia*, 8th ed. Philadelphia, PA: Elsevier; 2015.

15. Multiple alternative and complementary therapies are available for postoperative pain management. To be effective, which of the following techniques requires patient susceptibility?

    (A) TENS
    (B) cryotherapy
    (C) acupuncture
    (D) hypnosis
    (E) ultrasound

    Alternative and complementary therapies for the management of postoperative pain include TENS (transcutaneous electrical nerve stimulation), cryotherapy, acupuncture, hypnosis, and ultrasound. Research proving efficacy is limited and sometimes contradictory. Hypnosis requires active participation, and if the patient is not susceptible, hypnosis will not work.

    Ref: Hadzic A. *NYSORA Textbook of Regional Anesthesia and Acute Pain Medicine*, 1st ed. New York, NY: McGraw Hill; 2007.

16. Of the following alternative and complementary therapies for postoperative pain management, which is postulated to work via release of endorphins?

    (A) acupuncture
    (B) hypnosis
    (C) cryotherapy
    (D) ultrasound
    (E) therapeutic touch

    The mechanism of action for many complementary therapies for postoperative pain is not fully understood. Acupuncture may work for postoperative pain by increasing production of endorphins. Other proposed mechanisms for acupuncture also include the "gate control" theory of pain.

    Hypnosis alters the perception of pain, but the underlying mechanism is unclear. Cryotherapy acts to slow nerve conduction and reduce tissue inflammation. Ultrasound acts to increase blood flow and promote soft tissue healing. Therapeutic touch is supposed to alter the energy field around a patient.

    Refs: Hadzic A. *NYSORA Textbook of Regional Anesthesia and Acute Pain Medicine,* 1st ed. New York, NY: McGraw Hill; 2007.
    Furlan AD, van Tulder MW, Cherkin D, et al. Acupuncture and dry-needling for low back pain. *Cochrane Database Syst Rev* 2005;1(CD001351), doi: 10.1002/14651858. CD001351.pub2.

17. Atelectasis is diagnosed as the cause of a patient's postoperative hypoxemia. Which of the following is the most likely mechanism for postoperative hypoxemia in a patient with atelectasis?

    (A) hypoventilation
    (B) diffusion impairment
    (C) V/Q mismatch
    (D) right-to-left shunt
    (E) hypoxic pulmonary vasoconstriction

    Postoperative atelectasis may result in hypoxemia due to a right-to-left shunt. A right-to-left shunt occurs when parts of the lung are not ventilated due to atelectasis or consolidation (pneumonia, ARDS). Unlike a V/Q mismatch, a shunt may not be easily overcome by increasing the oxygen concentration. Perioperatively, atelectasis may be reduced with the application of PEEP, recruitment maneuvers, and minimizing gas resorption by using a lower FiO_2.

Hypoventilation may occur postoperatively when the minute ventilation is low relative to metabolic demand.

Diffusion impairment can occur in conditions such as pulmonary fibrosis and systemic vascular diseases.

Dead space is usually ~30% of tidal volume. Dead space can increase in situations where either ventilation ("V") *increases* or blood flow (perfusion, "Q") *decreases*. Ventilation-perfusion mismatch (V/Q mismatch) is the term used to describe this increase in dead space. Examples of V/Q mismatch include pulmonary emboli and obstructive lung disease such as asthma, emphysema, and chronic bronchitis. Atelectasis can cause hypoxic pulmonary vasoconstriction, but it is a consequence rather than a cause of postoperative hypoxemia. Hypoxic pulmonary vasoconstriction acts to divert venous blood from poorly ventilated areas of the lung.

Ref: Levitzky MG. *Pulmonary Physiology*, 8th ed. New York, NY: McGraw Hill; 2013.

18. Perioperatively, a number of factors may contribute to a decline in functional residual capacity (FRC). A patient is anesthetized and positioned for surgery: they are placed in the supine position, anesthesia is induced, followed by muscle paralysis, then the patient is placed in > 30-degree Trendelenburg position and nonlaparoscopic upper abdominal surgery is started. Which of the following factors is LEAST LIKELY to decrease FRC?

(A) patient in supine position
(B) induction of general anesthesia
(C) addition of muscle paralysis
(D) > 30-degree Trendelenburg position
(E) nonlaparoscopic upper abdominal surgery

The addition of muscle paralysis (and mechanical ventilation) does not significantly decrease FRC in an already anesthetized patient.

When a patient changes position from upright to supine, FRC decreases by 0.8 to 1.0 L. After induction of anesthesia, FRC decreases a further 0.4 to 0.5 L. Steep Trendelenburg position (>30-degree headdown) may further reduce FRC. Upper abdominal surgical procedures typically reduce FRC by 60% to 70% with the effects lasting 7 to 10 days.

Ref: Butterworth JF IV, Mackey DC, Wasnick JD. *Morgan & Mikhail's Clinical Anesthesiology*, 5th ed. New York, NY: McGraw Hill; 2013.

19. Postoperatively, a patient is noted to have significant systemic hypertension. Which of the following is the greatest risk factor for postoperative hypertension?

(A) history of essential hypertension
(B) increased sympathetic nervous system activity due to pain
(C) increased sympathetic nervous system activity due to hypercapnia
(D) shivering
(E) hypervolemia

A history of essential hypertension is the great risk factor for significant hypertension in the PACU. The differential diagnosis of postoperative hypertension is broad and includes:

• increased sympathetic nervous system activity due to:
  • pain
  • agitation
  • hypercapnia
  • bowel distention/urinary retention
• arterial hypoxemia
• hypervolemia
• shivering
• increased intracranial pressure—drug rebound
• emergence excitement

Ref: Miller RD. *Miller's Anesthesia*, 8th ed. Philadelphia, PA: Elsevier; 2015.

20. After an exploratory laparotomy for a bowel perforation, a patient is transferred to the postanesthesia care unit (PACU), and persistent hypotension is noted. Initial treatment consists of intravenous crystalloids. The hypotension is not corrected with fluid resuscitation. No ECG changes are noted; BP = 95/42; mean arterial pressure (MAP) = 60 mm Hg; HR = 96/min; CVP = 8 mm Hg, CO = 8.4 L/min. Based on this information, which of the following interventions is recommended?

(A) continue IV fluids only
(B) add infusion of dobutamine
(C) add infusion of vasopressin
(D) add infusion of norepinephrine
(E) add infusion of epinephrine

The addition of an infusion of norepinephrine is recommended for a hypotensive patient with suspected septic shock (suspected infection, hypotension not reversed with fluid resuscitation). The surviving sepsis guidelines recommend fluid resuscitation with crystalloid as the initial therapy, with target goals of central venous pressure (CVP) 8 to 12 mm Hg, mean arterial pressure (MAP) >65 mm Hg, urine output >0.5 mL/kg/hr, superior vena cava oxygenation saturation (SCVO$_2$) 70%. Vasopressors should be added to target MAP of 65 mm Hg. Norepinephrine is the first choice of vasopressor, while vasopressin and epinephrine are recommended when additional agents are required to maintain blood pressure.

Postoperatively, the differential diagnosis for hypotension is broad and includes:

- decreased preload (hypovolemia, hemorrhage, third-space losses)
- decreased afterload (sepsis, anaphylaxis, sympathectomy)
- cardiogenic causes affecting rate, rhythm, and contractility (myocardial ischemia, cardiomyopathy, valvular disease, arrhythmias)
- obstructive causes (tension pneumothorax, cardiac tamponade, massive pulmonary embolism)

Shock is the term for uncorrected hypotension resulting in impaired organ perfusion. Decreased preload is managed with crystalloids, colloids, or blood products as indicated. Decreased afterload is managed with vasopressors such as phenylephrine, norepinephrine, and vasopressin. Epinephrine is the treatment of choice for anaphylactic reactions. Decreased cardiac output can be increased with a positive inotrope such as dobutamine. Depending on the underlying cause of the decrease in cardiac output, other therapies may be warranted, including emergent interventional cardiac care, placement of an intra-aortic balloon pump, or pacing/cardioversion. A high index of suspicion is required to diagnose obstructive conditions such as tension pneumothorax, cardiac tamponade, or pulmonary embolus. Rapid assessment with bedside ultrasound is becoming a popular method to quickly assess and guide patient care.

Treatment algorithms for persistent hypotension generally recommend immediate evaluation of airway, breathing, and circulation; placement of adequate IV access; and fluid replacement. If blood pressure remains low, assessment of hemodynamic data with echocardiography/ultrasound assessment, pulmonary artery catheter, or arterial line with cardiac output measure should quickly follow. This additional data should allow for discrimination between the broad classes of hypotension/shock:

- hypovolemia is characterized by decreased stroke volume (SV), compensatory tachycardia, decreased central venous pressure (CVP), decreased cardiac output (CO), and increased systemic vascular resistance (SVR)
- decreased afterload (distributive shock) is characterized by decreased SVR, decreased SV, decreased CVP, and normal or increased CO
- cardiogenic hypotension/shock is characterized by decreased CO, increased CVP, and increased SVR
- obstructive hypotension/shock is characterized by similar findings as cardiogenic causes with decreased CO, increased CVP, and increased SVR. Ultrasound assessment may be a useful tool to discriminate between possible causes.

Ref: Miller RD. *Miller's Anesthesia*, 8th ed. Philadelphia, PA: Elsevier; 2015.

21. Multiple patient factors independently predict the risk of postoperative nausea and vomiting (PONV) in adults. Which of the following factors is LEAST likely to predict PONV?

   (A) female sex
   (B) nonsmoking
   (C) history of motion sickness
   (D) obesity
   (E) patient <50 years old

According to the 2014 Society for Ambulatory Anesthesiology consensus guidelines for the management of PONV, there are multiple independent risk factors for PONV in adults:

- female sex
- history of PONV or motion sickness
- younger age (<50 years)
- general anesthesia rather than regional anesthesia
- use of volatile anesthetics and nitrous oxide
- postoperative opioids
- duration of anesthesia
- type of surgery (laparoscopic, gynecologic, and cholecystectomy)

Disproven risk factors (or those with limited clinical relevance) for PONV in adults include:

- obesity
- anxiety
- nasogastric tube
- supplemental oxygen

- perioperative fasting
- migraine

Ref: Gan TJ, Diemunsch P, Habib AS, et al. Consensus guidelines for the management of postoperative nausea and vomiting. *Anesth Analg* 2014;118(1):85–113.

22. The brainstem's vomiting centers may receive stimulation from all of the following EXCEPT:

    (A) the chemoreceptor trigger zone
    (B) vagal afferents of the gastrointestinal tract
    (C) the vestibular system
    (D) visceral and somatic nuclei
    (E) the cerebral cortex

    In the pathway for nausea and vomiting, visceral and somatic nuclei are "downstream" from the vomiting centers. Activation of visceral and somatic nuclei by the vomiting center results in sympathetic and vagal symptoms and vomiting. The vomiting centers are influenced by the chemoreceptor trigger zone, the vestibular system, vagal afferents of the gastrointestinal tract, and possibly the cerebral cortex.

    Ref: Miller RD. *Miller's Anesthesia*, 8th ed. Philadelphia, PA: Elsevier; 2015.

23. There are many prevention strategies to reduce the baseline risk of postoperative nausea and vomiting (PONV) in adults. Which of the following strategies is most helpful?

    (A) avoid the use of neostigmine
    (B) use nitrous oxide instead of volatile anesthetic
    (C) use supplemental oxygen
    (D) routine gastric decompression
    (E) adequate hydration

    Guidelines recommend the following strategies to reduce baseline risk factors for PONV:

    - avoid general anesthesia and use regional anesthesia where appropriate
    - avoid nitrous oxide and volatile anesthetics
    - use propofol for induction and maintenance
    - minimize perioperative opioids with multi-modal analgesia
    - adequate hydration

    Evidence is contradictory that minimizing or avoiding neostigmine can reduce the risk of PONV. Supplemental oxygen does not have an effect on nausea or

overall vomiting (but it may reduce the risk of early vomiting). Routine gastric decompression is not a recommended strategy to prevent PONV.

Ref: Gan TJ, Diemunsch P, Habib AS, et al. Consensus guidelines for the management of postoperative nausea and vomiting. *Anesth Analg* 2014;118(1):85–113.

24. The act of vomiting is associated with which of the following physical signs?

    (A) decreased salivation
    (B) diaphragm contraction
    (C) small intestine peristalsis
    (D) bradycardia
    (E) abdominal muscle relaxation

    Nausea is an unpleasant sensation, while vomiting is the forceful expulsion of stomach contents. During the act of vomiting:

    - the diaphragm contracts
    - salivation *increases*
    - *retroperistalsis* of the small intestine
    - tachycardia
    - abdominal muscles *contract*
    - fundus and cardia of stomach relax
    - antrum of stomach contracts

    Ref: Miller RD. *Miller's Anesthesia*, 8th ed. Philadelphia, PA: Elsevier; 2015.

25. Which of the following medications is NOT indicated for prophylaxis and/or treatment of PONV?

    (A) dexamethasone
    (B) scopolamine
    (C) esomeprazole
    (D) haloperidol
    (E) perphenazine

    Proton pump inhibitors (e.g., esomeprazole, pantoprazole, lansoprazole) are not indicated for prophylaxis or treatment of PONV. Proton pump inhibitors are indicated for treatment of duodenal ulcer, GERD, and Zollinger-Ellison syndrome, and may be used preoperatively to reduce gastric volume and acidity.

    Pharmacotherapy for prophylaxis and/or treatment of PONV may include:

    - NK-1 antagonists (aprepitant)
    - antihistamines (dimenhydrinate, meclizine)
    - 5-HT3 antagonists (ondansetron, etc.)

- corticosteroids (dexamethasone)
- propofol (maintenance anesthesia, subhypnotic doses)
- butyrophenones (droperidol)
- anticholinergics (scopolamine)
- phenothiazines (perphenazine)

Refs: Gan TJ, Diemunsch P, Habib AS, et al. Consensus guidelines for the management of postoperative nausea and vomiting. *Anesth Analg* 2014;118(1):85–113.

American Society of Anesthesiologists: Practice guidelines for preoperative fasting and the use of pharmacologic agents to reduce the risk of pulmonary aspiration: application to healthy patients undergoing elective procedures. An updated report by the American Society of Anesthesiologists Task Force on Preoperative Fasting. *Anesthesiology* 2011;114:495–511.

26. Which of the following H1-receptor antagonists is indicated for treatment of postoperative nausea and vomiting (PONV) in adults?

    (A) fexofenadine
    (B) loratadine
    (C) **dimenhydrinate**
    (D) cetirizine
    (E) chlorpheniramine

    Dimenhydrinate is an H1-receptor antagonist that is indicated for treatment of PONV in adults. Other H1-receptor antagonists that are useful for treatment of PONV include diphenhydramine, promethazine, and hydroxyzine. Second-generation antihistamines such as loratadine, fexofenadine, and cetirizine do not cross the blood-brain barrier and are not effective antiemetics. Chlorpheniramine is a first-generation antihistamine that is not an effective antiemetic.
    Ref: Butterworth JF IV, Mackey DC, Wasnick JD. *Morgan & Mikhail's Clinical Anesthesiology,* 5th ed. New York, NY: McGraw Hill; 2013.

27. Which of the following medications is the LEAST effective at reducing postoperative nausea and vomiting (PONV)?

    (A) ondansetron 4 mg IV
    (B) aprepitant 40 mg PO
    (C) dexamethasone 8 mg IV
    (D) droperidol 1.25 mg IV
    (E) **metoclopramide 10 mg IV**

    Although metoclopramide 10 mg IV is commonly used to prevent PONV, this dose is *not* effective. Higher

doses of metoclopramide (25–50 mg IV) are efficacious but have a higher incidence of extrapyramidal side effects. Ondansetron 4 mg IV, aprepitant 40 mg PO, dexamethasone 8 mg IV, and droperidol 1.25 mg IV are all effective at reducing PONV. Droperidol is less popular with many clinicians due to a "black box" warning from the FDA regarding QTc prolongation.

Ref: Gan TJ, Diemunsch P, Habib AS, et al. Consensus guidelines for the management of postoperative nausea and vomiting. *Anesth Analg* 2014;118(1):85–113.

28. In order to reduce postoperative nausea and vomiting (PONV) most effectively, when should ondansetron (5-HT3 antagonist) be administered?

    (A) induction of anesthesia
    (B) **end of surgery**
    (C) prior evening before surgery
    (D) 2 hours before induction of anesthesia
    (E) during maintenance phase of anesthesia

    Most 5-HT3 antagonists, including ondansetron, granisetron, dolasetron, and tropisetron, require administration at the end of surgery for effective PONV prophylaxis. Palonosetron, also a 5-HT3 antagonist, is an exception and is usually given at induction of anesthesia.
    Aprepitant (NK-1 antagonist) is typically given just prior to induction of anesthesia. Transdermal scopolamine (anticholinergic) is typically given the prior evening before surgery or at least 2 hours before surgery. Droperidol (butyrophenone) is typically given at the end of surgery.

    Ref: Gan TJ, Diemunsch P, Habib AS, et al. Consensus guidelines for the management of postoperative nausea and vomiting. *Anesth Analg* 2014;118(1):85–113.

29. Despite initial prophylactic therapy with ondansetron, 4 hours after surgery a patient has significant PONV. For this patient, PONV rescue therapy may include all of the following EXCEPT:

    (A) dimenhydrinate
    (B) **ondansetron**
    (C) droperidol
    (D) transdermal scopolamine
    (E) dexamethasone

    Four hours postsurgery, a symptomatic patient previously given ondansetron should not receive a rescue dose of ondansetron. It is not recommended to repeat the same class of antiemetic unless >6 hours have passed in recovery.

Options for PONV rescue therapy include:

- an antiemetic from a different class than original prophylactic medication
- readminister the same antiemetic as prophylactic medication if >6 hours in recovery
- nonpharmacologic techniques such as P6 acupressure may be another option for rescue therapy
- do not readminister scopolamine or dexamethasone. Transdermal scopolamine and dexamethasone have a relatively slow onset of action of (~2–4 hours for scopolamine) and a long duration of action.

Refs: Miller RD. *Miller's Anesthesia*, 8th ed. Philadelphia, PA: Elsevier; 2015.

Gan TJ, Diemunsch P, Habib AS, et al. Consensus guidelines for the management of postoperative nausea and vomiting. *Anesth Analg* 2014;118(1):85–113.

30. PONV management may include the use of droperidol. In 2001, the FDA published a "black box" warning regarding the use of droperidol. According to this warning, if droperidol administration is considered, which of the following measures is recommended?

(A) avoid droperidol for patients with hyperkalemia

(B) avoid droperidol for patients with tachycardia

(C) droperidol only for prophylaxis of PONV

(D) **after droperidol, monitor ECG for 2 to 3 hours**

(E) after droperidol, monitor for extrapyramidal side effects

If droperidol is administered, the ECG should be monitored afterwards for 2 to 3 hours to assess for arrhythmias. The concern with droperidol is it may cause QT prolongation and potentially serious arrhythmias, including torsades de pointes. The FDA black box warning also includes other recommendations:

- only use droperidol if a patient fails to respond to other antiemetics; not as prophylaxis.
- if droperidol is considered, all patients should have a 12-lead ECG to assess the QT interval. If the QT interval is prolonged, then droperidol should not be administered.
- droperidol should be administered with "extreme caution" to patients at risk of prolonged QT interval,

including patients with bradycardia, congestive heart failure, hypokalemia, or hypomagnesemia.

Droperidol can cause extrapyramidal side effects, but this is not part of the FDA black box warning.

Ref: http://www.fda.gov/Safety/MedWatch/SafetyInformation/SafetyAlertsforHumanMedicalProducts/ucm173778.htm

31. Multi-modal therapy is selected for a patient at high risk of PONV. Compared to monotherapy, which of the following combinations is LEAST effective at reducing PONV?

(A) ondansetron + dexamethasone

(B) ondansetron + droperidol

(C) ondansetron + casopitant

(D) **dexamethasone + metoclopramide**

(E) dexamethasone + droperidol

Compared to monotherapy with dexamethasone, the addition of metoclopramide does not further reduce the incidence of PONV. Other combinations of multimodal therapy that demonstrate superior effectiveness compared to monotherapy include:

- ondansetron + dexamethasone
- ondansetron + droperidol
- dexamethasone + droperidol
- ondansetron + casopitant

Refs: Gan TJ, Diemunsch P, Habib AS, et al. Consensus guidelines for the management of postoperative nausea and vomiting. *Anesth Analg* 2014;118(1):85–113.

Miller RD. *Miller's Anesthesia*, 8th ed. Philadelphia, PA: Elsevier; 2015.

32. Best evidence suggests which of the following non-pharmacologic modalities as most effective at reducing the incidence of postoperative nausea and vomiting (PONV)?

(A) music therapy

(B) ginger

(C) hypnosis

(D) **P6 acupoint stimulation**

(E) aromatherapy with isopropyl alcohol

Best evidence suggests that P6 acupoint stimulation with a variety of techniques including acupuncture, transcutaneous nerve stimulation, and acupressure is an effective method of PONV prophylaxis. Meta-analysis of multiple studies concludes that P6 stimulation is as effective as pharmacotherapy using ondansetron or droperidol. Nonpharmacologic modalities that are not effective for PONV prophylaxis include music therapy and aromatherapy with isopropyl alcohol. Nonpharmacologic modalities with insufficient evidence include hypnosis and ginger.

Refs: Gan TJ, Diemunsch P, Habib AS, et al. Consensus guidelines for the management of postoperative nausea and vomiting. *Anesth Analg* 2014;118(1):85–113.

Miller RD. *Miller's Anesthesia*, 8th ed. Philadelphia, PA: Elsevier; 2015.

33. After a general anesthetic with the use of neuromuscular blocking drugs, a patient is awake and recovering in the postanesthesia care unit (PACU). The patient seems to have upper airway obstruction with a paradoxical breathing pattern. Residual neuromuscular blockade is considered in the differential diagnosis. In this situation, which of the following methods to assess for the ability to maintain and protect the airway is preferred?

(A) train-of-four stimulation

(B) tetanic stimulation

(C) grip strength

(D) **sustained head lift**

(E) tongue protrusion

In an awake patient, clinical evaluation is preferred over the use of painful train-of-four or tetanic stimulation to assess for residual neuromuscular blockade. Sustained head lift for 5 seconds is the standard to assess for the ability to maintain and protect the airway. Other clinical assessments include tongue protrusion and grip strength. Another clinical measure that correlates with pharyngeal muscle tone is the ability to oppose the incisor teeth against a tongue depressor.

Ref: Miller RD. *Miller's Anesthesia*, 8th ed. Philadelphia, PA: Elsevier; 2015.

34. Postoperatively, which of the following complications is most common?

(A) upper airway obstruction

(B) hypotension

(C) hypertension

(D) altered mental status

(E) **nausea and vomiting**

Postoperatively, the most common complication is nausea and vomiting. Other common complications include upper airway obstruction, hypotension, arrhythmias, hypertension, and altered mental status. With respect to malpractice claims and serious adverse events, cardiovascular and respiratory incidents are most significant.

Ref: Miller RD. *Miller's Anesthesia*, 8th ed. Philadelphia, PA: Elsevier; 2015.

35. A physically fit, 30-year-old male patient undergoes an inpatient surgical procedure. His airway management includes the use of a defasciculating dose of rocuronium and succinylcholine. He is ambulatory shortly after the procedure but notes significant myalgias (muscle stiffness) for 3 days postoperatively. Which of the following factors IS associated with postoperative myalgias?

(A) patient with greater muscle mass

(B) male sex

(C) inpatient surgery

(D) **early ambulation**

(E) use of defasciculating dose of rocuronium

Early ambulation after the use of succinylcholine is associated with a higher risk of postoperative myalgias.

Postoperative myalgias are reported to occur in 0.2% to 89% of patients after the use of succinylcholine. Risk factors for the development of succinylcholine-associated postoperative myalgias include:

• minor, ambulatory surgery

• female sex

• patients with less muscle mass (e.g., bedridden)

• early ambulation after surgery

There are many published methods to reduce the incidence of succinylcholine-associated myalgias, including lidocaine, NSAIDs, and defasciculating doses of nondepolarizing neuromuscular blocking drugs. Unfortunately the evidence is conflicting. Some studies suggest that pretreatment with a nondepolarizing neuromuscular blocker to prevent succinylcholine-induced fasciculations may reduce the incidence of postoperative myalgias by ~30%. Other studies suggest that although succinylcholine-induced fasciculations can be prevented, pretreatment with a nondepolarizing neuromuscular blocker does not reduce the incidence of myalgias.

Refs: Miller RD. *Miller's Anesthesia*, 8th ed. Philadelphia, PA: Elsevier; 2015.

Wong SF, Chung F. Succinylcholine-associated postoperative myalgia. *Anaesthesia* 2000; 55:144–152.

36. Which of the following is a risk factor for postoperative cognitive dysfunction (POCD)?

    (A) general anesthesia
    (B) patient's age
    (C) intraoperative episodes of hypotension
    (D) intraoperative episodes of hypoxemia
    (E) ambulatory surgery

    Risk factors for the development of postoperative cognitive dysfunction (POCD) include increasing age, duration of anesthesia, second operation, presence of infectious and respiratory complications, and level of patient education. Type of anesthesia, intraoperative hypotension, and hypoxemia are not correlated with POCD, while ambulatory surgery has a lower rate of POCD compared to inpatient surgery.

    Refs: Silverstein JH, Timberger M, Reich DL, et al. Central nervous system dysfunction after noncardiac surgery and anesthesia in the elderly. *Anesthesiology* 2007;106: 622–628.
    Miller RD. *Miller's Anesthesia*, 8th ed. Philadelphia, PA: Elsevier; 2015.

37. For an adult, which of the following is a risk factor for the development of postoperative delirium?

    (A) decreased functional status
    (B) intraoperative use of nitrous oxide
    (C) intraoperative hematocrit <35%
    (D) age >40 years
    (E) general anesthesia

    Preoperatively, a patient with decreased functional status is at increased risk of postoperative delirium.

    Delirium is defined as an acute change in "cognition or disturbance of consciousness that cannot be attributed to a preexisting medical condition, substance intoxication, or medication." Other patient risk factors include age >70 years, previous history of delirium, preexisting cognitive deficit, and alcohol abuse. Intraoperative risk factors include hematocrit <30%, amount of surgical blood loss, and number of blood transfusions. Anesthetic technique, use of nitrous oxide, and intraoperative hypotension are not associated with increased risk of delirium.

    Ref: Miller RD. *Miller's Anesthesia*, 8th ed. Philadelphia, PA: Elsevier; 2015.

38. Within 8 hours of surgery, a patient's mental function is notably altered. The patient, who previously exhibited no cognitive deficits, now exhibits altered level of attention and altered level of consciousness. The symptoms resolve after approximately 1 week. Which of the following is the best term to describe these findings?

    (A) postoperative cognitive dysfunction
    (B) postoperative delirium
    (C) emergence excitement
    (D) dementia
    (E) delayed awakening

    Postoperative delirium presents with impaired attention and altered level of consciousness, and is usually reversible. Postoperative delirium is characterized by acute onset (hours to days), with a duration of days to weeks.

    Postoperative cognitive dysfunction (POCD) is characterized by subtle onset (weeks to months), with a duration of weeks to months. POCD is also associated with impaired attention, but level of consciousness is normal. POCD is usually reversible but it can be long lasting.

    Emergence delirium occurs immediately after emergence from general anesthesia and typically resolves within minutes to hours.

    Dementia is a syndrome associated with disturbed memory, learning, language, and judgment. It is progressive in nature and not associated with altered consciousness. Delayed awakening describes a patient who does not respond to stimulation after discontinuation of anesthesia (usually response should occur within 60–90 minutes).

    Ref: Miller RD. *Miller's Anesthesia*, 8th ed. Philadelphia, PA: Elsevier; 2015.

39. A patient undergoing a laparoscopic sigmoid resection receives a general anesthetic. Sevoflurane, fentanyl, and rocuronium are selected for maintenance of anesthesia. Post-surgery, the patient fails to regain consciousness 60 minutes after the discontinuation of general anesthesia. Typically, what is the most likely explanation of this delayed emergence?

    (A) residual effects of sedative drugs
    (B) residual neuromuscular blockade
    (C) hypothermia
    (D) perioperative stroke
    (E) hypoglycemia

The most common cause of delayed emergence is due to the residual effects of sedative drugs (volatile anesthetics, induction agents, opioids, benzodiazepines). Although the time period for awakening after anesthesia may vary considerably from one patient to another, delayed emergence after general anesthesia is usually defined as failure to regain consciousness within 30 to 90 minutes after the discontinuation of anesthesia. Other possible causes of delayed emergence include:

- prolonged neuromuscular blockade
- neurologic complications, including stroke
- metabolic disturbances such as hypo- or hyperglycemia, hypo- or hypernatremia, hypercalcemia, or hypermagnesemia
- hypothermia
- respiratory failure

A suggested approach for a patient with delayed emergence includes assessing vital signs and level of consciousness; followed by review of perioperative medications and use of reversal agents as indicated; assessment of glucose, temperature, and arterial blood gas; and other tests including chest X-ray and CT head as indicated.

Refs: Miller RD. *Miller's Anesthesia*, 8th ed. Philadelphia, PA: Elsevier; 2015.

Butterworth JF IV, Mackey DC, Wasnick JD. *Morgan & Mikhail's Clinical Anesthesiology*, 5th ed. New York, NY: McGraw Hill; 2013.

CHAPTER 30

Special Problems or Issues in Anesthesiology

1. In order to reduce fatigue and sleep deprivation, resident work hours are regulated. Fatigue can be an important cause of performance errors. A performance error due to sleep vulnerability is most likely to occur at what time of day?

   (A) between 0200 and 0700
   (B) between 0700 and 1200
   (C) between 1200 and 1700
   (D) between 1700 and 2200
   (E) between 2200 and 0200

2. Human performance in the operating room may be affected by many different factors. Best evidence shows which of the following is potentially the MOST detrimental to an anesthesiologist's performance in the operating room?

   (A) reading in the operating room
   (B) playing music in the operating room
   (C) ingestion of a single alcoholic beverage 8 hours prior to working
   (D) 4 hours of sleep within the last 24 hours
   (E) occupational exposure (time-weighted average) to 25 ppm nitrous oxide

3. According to the ASA Task Force on Chemical Dependence, which of the following descriptions is MOST characteristic of an addicted anesthesiologist?

   (A) most abuse propofol
   (B) most are in academic practice
   (C) most have a family history of addiction
   (D) most are usually detected within 2 years
   (E) most are anesthesiology residents

4. Unfortunately, identification of a physician who is chemically dependent usually occurs at a late stage. Awareness of the signs and symptoms of chemical dependency may prompt earlier intervention. Which of the following may be a work-related sign or symptom of opioid dependence?

   (A) meticulous charting
   (B) unwillingness to take call
   (C) weight gain
   (D) preference for working alone
   (E) unwillingness to relieve others

5. An impaired physician is identified and agrees to undergo treatment for opioid dependency. After completion of the treatment program, the physician requests to return to the workplace. The Americans with Disabilities Act (ADA) may offer some protection for physicians with a history of chemical dependency. In general, which of the following scenarios is in agreement with the ADA?

   (A) The employer must make accommodation for the recovering physician to reenter the workplace.
   (B) A physician currently using drugs is protected from losing their job.
   (C) The employer may offer a modified work schedule for the recovering physician.
   (D) The employer must provide ongoing treatment for the recovering physician.
   (E) The returning physician must complete at least 6 months of naltrexone treatment before reentry into the workplace.

6. An anesthesiologist performs an interscalene block on the patient's wrong side. A medical malpractice suit is brought against the anesthesiologist. Which of the following is the most likely cause of action?

(A) abandonment

(B) criminal negligence

(C) vicarious liability

(D) battery

(E) assault

7. A demented, geriatric patient requires a surgical procedure. The patient has an advance directive: a do-not-resuscitate (DNR) order. The morning of surgery, the patient's surrogate decision maker states that the DNR order SHOULD NOT BE SUSPENDED during anesthesia and surgery. Which of the following is correct?

(A) The anesthesiologist should obtain a court order to suspend the DNR order.

(B) Irrespective of the instructions of the surrogate decision maker, the DNR order is automatically suspended during anesthesia and surgery.

(C) The anesthesiologist should review any exceptions to the DNR order.

(D) The anesthesiologist must participate in the care of the patient.

(E) The DNR order is not legally binding in the operating room.

8. A professional opera singer undergoes a surgical procedure that requires general anesthesia and endotracheal intubation. Given the patient's profession, the informed consent process includes a lengthy discussion regarding the risks of endotracheal tube placement and potential vocal cord injury. Which of the following aspects of informed consent best describes this disclosure?

(A) reasonable person standard

(B) subjective standard

(C) professional standard

(D) therapeutic privilege

(E) paternalism

9. An anesthesiologist is sued for negligence related to the informed consent process. The case involves a parturient who received an epidural for labor and delivery. The patient claims the consent for the epidural was not valid because she was in too much pain during the informed consent process. According to the patient, which of the following components of the informed consent for anesthesia was lacking?

(A) voluntariness

(B) disclosure

(C) recommendation

(D) understanding

(E) autonomous authorization

10. After reviewing a medication error, a hospital safety committee attempts to design a system to prevent future medication errors. Such a system should include which of the following processes?

(A) Have physicians prepare intravenous solutions in patient care areas.

(B) Use the same procedures for all types of medication.

(C) Reduce use of pharmacists during bedside rounds.

(D) Implement computerized order entry.

(E) Improve visibility of dangerous medications in patient care areas.

11. During surgery an anesthesiologist gives the patient a wrong unit of packed red blood cells (PRBCs). An acute hemolytic transfusion reaction occurs. The patient recovers uneventfully. Which of the following should occur?

(A) document in chart; no disclosure to patient required as no long-term harm occurred

(B) disclosure to patient is mandatory

(C) initial disclosure should occur only after a thorough review of the error

(D) risk management personnel, rather than the anesthesiologist, should disclose to patient

(E) disclosure to patient should include speculation as to who was at fault

Answers and Explanations:
Special Problems or Issues in Anesthesiology

1. In order to reduce fatigue and sleep deprivation, resident work hours are regulated. Fatigue can be an important cause of performance errors. A performance error due to sleep vulnerability is most likely to occur at what time of day?

   (A) **between 0200 and 0700**
   (B) between 0700 and 1200
   (C) between 1200 and 1700
   (D) between 1700 and 2200
   (E) between 2200 and 0200

   The time between 0200 and 0700 (2 am and 7 am) represents the time when a person is most vulnerable to sleep (the second most vulnerable time is from 2 pm to 6 pm). In order the reduce the potential risk for performance errors due to sleep deprivation and fatigue, there are regulations set by the Accreditation Council for Graduate Medical Education (ACGME) that limit resident work hours.

   Ref: Miller RD. *Miller's Anesthesia*, 8th ed. Philadelphia, PA: Elsevier; 2015.

2. Human performance in the operating room may be affected by many different factors. Best evidence shows which of the following is potentially the MOST detrimental to an anesthesiologist's performance in the operating room?

   (A) reading in the operating room
   (B) playing music in the operating room
   (C) ingestion of a single alcoholic beverage 8 hours prior to working
   (D) **4 hours of sleep within the last 24 hours**
   (E) occupational exposure (time-weighted average) to 25 ppm nitrous oxide

   Ideally, typical adults require 7 to 8 hours of sleep each night. Sleep deprivation of just 2 hours less sleep per night can have a detrimental effect on performance.

   Unfortunately sleep debts are very common throughout society and are a source of not only medical errors but also other industrial accidents.

   Reading may distract from overall vigilance in the OR; the degree to which this affects overall performance is not known. Often the issue with reading in the OR focuses on professionalism and the negative perceptions of surgeons and patients.

   In general, noise can negatively affect performance. However, with respect to music in the OR, there is conflicting evidence as to whether music promotes a relaxed atmosphere or interferes with work in the OR.

   There is no clear-cut evidence for a threshold at which occupational exposure to anesthetic waste gases impairs performance.

   With respect to alcohol consumption, there is little evidence regarding performance in the medical domain. Occupational studies from other fields suggest that a "hangover" can affect performance even after there is no detectable blood alcohol level.

   Ref: Miller RD. *Miller's Anesthesia*, 8th ed. Philadelphia, PA: Elsevier; 2015.

3. According to the ASA Task Force on Chemical Dependence, which of the following descriptions is MOST characteristic of an addicted anesthesiologist?

   (A) most abuse propofol
   (B) **most are in academic practice**
   (C) most have a family history of addiction
   (D) most are usually detected within 2 years
   (E) most are anesthesiology residents

   The ASA Task Force on Chemical Dependence has identified a number of characteristics of addicted anesthesiologists:

   • most abuse opioids (fentanyl abuse is most common)
   • most are in academic practice
   • most have no family history of addiction

- although residents are relatively overrepresented, most are attending anesthesiologists
- approximately half are younger than 35 years

Most addicted anesthesiologists are detected within 1 year of abuse. This is likely due to the potency of drugs abused (particularly fentanyl and sufentanil). In contrast, detection of alcohol abuse may take many years.

Refs: Arnold WP, Bogard TD, Harter RL, et al. Model curriculum on drug abuse and addiction for residents in anesthesiology, American Society of Anesthesiologists, Committee on Occupation Health, Task Force on Chemical Dependence, http://www.asahq.org/.../Practice Management/modelcurriculum/en/1.

Miller RD. *Miller's Anesthesia*, 8th ed. Philadelphia, PA: Elsevier; 2015.

4. Unfortunately, identification of a physician who is chemically dependent usually occurs at a late stage. Awareness of the signs and symptoms of chemical dependency may prompt earlier intervention. Which of the following may be a work-related sign or symptom of opioid dependence?

   (A) meticulous charting
   (B) unwillingness to take call
   (C) weight gain
   (D) **preference for working alone**
   (E) unwillingness to relieve others

Although none of the signs of chemical dependency may be pathognomonic (except for witnessed self-administration), opioid dependence may be associated with a preference for working alone.

   Other signs of opioid dependence may include:

- withdrawal from outside interests
- unusual changes in behavior (e.g., wide mood swings)
- unexplained absences
- careless charting
- frequent bathroom breaks
- unusual willingness to take call
- unusual willingness to relieve others
- difficult to find when on call
- apparent increase in opioid use for anesthetics, yet excessive postoperative pain in patients

Other signs and symptoms are specifically related to the drug of choice and withdrawal syndromes. For opioids, weight loss, pinpoint pupils, chills, or diaphoresis may be noticeable.

When taken together, the picture of an opioid-dependent physician is one who struggles to maintain normal work-home relationships, seeks opportunities to divert drugs, and may show signs of withdrawal. Unfortunately, denial may delay intervention until the physician is found dead.

Ref: Miller RD. *Miller's Anesthesia*, 8th ed. Philadelphia, PA: Elsevier; 2015.

5. An impaired physician is identified and agrees to undergo treatment for opioid dependency. After completion of the treatment program, the physician requests to return to the workplace. The Americans with Disabilities Act (ADA) may offer some protection for physicians with a history of chemical dependency. In general, which of the following scenarios is in agreement with the ADA?

   (A) The employer must make accommodation for the recovering physician to reenter the workplace.
   (B) A physician currently using drugs is protected from losing their job.
   (C) **The employer may offer a modified work schedule for the recovering physician.**
   (D) The employer must provide ongoing treatment for the recovering physician.
   (E) The returning physician must complete at least 6 months of naltrexone treatment before reentry into the workplace.

The Americans with Disabilities Act (ADA) considers a physician with a history of chemical dependence as having a disability. The ADA requires that an employer make "reasonable accommodation" for the disabled individual. A modified work schedule for the recovering physician is in agreement with the ADA.

   The ADA *does not* protect a physician who is currently abusing drugs. The ADA also does not specify that the employer provide ongoing treatment for the recovering physician. The employer also does not have to accommodate the recovering physician if "undue hardship" (e.g., excessive cost) would result. Although many treatment programs (and state regulations) require at least 6 months of naltrexone treatment for opioid-dependent physicians, this is not part of the ADA requirements.

Ref: Miller RD. *Miller's Anesthesia*, 8th ed. Philadelphia, PA: Elsevier; 2015.

6. An anesthesiologist performs an interscalene block on the patient's wrong side. A medical malpractice suit is brought against the anesthesiologist. Which of the following is the most likely cause of action?

   (A) abandonment
   (B) criminal negligence
   (C) vicarious liability
   (D) battery
   (E) assault

Wrong-sided surgery may bring action against an anesthesiologist for a number of different reasons including lack of informed consent, medical negligence, and battery. Since the patient did not discuss having a procedure on the wrong-sided site, there cannot be informed consent. Touching a patient without consent is battery (assault is the attempt to touch another person). Medical negligence is a breach of duty causing harm. If care is far from the standard of care, criminal negligence may be prosecuted. Abandonment can result if an anesthesiologist fails to provide continuity of care once they have assumed responsibility for the patient. Vicarious liability can result if an anesthesiologist fails to provide reasonable oversight of those working for them.

Ref: Miller RD. *Miller's Anesthesia*, 8th ed. Philadelphia, PA: Elsevier; 2015.

7. A demented, geriatric patient requires a surgical procedure. The patient has an advance directive: a do-not-resuscitate (DNR) order. The morning of surgery, the patient's surrogate decision maker states that the DNR order SHOULD NOT BE SUSPENDED during anesthesia and surgery. Which of the following is correct?

   (A) The anesthesiologist should obtain a court order to suspend the DNR order.
   (B) Irrespective of the instructions of the surrogate decision maker, the DNR order is automatically suspended during anesthesia and surgery.
   (C) The anesthesiologist should review any exceptions to the DNR order.
   (D) The anesthesiologist must participate in the care of the patient.
   (E) The DNR order is not legally binding in the operating room.

Advance directives, including DNR orders, are NOT automatically suspended for surgery and anesthesia. According to ASA guidelines for care of patients with a DNR order, the required preoperative discussion for a patient with a DNR order includes:

• review of the DNR order with clarification or modification as required
• review of any exceptions to the DNR order
• a review of plan for reinstating DNR order after recovery from anesthesia

After discussion, the DNR order may be continued, modified, or revoked, and as required, the anesthesiologist should document consent for specific resuscitative measures.

   Under certain circumstances, an anesthesiologist may refuse to treat a patient with an active DNR order, with the provision that alternative care is arranged.

Refs: Miller RD. *Miller's Anesthesia*, 8th ed. Philadelphia, PA: Elsevier.
Kelly RJ. *Perioperative Do-Not-Resuscitate Orders. ASA Monitor* 2014;78(3):14–47.

8. A professional opera singer undergoes a surgical procedure that requires general anesthesia and endotracheal intubation. Given the patient's profession, the informed consent process includes a lengthy discussion regarding the risks of endotracheal tube placement and potential vocal cord injury. Which of the following aspects of informed consent best describes this disclosure?

   (A) reasonable person standard
   (B) subjective standard
   (C) professional standard
   (D) therapeutic privilege
   (E) paternalism

In this situation a patient with a special need (as an opera singer) requires specific information to be disclosed (risk of vocal cord injury) in order to fully weigh the risks of endotracheal intubation and consent to the anesthetic technique. This is known as the "subjective standard."

   Informed patient consent requires the physician to disclose medical information. There are two main standards: the aforementioned "subjective standard" for specific information, and the "reasonable person" standard. The "reasonable person" standard requires the physician to disclose all information a "reasonable person" would desire.

   The "professional standard," which is not typically recognized, requires disclosure of information that a physician would disclose to another physician of the same specialty. Rarely used, therapeutic privilege is avoidance of a medical disclosure in order to avoid psychological or physical harm of a patient.

Paternalism is a belief that the physician inherently knows what is best for the patient. Current practice of informed consent affirms patient autonomy to make their own decisions.

Ref: Miller RD. *Miller's Anesthesia*, 8th ed. Philadelphia, PA: Elsevier; 2015.

9. An anesthesiologist is sued for negligence related to the informed consent process. The case involves a parturient who received an epidural for labor and delivery. The patient claims the consent for the epidural was not valid because she was in too much pain during the informed consent process. According to the patient, which of the following components of the informed consent for anesthesia was lacking?

(A) voluntariness

(B) disclosure

(C) recommendation

(D) understanding

(E) autonomous authorization

Modern informed consent has seven components:

1. Decision-making capacity—this is relevant for a specific decision at a specific time. Patients need to understand treatment options and repercussions of refusing treatment.

2. Voluntariness—patients must willingly participate in care without coercion.

3. Disclosure—relevant information for the patient to make a decision.

4. Recommendation—anesthesiologist's opinion of advantages and disadvantages of each treatment option.

5. Understanding—of risks and benefits. Despite the patient's claims, pain DOES NOT inhibit the ability to recall risks and DOES NOT prevent informed consent.

6. Decision—patient's decision of anesthetic technique.

7. Autonomous authorization—patient intentionally authorizes specific procedure (e.g., surgical consent form or separate anesthesia consent form).

Ref: Miller RD. *Miller's Anesthesia*, 8th ed. Philadelphia, PA: Elsevier; 2015.

10. After reviewing a medication error, a hospital safety committee attempts to design a system to prevent future medication errors. Such a system should include which of the following processes?

(A) Have physicians prepare intravenous solutions in patient care areas.

(B) Use the same procedures for all types of medication.

(C) Reduce use of pharmacists during bedside rounds

(D) Implement computerized order entry

(E) Improve visibility of dangerous medications in patient care areas.

Reduction in medication errors requires evaluation of all involved systems including:

- prescription
- documentation
- transcription
- dispensing
- administration
- monitoring

Safe practice also includes built-in redundancies so a medication is reviewed and confirmed before administration. Suggested best practice recommendations to reduce medication errors include:

- technology-based systems such as computerized order entry, computerized dosage and allergy review, computerized medication tracking, and bar code readers for medication preparation and administration

- have pharmacists, rather than physicians, prepare intravenous solutions

- develop special procedures for high-risk drugs, rather than use the same procedure for all types of medication

- increase accessibility of pharmacists for bedside clinicians

- improve medication education for physicians, nurses, and patients—remove potentially dangerous medications from patient care areas

Ref: Brunton LL, Chabner BA, Knollman BC. *Goodman & Gilman's the Pharmacological Basis of Therapeutics*, 12th ed. New York, NY: McGraw Hill; 2011.

11. During surgery an anesthesiologist gives the patient a wrong unit of packed red blood cells (PRBCs). An acute hemolytic transfusion reaction occurs. The patient recovers uneventfully. Which of the following should occur?

(A) document in chart; no disclosure to patient required as no long-term harm occurred

(B) **disclosure to patient is mandatory**

(C) initial disclosure should occur only after a thorough review of the error

(D) risk management personnel, rather than the anesthesiologist, should disclose to patient

(E) disclosure to patient should include speculation as to who was at fault

According to the Joint Commission on Accreditation of Healthcare Organizations (JCAHO), all patient outcomes, both anticipated and unanticipated, require disclosure. Despite this requirement to disclose medical errors to patients, often incomplete or no information is provided. This is often due to medico-legal concerns and incomplete knowledge as to what to disclose and how to do it. In general, the initial disclosure should be made in a timely manner. It should include an explanation of what occurred, without speculation, and an apology or admission of liability is not required. In general, the responsible physician should disclose to the patient; however, in certain situations, risk management personnel may offer assistance. Ongoing communication with the patient's family should be established to provide additional information as the patient safety review process is completed.

Refs: Longnecker DE, Brown DL, Newman MF, Zapol WM. *Anesthesiology*, 2nd ed. New York, NY: McGraw Hill; 2012.

Gallagher TH, Denham CR, Leape LL, et al. Disclosing unanticipated outcomes to patients: the art and practice. *J Patient Saf* 2007;3:158–165.

Index

CPSIA information can be obtained
at www.ICGtesting.com
Printed in the USA
FSHW020725190421
80524FS